Neurology

Mark Mumenthaler, M.D.

Professor Emeritus of Neurology
Former Head of the Department
of Neurology
Berne University, Inselspital
Berne, Switzerland

Heinrich Mattle, M.D.

Professor of Neurology
Berne University
Inselspital
Berne, Switzerland

Translated and adapted by
Ethan Taub, M.D.

4th revised and enlarged edition

438 illustrations
210 tables

Georg Thieme Verlag
Stuttgart · New York

Library of Congress Cataloging-in-Publication Data

This book is an authorized and revised translation of the 11th German edition published and copyrighted 2002 by Georg Thieme Verlag, Stuttgart, Germany. Title of the German edition: Neurologie

Translator: Ethan Taub, M.D., Klinik Im Park, Zurich, Switzerland

1st German edition 1967
2nd German edition 1969
3rd German edition 1970
4th German edition 1973
5th German edition 1976
6th German edition 1979
7th German edition 1982
8th German edition 1986
9th German edition 1990
10th German edition 1997
1st English edition 1977
2nd English edition 1983
3rd English edition 1990
1st Czech edition 2001
1st French edition 1974
1st Greek edition 1990
1st Hungarian edition 1989
1st Indonesian edition 1995
1st Italian edition 1975
2nd Italian edition 1984
1st Japanese edition 1983
1st Polish edition 1972
2nd Polish edition 1979
3rd Polish edition 2001
1st Portuguese edition 1997
1st Spanish edition 1976
2nd Spanish edition 1982
1st Turkish edition 1984

© 2004 Georg Thieme Verlag,
Rüdigerstrasse 14, 70469 Stuttgart,
Germany
http://www.thieme.de
Thieme New York, 333 Seventh Avenue,
New York, NY 10001 USA
http://www.thieme.com

Cover design: Cyclus, Stuttgart
Typesetting by Mitterweger, Plankstadt
Printed in Germany by Grammlich,
Pliezhausen

ISBN 3-13-523904-7 (GTV)
ISBN 1-58890-045-2 (TNY)
1 2 3 4 5

Important note: Medicine is an ever-changing science undergoing continual development. Research and clinical experience are continually expanding our knowledge, in particular our knowledge of proper treatment and drug therapy. Insofar as this book mentions any dosage or application, readers may rest assured that the authors, editors, and publishers have made every effort to ensure that such references are in accordance with **the state of knowledge at the time of production of the book.** Nevertheless, this does not involve, imply, or express any guarantee or responsibility on the part of the publishers in respect to any dosage instructions and forms of applications stated in the book. **Every user is requested to examine carefully** the manufacturers' leaflets accompanying each drug and to check, if necessary in consultation with a physician or specialist, whether the dosage schedules mentioned therein or the contraindications stated by the manufacturers differ from the statements made in the present book. Such examination is particularly important with drugs that are either rarely used or have been newly released on the market. Every dosage schedule or every form of application used is entirely at the user's own risk and responsibility. The authors and publishers request every user to report to the publishers any discrepancies or inaccuracies noticed.

For Regula, Sarah, and Sofia-Rebecca
from M. Mumenthaler

**For Rösly, Stephanie, Selina,
and Regula**
from H. Mattle

Preface to the Fourth English Edition

Since this book first appeared in German in 1967, the reading and study habits of medical students and physicians have changed dramatically. As foreign travel is now commonplace, many young physicians take part of their training abroad and thereafter continue to enjoy a lively exchange of experiences with colleagues in different countries. International communication, of course, requires a common language, and English has gradually become the predominant language for this purpose. The authors and publisher therefore decided to arrange a translation of the 11th German edition into English.

The book is now 3 times its original length; since 1967, the number of illustrations has risen sixfold from 70 to 438, the number of tables from 30 to 210, and the number of references from 640 to about 2000. Its scope having widened over the years, this text, originally intended for beginning medical students, has come to be more suitable for advanced medical students with a special interest in neurology, for resident trainees, and for physicians in practice.

As a logical consequence of this development, the authors and publisher have decided to tailor the current edition for practicing physicians. Thus, we have omitted the sections concerning the basic neurological examination and ancillary tests in neurology, while introducing a substantial amount of new material and providing greater detail on many of the topics previously covered. We have entirely rewritten the chapters on epilepsy, disorders of cerebral perfusion, extrapyramidal motor disorders, polyneuropathies, and myopathies. We have also considerably enlarged the sections on treatment in each chapter, as requested by readers of previous editions.

In order to keep the book from becoming unwieldy through the addition of so much material, we have not printed the reference list in the book, but have published it instead on the Thieme Internet site (http://www.thieme.com/mm-refs), where the abstracts of most references can also be read. The didactic aspects of the text and its graphic presentation have been brought up to date with the help of Ms. Susanne Huiss of Georg Thieme Verlag.

We have tried to make the book comprehensive, though not complete (which would be impossible in any case), aiming at a clear and understandable presentation of what we think are the more important aspects of neurological disease. We encourage readers to consult the amply cited references for more detail on particular matters of interest.

Many of the illustrations show imaging studies of the kinds that are now indispensable in clinical neurology. Physicians should order such studies, in our opinion, mainly to confirm a diagnosis that has already been formulated on the basis of the case history and physical examination. It should be possible to arrive at a single diagnosis or a narrow differential diagnosis through a critical assessment and logical combination of these elements, in the light of an understanding of topical neurologic diagnosis and of the patterns of neurologic disease, which is what this book seeks to impart.

We have also written another, less comprehensive text, Grundkurs Neurologie (soon to be available in English as Fundamentals of Neurology), which provides an introduction to clinical neurology for medical students and allied health professionals. That text, unlike this one, includes introductory chapters on the neurological examination and on ancillary testing.

We are glad to have secured the collaboration of Dr. Ethan Taub, an American-trained and certified neurosurgeon practicing in Switzerland, for this English edition. He has not only produced an accurate translation of fine literary quality, but has also, through his familiarity with American medicine, succeeded in adapting this edition optimally to the standard practice and terminology of English-speaking physicians.

We would like to thank Dr. Thomas Scherb, Dr. Thorsten Pilgrim, Susanne Huiss, M.A., and Rolf Dieter Zeller of Georg Thieme Verlag for designing and producing the German edition with such great care, and Dr. Clifford Bergman and Gert Krüger of Thieme International for managing production the English edition. We also thank all of the readers and friends whose critical advice has helped us eliminate errors and maximize the accuracy of the text. We gratefully look forward to more such advice in the future.

Many people have helped us obtain references and illustrations, reviewed parts of the manuscript critically, and participated in the technical aspects of book production. We would like to express our particular thanks in this regard to Professor G. Schroth, Dr. L. Remonda, Dr. K. Lövblad, Dr. F. Donati, Dr. K. Gutbrod, Professor Ch. W. Hess, Dr. G. Jenzer, PD Dr. K. Rösler, PD Dr. J. Mathis, Prof. C. Bassetti, Dr. A. Nirkko, and Dr. P. Imesch, as well as Dr. sc.nat. Karin Hänni and Dr. phil. Annelies Blum.

We hope that this translation of the book into the lingua franca of modern medicine will make it accessible to a wider audience, in the English-speaking countries and throughout the world.

Mark Mumenthaler
Heinrich Mattle
Zurich and Berne, Switzerland
Autumn 2003

Translator's Note

This textbook of neurology has been translated into many languages since its original publication in German in 1967 and has earned the appreciation of generations of readers all over the world. It has covered the field of neurology in greater depth with each new edition, while incorporating the latest clinical and scientific advances, and has thus doubled in size since it last appeared in English (the 3rd edition of 1990, translated by E. H. Burrows from the 9th German edition). Yet, thanks to the skill of the authors, the book has not become unwieldy and remains eminently readable for both study and reference.

In translating and adapting the 11th German edition to produce this English version, I have worked directly from the current German text, but have occasionally borrowed words and phrases from the previous English edition when I found they could

not be improved on. The text mostly corresponds to the German, paragraph by paragraph, and even page by page for long stretches toward the beginning of the book. I have sparingly added words of explanation wherever this might help the reader, especially in passages touching on my own specialty (neurosurgery), but have otherwise done my best to convey the sense of the original unaltered. Needless to say, the opinions and expert judgments expressed in the book are those of the authors.

I have learnt much in the process of translation and am grateful to Professors Mumenthaler and Mattle, and to Georg Thieme Verlag, for the privilege of helping them put this book before an English-speaking audience.

Ethan Taub, M.D.
Zurich, Switzerland, Autumn 2003

Contents

3 Diseases Mainly Affecting the Spinal Cord 389

4 Autonomic and Trophic Disorders 449

5 Demyelinating Diseases 465

6 Injury to the Nervous System by Specific Physical Agents 487

7 Epilepsy, Other Episodic Disorders of Neurologic Function, and Sleep Disorders 493

8 Polyradiculitis and Polyneuropathy 575

9 Diseases Affecting the Cranial Nerves 617

10 Spinal Radicular Syndromes 717

13   Pain Syndromes of the Limbs and Trunk   833

14   Myopathies   851

15   References   925

See also http://www.thieme.com/mm-refs

Appendix 927

Scales for the Assessment of Neurologic Disease 928

Clinical
Syndromes

1 Clinical Syndromes in Neurology

Because of the anatomical construction of the nervous system and the manner in which functions are assigned to its components, lesions in specific areas of the central or peripheral nervous system are regularly associated with characteristic symptoms and signs. An acquaintance with these recurring patterns allows one to trace individual findings or constellations of findings back to the responsible dysfunctional component of the nervous system (Table 1.1).

Table 1.1   Components of the nervous system

Central	Peripheral
Brain (not including cranial nerve nuclei)	Cranial nerve nuclei
Spinal cord (not including anterior horn ganglion cells)	Anterior horn ganglion cells Nerve roots Brachial and lumbar plexuses Peripheral nerves Motor end plates Muscles

The following discussion will concern the most important typical constellations of findings (syndromes):
- central paresis,
- peripheral paresis,
- monoparesis,
- hemiparesis,
- paraparesis,
- quadriparesis,
- anterior horn lesion,
- radicular lesion,
- polyradiculopathy,
- polyneuropathy,
- plexus lesion,
- lesion of a single peripheral nerve,
- dysfunction of the neuromuscular junction (motor end plate),
- myopathy.

Differentiation of Central and Peripheral Paresis

Central and peripheral forms of paresis may be differentiated from each other by the criteria listed in Table 1.2.

Table 1.2 Characteristics of central and peripheral paresis

Feature	Central paresis	Peripheral paresis
Proprioceptive muscle reflexes	Increased	Decreased
Exteroceptive muscle reflexes	Decreased	Decreased
Babinski sign	Present	Absent
Muscle atrophy	Absent (or mild atrophy of disuse)	Present
Muscle tone	Increased (i.e., spasticity; not yet present in acute phase)	Decreased

Bodily Distribution of Paresis

The distribution of paresis in the body enables a number of inferences to be made about the nature and anatomical localization of the responsible lesion.

Monoparesis

Monoparesis is defined as isolated weakness of an entire limb or of a major part of it. Possible causes are listed in Table 1.3.

Table 1.3 Sites of lesions causing monoparesis, and corresponding clinical features

Site of lesion	Clinical features
Central nervous system	Spastic paresis (increased muscle tone, increased reflexes) No muscle atrophy Possibly a purely motor deficit (e.g., contralateral leg paresis due to ischemia in the territory of the anterior cerebral artery)
Anterior horn of spinal cord (chronic lesion)	Paresis of individual muscles with accompanying atrophy and decreased tone No sensory deficit Possibly accompanied by fasciculations Decreased proprioceptive muscle reflexes (but may be increased in amyotrophic lateral sclerosis)
Brachial or lumbar plexus	Mixed sensory and motor deficit Decreased muscle tone Muscle atrophy, decreased proprioceptive muscle reflexes Sensory deficit for all modalities
Multiple peripheral nerves	Same as in plexus lesions in a single limb
Muscle	Hardly ever a pure monoparesis; if so, then flaccid Purely motor deficit, sometimes with muscle atrophy

Hemiparesis

Hemiparesis may be due to any of the causes listed in Table 1.**4**.

Para- and Quadriparesis

Paraparesis is weakness affecting both lower limbs, and quadriparesis is weakness affecting all four limbs (but sparing the head). These may be due to any of the causes listed in Table 1.**5**.

Table 1.**4**   Sites of lesions causing hemiparesis, and corresponding clinical features

Site of lesion	Clinical features
Cerebrum	Spastic hemiparesis, possibly also involving facial muscles, characterized by: Increased muscle tone Increased reflexes Pyramidal tract signs No atrophy Usually associated with a sensory deficit
Brain stem	Spastic hemiparesis, as above Face involved or not, depending on level of lesion Cranial nerve deficits contralateral to hemiparesis
Upper cervical spinal cord	Spastic hemiparesis, as above Face spared Possible ipsilateral loss of position and vibration sense and contralateral loss of pain and temperature sense below the level of the lesion (Brown-Séquard syndrome)

Table 1.**5**   Sites of lesions causing para- or quadriparesis, and corresponding clinical features

Site of lesion	Clinical features
Cerebrum (bilateral lesion)	Clinical picture of "bilateral hemiparesis," or paraparesis due to a bilateral parasagittal cortical lesion
Corticobulbar pathways in the brain stem (bilateral lesion) (e.g., lacunar state, p. 178)	Bilateral spasticity with only mild weakness Spastic, small-stepped gait hyperreflexia, pyramidal tract signs No sensory deficit Usually accompanied by pseudobulbar signs (dysarthria, hyperreflexia of the facial musculature)
Corticospinal pathways in the spinal cord (bilateral lesion)	Para- or quadriparesis Face spared Hyperreflexia, pyramidal tract signs No sensory deficit Only mild weakness

Lesions Affecting the Anterior Horn Ganglion Cells

Lesions selectively affecting the efferent neurons (ganglion cells) of the anterior horn of the spinal cord (p. 425 ff.) produce the characteristic clinical findings listed in Table 1.**6**.

Table 1.**6**   Clinical features of an isolated lesion of the anterior horn ganglion cells

Muscle atrophy
Weakness
Fasciculations (in chronic phase)
Intact sensation
Decreased or absent reflexes
But: hyperreflexia and pyramidal tract signs in amyotrophic lateral sclerosis, which involves not only the anterior horns but also the corticospinal pathways (thus the term "lateral" sclerosis, as these pathways are lateral in the spinal cord)

Lesions Affecting a Spinal Nerve Root

Lesions affecting a spinal nerve root (p. 717 ff.) always produce both motor and sensory deficits. Individual spinal nerve roots always supply more than one muscle, and no muscle is supplied exclusively by a single root. Thus, the motor deficit produced by a monoradicular lesion has the following characteristics:

- There is always more than one affected muscle.
- No affected muscle is ever totally paralyzed.

Nevertheless, certain muscles are predominantly supplied by a single root and are, therefore, weakened to a particularly severe degree by a corresponding monoradicular lesion. Proprioceptive muscle reflexes partially subserved by the affected root may be decreased or even absent (cf. Table 1.4). The sensory deficit lies within the corresponding sensory dermatome (cf. Table 1.1) and thus usually has a band-like cutaneous distribution. Pain, if present, is referred into the dermatome of the affected root. Although the deficit is mixed (both motor and sensory), the clinical picture may be dominated by either the motor deficit or the sensory deficit in individual cases. Atrophy of the affected muscles is evident about 3 weeks after the onset of weakness.

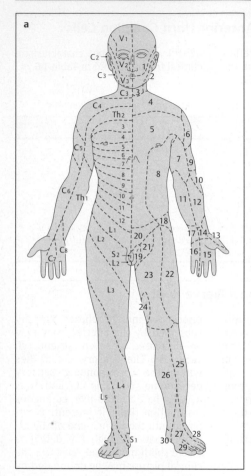

Fig. **1.1a**
1   Trigeminal n.
2   Great auricular n.
3   Transverse cutaneous n.
4   Supraclavicular nn.
5   Anterior cutaneous branches of the intercostal nn.
6   Superior lateral cutaneous n. of the arm (a branch of the axillary n.)
7   Medial cutaneous n. of the arm
8   Lateral cutaneous branches of the intercostal nn.
9   Posterior cutaneous n. of the arm (a branch of the radial n.)
10   Posterior cutaneous n. of the forearm
11   Medial cutaneous n. of the forearm
12   Lateral cutaneous n. of the forearm
13   Superficial branch of radial n.
14   Palmar branch of median n.
15   Median n.
16   Common palmar digital nn.
17   Palmar branch of ulnar n.
18   Iliohypogastric n. (lateral cutaneous branch)
19   Ilioinguinal n. (anterior scrotal nn.)
20   Iliohypogastric n. (anterior cutaneous branch)
21   Genitofemoral n. (femoral branch)
22   Lateral femoral cutaneous n.
23   Femoral n. (anterior cutaneous branches)
24   Obturator n. (cutaneous branch)
25   Lateral sural cutaneous n.
26   Saphenous n.
27   Superficial peroneal n.
28   Sural n.
29   Deep peroneal n.
30   Tibial nerve (calcanean branches)

Fig. **1.1a–g   Cutaneous sensation.**
Fields of sensory innervation of peripheral nerves and spinal nerve roots, depicted on the left and right sides of the body, respectively.

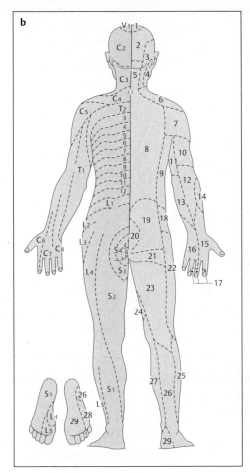

1 Frontal n. (V_1)
2 Greater occipital n.
3 Lesser occipital n.
4 Great auricular n.
5 Dorsal branches of the cervical nn.
6 Supraclavicular nn.
7 Superior lateral cutaneous n. of the arm (a branch of the axillary n.)
8 Dorsal branches of the cervical, thoracic, and lumbar spinal nn.
9 Lateral cutaneous branches of the intercostal nn.
10 Posterior cutaneous n. of the arm
11 Medial cutaneous n. of the arm
12 Posterior cutaneous n. of the forearm
13 Medial cutaneous n. of the forearm
14 Lateral cutaneous n. of the forearm
15 Superficial branch of radial n.
16 Dorsal branch of ulnar n.
17 Median n.
18 Iliohypogastric n. (lateral cutaneous branch)
19 Superior cluneal nn.
20 Middle cluneal nn.
21 Inferior cluneal nn.
22 Lateral femoral cutaneous n.
23 Posterior femoral cutaneous n.
24 Obturator n. (cutaneous branch)
25 Lateral sural cutaneous n.
26 Sural n.
27 Saphenous n.
28 Lateral plantar n.
29 Medial plantar n.

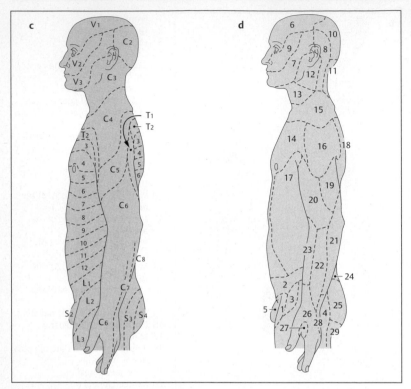

Fig. 1.**1c**   Radicular innervation: lateral view.
Fig. 1.**1d** Peripheral innervation: lateral view.

1 Ilioinguinal n.
2 Iliohypogastric n.
3 Genitofemoral n. (femoral branch)
4 Lateral femoral cutaneous n.
5 Dorsal n. of penis (pudendal n.)
6 Ophthalmic n. (V_1)
7 Mandibular n. (V_3)
8 Lesser occipital n.
9 Maxillary n. (V_2)
10 Greater occipital n.
11 Dorsal branches of cervical nn.
12 Great auricular n.
13 Transverse cutaneous n.
14 Anterior cutaneous branches of the intercostal nn.
15 Supraclavicular nn.
16 Superior lateral cutaneous n. of the arm
   (a branch of the axillary n.)

17 Intercostobrachial nn. (intercostal nn.)
18 Dorsal branches of the thoracic nn.
19 Posterior cutaneous n. of the arm
20 Lateral cutaneous n. of the arm
21 Posterior cutaneous n. of the forearm
   (a branch of the radial n.)
22 Superior lateral cutaneous n. of the
   forearm
23 Medial cutaneous n. of the forearm
24 Lateral cutaneous branch of the iliohypogastric n.
25 Superior cluneal nn.
26 Superficial branch of radial n.
27 Autonomous area of superficial branch
   of radial n.
28 Dorsal branch of ulnar n.
29 Inferior cluneal n.

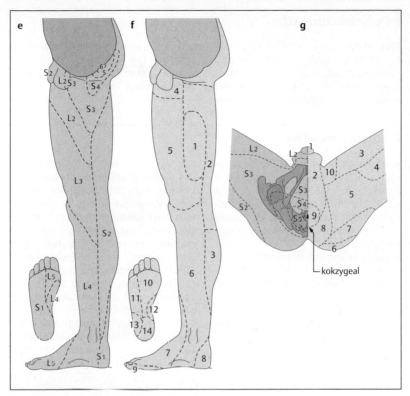

Fig. 1.**1e, f**
1 Cutaneous branch of obturator n.
2 Posterior femoral cutaneous n.
3 Lateral sural cutaneous n.
4 Ilioinguinal n. and genital branch of genitofemoral n.
5 Anterior cutaneous branches of femoral
   n.
6 Medial cutaneous branches of the saphenous n.
7 Medial dorsal cutaneous n. (superficial
   peroneal n.)
8 Medial calcaneal branches
9, 10 Medial plantar n.
11 Lateral plantar n.
12 Medial cutaneous branches of the saphenous n.
13 Sural n.
14 Medial calcaneal branches

Fig. 1.**1g**
1 Dorsal n. of the penis or clitoris (pudendal n.)
2 Posterior scrotal or labial nn.
3 Anterior cutaneous branches of the
   femoral n.
4 Obturator n.
5 Posterior femoral cutaneous n.
6 Superior cluneal nn.
7 Inferior cluneal nn.
8 Middle cluneal nn.
9 Anococcygeal nn.
10 Ilioinguinal n. and genital branch of genitofemoral n.

Polyradiculopathy

Polyradiculopathy (p. 575 ff.) is manifested by a rapidly progressive and symmetric bilateral paresis, which usually begins in the lower limbs. The motor deficits dominate the clinical picture in most forms of polyradiculopathy. The affected muscles are flaccid, and reflexes are absent. Micturition is not impaired.

Polyneuropathy

The clinical picture of polyneuropathy (p. 582 ff.) usually develops very slowly, over the course of several years. The initial symptoms are practically always confined to the lower limbs. Only sensory abnormalities are present at first:
• paresthesiae and formication in the toes,
• abnormal sensation in the soles of the feet,
• burning sensations,
• (occasionally) the feeling of walking on cotton wool.

Shortly after these symptoms arise, the Achilles reflex disappears, furnishing the first objective clinical sign. Vibration sense is impaired, more so distally than proximally. Weakness first manifests itself as an inability to spread the toes, and, when the toes are dorsiflexed, the examiner feels no contraction of the extensor digitorum brevis muscles on the dorsum of the foot. Later, cutaneous sensation to touch is impaired, and the proximal calf muscles become weak. Finally, severe bilateral foot drop appears and leads to a characteristic bilateral steppage gait.

Plexus Lesions

Plexus lesions (p. 749 and 780 ff.) always give rise to a mixed motor and sensory deficit. The involved muscles and the distribution of the sensory deficit do not correspond to the field of innervation of a single peripheral nerve, but rather to that of a combination of nerves. There is a flaccid paresis, and the reflexes subserved by the affected nerves are absent. The sensory deficit is sharply delimited and complete and involves all modalities. Sweating is absent in the area of the sensory deficit. Muscle atrophy becomes evident a few weeks after the onset of weakness.

Lesions of a Single Peripheral Nerve

A lesion of a single peripheral nerve (p. 741 ff.) produces a characteristic motor deficit in the muscles it supplies, and a characteristic sensory deficit in its field of sensory innervation. Lesions of purely motor or purely sensory nerves (or nerve branches) will obviously produce purely motor or purely sensory deficits. Sweating is absent in the area of a sensory deficit, and any reflex that is subserved by the affected nerve is absent. There is a flaccid paresis, and muscle atrophy becomes evident 2–3 weeks after the onset of weakness.

Dysfunction of the Neuromuscular Junction

In dysfunction of the neuromuscular junction (motor end plate) (pp. 875 ff.), there is a purely motor paresis of variable severity. However, as in the (other) myopathies (see below), sensation remains intact. There is no muscle atrophy.

Myopathy

Myopathy (p. 815 ff.) is characterized by paresis in the absence of a sensory deficit, because the lesion lies within the striated muscle itself. The clinical picture is thus comparable to that of an anterior horn lesion (see above). Most myopathies progress very slowly and affect both sides of the body symmetrically. The paresis is flaccid and the muscles become atrophic, albeit usually less severely than is seen with anterior horn or peripheral nerve lesions. The corresponding reflexes are decreased or absent in advanced stages of the illness. Fasciculations do not occur, in contrast to anterior horn lesions.

Clinical
Neurology

2 Diseases Mainly Affecting the Brain and its Coverings

Characteristics of Diseases of the Brain

Definition:
Diseases of the brain are characterized by both *general* and *localizing* manifestations. *General symptoms and signs* include headache, disturbances of consciousness, (generalized) epileptic seizures, an organic mental syndrome, meningism, and signs of elevated intracranial pressure (vomiting, bradycardia). *Localizing signs* include focal neurological and neuropsychological deficits, visual disturbances, cranial nerve deficits, and focal epileptic seizures. None of these features are obligatory for diagnosis, and they may be present in varying combinations and degrees of severity.

Congenital and Perinatally Acquired Diseases of the Brain

Definition:
Both *genetic defects* and *disturbances occurring during pregnancy* may lead to developmental disorders of the brain (and of the remainder of the nervous system, as well as other organs of the body). These may already be evident in the newborn infant (e.g., microcephaly), or they may become evident only in the course of further development. The same is true of *brain injuries occurring during delivery,* which are of two types: hemorrhages, and more or less diffuse hypoxic injuries. The more common *modes of presentation* in the early postnatal phase are abnormalities of muscle tone and pathological reflexes. Later manifestations include delayed psychomotor development, motor deficits (para- or hemiparesis) and involuntary movements (e.g., athetosis). Epileptic seizures in children and adolescents are not uncommonly an expression of a congenital or perinatally acquired disease of the brain.

The Neurological Examination in Infancy and Early Childhood

Techniques used in the neurological examination of adults are generally not applicable to infants and very young children. Information about the child's functional state is more usefully derived from observation of spontaneous behavior and of complex motor reflexes (104, 311).

In the infant, *spontaneous posture* should be noted, as well as any bodily asymmetries or constantly maintained postures. It should also be noted whether the head is asymmetric (plagiocephalic) or otherwise abnormal in shape (p. 44). The head circumference, body weight, and body length should be measured, entered into a table for future reference, and compared with normal values for age and sex (Fig. 2.1).

Primitive motor function in children is initially governed by a number of *reflex mechanisms*. These are listed in Table 2.1, and their temporal development and clinical significance are briefly described.

The *stages of normal motor development* are shown in Fig. 2.2.

In the initial months of life, the following motor abnormalities may indicate the presence of a cerebral movement disorder (cerebral palsy):

- feeding problems,
- hypotonia,
- paucity of movement,
- spastic extension of the legs when the child is lifted,
- intense adductor spasms—e.g., during diaper changes,
- absence of head lifting while prone persisting into the 3rd month of life,

- an abnormally brisk hand grasp reflex,
- increased tonic reflexes,
- increased neck reflexes,
- en bloc rotation on testing of the trunk postural reflex and the head-on-trunk reflex.

By the end of the 4th month, the infant should be able to control its head while sitting, lift its head while prone, and use both hands for play. The Moro reflex fades, and the Landau and parachute reflexes make their first appearance. The phenomena listed above are pathological in this stage also.

By the end of the 6th month, the following findings are highly suggestive or, if pronounced, definitely indicative of a cerebral movement disorder: retained tonic neck reflex and Moro reflex, and absent Landau, labyrinthine positional, and parachute reflexes. The child should be able to lift its head while supine, turn from supine to prone, sit up with support, turn toward an external noise, and use the whole hand, including the thumb.

By the end of the 9th month, the child should be able to sit unaided, and the lumbar kyphosis becomes less pronounced. The following findings are suggestive of a cerebral movement disorder, in addition to the pathologic reflexes already mentioned: absence of the body righting and limping reactions, and presence of a trunk postural reflex.

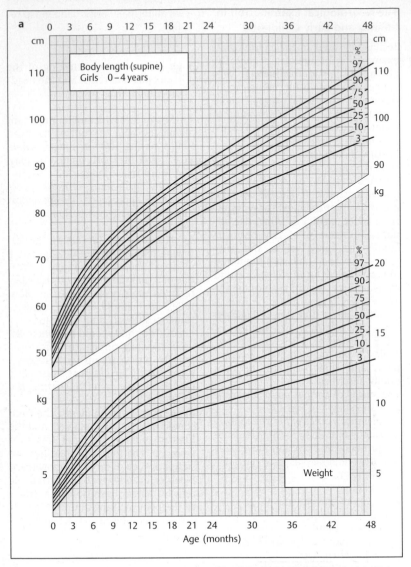

Fig. 2.**1a–h   Head circumference, body length, and weight in childhood and adolescence.** (Adapted from: *Berner Datenbuch der Pädiatrie: Praktische Richtlinien, Therapie, Ernährungsgrundlagen, Referenzwerte,* 4th ed., Stuttgart: Fischer, 1992).

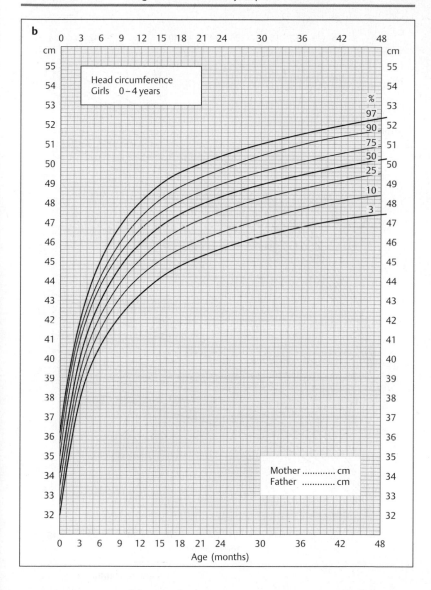

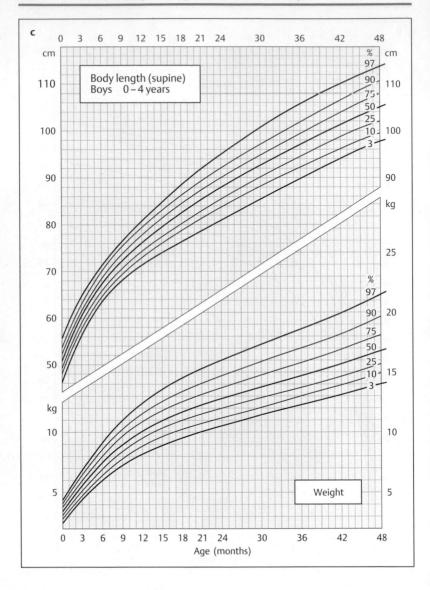

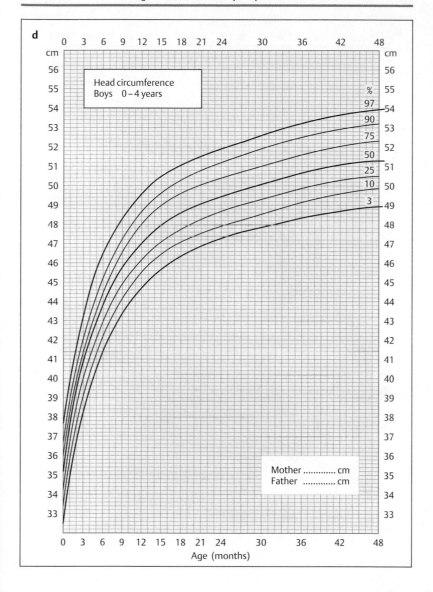

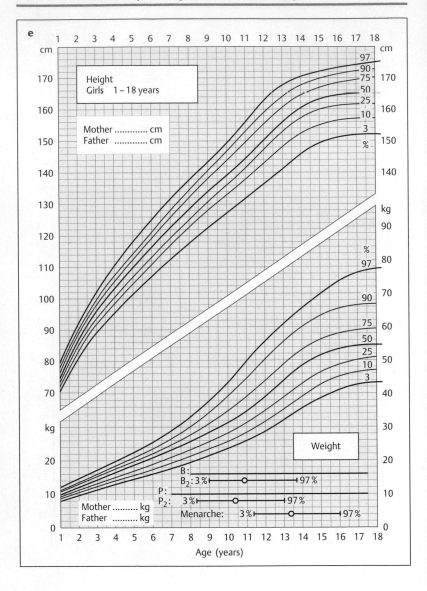

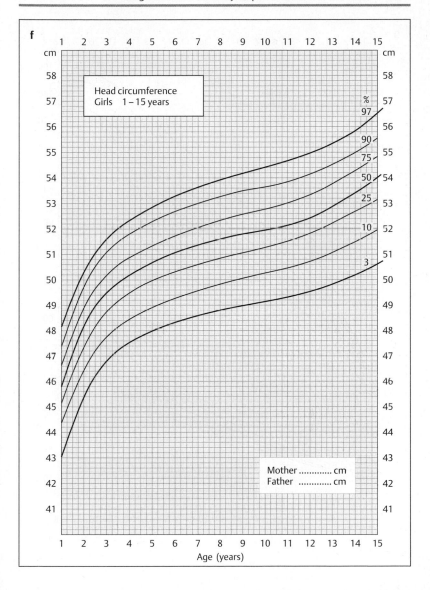

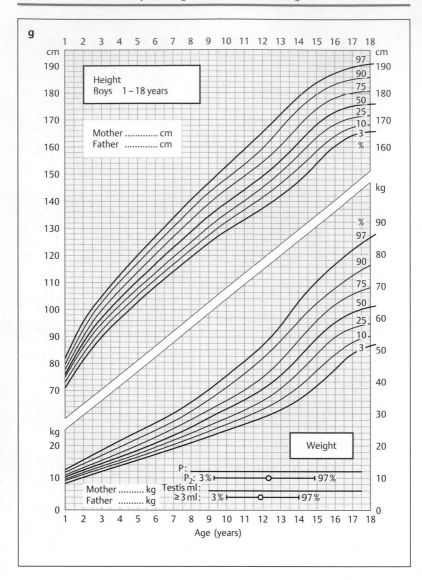

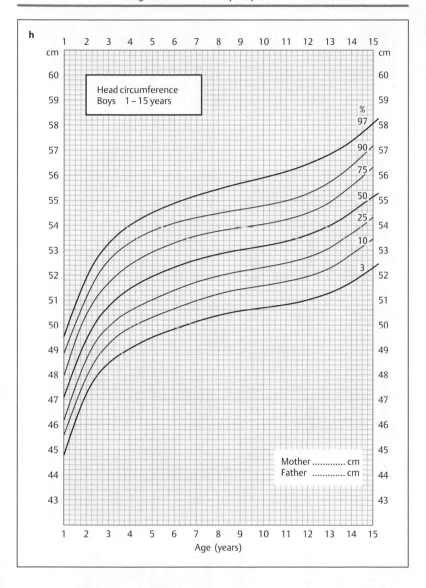

Table 2.1 Reflexes in infancy and childhood

	Reflex	Mode of testing and response	Time normally present	In cerebral palsy	Remarks
Postural reflexes	Doll's eyes phenomenon	Infant awake and recumbent, passive turning of the head. Gaze stays in the original direction	Birth to 10th day	Persistent	
	Step reflex	Child held up under axillae, with soles lightly touching the ground. Stepping movements, body carried along by examiner	First few weeks of life		
	Crossed stretch reflex	Child supine, passive maximal flexion of one hip and knee. Extension of opposite leg and foot	Always abnormal	Note tone in foot	Spinal reflex
	Crossed flexion reflex	Child supine, passive maximal flexion of one hip and knee. Flexion of opposite leg	Birth to 7th–12th month	Abnormal only after the first year	Differential diagnosis: movement accompanying hip contracture of other etiology
Positional reactions	Support reactions	Legs: standing the child up on its feet, or the examiner's pressing on the soles of the feet, induces extension of legs. Arms: pressure induces extension	Increasing from birth to 4th–6th month	Increased, persistent	Physiological astasia in 2nd and 3rd month
	Foot placing reflex	Child held up under axillae, dorsum of foot lightly touches edge of table. Child actively raises leg and plants foot on table	Only in the first few weeks of life		

	Reflex	Stimulus and response			
Positional reactions / **Postural reflexes**	Tonic hand grasp reflex	Examiner touches palm with finger. Clenching of fist	Birth to 3rd month	Increased after 3rd month	Possibly abnormal after 3rd month, definitely abnormal after 6th month
	Tonic foot grasp reflex (toe reflex)	Touching the sole of the foot induces clawing of the toes	Birth to 12th month	Absent at birth, later increasing	Marked clawing of the toes may impair gait
	Tonic spine reflex	Child prone, examiner strokes the skin of the back. Child turns to stroked side, extends ipsilateral leg, and flexes contralateral leg	First few months of life	Increased	Usually barely perceptible
	Tonic neck reflex, asymmetric	Child prone or supine, head slowly passively turned. Altered posture or tone. On the side to which the head is turned, the arm is extended and the leg is extended at the knee and ankle. On the opposite side, the arm is flexed and the leg is flexed in all joints	Birth to 5th–6th month; absent during sleep	Increased; present in sleep after 6th month	
	Tonic neck reflex, symmetric	Child supine, head passively flexed. Flexion of both arms and flexion of both legs at hips, possibly also at other joints	Birth to 5th–6th month; absent during sleep	Increased; present in sleep after 6th month	
	Tonic labyrinthine reflex	Child supine, head passively flexed. Active retraction of head and shoulders, contraction of trunk and hip extensors, opening of mouth	Never pure	Increased	Spastic children do not like to lie prone!
		Child prone, head passively flexed. Flexion of head, flexion and adduction of arms and legs	Rarely pure	Increased	

Table 2.1   Reflexes in infancy and childhood (Cont.)

	Reflex	Mode of testing and response	Time normally present	In cerebral palsy	Remarks
Righting reflexes	**Labyrinthine postural reflex (head)**	Child turned prone or held upside-down by the feet. Retraction of head	Appears in 2nd month; from 3rd–4th to 6th month	Absent Delayed	
		Child sitting, trunk flexed to one side: head kept vertical	Persistent from the 3rd or 4th month onward, though masked by other movements		Sometimes asymmetrical (in presence of hemiparesis)
	Landau reflex	Child held horizontal in abdominal suspension: head retracted, trunk and legs extended. Passive flexion of head: all joints flexed	4th–18th month	Absent, delayed, sometimes prolonged	
	head-on-trunk reflex	Child supine, head turned passively and rapidly to one side. After 1/3 rotation, the trunk follows with a torsional movement	Birth to 12th month	Delayed, protracted, rotation en bloc	Rotation en bloc requires treatment
	Trunk postural reflex	Child supine, shoulder (or pelvis) passively rotated. 1st stage: the trunk follows en bloc. 2nd stage: the trunk follows with torsion Supine position, hips flexed to right angle, rotation of trunk on thighs	Birth to 4th–6th month 4th–6th to 14th month; birth to 6th month	Increased, sometimes prolonged	Test is negative when the pelvis begins to rotate only after 80° of shoulder rotation

	Reflex	Description	Age		
Balance reactions	**Moro reflex**	Child supine. A sudden blow on the bed induces movement of the arms to the sides and then forwards, as if in an embrace, with hands open. The same response occurs when the patient is held supine in the air and the head is suddenly let go	Birth to 4th–7th month	Positive for longer period	Absent in the first few months in cases of severe brain injury
	Body righting reaction	Attempting to push the child out of any body position induces contraction of the ipsilateral muscles	When sitting, from 7th month onward	Delayed, absent or deficient	
	Limping reaction	Attempting to push the child out of any body position induces a buttressing movement, possibly across the midline	When sitting, from 7th month onward	Delayed, absent or deficient	When standing, better toward the affected side; when sitting, child may use unaffected arm across midline to affected side
	Parachute reflex	Child in ventral suspension or kneeling position and suddenly pushed forward. Extension of arms, palms open	From the 6th to 9th month onward	Absent, delayed, or incomplete	An abnormal reflex, even if asymmetric or if the hands are clenched; a statokinetic reaction

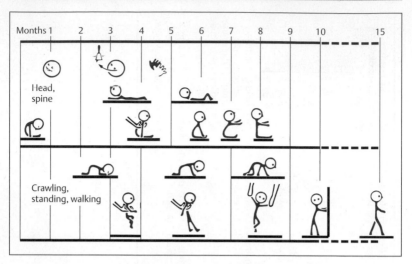

Fig. 2.**2**   **Normal motor development in infancy and early childhood.**

Cerebral Movement Disorders, Infantile Cerebral Palsy, Psychomotor Retardation (311, 661, 926)

Definition:
These terms are used more or less synonymously to denote any delay of motor development that becomes evident in early childhood, regardless of etiology. In most cases, such disorders are already evident in the first year of life and are accompanied by delayed mental development.

Etiology and Pathogenesis

Problems during pregnancy and delivery, premature birth, and birth weight under 2000 g or over 4000 g often cause hypoxic injury to the brain and thereby lead to a cerebral movement disorder. The Apgar scale is a measure of the infant's neurological and general medical condition at birth (Table 2.**2**). Congenital malformations (p. 32), infectious and toxic conditions affecting prenatal development of the brain (p. 36), and severe neonatal jaundice (p. 38) are

further causes of cerebral movement disorders.

Clinical Features

A cerebral movement disorder may be manifested at birth by cyanosis or a delayed first cry, or in the first few weeks of life by feeding difficulties, hypotonia or a fixed arching of the back, a tendency to opisthotonus, and spasticity, which may make diaper changes difficult. Strabismus and left-handedness are also more common

Table 2.**2** The Apgar scale

Criterion	Finding	Score	Score of neonate, recorded 1, 5, and 10 min after birth
Pulse	None	0	
	< 100/min	1	
	> 100/min	2	
Respirations	Absent or slow	0	
	Irregular	1	
	Loud cry	2	
Muscle tone	Absent	0	
	Weak	1	
	Strong, active movements	2	
Reflexes (in response to stimulation, e.g., of sole of foot)	Absent	0	
	Grimace	1	
	Cry	2	
Skin color	Generalized cyanosis or pallor	0	
	Trunk pink, limbs blue	1	
	Entire body pink	2	
	Overall score:		

An Apgar score of 4 or less 1 minute after birth, or 6 or less 5 minutes after birth, indicates hypoxia.

in infants with cerebral movement disorders.

For a discussion of the clinical features of cerebral movement disorders in the first year of life, see p. 15. Motor development in infancy and early childhood is depicted in Fig. 2.**2**, and reflexes in infancy and early childhood (104) are described in detail in Table 2.**1**.

Findings on Examination

At first, *hypotonia* may be present, for as long as 6 months ("floppy infant"). There follows a period of several months characterized by dystonic, fluctuating, position-dependent and stimulus-related *increasing muscle tone*, after which true *spasticity* appears. Involuntary movements (athetosis, chorea, choreoathetosis, torsion dystonia, tremor), ataxia, and rigidity are also frequently present, with or without spasticity. Epileptic seizures occur in some cases.

Intellectual ability may be more or less severely impaired. The term *oligophrenia* denotes a significant impairment of intellectual ability that is either congenital, or acquired in early childhood.

In some children, varying degrees of agnosia and apraxia may produce *disturbances of fine motor control*, of drawing, and of the appreciation of spatial relationships. These children are often not only clumsy, but also restless and *hyperkinetic*. They often have choreiform movements, which can, however, be suppressed at will or by voluntary movement. Poor performance on tests of practical manual skills contrasts with relatively high verbal intelligence. There is a complex relationship to dyslexia. The mental status examination is normal, but the EEG is almost always diffusely abnormal. The term "clumsy child" is sometimes used as a shorthand description of this condition, which is also called "débilité motrice" (motor debility).

This condition is almost always due to a relatively minor congenital abnormality of, or perinatal injury to, the brain. Some of its clinical features may reflect an abnormality of cortical organization occurring during fetal development. Table 2.3 provides an overview of cerebral movement disorders.

Course

About 25% of cases improve spontaneously, and a further 50% can be helped to a greater or lesser extent by early therapeutic intervention. Early detection is, therefore, essential. Much can be achieved at present with exercise therapies (e.g., those of Bobath or Vojta) that are specifically tailored to the abnormal reflex activity of these children. 25% do, however, remain severely impaired.

Malformations of the Brain

Most of the conditions listed in Table 2.4 become evident at birth or shortly thereafter.

Table 2.3   The most important cerebral movement disorders

Name of disorder	Clinical features	Pathoanatomical substrate	Causes
Infantile spastic diplegia (Little's disease)	Spasticity, predominantly in the legs; pes equinus, scissor gait, often mentally normal	Pachymicrogyria, lobar sclerosis	Perinatal injury (disturbance of cerebral development, embryopathy, severe neonatal jaundice)
Congenital cerebral monoparesis	Usually, paresis of arm and face	Porencephaly, localized atrophy	Birth trauma (asphyxia, hemorrhage)
Congenital hemiparesis	Arms more severely affected than legs, seizures in ca. 50%, usually mentally impaired	Porencephaly	Birth trauma (asphyxia, hemorrhage)

Table 2.3   The most important cerebral movement disorders *(Cont.)*

Name of disorder	Clinical features	Pathoanatomical substrate	Causes
Congenital quadriparesis (bilateral hemiparesis)	Arms more severely affected than legs, occasionally bulbar signs, seizures; severe mental impairment	Porencephaly, bilateral; often hydrocephalus	Birth trauma (asphyxia, hemorrhage), also prenatal injury
Congenital pseudobulbar palsy	Dysphagia to liquids, dysarthria, usually not mentally impaired	Bilateral lesions of the corticobulbar pathways	Prenatal injury or birth trauma, malformation (syringobulbia)
Atonic–astatic syndrome (Foerster)	Generalized flaccid weakness, inability to stand, impaired coordination, severe mental impairment	Frontal lobe atrophy? Cerebellar defects?	
Bilateral athetosis (athétose double) and congenital chorea (choreoathetosis)	Athetotic or other involuntary movements, often combined with spastic paresis	Basal ganglionic defects, status marmoratus (Vogt); status dysmyelinisatus in cases of later onset	Disturbance of cerebral development, perinatal injury, esp. severe neonatal jaundice
Congenital rigor	Rigor without involuntary movements, postural abnormalities, no pyramidal tract signs, severe mental impairment, seizures	Status marmoratus	Disturbance of cerebral development, perinatal injury, esp. severe neonatal jaundice
Congenital cerebellar ataxia	Gait ataxia, intention tremor and impaired coordination, motor developmental retardation, dysarthria, possibly in combination with other motor syndromes	Cerebellar defect	Disturbance of cerebellar development

Table 2.4   The most important malformations of the brain

Dysgenesis or agenesis of parts of the brain:	
• Micropolygyria	Focally abnormal gyral pattern: gyri abnormally narrow and abnormally numerous
• Pachygyria	Abnormally few secondary convolutions
• Agyria	Absence of convolutions (smooth brain)
• Lissencephaly	(See agyria)
• Double cortex syndrome (348a)	Cortical cells in two layers (genetically determined)
• Arrhinencephaly	Absence of olfactory nerves and tracts, (sometimes) agenesis of the corpus callosum, other abnormalities
• Cyclopia	Single orbit
• Holotelencephaly	Single ventricle in rostral portion of cerebrum
• Dandy-Walker syndrome	Cystic dilatation of the fourth ventricle, hydrocephalus
• Arnold-Chiari malformation	Caudal displacement of the cerebellar tonsils, sometimes associated with syringomyelia and other anomalies of the craniocervical junction
Microcephaly	Small head and brain
Neural tube defects:	Incomplete closure of the neural tube
• Spina bifida occulta • Meningocele • Myelomeningocele • Myelomeningocystocele • Open anencephaly	
Sinus pericranii	Vascular malformation communicating with a venous sinus, usually frontal
Cranial dermal sinus	In the midline, usually occipital, often associated with a dermoid cyst
Phakomatoses	Malformations affecting multiple systems including the central nervous system (see Table 2.5)

■ Agenesis or Dysgenesis of Parts of the Brain
See Table 2.4.

■ Microcephaly
A variety of prenatal influences can result in microcephaly, particularly cytomegalovirus (p. 37), but also genetic factors in 15% of cases.

■ Meningoencephalocele and Meningomyelocele
The following defects of the brain and spinal cord may occur:
• Incomplete closure of bone over the central nervous structures: *cranium bifidum occultum (spina bifida occulta)*.
• Emergence of the meninges through the bony defect, covered by skin: *meningocele*.

- Emergence of the meninges and of brain or spinal cord parenchyma through the bony defect: *encephalomeningocele (myelomeningocele)*.
- The emerging portion of the central nervous system includes part of the fluid-filled ventricular system: *encephalomeningocystocele (myelomeningocystocele)*.
- The neural tube has failed to close, so that the malformed primordial brain lies uncovered as an open neural plate: *anencephaly (complete rachischisis)*.

■ **Phakomatoses**

The abnormalities associated with the phakomatoses (Table 2.**5**) are found not only in the brain, but also in the skin, the peripheral nerves, and other internal organs.

■ **Tuberous Sclerosis (Bourneville's Disease)**
Genetics and Pathogenesis
This multifaceted disorder of histogenesis is transmitted in an autosomal-dominant inheritance pattern with a high rate of spontaneous mutation.

Clinical Features
The illness is clinically characterized by feeblemindedness, cutaneous manifestations (particularly adenoma sebaceum), nodular tumors of the heart, kidneys, and retina, epileptic seizures, and nodular intracranial tumors ("tubers"), which are frequently calcified.
The *intellectual deficit* becomes evident within the first 2 years of life. *Hypopigmented macules* ("white spots") are seen in only three-quarters of cases; the presence of more than 54 such spots should arouse clinical suspicion of the dis-

■ **Prevention and Treatment** ■
The risk of an open neural tube defect is reduced by 70% or more if the mother takes at least 0.4 mg of folic acid around the time of conception, and other vitamins and minerals may also be protective (124b, 200a). Of the malformations of the brain listed above, only meningocele and encephalomeningocele are, in principle, operable; for myelomeningocele, see p. 393. If a surgical repair is to be performed, it should be done in the first few hours after birth. The decision whether to operate should be based on careful consideration of what is likely to be achieved thereby for the newborn and its family. The parents' attitude, and any accompanying spinal malformations or hydrocephalus, should be taken into account.
Prenatal detection of malformations of the brain and spinal cord is at least as important as treatment. The concentration of fetally derived protein (α-fetoprotein) in maternal blood is measured. A normal αFP level is associated with a risk of only one in 10,000 that the newborn will have a neural tube defect. If the αFP level is elevated, the risk rises to 1 in 15.

ease. *Adenoma sebaceum* (Pringle's nevus) often becomes visible at some time in early childhood. *Intracranial calcifications* are often visible on radiological images from the age of 2–4 years onward.
Seizures practically always begin in the first 2 years of life, at first often as salaam spasms (p. 515).
Nodular tumors are found in the heart, kidneys, and retina, and so-

Table 2.5   The most important phakomatoses

Disease	Neurological abnormalities	Further characteristics	Inheritance
Tuberous sclerosis (Bourneville's disease)	Feeble-mindedness, seizures, white spots, adenoma sebaceum	Nodular tumors in heart, kidney, and retina, and tubers in the brain, often calcified	Autosomal dominant
Encephalofacial angiomatosis (Sturge-Weber disease)	Seizures, feeble-mindedness, possibly hemiparesis, nevus flammeus of the face	"Railroad-track" intracranial calcifications	Sporadic or dominant, with variable penetrance
von Hippel-Lindau disease	Progressive cerebellar signs in middle age, signs of elevated intracranial pressure	Retinal angiomatosis, cystic cerebellar hemangioblastoma, rarely tumors of other internal organs	Autosomal dominant
Neurofibromatosis (von Recklinghausen's disease)	Progressive peripheral neuropathy or radiculopathy, vestibular schwannoma, meningioma, spinal cord tumors	Cutaneous neurofibroma, café-au-lait spots, axillary freckling	Autosomal dominant, often a new mutation; malignant degeneration may occur
Ataxia telangiectasia (Louis-Bar syndrome)	Progressive cerebellar ataxia beginning in infancy, sometimes with chorea	Later, telangiectasia, particularly of the conjunctiva; frequent pulmonary and ear infections	Autosomal recessive

called *tubers* in the brain (subependymal giant-cell astrocytomas), which are often calcified. When the diagnosis is suspected, it should be confirmed by CT or MRI of the brain in the first few months of life, to enable appropriate genetic counseling of the parents.

■ Encephalofacial Angiomatosis (Sturge-Weber Disease)
Genetics
This disease is mostly found in individuals without relevant family history, but is probably transmitted in autosomal-dominant fashion with variable penetrance.

Clinical Features
It is characterized by the combination of a facial nevus ("nevus flammeus") in the distribution of one or more branches of the trigeminal nerve with (focal) epilepsy, intellectual deficiency, and sometimes contralateral hemiparesis.

Diagnosis
Radiologic studies reveal "railroad-track" calcifications of the cerebral cortex, corresponding to abnormal, serpentine vessels (mostly capillaries and small veins) in the meninges covering the parieto-occipital convexity.

■ Von Hippel-Lindau Disease
Genetics
Von Hippel-Lindau disease is of simple autosomal dominant inheritance.

Clinical Features
Retinal angiomatosis is found in combination with a single or, rarely, multiple hemangioblastoma of the cerebellum. Syringomyelia may also be present. The cerebellar tumor usually arises in middle age and consists of a cyst with a mural nodule. It may become manifest through cerebellar dysfunction, signs of intracranial hypertension, or signs of syringomyelia.

Treatment
The treatment consists of the complete neurosurgical removal of the mural nodule of the cerebellar hemangioblastoma. Early diagnosis and treatment confer a good prognosis.

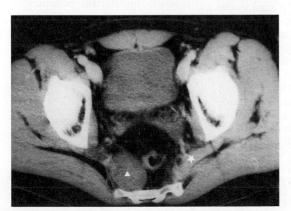

Fig. 2.**3   Neurinoma (▲) of the sciatic nerve in von Recklinghausen's neurofibromatosis.** CT of the pelvis. The star indicates the piriformis muscle, which divides the sciatic foramen into supra- and infrapiriform compartments.

■ Neurofibromatosis (von Recklinghausen's Disease)

Clinical Features

This phakomatosis is characterized by the presence of numerous neurofibromas, which develop from connective tissue nerve sheaths. These may affect either *peripheral nerves* or *nerve roots,* giving rise to progressive mononeuropathies or radiculopathies, respectively (Fig. 2.**3**).

Neurofibromas within the spinal canal may lead to signs of spinal cord compression and paraplegia. A neurofibroma growing within an intervertebral neural foramen assumes a characteristic *dumbbell* shape because of the combination of intra- and extraspinal tumor mass (see Fig. 3.**5**). The intraspinal portion of the tumor causes neurologic symptoms and signs. Enlargement of the neural foramen itself may be demonstrable on plain roentgenograms of the spine (oblique view).

The most common *intracranial* tumor in this disease is a schwannoma affecting the vestibulocochlear nerve, usually (but inaccurately) termed "acoustic neuroma." These tumors are often bilateral and give rise to the typical clinical signs of a mass in the cerebellopontine angle (p. 68). Tumors are also found in association with the optic nerve and the retina, leading to visual disturbances, and occasionally within the brain itself, leading to epilepsy and other signs of space-occupying lesions. Neurofibromas may undergo malignant degeneration. Meningiomas are also found with increased frequency in this patient group.

Cutaneous lesions include neurofibromas, which may be very large, and pigmented patches (café-au-lait spots, freckles). Axillary freckling is typical. The pattern of inheritance is autosomal dominant, and 90% of cases represent new mutations.

■ Ataxia Telangiectasia

Ataxia telangiectasia may be considered one of the phakomatoses and is discussed on p. 280.

Infectious and Toxic Conditions Affecting Prenatal Development of the Brain (Table 2.6)

Table 2.**6**   Infectious and toxic conditions affecting prenatal development of the brain

Rubella embryopathy
Congenital toxoplasmosis
Congenital cytomegalovirus
Congenital syphilis
Congenital HIV infection
Alcohol embryopathy

■ Rubella Embryopathy

Rubella in the mother in the first trimester of pregnancy carries an approximately 10% risk of damage to the fetus; the later the maternal illness, the lower the risk. The more common defects are:

- cataract,
- deafness (abnormal development of the inner ear),
- microcephaly, and
- cardiac anomalies.

■ Congenital Toxoplasmosis

A maternal infection with toxoplasmosis in early pregnancy is followed in late pregnancy by generalized infection of the fetus, and then by florid encephalitis with general cerebral symptoms and signs, seizures, and hydrocephalus. The cerebrospinal fluid is abnormal (for serologic diagnosis, see p. 108).

■ Congenital Cytomegalovirus
This disease causes:
- premature birth and other disturbances of delivery,
- microcephaly (the leading sign),
- hydrocephalus,
- seizures,
- paralysis,
- intracerebral calcifications, particularly around the ventricles.

■ Congenital Syphilis
This form of neurosyphilis is more common when the mother is affected with an early stage of the disease. The syphilis-related serologic reactions in blood and cerebrospinal fluid are usually positive. Chorioretinitis is often seen. Tertiary manifestations, such as general paresis or tabes dorsalis, may appear years later (p. 112).

■ Congenital HIV Infection
Approximately 25% of HIV-positive pregnant women transmit the infection to their children either in utero, during labor, or through breast-feeding. The risk is much lower when delivery is by caesarean section and when antiretroviral therapy is given (p. 124). Documentation of infection is complicated by the presence of maternal HIV antibodies in neonatal blood, and therefore a direct demonstration of the virus itself should be attempted. The polymerase chain reaction (PCR) reveals infection at the age of 3 months in almost all cases. The manifestations are highly variable and include delayed psychomotor development and spasticity (with mortality over 50% in the first 3 years) and immunodeficiency. Infants with immunodeficiency but without encephalopathy have a better prognosis and may survive into the second decade of life.

■ Alcohol Embryopathy
Alcohol embryopathy is damage to the fetus caused by maternal alcohol consumption during pregnancy. The manifestations include small stature, psychomotor retardation, microcephaly, facial dysmorphia (small nose, thin lips, micrognathia), and a number of other structural abnormalities.

Brain Disorders Due to Birth Trauma

■ Subdural Hematoma
Subdural hematoma is the most common hemorrhagic complication resulting from trauma during delivery. The source of bleeding is either a torn venous sinus (often the transverse sinus) or one or more bridging veins.

Treatment
The treatment is neurosurgical and consists of repeated puncture with aspiration, and/or craniotomy.

■ Intracerebral and Intraventricular Hemorrhage
These hemorrhages are usually fatal, but the patient may survive a smaller hemorrhage (single or multiple) and develop the clinical picture of a cerebral movement disorder. The manifestations are comparable to those of diffuse brain damage from *neonatal asphyxia.* The pathological changes arising in such cases include thinning and sclerosis of the cerebral convolutions (*ulegyria*), the formation of large cystic spaces (*porencephaly*), and *status marmoratus* of the basal

ganglia. The last-named is due to an excess of myelinated fibers and is associated with athetosis or *athétose double*.

Severe Neonatal Jaundice ("Icterus Gravis Neonatorum")

Definition:
Maternal–fetal Rh-incompatibility leads to deposition of bilirubin in the brain, particularly in the basal ganglia, and thereby to paresis, dystonia, athetosis, deafness, and intellectual deficiency.

■ Pathoanatomy and Pathophysiology

When an Rh-negative woman has formed anti-Rh antibodies through previous pregnancy with an Rh-positive fetus (or transfusion of Rh-positive blood) and then becomes pregnant with another Rh-positive fetus, the anti-Rh antibodies cross the placenta and induce the immunologic destruction of fetal erythrocytes. So-called "kernicterus" develops (German for "jaundice of the [deep cerebral] nuclei"), in which bilirubin is deposited in various portions of the basal ganglia.

■ Clinical Features

The neonate suffers from edema, anemia, erythroblastosis, and jaundice that rapidly worsens within a few days of birth. Kernicterus develops in about 20% of cases with erythroblastosis. Two to five days after the onset of jaundice, the neonate becomes apathetic, does not drink, and develops clonic movements, opisthotonus, and irregular breathing. Death ensues in severe cases in 3–7 days, but most of these children survive to suffer from a form of cerebral palsy with motor abnormalities, pareses, involuntary dystonic or athetotic movements, deafness, and intellectual deficiency.

In recent years, hemolytic disease of the newborn due to maternal–fetal Rh-incompatibility has become a preventable illness through the administration of anti-Rh immunoglobulin injections during pregnancy.

■ Diagnosis

The diagnosis is made by measurement of the serum bilirubin level.

Treatment

In milder cases (bilirubin concentration 10–20 mg/100 mL), *phototherapy*. In severe cases (greater than 20 mg/100 mL), *exchange transfusion*.

Hydrocephalus

Definition:
Enlargement of the internal and/or external cerebrospinal fluid spaces (see Table 2.7).

Table 2.7 Types and terminology of hydrocephalus

Internal hydrocephalus	Enlargement of the ventricles:
• Obstructive	Due to obstruction of CSF flow within the ventricular system (e.g., aqueductal stenosis) or at its exits (e.g., obstruction of foramina of Magendie and Luschka)
• Communicating	Nonobstructive internal hydrocephalus
• Malresorptive	A subtype of communicating hydrocephalus due to impaired CSF resorption (e.g., cisternal adhesions or dysfunction of the pacchionian granulations)
External hydrocephalus	Enlargement of the subarachnoid space over the cerebral convexities and/or in the cisterns
External and internal hydrocephalus	Combination of the above
Hydrocephalus ex vacuo	Widening of sulci and ventricles secondary to brain atrophy

■ Normal Physiology

The cerebrospinal fluid (CSF) is produced in the choroid plexus of the lateral, third, and fourth cerebral ventricles. It flows from the lateral ventricles through the interventricular foramina of Monro into the third ventricle, through the cerebral aqueduct of Sylvius into the fourth ventricle, and through the medial foramen of Magendie and lateral foramina of Luschka into the basal cisterns (cerebellomedullary cistern and lateral pontine cisterns, respectively) (Fig. 2.4). Having thus arrived in the perimedullary subarachnoid space, it flows over the entire surface of the brain and spinal cord and finally enters the bloodstream through the Pacchionian granulations (arachnoid villi) of the superior sagittal sinus. CSF is probably also independently produced within the subarachnoid space itself.

■ Pathogenesis

Hydrocephalus arises when the flow of CSF is impeded at any point along its pathway. A distinction is drawn between *communicating hydrocephalus,* in which the ventricles communicate with each other and with the subarachnoid space, and *obstructive (noncommunicating) hydrocephalus,* in which the flow of CSF is blocked at some point at or above the level of the fourth ventricular outflow. Causes of the latter include agenesis, gliosis, stenosis, or malformation of the cerebral aqueduct, posterior fossa tumors, and blockage of the foramina of Luschka and Magendie.

■ Congenital and Infantile Hydrocephalus
■ Clinical Features

Congenital and infantile hydrocephalus are characterized by an abnormally large and progressively increasing head circumference (see Fig. 2.1). The fontanelles are wide and may

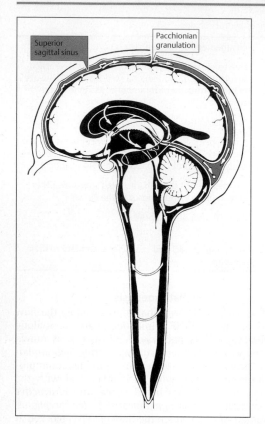

Fig. 2.**4   Circulation of the cerebrospinal fluid** (adapted from Gardner).

bulge. Percussion of the skull may yield a cracked-pot sound. The forehead bulges outward and the orbital plates are pushed downward, so that the sclera is visible above the iris of both eyes, which thus appears to dip below the lower lid ("setting-sun sign").

■ Ancillary Tests

Suspected hydrocephalus should be initially evaluated by ultrasound, as long as the fontanelle is still open. The diagnosis is revealed in other cases by CT or MRI. The only possible contraindication to further evaluation and treatment of hydrocephalus is a demonstrated, severe accompanying malformation of the brain.

■ Prognosis

Untreated hydrocephalus in childhood confers a mortality of more than 50%. Only a small minority of the surviving untreated individuals will develop normally. CSF shunting has reduced the overall mortality at 10 years after diagnosis to less than 10%, with an operative mortality under 1%. More than two-thirds of all children with treated isolated hydrocephalus (i.e., without accompanying malformation of the brain) go on to develop normally, both physically and mentally. If the brain parenchyma is less than 1.5 mm thick at the time of diagnosis, however, the prognosis for normal development is poor.

■ Differential Diagnosis

A large head frequently reflects familial microcephaly. Such children, who are typically larger and heavier than usual, are otherwise healthy and exhibit normal psychomotor development. The setting-sun phenomenon is absent, and the CT scan is normal. Serial measurement reveals tracking of the larger-than-normal head circumference along its percentile curve.

Treatment

The findings of the imaging studies determine the type of treatment. In rare cases, a direct reopening of a blocked passageway may be attempted (e.g., atresia of the foramina of Luschka and Magendie), but, much more commonly, a shunt operation will be performed.

Occlusive hydrocephalus was once most commonly treated by ventriculocisternostomy (the Torkildsen shunt), in which CSF was redirected through permanently implanted tubes from the posterior horns of the lateral ventricles into the cerebellomedullary cistern. This operation has now been entirely supplanted by the ventriculoperitoneal shunt.

Ventriculoatrial shunting, once commonly performed for communicating hydrocephalus, has also been largely replaced by ventriculoperitoneal shunting.

In recent years, neuroendoscopic surgery has been introduced for the treatment of occlusive hydrocephalus. A hole is made in the floor of the third ventricle to enable flow of CSF from the ventricles into the subarachnoid space (endoscopic third ventriculostomy). A permanent, indwelling foreign body (shunt catheter) is thus unnecessary. Further experience with this technique, and long-term follow-up of treated patients, will reveal whether it truly provides comparable or better results than the conventional ventriculoperitoneal shunt.

■ Otitic Hydrocephalus

This rather imprecise term denotes an elevation of intracranial pressure caused by thrombosis of a venous sinus, usually the transverse sinus, which impedes the resorption of CSF from the subarachnoid space into the bloodstream. This syndrome may occur as a consequence of otitis media (more commonly on the right side) or of other primary processes. It is characterized by:
- headache,
- vomiting,
- papilledema, and
- abducens palsy, often bilateral.

Most of the affected patients are children. The prognosis is good if the primary process is appropriately treated.

■ Normal-Pressure Hydrocephalus (Nonresorptive Hydrocephalus, Malresorptive Hydrocephalus)

■ Clinical Features

Normal-pressure hydrocephalus affects adults, but is considered in this section along with the other hydrocephalus syndromes. Its clinical features are listed in Table 2.**8**.

Table 2.8   Clinical features of normal-pressure hydrocephalus

Symptoms	Clinical findings	Ancillary tests	Etiology
Progressive gait disturbance, urinary incontinence, fluctuating psycho-organic changes	Spasticity in the lower extremities, pyramidal tract signs, psycho-organic syndrome, transient improvement after lumbar puncture	CT: dilatation of lateral ventricles and narrowing of the subarachnoid space. Radioisotope cisternography: activity in the lateral ventricles. Continuous ICP monitoring (24 hours): pressure spikes. Intrathecal infusion test: reduced compliance.	Subarachnoid hemorrhage, traumatic brain injury, meningitis, venous sinus thrombosis; rarely cryptogenic

■ Causes

Adhesions in the subarachnoid space or impaired CSF resorption through the Pacchionian granulations leads to the development of normal-pressure hydrocephalus. Common etiologies include a previous traumatic or aneurysmal subarachnoid hemorrhage, meningitis, and, more rarely, borreliosis (Lyme disease). The syndrome may also arise without any discernible cause.

■ Ancillary Tests

CT and MRI scans reveal symmetrical enlargement of the cerebral ventricles with normal, or constricted, external CSF spaces. A typical MRI finding is abnormal signal intensity adjacent to the poles of the lateral ventricles, so-called "polar capping." A characteristic clinical feature is rapid and dramatic improvement after lumbar puncture and withdrawal of CSF.

Radioisotope cisternography with labeled albumin may be used to trace the abnormally slow flow of CSF from the subarachnoid space into the ventricles.

An important diagnostic aid is continuous monitoring of intracranial pressure or of lumbar CSF pressure. A constant or intermittent mild elevation of pressure distinguishes so-called normal-pressure hydrocephalus from hydrocephalus ex vacuo (in which the pressure is truly normal). A CSF infusion test can provide a direct measure of resorptive capacity.

A further aid to differential diagnosis is the glycosphingolipid (sulfatide) concentration in CSF, which is elevated in hydrocephalus ex vacuo on an atherosclerotic basis, but not in normal-pressure hydrocephalus (956a).

■ Diagnosis

In the last 30 years, this syndrome has been too frequently diagnosed, and too many shunt operations have been performed. Surgical treatment should only be considered when typical signs, such as gait ataxia, are present (though the associated dementia may be no more than mild), when the CT or MRI findings are consistent, and when an appropriate etiology can be determined (974, 974a).

███ **Treatment** ███

Treatment is highly beneficial in properly selected cases and consists of a ventriculoperitoneal or ventriculoatrial shunt operation (see above). Those patients benefit most who exhibit the full neurological and psychopathological syndrome and in whom a prior etiological event can be clearly identified. Only one-third to two-thirds of patients will actually improve after the operation. Shunting should not be performed in cases of progressive psycho-organic syndrome or progressive spasticity without identifiable cause, even if the radioisotope cisternogram is abnormal.

Craniostenosis (Craniosynostosis)

Premature closure of one or more cranial sutures upsets the coordinated enlargement of the skull in step with the growing brain (218). The clinical subtypes of craniostenosis are listed in Table 2.**9**. At first, the proportions of the growing skull are distorted. Later, in many cases, intellectual development is impaired, and there may be seizures and signs of intracranial hypertension.

███ **Treatment** ███

The treatment is neurosurgical and consists of excision of strips of bone incorporating the abnormally closed suture(s). For best results, surgery should be performed early, before the age of 4 months if possible.

Anomalies of the Craniocervical Junction

■ Classification

The following malformations may be present, singly or in combination:
- atlanto-occipital assimilation,
- os odontoideum,
- atlantoaxial instability,
- occipital vertebra,
- spina bifida of the atlas,
- platybasia,
- basilar impression.

In basilar impression, the lateral skull roentgenogram shows the tip of the dens projecting more than 5 mm above either Chamberlain's line (from the posterior rim of the hard palate to the posterior rim of the foramen magnum) or McGregor's line (from the posterior rim of the hard palate to the most caudal point of the occiput).

Block vertebrae (the Klippel-Feil anomaly) may be present in the cervical spine. These skeletal anomalies are sometimes accompanied by anomalies of the brain itself, such as the Arnold-Chiari malformation (p. 32).

■ Clinical Features

Patients with anomalies of the craniocervical junction often have a short neck and a low hairline. Neurological symptoms generally begin in adulthood and progress slowly. The typical clinical picture is a combination of lower cranial nerve palsies, brainstem signs (nystagmus) and long tract signs (bilateral pyramidal tract signs and sensory disturbances, which may be dissociated).

Treatment

The optimal form of treatment has yet to be defined. It is not yet clear whether wide occipital decompression or a shunt operation is beneficial. If a bony decompression is performed for this indication (in the presence or absence of an associated Arnold-Chiari malformation), a duraplasty should be performed as well to enlarge the space available for the brain, and retroflexion of the head should be avoided during the procedure (271).

Table 2.**9**   Clinical types of craniosynostosis

Name	Fused suture	Shape of head	Remarks
Scaphocephaly (= dolichocephaly)	Sagittal suture	Long, narrow ("boat-shaped")	Most common form
Acrocephaly	Coronal suture	High, broad on top; flat forehead	
Oxycephaly	Sagittal, coronal, and lambdoid sutures	Pointed	Second most common form
Brachycephaly	Coronal and lambdoid sutures	Short, broad	
Plagiocephaly	Premature fusion (or incomplete fusion) of a coronal suture	Asymmetrical (e.g., flattened on one side)	More often due to asymmetrical muscle tone in cerebral palsy
Crouzon's disease (craniofacial dysostosis)	Primarily the coronal suture, and maxillary sutures in the face	Broad skull and face, jutting forehead, exophthalmos, hypertelorism, hook nose, prognathism	Sometimes with airway compromise

Table 2.**9** Clinical types of craniosynostosis *(Cont.)*

Name	Fused suture	Shape of head	Remarks
Trigonocephaly	Metopic suture	Forehead pointed in front	
Platycephaly	Lambdoid suture	Broad occiput	

Traumatic Brain Injury (253)

Definition:

An external force acting on the head, depending on its intensity, may lead to a simple brain contusion without discernible clinical manifestations, or to varying degrees of more severe injury, up to a deep laceration of the brain. Loss of consciousness commonly occurs at the moment of impact and may be brief or prolonged, depending on the severity of the injury. Amnesia for events occurring before the injury *(retrograde amnesia)* and for events occurring afterward *(anterograde amnesia)* is often present once consciousness is regained; the duration of time for which memory is lost is an index of the severity of the injury. There may be intracranial hemorrhage (epidural, subdural, or intracerebral). Neurological deficits present in the early post-traumatic phase of a brain contusion may persist. Treating personnel are often insufficiently aware of lasting neuropsychological deficits and a generalized psycho-organic syndrome that may impair reintegration into everyday life and occupational activities. Posttraumatic epilepsy may arise, sometimes long after the injury. There are often major *permanent sequelae.*

Frequency

Traumatic brain injury is steadily becoming more common, largely because of motor vehicle accidents. In industrial countries, the incidence is ca. 8000 cases per million persons per year, of which approximately half require hospitalization. Some 2.5–5% of patients later require rehabilitation.

Classification

The following types of injury are distinguished, in increasing order of severity:

- *scalp contusion* without brain injury and no evidence of concussion (this condition requires no further discussion here);
- *brain concussion* (with or without skull fracture);
- *brain contusion* (not always accompanied by a fracture, and occurs in exceptional cases without signs of concussion), due to indirect trauma;
- *brain laceration:* a direct trauma to the brain, always associated with bony injury;
- early and late posttraumatic sequelae, sometimes involving *brain compression.*

The boundary between simple scalp trauma and concussion, and that between concussion and brain contusion, are not always easy to define. The presence or absence of a skull fracture says nothing about the severity of the associated brain injury.

History and Physical Examination in Traumatic Brain Injury

Accident History

The following points should be noted:

- the exact time and nature of the accident, including the direction of the blow;
- head covering, if any;
- the patient's recollection of the accident;
- the presence and duration of retro- or anterograde amnesia;
- nausea and vomiting.

Physical Examination

Examination immediately following craniocerebral trauma should include the following:

- level of consciousness;
- external injuries, particularly of the head;
- bleeding or flow of cerebrospinal fluid from the nose or ears, or in the throat;
- injuries of the cervical spine;
- periorbital and/or retroauricular hematoma;
- general medical condition, and particularly circulatory state (shock!);
- neurological findings (in particular, pupils, visual function, nystagmus, hearing, paresis, and pyramidal tract signs);
- cervical spine roentgenogram in the unconscious patient, and in any patient whose mechanism of injury suggests the possibility of cervical spine trauma;
- CT for immediate documentation of acute anatomical injuries, esp. hemorrhage. The CT scan often reveals more lesions 24–48 hours after the trauma than on the initial examination. MRI is particularly useful for the documentation of infratentorial injuries. T2-weighted MRI also reveals axonal shear injuries, which are most common in the corpus callosum and in the frontal white matter (see Fig. 2.**6**).

Mild Traumatic Brain Injury (Concussion)

Definition:
Brain concussion is not accompanied by any macroscopically evident anatomic brain injury and is accordingly not followed by any lasting neurologic deficit. Histological examination, however, reveals disruptions of axonal continuity caused by a shearing effect; corresponding abnormalities may be seen on T2-weighted MRI (see below). The clinical features of concussion include loss of consciousness, which may be very brief, retrograde amnesia, vomiting, headache, vertigo, and transient mental impairment. Practically all significant injuries to the skull, not including simple scalp contusions, are accompanied by (at least) a concussion of the brain.

Clinical Features

Impairment of consciousness is a defining feature of concussion, but may be very brief. Witnesses to the accident may fail to note a loss of consciousness (e.g., the victim may stand up immediately), but there is practically always a discernible gap in the patient's memory for events either before or after the accident, or both. *Retrograde amnesia* is common, but not obligatory. The period of *anterograde amnesia* is not limited to that of loss of consciousness, but rather largely corresponds to that of the *posttraumatic twilight state.*

As a rule, the unconsciousness of simple brain concussion lasts no longer than 15 minutes, and the twilight state no longer than 1 hour. If the former lasts more than 1 hour or the latter more than 24 hours, a brain contusion is likely to be present.

Vomiting occurs commonly in brain concussion. It has been found that vomiting is four times more common in the presence of a skull fracture, although, even when a skull fracture is present, only one-third of patients with concussion will vomit (699b). In children, even very mild trauma leads not uncommonly to initially quite dramatic manifestations, including loss of consciousness and confusion, which then regress spontaneously and completely.

Examination

Physical examination reveals no general medical or focal neurological abnormalities, and the findings of lumbar puncture and EEG are normal.

Postconcussional Complaints

These generally arise immediately after the injury and gradually regress over a variable interval. *Headaches* are prominent, usually diffuse, occasionally present in the morning, but often developing only in the course of the day, in response to stress. They are regularly aggravated by exposure to the sun or consumption of alcohol, sometimes also by frequent bending and standing up. They are thoroughly genuine and occur whether or not the patient has a claim to compensation for his injury (287b). Occasionally, a more localized and intensively boring headache is present, which may prompt suspicion of a meningeal scar. Genuine posttraumatic migraine may occur, even as the result of a relatively minor injury (692c) (p. 807).

Vertigo is often present, generally of nonspecific type, leading to instability of gait, particularly when rapid movements are made and when the patient looks up and down (as when climbing stairs). Benign paroxysmal positional vertigo is also common. These complaints are approximately equally common in patients with and without claims to compensation for their injury (219a).

Patients further complain of a generalized *mental impairment* including memory difficulties (particularly for names), lack of concentration, easy fatigability, and irritability.

These complaints may persist for weeks or months, depending not only on the severity of the injury, but also on the personality and attitude of the patient. Although accident neurosis undoubtedly occurs with some frequency in insured trauma victims, it should be remembered that genuine complaints persist in many cases for months, or even years. Genuine complaints, however, do not automatically imply disability or entitlement to compensation.

Treatment

Bed rest for a few days at most, then *neurovegetative stabilization with medications*, as indicated. Overtreatment should be avoided, and the physician should project an optimistic attitude.

Brain Contusion and Penetrating Injuries of the Brain

Definition:

Brain contusion involves macroscopically evident anatomical injury to the brain. The associated loss of consciousness and post-traumatic twilight state generally last longer than those of concussion. In exceptional cases, however, there may be "contusion without concussion," i.e., a macroscopic injury unaccompanied by loss of consciousness, usually as the result of a localized blow to a small area. Common loci of brain contusion include the orbital gyri, the frontal poles, and, more rarely, the parasagittal cortex, lateral portions of the brainstem, and the caudal portion of the cerebellum.

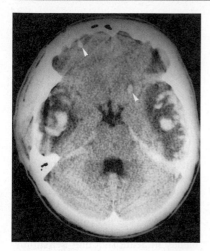

Fig. 2.**5 CT image of posttraumatic brain contusions.** Hemorrhagic contusions are seen in both temporal lobes. Smaller ones are also seen in the frontal lobes (arrow).

Clinical Features (335)

Neurologic signs are usually present from the start and indicate an underlying focal brain injury. The level of consciousness is assessed by means of the Glasgow Coma Scale (GCS; see Table 2.**54**). Cardiac dysrhythmias commonly accompany brain contusion, just as they commonly accompany brain ischemia (p. 188). Lumbar puncture yields bloody or xanthochromic cerebrospinal fluid, and CT usually reveals a focus of contusion (Fig. 2.**5**) but may be entirely normal within weeks or months of the injury.

Post-traumatic Complaints

Epileptic seizures always indicate an established cerebral contusion (see below). Traumatic anosmia (p. 53) is more common with more severe injuries and is practically always an ac-

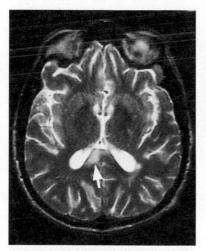 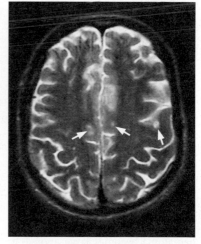

Fig. 2.**6a, b   MRI of axonal shear injury.**
The patient is a 50-year-old man still comatose 2 weeks after a severe traumatic brain injury. The T2-weighted spin-echo images reveal multiple shear injuries.
a Shear injury in the splenium of the corpus callosum (arrow).
b Subcortical shear injuries (arrows).

companiment of an established cerebral contusion. Other subjective complaints after brain contusion resemble those of concussion and are often, though not always, more severe. Additionally, there are symptoms and signs relating to the focal lesion (e.g. paresis, gait disturbance, dysphasia, visual disturbance). Often, a post-traumatic encephalopathy is present (see below).

Post-traumatic Complications and Late Sequelae

The complications of traumatic brain injury are shown schematically in Fig. 2.7.

■ Intracranial Hematoma

An intracranial hematoma may be an early or late complication. Careful observation of the patient is necessary in the acute phase because of the risk of secondary brain compression from a hematoma.

■ Epidural Hematoma

Epidural hematoma is usually the result of tearing of a meningeal artery, so that blood accumulates between the dura mater and the skull and compresses the brain. If the initial injury is severe, the patient may be unconscious from the moment of injury or awaken only briefly thereafter (absent or brief lucid interval). In the classic case, however, epidural hematoma occurs in association with absent or mild initial brain injury, so that a long lucid interval may be present (up to several hours). Secondary coma may develop rapidly once the hematoma becomes large enough to compress the brain.

The decisive factor for neurologic recovery is immediate surgical evacuation of the hematoma. Depending on the availability of transport, this may need to be performed outside a specialized neurosurgical center. Figure 2.8 shows a subdural and an epidural hematoma.

■ Acute Subdural Hematoma

An acute subdural hematoma generally arises as a contusional hemorrhage accompanying a severe traumatic brain injury, and there is thus often no lucid interval after the initial loss of consciousness. Nonetheless, a clear-cut differentiation of subdural and epidural hematoma is often not possible on clinical grounds alone. The cerebrospinal fluid is always bloody in acute subdural hematoma, but it may also be so in cases of simple brain contusion and of contusion with epidural hematoma. A hematoma producing mass effect on the brain should be suspected when the level of consciousness declines after a more or less lucid interval, or when it fails to improve for an unusually long time after the initial injury.

■ Chronic Subdural Hematoma

It is not possible to distinguish post-traumatic and nontraumatic chronic subdural hematoma on clinical grounds alone. The existence of the latter entity, a chronic subdural hematoma without any prior trauma whatsoever (earlier known as *pachymeningosis hemorrhagica interna*), is questioned by neurosurgeons, as the responsible trauma may be so slight as to escape the patient's notice. A history of trauma is present in approximately three-quarters of cases. Anticoagulated patients complaining of headache should always be evaluated for the presence of a chronic subdural hematoma, which is frequently bilateral in such cases.

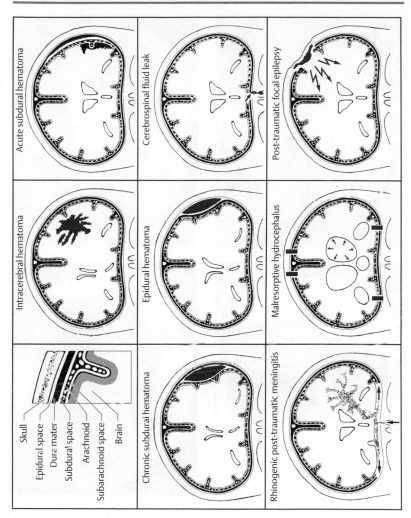

Fig. 2.**7** **Complications of traumatic brain injury.**

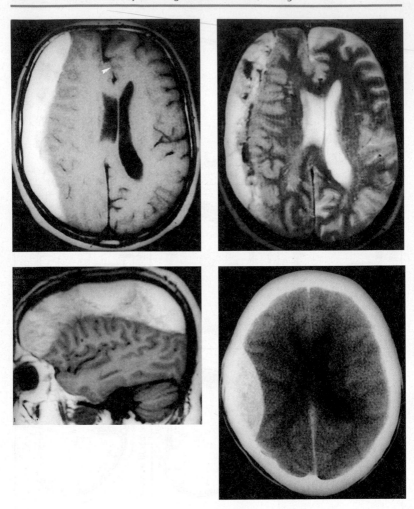

Fig. 2.**8a–d   Subdural hematoma and epidural hematoma.** MRI of a subacute subdural hematoma (a few days old) and CT of an acute epidural hematoma. **a** Axial T1-weighted spin-echo image. **b** Axial T2-weighted spin-echo image. **c** Parasagittal T1-weighted spin-echo image. Typical for a hematoma is the simultaneous appearance of areas of increased and decreased signal (**b**). Note that the hematoma extends over the entire surface of the hemisphere. In Figures 2.**8a** and **b**, a significant midline shift is evident. The cingulate gyrus is displaced to the opposite side (arrowhead in **a**). **d** CT image of an acute epidural hematoma. The hematoma is lens-shaped. Epidural hematomas generally do not cross suture lines and thus, unlike subdural hematomas, do not extend over the entire hemisphere.

Clinical Features

After an initial period that may be entirely asymptomatic, the major symptoms arise several weeks after a mild initial trauma and usually reach their peak after 2 or 3 months. Most patients are elderly, and men are more commonly affected than women. The characteristic initial symptoms are headache and an initially fluctuating and then progressive impairment of consciousness. Deep somnolence may set in, often in the absence or near-absence of focal neurologic signs, though hemiparesis or dysphasia may provide a clue to the side of the hematoma.

Diagnosis

The diagnosis is supported by the finding of xanthochromic cerebrospinal fluid under normal or low pressure and confirmed by CT or MRI, which reveals a biconvex, hypodense hematoma displacing the brain from the inner surface of the skull (Fig. 2.**8**).

▀ Treatment ▀

Larger hematomas are surgically evacuated through burr holes or (when multiple loculations are present) an osteoplastic craniotomy. Small hematomas may resolve spontaneously and are often initially treated by observation.

■ Subdural Hygroma

A subdural hygroma is a collection of cerebrospinal fluid in the subdural space over the cerebral convexity. In adults, subdural hygromas are usually thin and may arise without prior trauma, sometimes in connection with a low pressure syndrome (p. 819). The clinical features and treatment of larger hygromas are analogous to those of chronic subdural hematoma. In infants and children, bilateral subdural hygromas are often found days or weeks after the onset of meningitis. An unsatisfactory course of meningitis in a small child should provoke a diagnostic evaluation for subdural hygroma, which can be treated with repeated aspiration or surgical evacuation if found.

■ Intracerebral hematoma

An intracerebral hematoma exerts an effect on the surrounding brain both by occupying space and by inducing collateral edema. The clinical findings include focal neurologic signs, impairment of consciousness, and bloody or xanthochromic cerebrospinal fluid. CT or MRI establishes the diagnosis.

■ Cranial Nerve Palsies

Injury to the olfactory nerve results in uni- or bilateral anosmia, which is permanent in two-thirds of cases (p. 623). Injury to the optic nerve is also usually permanent, while traumatic third, fourth or sixth nerve palsy often resolves over ca. 3–4 months. Nonspecific visual disturbances may be due to a latent strabismus that manifests itself transiently in connection with the trauma. Lesions of the visual system itself can be ruled out with a normal visual evoked potential study. For traumatic arteriovenous fistula in the cavernous sinus, see p. 213; for post-traumatic facial nerve palsy, see p. 286.

Traumatic disturbances of hearing may be caused by skull base fractures through injury to the inner ear or, more commonly, the vestibulocochlear nerve itself. Injuries of the latter type cannot be surgically repaired and carry a correspondingly poor prognosis.

A skull base fracture extending into the jugular foramen may injure the ninth, tenth, and eleventh cranial nerves, which exit the cranial cavity here. The Siebenmann syndrome ("syndrome du trou déchiré postérieur") is characterized by palatal paralysis, dysphagia, hoarseness, and weakness of the sternocleidomastoid muscle and of the upper portion of the trapezius.

■ Focal Brain Injury

A focal brain injury may produce hemiparesis, central sensory disturbances, visual field defects, dysphasia, and other neuropsychological deficits.

Pseudobulbar manifestations are uncommon. Diabetes insipidus (urine specific gravity < 1.005) may develop a few days after a severe traumatic brain injury, often involving a basilar skull fracture, and usually regresses spontaneously in surviving patients. Diabetes insipidus must be distinguished from polyuria with high specific gravity due to the Schwartz-Bartter syndrome.

The focal injury is generally revealed by CT or MRI scan. Late images show focal atrophy.

■ Lhermitte's Sign

Lhermitte's sign (p. 470) may not appear till weeks or months after a traumatic brain injury. It should disappear within a few months as long as the neurological examination and radiologic studies, including views of the cervical spine in flexion and extension, are normal.

■ Cerebral Fat Embolism

Clinical signs of fat embolism are found in 1–5% of cases of traumatic brain injury, particularly when there is an associated long bone fracture. Neurologic abnormalities are present in 80% of cases, arising 12 hours to 3 days after the traumatic event. The typical picture is of diffuse brain injury, possibly manifesting as prolongation of an initial post-traumatic coma. The diagnosis is supported by the appearance of the chest roentgenogram and the finding of petechiae in the skin and fat emboli in the retinal vessels.

■ Cerebrospinal Fluid Leak, Meningitis, Brain Abscess

Cerebrospinal fluid leak. A basilar skull fracture may tear the dura mater and result in leakage of cerebrospinal fluid out of the cranial cavity, most frequently into the nasal cavity. The diagnosis is confirmed by collection and testing of the suspect fluid (the concentration of glucose in cerebrospinal fluid is above 30 mg/100 mL, and β_2-transferrin is present). Compression of the jugular veins increases the rate of flow. Isotope cisternography confirms the presence of contrast in the nasal cavity and may pinpoint the site of the leak. Cerebrospinal fluid rhinorrhea usually resolves spontaneously, but persistent cases must be treated surgically within 2–3 weeks to prevent meningitis. The dural defect is usually repaired with a pericranial or fascia lata graft.

Meningitis. The most important complication of a cerebrospinal fluid leak is ascending bacterial meningitis, which is generally pneumococcal in origin, and often recurs despite antibiotic treatment. There may be an interval of up to several years between the initial trauma and the meningitis.

Brain abscess. A post-traumatic brain abscess may be the result of a persistent cerebrospinal fluid leak or of a penetrating injury to the brain.

■ **Benign Post-traumatic Intracranial Hypertension**

This condition, which follows a mild or moderately severe traumatic brain injury, is probably caused by venous sinus thrombosis, which impairs CSF resorption and thus leads to intracranial hypertension. It may arise within days or months of the injury and is characterized by headache, nausea, blurred vision, papilledema, and (occasionally) abducens palsy, but no other focal neurologic signs. The cerebrospinal fluid pressure is elevated. The signs and symptoms regress spontaneously.

■ **Post-traumatic Encephalopathy**

The longer the initial loss of consciousness lasts, the greater the likelihood of permanent brain damage. In addition to the initial injury, pathogenetic factors include brain necrosis remote from the initial contusion, brain hemorrhage, brain infarction due to arterial or venous compromise, and diffuse axonal injury. Post-traumatic encephalopathy is characterized by neuropsychological deficits, including impairment of memory and attention, easy fatigability, disturbances of motivation and impulse control, and often marked personality changes, which may lead to severe disability. An accurate assessment of permanent deficits is usually not possible until 2 or more years after the injury. A seemingly paradoxical late progression of clinical mani-

festations may occur, sometimes on the basis of progressive communicating hydrocephalus. The latter arises when there is a disturbance of cerebrospinal fluid resorption consequent upon traumatic subarachnoid hemorrhage (p. 41). Of all sequelae of traumatic brain injury, the neuropsychological deficits produce the most severe social impairment.

■ **Post-traumatic Epilepsy**

Posttraumatic epilepsy occurs almost exclusively after severe traumatic brain injury and usually arises in the first few weeks and months after the trauma. It is discussed in greater detail on p. 531.

■ **Subjective Complaints after Traumatic Brain Injury**

We use this term to designate a complex of symptoms not associated with any positive finding on clinical examination or ancillary testing. These include fatigability, impairment of memory, attention, and concentration, dizziness (219a), and headaches (287b, 504a).

True post-traumatic migraine is rare (p. 807). Post-traumatic headache is thoroughly genuine and is more common after mild than after severe traumatic brain injury (777c). The headache generally regresses within a few months. Persistent, disabling headache often raises the question of causality, which may have to be addressed in the context of a medicolegal evaluation requested by an insurer. This matter must be considered individually for each patient with attention to the antecedent history, the severity of the injury, the temporal relationship of the injury to the symptoms, and the patient's personality and psychosocial situation.

Intracranial Hypertension and Brain Tumors

Definition:
An elevation of intracranial pressure (intracranial hypertension) may be caused by various types of intracranial process, particularly brain tumors. In addition to the focal signs produced by the underlying process itself, intracranial hypertension manifests itself initially by headache, then by progressive impairment of consciousness and vegetative signs such as vomiting, bradycardia and arterial hypertension. The objective findings include papilledema, oculomotor palsy, pupillary abnormalities, disturbances of respiration and other vital functions, and, finally, coma, when the elevated intracranial pressure has led to herniation through the tentorial notch or the foramen magnum (p. 223).

Signs of Intracranial Hypertension and Pseudotumor Cerebri

The main signs of intracranial hypertension are listed in Table 2.**10**.

■ Altitude Sickness
Too rapid ascent may be associated with pulmonary edema, retinal hemorrhages, coronary hypoperfusion, paresthesias in the hands and feet, headache, and cerebral edema. Immediate descent and treatment for intracranial hypertension (see below) are essential for recovery.

Table 2.**10**   Clinical manifestations of intracranial hypertension

Subjective	Headache (diffuse and persistent, most severe in the morning), vomiting (fasting, projectile), apathy
Signs of impending herniation	Confusion, respiratory disturbance, bradycardia, hypertension, cerebellar fits (opisthotonus and extensor spasms of arms and legs), dilated pupils
Ocular findings	Papilledema (may appear within hours), enlarged blind spot, attacks of amblyopia, oculomotor palsy, occasionally abducens palsy
Skull radiograph	Increased digitate markings, enlarged sella turcica with demineralized dorsum sellae, diastasis of sutures in children
CT/MRI	Slit ventricles (when elevation of ICP is due to cerebral edema), periventricular signal change, possible causative lesion (e.g., tumor, hemorrhage)
EEG	Diffusely abnormal, nonspecific
Lumbar puncture	Contraindicated when a dangerous elevation of ICP is suspected! Pressure over 200 mmH$_2$O; may be normal, however, if CSF flow is blocked at the occipitocervical or spinal level

Table 2.**11** Causes of intracranial hypertension

Category	Specific entities	Clinical features	Remarks
Intracranial mass	Brain tumor, subdural hematoma, intracerebral hematoma	Focal neurological and neuropsychological deficits, headache	
Infection	Encephalitis, meningitis	Fever, meningism	E.g., neurobrucellosis, syphilis
Traumatic brain injury	Contusion, brain edema, intracerebral hematoma	Progression of brain edema, focal seizures	
Impairment of cerebrospinal fluid resorption	Intraventricular tumors, aqueductal stenosis, malresorptive hydrocephalus	Headache (possibly ictal), vomiting; in malresorptive hydrocephalus spasticity of legs, urinary incontinence, psychoorganic syndrome	Intermittent elevation of cerebrospinal fluid pressure, prior subarachnoid hemorrhage or meningitis
Elevation of cerebrospinal fluid protein	E.g. in polyradiculitis, spinal tumors (esp. schwannoma)	Lumbar puncture yields cerebrospinal fluid with elevated protein	
Toxic processes	Lead poisoning, insecticide poisoning	Psycho-organic syndrome, anemia, lead line (on gums)	
Iatrogenic	Steroids, oral contraceptives, tetracycline		
Altitude sickness	On rapid ascent	Headache, pulmonary edema, retinal hemorrhage, angina pectoris	Descend immediately!
Pseudotumor cerebri		Usually affects obese young women; slit ventricles, often papilledema	A diagnosis of exclusion; see Table 2.**12**
Empty sella syndrome		CT shows an apparently empty sella turcica containing air	May be associated with visual disturbances

■ Pseudotumor Cerebri (Benign Intracranial Hypertension)

Cases of intracranial hypertension that are not due to any of the entities listed above or to any other discernible organic intracranial process are designated as pseudotumor cerebri or benign intracranial hypertension. This diagnosis of exclusion is most commonly made in obese young women. The neurological examination and neuroimaging studies are normal except for papilledema, an enlarged blind spot, and (occasionally) very narrow cerebral ventricles ("slit ventricles"). The cerebrospinal fluid is under elevated pressure but of normal composition. The clinical features are summarized in Table 2.**12**.

Causative factors are found in only about three-quarters of cases of intracranial hypertension not associated with an intracranial space-occupying lesion (see above). Approximately one-quarter are associated with otitis media. Other causes include neuro-

Table 2.**12** Characteristics of pseudotumor cerebri

Usually diffuse headache
Young women
Often obese
Relatively common in pregnancy
Vomiting (moderately common)
Dizziness and tinnitus (common)
Nystagmus (moderately common)
Papilledema (common)
Enlarged blind spot
Slit ventricles on CT
Elevated cerebrospinal fluid pressure

syphilis and vitamin A deficiency (246a).

Spontaneous recovery is the rule, and recurrence is rare. 8% of these patients suffer permanent visual impairment as a consequence of papilledema; the risk is particularly high in patients concomitantly suffering from arterial hypertension. Gradual shrinkage of the blind spot on visual field testing is an excellent indicator of a positive response to treatment.

Treatment

Serial therapeutic lumbar punctures. If cerebral edema is present, high-dose dexamethasone or prednisone should be given intravenously at first, and then orally. Mannitol or furosemide, 40 mg i.v. b.i.d. or t.i.d., may also be given. A commonly used treatment is with the carbonic anhydrase inhibitor acetazolamide, 250–750 mg/day. Obese patients should be put on a reducing diet.

■ Empty Sella Syndrome

The subarachnoid space may extend into the sella turcica in the presence or absence of intracranial hypertension when the diaphragma sellae inadequately separates the intrasellar and suprasellar compartments. CT reveals a seemingly empty sella with Hounsfield values approximating those of air. In cases of pseudotumor cerebri, an empty sella is associated with a higher frequency of visual disturbances.

■ Brain Tumors
(97c, 221b, 520a, 851a)

Epidemiology

One in 10,000–20,000 people will develop a brain tumor. Perhaps an additional one-quarter of this number harbor an asymptomatic cerebral metastasis of a malignant tumor elsewhere in the body. Primary brain tumors are much more common among psychiatric inpatients (prevalence 1%) than in the general population. In an epidemiologic study performed at the Mayo Clinic over a period of 40 years, the overall incidence of brain tumors was 19.1 per 100,000 persons per year (778a).

Causes

Brain tumors are thought to result from the interaction of a nonlocalized *"humoral" factor* with a *local factor* related to embryonic histogenesis, which is responsible for the typical locations of various particular types of tumor, and for the overall increased occurrence of brain tumors in the vicinity of the neural groove. *Genetic factors* also play a role; thus, the loss of tumor suppressor genes through mutation seems to play a role in the generation of glioblastoma multiforme. *Trauma* contributes to the generation of brain tumors exceedingly rarely, if at all.

■ General Clinical Manifestations of Brain Tumors

General Characteristics

The general characteristics of brain tumors are listed below and summarized in Table 2.**13**.

- The symptoms and signs are steadily progressive. (N.b., so may be those of inflammatory and (more rarely) vascular processes, while a sudden hemorrhage into a tumor may produce sudden, "apoplectiform" manifestations.)
- Headache is common (steady, diffuse, often both day and night with diminution over the course of the day); it may be an early symptom in ca. one-third of cases.
- Signs of intracranial hypertension may be present (see Table 2.**10**).
- Mental changes may include irritability, fatigability, memory impairment, and general and focal psycho-organic syndromes.
- Epileptic seizures are more commonly generalized than focal, and are the first symptom in ca. one-fourth of all cases.

Table 2.**13**   General characteristics of brain tumors

Symptoms and signs:	Course	Objective findings
Headache (early symptom in one-third)	Steady progression (exception: acute onset due to hemorrhage into tumor)	Focal neurologic deficits
General signs of intracranial hypertension (vomiting, bradycardia not always present)		Neuropsychological and psychopathological abnormalities
Epileptic seizures (initial symptom in one-fourth)		Cranial nerve palsies (sometimes)
Neuropsychological changes (apathy, irritability, memory impairment)		papilledema (common)

Focal signs and symptoms. These usually appear sooner or later in the course of the illness, accompanied by the general manifestations described above. They may provide a clue to the localization of the tumor.

Falsely localizing symptoms and signs. These may result from shifting of intracranial structures due to mass effect.

■ **Diagnostic Evaluation**

Imaging Studies

MRI and CT. MRI and CT are essential procedures in the diagnostic evaluation of brain tumors. An MRI should be performed when the CT is negative despite a high degree of clinical suspicion (e.g., of an infiltrative, low-grade astrocytoma), or when the clinical findings suggest a lesion in the posterior fossa. It should never be forgotten that a negative CT does not rule out a brain tumor, particularly an infiltrative, low-grade glioma. Thus, it may be necessary to repeat an initially negative study, particularly when the symptoms and signs are progressive.

Arteriography. This technique has vastly declined in importance since the introduction of CT and MRI, but may still be required as a complementary preoperative study in some cases. In yet other cases, a decision to remove the tumor surgically or to administer radiation therapy can only be made after a diagnostic stereotactic biopsy.

EEG. EEG no longer plays a role in the diagnostic evaluation of brain tumors.

Cerebrospinal fluid examination. The cerebrospinal fluid is normal or else shows an elevation of protein and cell count, particularly when the tumor abuts the ependymal or pial surface. Acoustic neuromas are characteristically accompanied by an elevation of cerebrospinal fluid protein. Tumor cells are sometimes noted on cytological examination of the cellular sediment.

Plain skull roentgenogram. Plain skull roentgenograms may reveal evidence of intracranial hypertension: increase of the digitate markings, enlarged sella turcica, demineralized dorsum sellae (note the distinction between this finding and that of an intrasellar tumor!), diastasis of the sutures in young children, or, in posterior fossa tumors, an increased vertical height of the posterior fossa with thinning of the occipital bone. The pineal calcification or falcine calcification (if present) may be displaced to the side opposite the tumor. The skull may be locally sclerotic (meningioma) or destroyed (metastasis). Meningiomas may also be associated with abnormally deep vascular grooves, reflecting the meningeal blood supply to the tumor. Some tumors may be calcified (meningioma, oligodendroglioma, craniopharyngioma, choroid plexus papilloma, lipoma of the corpus callosum), but this finding is not pathognomonic for tumor, as various kinds of inflammation may also be calcified (e.g., tuberculoma). Large intracranial aneurysms may display sickle-shaped calcifications.

ECG. Potentially misleading **ECG** abnormalities (QT prolongation, sinus tachy- or bradycardia, pathological U wave, and ST elevation or depression) are found in association with 40%

of tumors involving the temporal lobe (529).

■ Individual Types of Brain Tumor

The most important types of brain tumor and their frequency in a neurosurgical patient base are listed in Table 2.**14**.

■ Astrocytic Tumors (Gliomas)

The loss of tumor suppressor genes is a contributing factor in the generation of astrocytic tumors (e.g., LOH 10 in glioblastoma). Mutations of the

Table 2.**14** Frequency of different types of brain tumors in a group of neurosurgical patients

Tumor	Percent
Gliomas:	
• Glioblastoma multiforme (= astrocytoma, grade IV)	20
• Astrocytoma, grades I–III	10
• Ependymoma	6
• Medulloblastoma	4
• Oligodendroglioma	5
Meningioma	15
Pituitary adenoma	7
Schwannoma (= neurinoma)	7
Metastasis	6
Craniopharyngioma, dermoid, epidermoid, teratoma	4
Angioma	4
Sarcoma	4
Unclassifiable	5
Other, rarer tumors (pinealoma, chondroma, granuloma, etc.)	3
Total	100

tumor suppressor genes primarily affect protein phosphorylation and phosphatase activity.

Grade IV astrocytoma (glioblastoma multiforme). Grade IV astrocytomas grow very rapidly and are highly malignant. Histologically, they are characterized by necrosis and vascular proliferation. They are the most common primary brain tumor, appearing mainly in the fifth and sixth decades of life, and they grow by infiltrating into the brain substance. They usually arise in a cerebral hemisphere but may cross the corpus callosum to involve both sides ("butterfly glioma") or grow downward into the basal ganglia (Fig. 2.**9**). They account for approximately 90% of all cerebral gliomas in adults. The patients generally come to medical attention because of neurologic deficits within weeks or, at most, a few months of their first symptom. Apart from general tumor symptoms and signs, focal deficits such as hemiparesis and dysphasia are usually present. Even after gross total neurosurgical resection of the tumor, patients generally die of tumor recurrence within a few months to, at most, 2 years. A combination of surgery, radiotherapy, and chemotherapy improves the prognosis only slightly. Wafers containing the cytostatic agent BCNU bound to a polymer are sometimes surgically implanted in the tumor cavity when a recurrent tumor is resected, although this has been found to prolong survival by no more than a few weeks (136). Temozolomide has also been recommended recently for chemotherapy of recurrent tumors. The only beneficial prognostic factor for a grade IV astrocytoma is a younger age of onset of the disease.

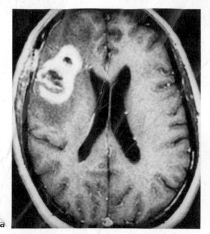
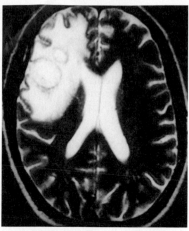

a

b

Fig. 2.**9a, b Grade IV astrocytoma (glioblastoma multiforme).** The T1- and T2-weighted spin-echo images (**a** and **b**, respectively) reveal a polycystic tumor surrounded by marked edema. The peripheral portion of the tumor is strongly contrast-enhancing (**a**).

Grade I–III astrocytoma (972a). These astrocytomas of the cerebrum arise most commonly in the fourth decade of life. They generally grow slowly and are sometimes well circumscribed, but often infiltrate into the white matter of the frontal and temporal lobes. Pilocytic astrocytoma is a subtype of grade I astrocytoma, while astrocytomas of grades I and II are sometimes termed "low-grade astrocytomas"; grade II tumors differ from grade I tumors in the degree of cellular abnormality. An increased mitotic rate is found in grade III tumors (so-called anaplastic astrocytoma). Well-differentiated tumors may reside in the cerebral white matter for years while they slowly grow and produce progressive clinical manifestations. The most common of these are cognitive changes, slowly progressive hemiparesis, ataxia, papilledema, headache, and epileptic seizures. The tumor is often initially detectable only on MRI, and not on CT. Well-circumscribed fibrillary astrocytomas that have been macroscopically totally resected may not recur till years afterward (792a), and permanent surgical cures are occasionally seen. In many cases, however, the tumor eventually transforms itself into a glioblastoma. Sometimes the tumor appears to be multifocal, with a highly heterogeneous degree of malignity; in such cases, one may speak of gliomatosis of the brain.

Cerebellar astrocytoma (pilocytic astrocytoma of the cerebellum). These tumors have a much better prognosis than supratentorial astrocytomas. They usually arise between the ages of 5 and 15 and account for 25% of all brain tumors of childhood and adolescence. They are well-circumscribed, often cystic tumors that usually reside in the cerebellar hemispheres but may also be found in the vermis or pons. They give rise to slowly progressive cerebellar signs

such as ataxia, dysequilibrium, nystagmus, and sometimes intracranial hypertension as an early manifestation. Neurosurgical resection may be difficult because of the location of the tumor, but a total resection, if achieved, can be curative.

Ependymoma. These tumors, too, generally affect children and adolescents, and only rarely adults. They arise from ependymal cells that lie abnormally deep within the tissue substance, rather than at the ependymal surface. The arrangement of tumor cells into perivascular pseudorosettes is the histologic hallmark of this tumor. It is found in the vicinity of the ventricular system, more often below the tentorium than above it; the commonest site is the area around the fourth ventricle. *Intramedullary ependymomas* are most commonly found in the conus medullaris of the spinal cord (cf. Fig. 3.**4e, f**). Ependymomas of the posterior fossa produce focal cerebellar signs as well as obstructive hydrocephalus, which often dominates the clinical picture. Unusual (persistent) headache in a child should arouse suspicion of an ependymoma. Such tumors also manifest themselves on occasion by focal signs of the pons or medulla, e.g., hemifacial spasm (p. 678) (780a). They are relatively benign, and the patient may survive many years after the initial resection; the older the child at first manifestation of the tumor, the better the prognosis. Radical resection may be impossible if the tumor involves the floor of the fourth ventricle. Surgery should always be followed by radiation therapy, which should encompass not only the brain, but also the entire spinal cord. The combination of surgery and radiation

yields a 10-year survival rate of nearly 70%.

Medulloblastoma. This malignant tumor of childhood and adolescence accounts for 20% of brain tumors in this age group. It is found in the inferior portion of the vermis in nine out of 10 cases but may also arise in the cerebellar hemispheres or the pons. It grows by infiltration and often fills the fourth ventricle, thereby obstructing cerebrospinal fluid flow and sending drop metastases caudally along the cerebrospinal fluid pathway into the spine. These may lead to clinical findings relating to the spinal cord or cauda equina. In general, medulloblastomas cause symptoms and signs similar to those of cerebellar astrocytoma (see above). Much less commonly, a medulloblastoma may appear in adulthood, practically always in the posterior fossa. Even after appropriate treatment, these tumors usually recur and go on to metastasize to other locations in the central nervous system and other organs (756). Macroscopically radical resection combined with radiation therapy, to which this tumor has a high rate of response, still cannot prevent recurrences, which frequently appear within months or years, in both older and younger patients. In one study, 58 patients with a mean age of 17 years underwent surgical resection followed by radiation therapy (331). The rates of survival and of recurrence-free survival were 50%/46% at 5 years, and 32%/32% at 10 years. Positive prognostic factors included radical resection, radiation dose above 50 Gy, and radiation of the entire neuraxis. Further chemotherapy for the treatment of recurrence yielded a 2-year survival rate of 46%,

while the survival rate after tumor recurrence without further chemotherapy was zero.

Oligodendroglioma. These tumors most commonly appear between the ages of 35 and 45. They grow by displacement or infiltration of brain tissue in the cerebral hemispheres or basal ganglia or, particularly in younger patients, in the thalamus. More than half of all oligodendrogliomas are located in the frontal lobes. They grow very slowly, and, in the pre-CT era, there was usually an interval of several years between the appearance of the first symptom and the diagnosis. Epileptic seizures occur in 70% of patients and are the initial manifestation in 50%. Focal neurologic deficits develop over the ensuing months or years. Gross total resection is almost invariably followed by recurrence, but sometimes at a latency of 3–5 years, so that the median postoperative survival time of 5 years

is comparable to that of supratentorial astrocytomas of grades I–III. Oligodendrogliomas are responsive to PCV chemotherapy, which is recommended as an adjuvant treatment.
A study of 81 patients revealed a median survival time of 7.9 years for those who were treated with a combination of surgery and local radiation therapy at a dose of at least 50 Gy. 31% of these patients survived 10 years or more (867).

Brainstem glioma. The different histological types of glioma occurring in the brainstem may be considered together because of the typical clinical features associated with this location. They generally arise in the first two decades of life and cause progressive symptoms and signs through involvement of the pons and medulla oblongata, as summarized in Table 2.**15**.
These tumors are often difficult to distinguish from other brainstem tumors and vascular malformations, brainstem encephalitis, or the initial manifestations of multiple sclerosis. Surgical resection is only rarely possible and usually incomplete. The benefit of chemotherapy is uncertain. Ventricular shunting may be necessary if hydrocephalus develops. The median survival time is 1 year.

Optic and chiasmatic glioma. These tumors are found nearly exclusively in children and adolescents, and are twice as common in girls. Fourteen percent of cases are associated with neurofibromatosis. Their clinical manifestations are listed in Table 2.**16**. The diagnosis is made by CT or MRI, by means of which these tumors can be distinguished from pituitary tumors, intraorbital meningi-

Table 2.**15** Signs and symptoms of a brainstem tumor

Nuclear cranial nerve palsies with:
• Dysphagia • Trigeminal sensory and motor deficits • Peripheral facial nerve palsy
Hemifacial spasm
Oculomotor disturbances
Long tract manifestations: • Pyramidal tract signs • Hemiparesis • Ataxia • (possibly) dissociated sensory deficit • All of the above may be bilateral
Intracranial hypertension, if the aqueduct is occluded

oma, medial sphenoid wing meningioma, and the lesions of Hand-Schüller-Christian disease. The combination of surgery and radiation therapy yields a long-term survival rate of 85% for anterior tumors and 50% for posterior tumors.

Hypothalamic tumors. *Astrocytoma* is the most common histological type. These tumors lie in the rostral portion of the floor of the third ventricle and usually arise in the first 2 years of life. Their clinical hallmark is a progressive emaciation that leads to cachexia, despite normal food intake and otherwise normal behavior (Russell syndrome). This picture is to be distinguished from anorexia nervosa, which generally strikes older girls.
Colloid cysts are also found in the third ventricle and may lead to an obstruction of cerebrospinal fluid flow in one or both foramina of Monro, and thereby to uni- or bilateral hydrocephalus of the lateral ventricles. They are treated neurosurgically.

■ Meningioma

This is a benign tumor that arises from the dura mater and grows slowly over the years, compressing the adjacent brain tissue. Malignant transformation is rare, but there is a statistical association with other, malignant tumors, especially breast cancer. Meningioma is the most common intracranial tumor of mesodermal origin and most often becomes clinically evident between the ages of 40 and 50. It may also be encountered as an incidental finding at autopsy or on CT or MRI studies of the brain. In such cases, follow-up studies have shown highly variable annual growth rates, ranging from 1% to 21%; thus, slowly growing, asymptomatic meningio-

Table 2.**16**   Symptoms of optic and chiasmatic glioma

Almost exclusively in children and adolescents
Visual disturbances
Visual field defects
Exophthalmos
Late diencephalic manifestations:
• Polyuria
• Obesity
• Infantilism
• Arousal disturbances

mas can be treated by observation (301), particularly in elderly patients (709b). Larger tumors and those displaying hyperintensity on T2-weighted images are more likely to progress (709b). In general, meningiomas should be neurosurgically resected.
Although meningiomas may, in principle, arise from the dura mater at any site, they are preferentially found at a number of classic sites, which are listed in Table 2.**17**, together with some of the particularities associated with tumors at each site.
Figure 2.**10** shows an MR image of a meningioma.
The adjacent bony structures are thickened and demonstrate radially arranged bony spicules. Exostoses may also be present. Flat "en plaque" meningiomas may develop largely within the bone of the skull and give rise to a picture resembling fibrous dysplasia (287). Supratentorial meningiomas in any location are frequently associated with epileptic seizures, which may be their initial symptom.

Table 2.17   Preferential locations of meningioma, and associated clinical features

Site	Most common initial manifestations	Course	Special features
Olfactory groove	Anosmia	Seizures, headache, personality change with frontal features, possible involvement of optic nerve	The frontal branch of the temporal artery may be enlarged
Convexity	Seizures	Hemiparesis	
Parasagittal and falx	Lower extremity paresis, (sometimes) bilateral Babinski sign	Seizures	Rarely causes paraparesis
Sphenoid wing	Visual disturbances (when medially located, adjacent to optic nerve)	Exophthalmos, hemiparesis	Lateral tumors may be externally evident as temporal hyperostosis
Tuberculum sellae	Visual disturbances, pale optic disks	Progressive visual field defect	
Cerebellopontine angle	Deafness, vertigo	Facial and trigeminal nerve deficits, brainstem compression	Differential diagnosis: acoustic neuroma
Foramen magnum	Spastic quadriparesis, dysphagia, dysarthria	Lower cranial nerve deficits	Diagnosis difficult, clinical findings may be misleading
Intraventricular	Intermittent headaches and vomiting	Progressive hydrocephalus	Often found in trigone
Intraspinal	Progressive paraparesis	Paraplegia	

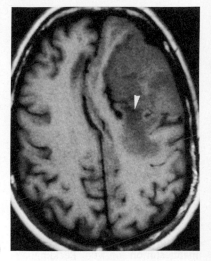

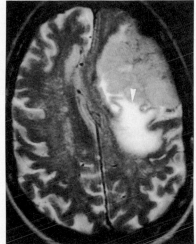

Fig. 2.**10a–c Meningioma.** An 85-year-old man who had had a slowly progressive right hemiparesis for 2 years.

a, b The T1- and T2-weighted spin-echo images (**a** and **b**, respectively) reveal a large left frontal convexity meningioma compressing the underlying brain tissue. Abnormal signal in compressed cortex (arrowhead); brain edema (T1-hypointensity and T2-hyperintensity).

c Marked contrast enhancement, typical for meningioma.

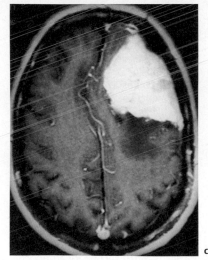

■ **Pituitary Adenoma**

Only about 10% of these tumors are associated with sellar enlargement and other signs of an intracranial space-occupying lesion. Adenomas mainly occur in patients between the ages of 30 and 50. Practically all cases exhibit endocrine disturbances:

• The rare *growth-hormone secreting tumors* (in older nomenclature, eosinophilic adenomas) cause acromegaly.

• *Nonsecreting tumors* (chromophobe adenomas) cause panhypopituitarism, with thin, wrinkled skin and secondary thyroid and sex hormone deficiencies.

• *Prolactinomas* (serum prolactin > 100 ng/mL) cause galactorrhea and secondary amenorrhea in women, and impotence in men.

Larger pituitary adenomas cause *visual field defects* (usually bitemporal hemianopsia or bitemporal upper quadrantanopsia) and *sellar enlargement,* which may be balloon-like or plate-like in radiological views. The degree of improvement of visual acuity and visual fields after surgical resection is highest in patients with milder impairment preoperatively, shorter duration of visual symptoms, and slower tumor progression.

ACTH-secreting tumors (basophil adenomas) are the responsible lesion in Cushing's disease. They cause symptoms not through mass effect, but rather through secondary adrenocortical hypersecretion of cortisol, which leads to truncal obesity, hypertension, osteoporosis, and hyperglycemia as well as abdominal striae, hirsutism, and (in women) secondary amenorrhea. Craniopharyngiomas may arise in the pituitary fossa and are described below on p. 69.

■ **Schwannoma (Neurinoma)**

Schwannomas are benign neoplasms arising from the Schwann cells. They most commonly affect the eighth cranial nerve, where they are familiarly but inaccurately known as acoustic neuromas. These usually appear in the fourth and fifth decades of life and give rise to the clinical syndrome of the *tumor of the cerebellopontine angle,* including progressive unilateral deafness, tinnitus, dysequilibrium, (later) trigeminal nerve deficits, facial palsy, and possibly (in advanced stages) cerebellar deficits, pyramidal tract signs, and signs of intracranial hypertension.

Acoustic neuroma is sometimes a manifestation of von Recklinghausen's neurofibromatosis (p. 86) and is then often bilateral.

The syndrome of the tumor of the cerebellopontine angle is more rarely produced by other processes, e.g., meningioma or epidermoid.

Acoustic neuroma is always associated with an elevation of the cerebrospinal fluid protein concentration. The diagnosis is established by CT or MRI (Fig. 2.11). Small, intracanalicular tumors are well seen on MRI but only with difficulty on CT; they may be seen more easily on CT after the introduction of positive or negative contrast (air) into the subarachnoid space, which outlines the tumor in the internal auditory canal. Microsurgical resection can usually be performed without injury to the facial and trigeminal nerves. Stereotactic radiosurgery (Gamma Knife) is rapidly becoming the treatment of choice for smaller tumors.

■ **Brain Metastases**

Some 10–15% of cancer patients eventually develop clinically evident

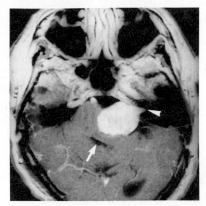

Fig. 2.11   Acoustic neuroma.
T1-weighted spin-echo MR image after the administration of intravenous contrast. Observe the marked displacement of the pons to the opposite side and the compression of the fourth ventricle (small arrow). The beak-like projection of the tumor into the internal auditory canal (arrowhead) and the marked contrast enhancement are typical features of acoustic neuroma.

brain metastases. The commonest brain metastases arise from carcinoma of the lung (in men) and breast (in women), followed by melanoma and renal cell carcinoma. In at least three-quarters of cases, brain metastases are already multiple by the time of clinical presentation; this fraction is even higher for melanoma, while metastatic renal cell carcinoma is more often solitary. Sometimes, a cancer outside the central nervous system may initially present as a brain metastasis; this occurs most commonly in lung cancer. According to the literature, brain metastases account for 4–20% of all brain tumors. The mean life expectancy after diagnosis of one or more brain metastases is only 1–2 months. Positive prognostic factors for survival include supra-

tentorial location, gross total resection, and advanced age. Only about 30% of cases are suitable for surgical treatment (71a). In one study, of 122 patients from whom apparently solitary brain metastases were removed, only 5% were alive 4 years later. In the overall group of 122 patients with apparently solitary brain metastases, the longest survival was attained by those who underwent gross total resection of the metastasis followed by whole-brain radiation therapy in the absence of other systemic evidence of disease. The median survival time in this group was 1.3 years; 41% were alive at 2 years, and 21% at 5 years (888). Whole-brain radiation therapy led to an improvement of symptoms in 80% of patients (71a).

For carcinomatous meningitis, see p. 410; for paraneoplastic encephalopathy, see p. 321.

■ Tumors of Maldevelopmental Origin

Craniopharyngioma. This tumor enters into the differential diagnosis of a pituitary tumor. It is diagnosed most commonly in children and adolescents, with peak incidence in the second decade of life, but older patients may also present with initial symptoms of craniopharyngioma, particularly visual disturbances. Endocrine disturbances are almost always present except in the less common cases of purely suprasellar tumor. Craniopharyngioma is far more likely than pituitary adenoma to extend into the diencephalon and third ventricle and produce the corresponding clinical signs (hydrocephalus, behavioral disturbances, diabetes insipidus, etc.). Craniopharyngiomas are often calcified and contain cholesterol. Although they are histologically benign,

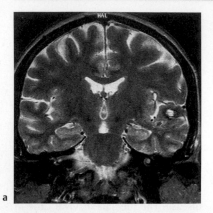

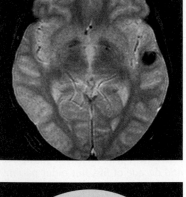

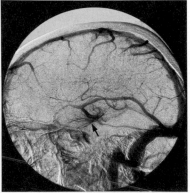

Fig. 2.12a–c Cavernoma (cavernous angioma).

A 59-year-old woman with temporal lobe epilepsy of increasing severity, despite anticonvulsant treatment. A neuroradiological evaluation after the first seizure (10 years previously) was normal. This follow-up study reveals a cavernoma combined with anomalous venous drainage. This finding suggests the possibility of treatment by neurosurgical resection of the cavernoma.

a The coronal, T2-weighted spin-echo image reveals a cavernoma in the left superior temporal gyrus. The hemosiderin ring around the lesion, seen as loss of signal, is typical.

b The hemosiderin ring is even more clearly seen in this axial gradient-echo image, because of signal loss due to a susceptibility effect.

c Venous phase angiogram. An anomalous venous drainage with caput medusae is seen (arrow). Anomalous venous drainage is frequently associated with cavernoma. The neurosurgeon need only resect the cavernoma.

their clinical management can be problematic, because they are often not radically resectable for technical reasons.

Other tumors of maldevelopmental origin. *Epidermoid and dermoid tumors* are derived from tissues not normally found within the central nervous system. Epidermoid tumors generally present between the ages of 25 and 45 and are most often located at the skull base and in the cerebellopontine angle. Dermoid tumors, on the other hand, are tumors of childhood and are most often located in the parapituitary, parapontine, and orbitomaxillary regions. They often present with visual disturbances (from involvement of the optic chiasm), lower cranial nerve palsies, brainstem compression, seizures, and (occasionally) behavioral abnormalities and signs of intracranial hypertension. Both of these types of tumor grow very slowly and compress, rather than invade, the adjacent nervous tissue. They are only rarely found in the spinal canal. Radical removal is associated with a good prognosis.

Cavernomas (cavernous angiomas) (564, 792, 879, 905) are a variety of hamartoma composed of abnormal blood vessels (Fig. 2.**12**). Pathological examination reveals a well-circumscribed mass of blood vessels without intervening nervous tissue, containing foci of calcification. Cavernomas may be found anywhere in the brain, brainstem, or spinal cord, but are most commonly found subcortically in the cerebral hemispheres. They are multiple in nearly one-fourth of all cases (674a) and may occur in families (679c). Approximately two-thirds cause epileptic seizures (188c), and 16% cause clinically apparent hemorrhage (674a). A cavernoma gene is found at the CCM 1 locus on chromosome 7 (367b). The commonest presenting manifestations are seizures, headache, and intracranial hemorrhage. In CT images, they appear as hyperdense regions with contrast enhancement; calcification may also be seen. MRI commonly reveals hemosiderin deposits reflecting previous, often clinically silent hemorrhage. The treatment consists of microsurgical removal and is advisable because these lesions tend to bleed with a frequency estimated at 0.7% per year, and somewhat higher in women (674a, 792). The risk of a symptomatic hemorrhage is particularly high when there has been a previous hemorrhage, but substantially lower when seizures are the only presenting feature or when the lesion is an incidental radiological finding (16).

Tumors of the pineal region are rarely derived from cells intrinsic to the pineal gland (pineocytoma, pineoblastoma), and belong somewhat more commonly to the glioma series (astrocytoma, ependymoma), but are most often of maldevelopmental origin (germinoma, teratoma, choriocarcinoma, embryonal cell carcinoma, endodermal sinus tumor). Any of these tumors may compress the aqueduct and cause obstructive hydrocephalus. Physical findings include paresis of upward gaze (sometimes a late sign) and wide pupils that contract on convergence, but not in response to light (all of these findings together constitute the Parinaud syndrome). Germ cell tumors of the pineal region occur predominantly in young men.

■ Other Brain Tumors

The following tumors are rare and will be mentioned only briefly.

Malignant lymphoma. Malignant lymphoma may occur as a solitary or multiple lesion anywhere in the cerebrum or cerebellum. These tumors grow rapidly and infiltrate the surrounding tissue. They are seen more commonly, but by no means exclusively, in immunocompromised persons, including AIDS patients. Their prevalence is approximately five per 10 million population, and they account for only about 1% of all brain tumors. They are clinically manifested by general signs of intracranial hypertension, seizures, and/or focal neurological and neuropsychological abnormalities. Simultaneous involvement of the cranial nerves and eyes is not uncommon. CT reveals one or more foci of tumor in the vicinity of the cerebral ventricles; these are initially hyperdense and enhance strongly on the administration of contrast. They are solitary in only one-third of cases (135). The treatment consists of whole-brain radiation therapy at a dose of 50 Gy and sometimes chemotherapy as well (448). Treatment is effective, but not curative (135). Brain lymphoma only rarely represents metastasis of extracerebral disease.

Intraventricular tumors. These tumors may intermittently obstruct the flow of cerebrospinal fluid. See the above discussion of *intraventricular meningioma* (p. 65) and *colloid cyst of the third ventricle* (p. 819).

Choroid plexus papilloma. These tumors are most common in the first decade of life, particularly in the first 2 years. They are most commonly located in the fourth ventricle, grow by compression rather than invasion, may become calcified, give rise to drop metastases, and are accessible to radical surgical resection (706).

Syphilitic gummata and tuberculomas. These intracranial masses are uncommon in Europe and North America. Suspicion of either should prompt a search for other manifestations of the underlying disease.

Hydatid cysts and cysticercosis. Hydatid cysts are quite rare lesions, but cysticercosis of the nervous system affects up to 4% of persons harboring the pork tapeworm *Taenia solium* in regions in which this infection is endemic. Neurocysticercosis evokes symptoms by mass effect in approximately half of affected individuals.

Differential Diagnosis of Brain Tumors

Other intracranial processes may produce clinical manifestations resembling those of brain tumor, either by mass effect or by other mechanisms. Table 2.**18** provides an overview of the differential diagnosis of brain tumors.

Treatment of Intracranial Hypertension and Cerebral Edema

The available means of treating intracranial hypertension and cerebral edema are most effective when these are due to brain tumor, but can also be used in cases of pseudotumor cerebri (p. 58), intracranial hemorrhage, and traumatic brain injury. *Dexamethasone (Decadron)* is given at an initial dose of 4 mg every 6 hours intravenously, later by mouth. 50–150 mg of soluble *prednisone* may be given instead. A 20% solution of *mannitol* can be given in an initial dose of 100 mL over 30–60 minutes, and thereafter up to eight times daily, as needed. *Furosemide (Lasix)* can be given as a diuretic in a dose of 40 mg intravenously up to three times a day. If either of the latter two medications are given to somnolent or comatose patients, a urinary catheter should be inserted.

Table 2.18 General differential diagnosis of brain tumors

Category	Example	Specific features	Important for differential diagnosis
Space-occupying lesion other than tumor	Chronic subdural hematoma	Headache (always), fluctuating mental changes, few neurological deficits	Prior head trauma (almost always)
	Brain abscess	Fever, high erythrocyte sedimentation rate, rapid progression	Febrile, acutely ill
	Arachnoid cyst	Most common in young males, on the left side, fronto-temporal	Skull asymmetry (common); often complicated by subdural hematoma after traumatic brain injury
Encephalitis	Herpes encephalitis	Involves temporal lobe	Fever, CSF pleocytosis and xanthochromia, positive CT or MRI
	Brainstem encephalitis	Brainstem signs, bilateral long tract signs	Positive MRI
	Multiple sclerosis	Progressive hemiparesis over a few days	Absence of general signs of intracranial hypertension; positive MRI
Vascular processes	Stroke in progress	Rapidly progressive hemiparesis without signs of intracranial hypertension	Vascular risk factors, possible demonstration of carotid stenosis by Doppler ultrasound
	Intracerebral hemorrhage	Headache (always), rapid progression, decline in level of consciousness	CT, MRI

Table 2.**18** General differential diagnosis of brain tumors (Cont.)

Category	Example	Specific features	Important for differential diagnosis
	Arteriovenous malformation	Seizures, (possibly) progressive focal manifestations, may bleed acutely	CT, MRI
	(Giant) aneurysm	Cranial nerve deficits, (rarely) hemiparesis	CT, MRI may show sickle-shaped calcification in wall of aneurysm
Other	Mill's paralysis	Hemiparesis slowly ascending from leg to arm (years)	CT, MRI (diagnosis of exclusion)
	Alzheimer's disease and Pick's disease	In rare cases, there may only be a focal progressive deficit (e.g., dysphasia) for several years	CT, MRI
Pseudotumor cerebri, benign intracranial hypertension		Manifestations of intracranial hypertension without focal deficit but possibly with papilledema	Young, obese women; CT shows symmetrical narrowing of the lateral ventricles

Infectious Diseases of the Brain and Meninges
(695, 835, 960, 1024)

Overview:

Pathogenic organisms may reach the central nervous system by hematogenous spread or local extension and cause infections of the meninges (meningitis), infections of the brain and spinal cord parenchyma (encephalitis, myelitis), focal purulent collections (brain abscess, subdural empyema, epidural abscess), or infections of the nerve roots (radiculitis, polyradiculitis). Depending on the causative organism, the infection may take an acute, subacute or chronic course and may be self-limiting or destructive and life-threatening. Prions are the causative agents of several neurodegenerative diseases. Many CNS infections can be treated if diagnosed in timely fashion. The cerebrospinal fluid examination, including culture, and neuroimaging studies (CT and MRI), together with the clinical findings, are generally sufficient to enable a differentiation among bacterial, viral, mycotic, and parasitic pathogens and a precise etiologic diagnosis. In general, antimicrobial therapy is given on an empirical basis until the causative organism is identified and the treatment can be tailored to it.

Meningitis is an infection of the pia-arachnoid and of the cerebrospinal fluid in the subarachnoid space. Because the subarachnoid space contains no anatomical barriers, meningitis can spread without hindrance over the entire surface of the brain and into the spinal canal and cerebral ventricles (ventriculitis). A more or less diffuse infection of the brain parenchyma is called encephalitis, and a focal collection of pus *cerebritis* (in the early stage) or *brain abscess* (in the late stage). A collection of pus in the (virtual) space between the dura mater and the arachnoid is called a *subdural empyema,* and one overlying the dura mater an *epidural abscess* (Fig. 2.**13**). As for infections affecting the spinal cord, see p. 414.

Infectious organisms reach the central nervous system by hematogenous spread, local extension, or, rarely, by direct (mechanical) inoculation, as in open head injuries. Systemic parameters of inflammation are almost always abnormal, but to differing degrees. Nearly all known infectious agents may involve the central nervous system. In this chapter, we discuss those that the neurologist encounters most frequently.

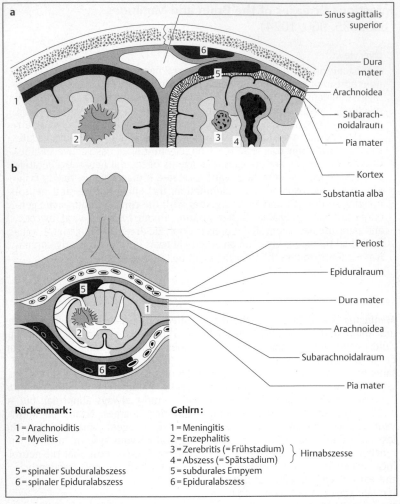

Rückenmark:

1 = Arachnoiditis
2 = Myelitis

5 = spinaler Subduralabszess
6 = spinaler Epiduralabszess

Gehirn:

1 = Meningitis
2 = Enzephalitis
3 = Zerebritis (= Frühstadium) ⎫
4 = Abszess (= Spätstadium)   ⎬ Hirnabszesse
5 = subdurales Empyem
6 = Epiduralabszess

Fig. 2.**13a, b   Localization and nomenclature of intracranial and spinal infections.**
a Intracranial infections.
b Spinal infections.

Ancillary Tests in the Evaluation of Suspected CNS Infection

■ Cerebrospinal Fluid Examination (308)

Definition:
The cerebrospinal fluid is examined for the diagnosis or exclusion of infectious or demyelinating diseases of the brain, meninges, spinal cord, and nerve roots, of subarachnoid hemorrhage, and of carcinomatous or sarcomatous meningitis. A sample of cerebrospinal fluid can be obtained by lumbar puncture or, in exceptional cases, by suboccipital puncture.

Indications

The indications for cerebrospinal fluid examination should be liberal, as imaging studies may fail to detect acute bacterial meningitis and "CT-negative" subarachnoid hemorrhage.

Contraindications

The following are *absolute contraindications* to lumbar and suboccipital puncture:

- clinical evidence of intracranial hypertension;
- platelet count under 5,000.

The following are *relative contraindications:*

- anticoagulation;
- platelet count 5,000–20,000;
- lumbar paraspinal abscess or other infection.

The *risks* of lumbar puncture are:

- transtentorial or transforaminal herniation, if the intracranial pressure is dangerously elevated;
- clinical worsening of paraparesis, if there is a partial block to the flow of cerebrospinal fluid;
- epidural, subdural, and subarachnoid hemorrhage.

The risk of bleeding after lumbar puncture in patients with normal coagulation status is less than 1%.

■ Lumbar Puncture

The most important consideration for a successful lumbar puncture is the positioning of the patient (Fig. 2.**14**).
The head should be at the same level as the puncture site. The shoulders should be vertically superimposed so that there is no torsion of the spine. If the patient is agitated or uncooperative, one or more assistants can hold the patient's head and knees from the front.

Orientation is facilitated by the line connecting the two posterior superior iliac spines, which usually intersects the spinous process of L4. The puncture may be one segment higher or one or two segments lower.

The physician wears sterile gloves. The skin is prepared with disinfectant and local anesthesia is injected at the intended puncture site. It is important to wait 1–2 minutes for this to take effect. The puncture is performed with an 8–10-cm long spinal needle with stylet, strictly in the midline and aiming approximately 30 degrees upward, through the tough interspinous ligament. If bony resistance is felt, the needle should be partially withdrawn and reintroduced in another direction, usually more cranial than before. Penetration of the ligamentum flavum is felt as a brief "pop" as the resistance to passage of

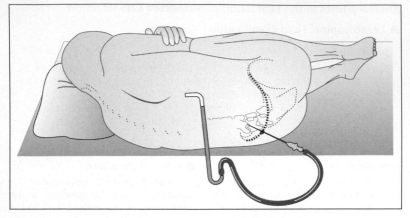

Fig. 2.**14   Lumbar puncture.**

the needle momentarily increases, then decreases.

After removal of the stylet, the cerebrospinal fluid should emerge spontaneously. If this is not the case, the angle of the opening at the needle tip should be changed by a partial rotation of the needle. If still no fluid is seen, the stylet should be reinserted and the needle introduced a bit farther. If the patient complains of a sudden pain radiating into the leg, it is because the needle has irritated a nerve root; it should be partially withdrawn and reintroduced at a new angle, away from the side on which pain was reported. The correct depth of insertion varies: in very obese patients, the needle may need to be inserted to the hilt, while infants rarely require an insertion deeper than 2.5 cm (119). If it is in proper position, but no fluid emerges, low cerebrospinal fluid pressure is a possibility and this should be checked by gently aspirating on the needle with a sterile syringe. Lumbar puncture may be particularly difficult in the presence of scoliosis, which is always associated with torsion of the spine; in such situations, an L5/S1 puncture is recommended, because torsion is least at this level. If difficulties are encountered for this or other reasons, the puncture can also be performed on the patient in the sitting position, and the patient can be laid horizontal again after successful puncture.

Once cerebrospinal fluid is seen emerging from the needle, its pressure should be measured in mmH$_2$O with a manometer. Compression of the jugular veins with a hand pressed flat against the neck impedes cerebrospinal fluid resorption and thus raises the intracranial pressure; this rise ought to be reflected in a corresponding rise of the lumbar cerebrospinal fluid pressure (Queckenstedt test). In a positive (normal) Queckenstedt test, the fluid column in the manometer promptly rises, demonstrating the patency of the spinal canal and the jugular veins; a negative test indicates the presence of an obstruction. External pressure on the abdomen or abdominal straining can raise the pressure in the lumbar spinal canal even if an obstruction to cerebrospinal fluid flow is present at a higher (cervical or thoracic) level, so this test cannot be used to rule out an obstruction. Poor needle position with partial misplacement of the opening at the tip of the needle may result in a falsely abnormal Queckenstedt test.

Once the pressure has been measured, a sufficient quantity of cerebrospinal fluid is collected for the desired diagnostic tests. For both medical and medicolegal reasons, the patient's informed consent should be obtained beforehand, and the procedure should be documented in the hospital chart.

The patient should lie prone for 1 hour and flat in bed for at least a further 8 hours after the procedure, to lessen the chance that cerebrospinal fluid will leak from the dural puncture site into the epidural space, producing a low fluid pressure syndrome (see p. 819). In general, this risk can also be reduced by the use of a finer needle. The risk is so low with the Sprotte needle (which is very fine, and has a blunt tip with a lateral opening) that the procedure can be performed on an outpatient basis.

■ Suboccipital Puncture

Suboccipital puncture is performed under fluoroscopic guidance by either of two possible approaches:

- Dorsomedian approach in the sitting or laterally recumbent patient. The cisterna magna is punctured between the lower rim of the occipital bone and the posterior arch of C1 (*cisternal puncture*).
- Lateral approach in the supine patient. The subarachnoid space is entered between C1 and C2 (lateral cervical puncture).

Indications

Suboccipital puncture is indicated only when:

- meningitis is suspected, but a lumbar puncture yields no cerebrospinal fluid for examination; or
- lumbar puncture is contraindicated by an infectious process in the lumbar region.

■ Laboratory examination of cerebrospinal fluid and interpretation of findings

Normal values for the most important cerebrospinal fluid tests are listed in Tables 2.**19** and 2.**20**.

Gross appearance. The cerebrospinal fluid is normally clear and colorless. Cloudy cerebrospinal fluid indicates meningitis, while bloody or xanthochromic fluid indicates subarachnoid hemorrhage. Bloody cerebrospinal fluid may also be the artefactual result of a traumatic puncture. Truly bloody cerebrospinal fluid can be differentiated from a "bloody tap" by the so-called three tube test, in which three tubes are filled with cerebrospinal fluid, one after the next. Truly bloody cerebrospinal fluid is equally bloody in all three tubes, while the fluid gradually clears from each tube to the next after a traumatic puncture. *Xanthochromia* of centrifuged cerebrospinal fluid may also be helpful in this regard: it is absent after a traumatic puncture, but present within 6–10 hours of a subarachnoid hemorrhage. By the same token, however, the absence of xanthochromia in the first few hours after the presenting event does not rule out a subarachnoid hemorrhage. Xanthochromia may be present in jaundiced patients, as well as those with extreme hyperproteinemia. Mild degrees of xanthochromia can be detected by spectroscopy if visual inspection is inconclusive.

Total and differential cell count. Normal cerebrospinal fluid contains no erythrocytes and up to four leukocytes per microliter. Lymphocytes predominate ($\geq 70\%$), and monocytes are rarer ($\leq 30\%$). An elevation of the total leukocyte count to 30 per microliter in the presence of a few neutrophils and macrophages may represent either a nonspecific inflammation or an actual infection; higher values practically always indicate meningitis. The cerebrospinal fluid picture of *acute inflammation* is dominated by *neutrophils*. In the *subacute phase*, there are fewer neutrophils; *monocytes and macrophages* (some of which contain phagocytosed neutrophils and lymphocytes) predominate, and eosinophils may herald the beginning of the regenerative response. The *chronic phase* is associated with a lymphocytic picture; many transformed lymphocytes and plasma cells are present.

Table 2.**19** Normal values in cerebrospinal fluid and serum in adults[1]

Cerebrospinal fluid	Serum	
Pressure	5–18 cmH$_2$O	
Volume	100–160 mL	
Osmolarity	292–297 mosm/L	285–295 mosm/L
Electrolytes		
• Na	137–145 mmol/L	136–145 mmol/L
• K	2.7–3.9 mmol/L	3.5–5.0 mmol/L
• Ca	1–1.5 mmol/L	2.2–2.6 mmol/L
• Cl	116–122 mmol/L	98–106 mmol/L
pH	7.31–7.34	7.38–7.44
Glucose	2.2–3.9 mmol/L	4.2–6.4 mmol/L
• CSF/serum glucose quotient	> 0.5–0.6	
Lactate	1.0–2.0 mmol/L	0.6–1.7 mmol/L
Total protein	0.2–0.5 g/L	55–80 g/L
• Albumin	56–75%	50–60%
• IgG	0.010–0.014 g/L	8–15 g/L
• IgG index [2]	< 0.65	
Leukocytes	< 4/µL	
Lymphocytes	60–70%	

1 Because serum and cerebrospinal fluid are in equilibrium, simultaneous measurement of values in both is recommended.

2 IgG index = CSF IgG (mg/dL) × serum albumin (g/dL) / serum IgG (g/dL) × CSF albumin (mg/dL).

Table 2.**20** Clinically useful investigations of cerebrospinal fluid

Routine investigations:
- Pressure, Queckenstedt test
- Color (turbidity? xanthochromia? bloody tinge?)
- Absolute and differential cell count
- Protein
- Glucose

Selectively applied investigations:
- Immunoglobulin
- IgG–albumin index
- Oligoclonal bands
- Specific testing for IgG, IgA, and IgM against *Borrelia*, parasites, and viruses
- Bacterial, fungal, viral, and mycobacterial culture
- Gram and Ziehl-Neelsen stain, touch prep
- VDRL and FTA tests for syphilis
- Cytological examination for malignant cells
- DNA amplification (PCR) for tuberculosis and viral pathogens
- Cystatin C in amyloid angiopathy (872)
- Antineuronal antibodies in paraneoplastic syndrome (207)

After a traumatically bloody lumbar puncture, the true lymphocyte count in the patient's cerebrospinal fluid (LC_P) may be approximately calculated on the basis of the measured lymphocyte and erythrocyte counts in the fluid obtained by lumbar puncture (LC_L and EC_L) and in the blood (LC_B and EC_B), as follows:

$$LC_P = LC_L - \frac{(LC_B \times EC_L)}{EC_B}$$

An *elevated cell count* of up to a few hundred cells per microliter is etiologically nonspecific. In general, an acutely inflammatory cerebrospinal fluid picture with a cell count of over 1000/µL indicates bacterial infection,

while a predominantly lymphocytic pleocytosis indicates viral infection. Nonetheless, the cerebrospinal fluid picture may be predominantly granulocytic in the initial phase of an acute viral meningitis. A chronically inflammatory cerebrospinal fluid picture is found in the healing phase of bacterial meningitis and in fungal and parasitic infections, borreliosis (Lyme disease), syphilis, and sarcoidosis. The presence of many eosinophils is a distinguishing feature of parasitic infection. In tuberculosis, the cellular picture is usually subacutely or chronically inflammatory. Erythrocytes may be a component of an inflammatory cerebrospinal fluid picture (hemorrhagic encephalitis) or may result from a subarachnoid hemorrhage of noninflammatory etiology. *Neoplastic cells* are shed into the cerebrospinal fluid by a number of primary brain tumors, including ependymoma, choroid plexus papilloma, germinoma of the pineal region, and medulloblastoma. The presence of carcinoma or sarcoma cells indicates meningeal metastatic spread, most commonly of breast cancer, lung cancer, or melanoma. Leukemia and lymphoma may also involve the meninges.

Cerebrospinal fluid protein. After the cell count, the protein concentration is the most important value to be determined (Table 2.**21**). An elevation of the protein concentration without any corresponding elevation in cell count (so-called "albuminocytologic dissociation") is a classic, albeit nonspecific, finding in Guillain-Barré syndrome and is also present in diabetes. An elevated IgG index (see Table 2.**20**) indicates intrathecal IgG production by an intrathecal inflam-

Table 2.**21**   Diseases associated with elevated cerebrospinal fluid protein concentration

Elevated protein with elevated cell count:
- Acute and chronic meningitides and encephalitides
- Bacterial
- Viral
- Fungal
- Spirochetal
- Parasitic
- Neoplastic
- Chemical/physical
- Poliomyelitis

Protein elevation ⩾ cell count elevation:
- Acute inflammatory polyradiculitis (Guillain-Barré syndrome)
- Chronic inflammatory demyelinating polyneuropathy (CIDP)
- Tabes dorsalis, meningovascular syphilis
- Myxedema
- Diabetes mellitus
- Schwannoma
- Chronic arachnoiditis
- Status post subarachnoid hemorrhage
- Cerebral venous (and venous sinus) thrombosis
- Brain tumors
- Metachromatic leukodystrophy
- Obstructed CSF flow at spinal level (Froin syndrome)
- Vitamin B_{12} deficiency
- Mitochondrial encephalomyelopathy

Elevated protein with or without elevated cell count:
- CNS vasculitis
- Gliomatosis cerebri
- Epidural abscess

Mildly elevated protein with or without mildly elevated cell count:
- Multiple sclerosis
- Epilepsy
- Brain infarct
- Abscess
- Uremia

matory process (588, 941). The gammaglobulins can be nonquantitatively separated by *electrophoresis* into mono-, poly- and (usually two to five) oligoclonal bands. *Isoelectric focusing* is a more sensitive test, based on the different isoelectric points of different proteins, which can be combined with *immune fixation* (the use of specific antisera) (938) for still greater sensitivity. Oligoclonal bands found in the cerebrospinal fluid, but not in an appropriately diluted serum sample tested alongside it, are indicative of an inflammatory process in the central nervous system. Such CSF-specific bands are found in more than 90% of patients with multiple sclerosis, and less commonly in patients with other types of central nervous disease.

Glucose. The concentration of glucose in the cerebrospinal fluid is 50–60% of that in serum. Thus, a CSF glucose concentration that is normal in absolute terms may be abnormally low if the serum glucose concentration is elevated, and a low CSF glucose concentration may be normal in hypoglycemia. Diseases associated with CSF pleocytosis lower the CSF glucose concentration, particularly chronic meningitides (Table 2.**22**).

■ **Brain Biopsy**

A biopsy is an invasive diagnostic procedure that should only be performed after a careful consideration of the indications and when all relevant noninvasive studies have failed to yield a diagnosis.

Brain biopsy is a neurosurgical procedure that can be performed either through an open craniotomy, or stereotactically under radiologic guidance. In most centers, its use is re-

Table 2.**22** Meningitic syndromes

Syndrome	Cell count	Protein	Glucose
Acute bacterial meningitis	× 100 – × 1000, mainly polynuclear	Elevated	Low or very low
Acute viral meningitis	× 100, more mono- than polynuclear	Normal or mildly elevated	Normal or mildly low
Chronic meningitis	× 100, mainly mononuclear	Elevated or mark- edly elevated	Low or very low

stricted to the diagnostic evaluation of radiologically identified abnormalities in the brain. Thus, a biopsy can provide histologic differentiation of tumors and inflammatory changes, which is important for the planning of further treatment. When a biopsy is performed, tissue specimens should be taken not only for histological examination, but also for culture, whenever a bacterial, mycotic, or mycobacterial infection is a diagnostic possibility.

■ **Neuroimaging Studies**

CT and MRI often provide critical diagnostic information about infections of the central nervous system. MRI, in particular, is indispensable for the diagnosis of abscess and encephalitis (p. 93). Inflammatory changes are often visible only after the administration of contrast. Contrast-enhanced scans are therefore recommended whenever a CNS infection is suspected.

Angiography may be of assistance in the diagnosis of vasculitis. Mycotic aneurysms are sometimes visible only on an angiogram.

Bacterial Infections

■ **Acute Bacterial Meningitis** (795)

Most cases of bacterial meningitis arise by hematogenous spread of a bacterial infection affecting the upper respiratory tract. Less commonly, they are caused by direct extension of pathogenic bacteria from purulent collections in the head, or else pathogens are directly inoculated into the intracranial cavity by traumatic brain injury, or iatrogenically by punctures and shunt operations.

The most common *pathogens* are:
- in the newborn: *Escherichia coli,* Group B streptococci;
- in children: *Haemophilus influenzae,* pneumococci, and meningococci;
- in adults: pneumococci and meningococci.

The risk of meningococcal infection increases in complement disorders or properdin deficiency, while that of pneumococcal meningitis increases after splenectomy. *Klebsiella, E. coli,* and *Pseudomonas aeruginosa* are the most common pathogens affecting aged persons, alcoholics, and persons who have suffered traumatic brain injuries or undergone neurosurgical procedures; *Listeria monocytogenes* may also cause meningitis at any age. Fewer than 1% of cases of meningitis involve multiple pathogens. Endemic and epidemic meningitis are a major public health problem in underdeveloped countries and are usually caused by *H. influenzae,* meningococci, and pneumococci.

Pathological Anatomy

A granulocytic infiltration of the meninges and subarachnoid space is observed. This may lead to disturbances of cerebrospinal fluid flow (hydrocephalus), vasospasm, arterial and venous thrombosis with consequent infarction, infection of the brain tissue (encephalitis, cerebritis, brain abscess), cerebral edema, and intracranial hypertension.

Clinical Features

The classic clinical triad of meningitis consists of:
- headache,
- fever, and
- meningism (nuchal rigidity).

Headache may be extremely intense and diffuse, commonly bioccipital. Back pain, myalgia, photophobia, nausea, and vomiting are further symptoms. As many as 40% of patients have epileptic seizures, and 10–20% have cranial nerve deficits. Such patients are usually somnolent or comatose and manifest a characteristic combination of hypertension and bradycardia. Papilledema may be present. Fever and meningism may be only mild in children, the elderly, and immune-suppressed patients, in whom headache and vomiting are the major manifestations of disease.

Diagnosis

Examination of the cerebrospinal fluid is critical for diagnosis (Table 2.**22**). If clinical signs of intracranial hypertension are present (bradycardia, hypertension, papilledema), an intracranial mass lesion should be ruled out by CT or MRI prior to lumbar puncture. The cerebrospinal fluid is turbid and contains 1,000–10,000 cells per microliter, and occasionally more. There is a predominantly granulocytic pleocytosis. The cerebrospinal fluid pressure and protein concentration are practically always elevated, and the glucose concentration low. Gram staining reveals the bacterial pathogen in 60–90% of cases. Cerebrospinal fluid cultures are positive in ca. 75% of cases, and blood cultures in 50–75%. Blood culture should be performed in all cases, as it may be positive even if the cerebrospinal fluid culture is negative. Partially treated bacterial meningitis and listerial meningitis may be associated with fewer than 1000 cells per microliter in the cerebrospinal fluid and should not be confused with viral meningitis.

Neuroimaging studies such as CT and MRI are generally not required for diagnosis, but they are helpful should complications arise. They are normal in the early stage of bacterial meningitis, but later show compression of the sulci and cisterns. Meningeal enhancement may be seen on MRI, and more rarely on CT (Fig. 2.**15**). (760). Bony defects of the base of the skull that may be of pathogenetic significance are usually seen in the bone window of a fine-section CT scan.

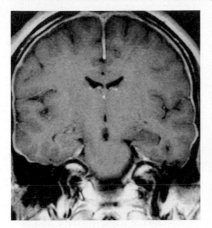

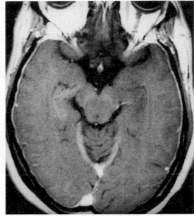

Fig. 2.**15a, b   Chronic meningitis.**
The patient is a 49-year-old woman. The pathogenic organism could not be identified. **a** Coronal T1-weighted MRI with contrast. **b** Axial T1-weighted MRI with contrast. Note the abnormal contrast enhancement in the meninges.

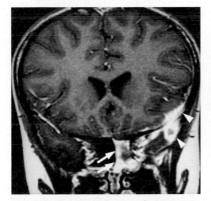

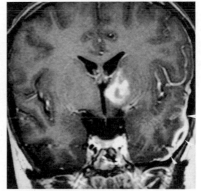

Fig. 2.**16a, b   Acute bacterial meningitis.**
The patient is a 10-year-old boy. **a** Coronal T1-weighted MRI with contrast demonstrates sphenoid sinusitis (arrows) spreading in the epidural space under the left temporal lobe and causing meningitis by direct extension with involvement of the temporal lobe (arrowheads). **b** T1-weighted MRI with contrast in a coronal section posterior to **a** shows a probable epidural empyema over the left temporal lobe (arrowheads). There is also extensive signal change in the left thalamus, probably due to an arterial infarction as a complication of meningitis.

Prognosis

The prognosis of acute bacterial meningitis depends on:

- the pathogenic organism,
- the severity of the infection,
- concomitant illnesses,
- the state of the immune system, and
- the type of treatment and time at which it is instituted.

Mortality is highest in the newborn (over 50%). Meningitis accompanied by meningococcal sepsis also confers a high mortality, because it is frequently complicated by bilateral adrenal hemorrhage and subsequent circulatory collapse (Waterhouse-Friderichsen syndrome). The mortality of other forms of meningitis is approximately 20% (1014). Surviving patients often suffer from permanent sequelae including deafness, malresorptive hydrocephalus, epilepsy, and intellectual deficits, particularly in children.

Treatment

(Fig. 2.**17**) (777a)

If a lumbar puncture cannot be performed immediately because of clinical signs of intracranial hypertension, "blind" parenteral antimicrobial treatment should be initiated at once, as *a few minutes may make the difference between life and death*. If the pathogenic organism is unknown, the antimicrobial treatment is chosen empirically (Table 2.**23**). It can then be modified in accordance with the findings of the cerebrospinal fluid and blood cultures, including sensitivity and resistance testing.

The *duration of treatment* is based on the findings of serial clinical examination and cerebrospinal fluid analysis. Some general recommendations are:

- for meningococci and *H. influenzae,* 7–10 days;
- for pneumococci, 10–14 days;
- for Listeria and Gram-negative aerobes, 3 weeks.

Steroids (dexamethasone 0.4 mg/kg every 12 hours in the first 2 days of treatment) favorably affect the course of the inflammatory process in children and probably also in adults, and should be given in addition to antimicrobial agents (560, 831).

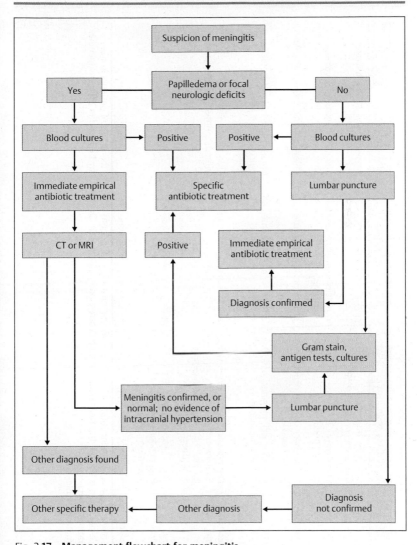

Fig. 2.**17 Management flowchart for meningitis.**
The essential element of treatment is immediate institution of antimicrobial therapy, at
first empirical and then tailored to the specific pathogen identified by culture.

Table 2.23   Antimicrobial therapy of bacterial meningitis (824, 831, 836)

Patient group	Most likely organism	Agent(s) of first choice[1]	Alternatives
Newborn	Group B streptococci, E. coli, Listeria monocytogenes	Ampicillin and cefotaxime[2]	Ampicillin and aminoglycoside
Infants 1–3 months	Same and H. influenzae, meningococci, pneumococci	Ampicillin and ceftriaxone or cefotaxime	Chloramphenicol and aminoglycoside
Infants > 3 months, toddlers	H. influenzae, meningococci, pneumococci	Ceftriaxone or cefotaxime	Chloramphenicol and ampicillin
Children and adults	Pneumococci, meningococci, Listeria monocytogenes	Ceftriaxone or cefotaxime and ampicillin or penicillin G	Chloramphenicol and ampicillin, vancomycin if penicillin-resistant
Adults > 60 years, alcoholics, patients with systemic disease	Pneumococci, E. coli, Haemophilus influenzae, Listeria monocytogenes, Pseudomonas aeruginosa, anaerobes[3]	Vancomycin and ceftriaxone[2] and rifampicin	Chloramphenicol and trimethoprim-sulfamethoxazole
Traumatic brain injury, neurosurgical procedures	Staphylococcus aureus, E. coli, Pseudomonas aeruginosa,[4] pneumococci	Vancomycin and ceftriaxone	
Cerebrospinal fluid leak	Pneumococci	Cefotaxime or ceftriaxone	

1 Unless otherwise specified, these recommendations are applicable to the most likely pathogens affecting the group of patients in question. If the responsible pathogen is known, the treatment should be correspondingly tailored. Dosages may be found in drug compendia.
2 Or other (third-generation) cephalosporin.
3 Chloramphenicol or metronidazole.
4 Add gentamicin.

Prevention

The administration of *Haemophilus* vaccine to infants confers 90% protection against this type of meningitis. Inoculation against the meningococcus is recommended for travelers to endemic areas. After exposure to *Haemophilus* or meningococcus, antimicrobial prophylaxis is recommended (10 mg/kg in children or 600 mg in adults, b.i.d. for 2 days).

■ Tuberculous Meningitis (1051)

Mycobacterium tuberculosis causes a chronic bacterial infection characterized by granuloma formation. The lung is usually affected. The meninges may become involved during the primary infection in children, or years afterward in adults. Meningitis comes about by reactivation of clinically silent granulomas and secondary deposits in the subarachnoid space, even in the absence of simultaneous pulmonary tuberculosis. HIV-positive persons are at particularly high risk of infection both by *M. tuberculosis* and by atypical mycobacteria.

Pathological Anatomy

An exudative basilar meningitis and vasculitis is found, particularly in the vicinity of the anterior and middle cerebral arteries. Meningeal involvement and vasculitis may lead to cranial nerve deficits and to cerebral infarction. Hydrocephalus is commonly seen.

Clinical Features

Over the course of several days or, more rarely, weeks, these patients exhibit progressive symptoms and signs including subfebrile temperature, fatigue, depression, personality changes, and (sometimes) confusion. One-third of patients develop headache, meningism, asymmetrical cranial nerve deficits, and ischemic stroke. Coma is a bad prognostic sign. For miliary tuberculosis, see p. 91.

Diagnosis

Cerebrospinal fluid examination reveals a picture of chronic meningeal inflammation with at first granulocytic and then monocytic pleocytosis of 100–500 cells, elevated protein concentration, and low glucose concentration. The diagnosis is confirmed by the demonstration of acid-fast bacilli by the Ziehl-Neelsen method or with auramine-rhodamine staining, either in the fresh cerebrospinal fluid sample or after 4–6 weeks of culture.

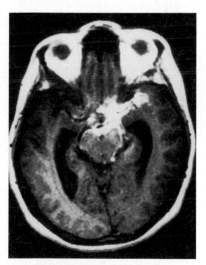

Fig. 2.18 Tuberculous meningitis.
This contrast-enhanced T1-weighted MR image reveals enhancement of the inflamed meninges at the basal cisterns and anterior to the brainstem. The asymmetrical extension of inflammation along the course of the middle cerebral artery is also typical.

In addition to the cerebrospinal fluid, the sputum, gastric juice, and urine should be examined and cultured for acid-fast bacilli. Contrast-enhanced CT and MRI reveal meningeal involvement at the skull base and along the course of the middle cerebral artery (151) (Fig. 2.**18**).

Differential Diagnosis

The differential diagnosis includes all types of chronic lymphocytic meningoencephalitis (see below).

▨ Treatment ▨

The treatment consists of a combination of four *tuberculostatic medications:* rifampicin, isoniazid, pyrazinamide, and ethambutol. At the same time, *steroids* and *vitamin B₆* should be given. The latter prevents the pyridoxine deficiency that may otherwise result from long-term use of isoniazid.

This therapy should be continued until the results of culture are available. If culture is positive for tubercle bacilli, a combination of three medications is given for a further 2 months, and then two medications for 8–10 months more. Once the culture results are negative and the cerebrospinal fluid picture has renormalized, treatment may be discontinued.

If the patient fails to improve on this regimen, other etiologies of chronic meningitis should be sought, and, even if cultures for *M. tuberculosis* are negative, it is prudent to continue the tuberculostatic therapy. The currently used tuberculostatic agents have only minor side effects even in long-term use.

Prognosis

Tuberculous meningitis is fatal if untreated, curable without sequelae if treated in time. The diagnosis should be made, and treatment initiated, before the onset of cranial nerve deficits or of impaired consciousness. Thus: *when tuberculous meningitis is strongly suspected, obtain fluid samples for culture and then begin antitubercular therapy immediately.*

■ Meningoencephalitis
■ Listeriosis (957, 959, 695b)

Listeria are aerobic or facultatively anaerobic bacilli that are usually ingested orally in food. They preferentially infect the newborn, diabetics, alcoholics, and aged or immune-suppressed persons. The clinical picture is generally that of a typical bacterial meningitis, but the cerebrospinal fluid cell count may be so low as to arouse suspicion of viral meningitis. Listeria also causes encephalitis, often with brainstem manifestations, as well as meningoencephalitis and cerebral or spinal abscesses (Fig. 2.**19**).

▨ Treatment ▨

The antimicrobial agents of first choice are *ampicillin* and *penicillin G.* An alternative is *trimethoprim/sulfamethoxazole.* Cephalosporins do not eliminate Listeria.

■ Brucella Meningitis (127)

Brucellosis is transmitted in milk or other animal products and usually presents nonspecifically with fever, arthralgias and myalgias, though it causes localized disease in some cases, and its manifestations are sometimes restricted to the central

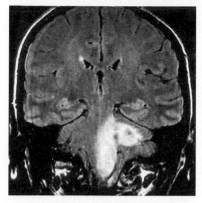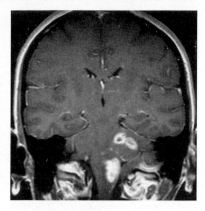

Fig. 2.**19** **Listeria meningoencephalitis.**
A 45-year-old woman with multiple cranial nerve deficits and left ataxia.
a The FLAIR sequence reveals a plate-like signal abnormality in the brainstem and left cerebellar hemisphere.
b The T1-weighted image shows several foci of contrast enhancement.

nervous system. These usually consist of subacute or chronic meningitis, more rarely meningoencephalitis, myeloradiculitis or neuritis.

Twenty to 500 cells are found in the cerebrospinal fluid. The diagnosis is confirmed by the demonstration of specific antibodies in the CSF.

> ### Treatment
> The treatment consists of doxycycline and rifampicin for 4 months, with surveillance of the cerebrospinal fluid.

■ Meningoencephalitis in Miliary Tuberculosis

In miliary tuberculosis, hematogenous spread of tubercle bacilli leads to the formation of millet-seed-sized granulomas throughout the body. The clinical manifestations are not specific to this disease but rather reflect

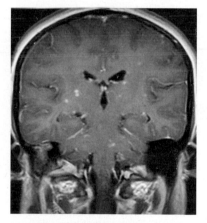

Fig. 2.**20** **Miliary tuberculosis.**
A 28-year-old woman with miliary tuberculosis. Cerebrospinal fluid examination revealed a mild monocytic pleocytosis, a markedly elevated protein concentration, and a low glucose concentration. The MRI reveals multiple pinhead-sized foci of contrast enhancement in the brain parenchyma and mild contrast enhancement of the meninges as well.

the predominantly involved organ(s). Symptoms and signs may include fever, night sweats, anorexia, generalized weakness and fatigue, hepatosplenomegaly, lymphadenopathy, and (if the brain is affected) headache and progressive impairment of consciousness. Miliary tuberculosis usually affects the brain parenchyma more than the meninges. The cerebrospinal fluid findings are the same as for tuberculous meningitis, except that pleocytosis is usually only mild. MRI reveals multiple pinhead-sized, contrast-enhancing nodules (Fig. 2.**20**).

For diagnosis and treatment, see "Tuberculous meningitis," above (p. 90).

■ Focal Embolic Encephalitis (148, 315, 819)

Neurological symptoms and signs develop in at least one-third of patients with infectious endocarditis and may be the presenting manifestations of the disease.

Streptococcus is the most common pathogen, followed by staphylococcus and Gram-negative bacilli. Central nervous manifestations arise by several different *pathogenetic mechanisms:*

- occlusion of cerebral arteries by septic and thrombotic emboli arising from heart valve vegetations;
- infection of the meninges, brain parenchyma, or vascular walls by septic emboli or by bacteremia;
- "toxic" and probably also immune-mediated injury.

Pathological Anatomy

There may be bland or hemorrhagic cerebral infarcts, intracerebral, subarachnoid or subdural hemorrhage, meningitis, abscesses, mycotic aneurysms, or any combination of these entities.

Clinical Features

The symptoms and signs depend on the pathological processes occurring in each individual case. Embolic events are prominent in 20% of cases, encephalitis due to multiple micro-emboli and microabscesses in 10%, hemorrhage due to mycotic aneurysms in 5%, and meningitis in 5%. Emboli produce focal manifestations, while the other types of lesion cause a diffuse encephalopathy with behavioral and cognitive disturbances, impairment of consciousness, focal or generalized seizures, and sometimes headache and meningism. Important diagnostic clues include subfebrile or (in acute endocarditis) septic temperature, a feeling of severe illness and prostration, anemia, splenomegaly, subungual, palmar and retinal petechiae, and heart murmur.

Diagnosis

The complete blood count reveals acute inflammation, and the erythrocyte sedimentation rate and C-reactive protein are elevated. The responsible organism can usually be demonstrated by *blood culture,* and endocarditis by *transesophageal echocardiography* (212). The cerebrospinal fluid may be sterile, purulent or hemorrhagic, depending on the nature of CNS involvement (772).

MRI is particularly useful for the demonstration of embolic and infectious processes affecting the central nervous system. *Angiography* is the most reliable way to demonstrate mycotic aneurysms, but need not be performed routinely in every patient (819).

Treatment

The most important initial step is the prompt institution of empiric *antimicrobial treatment*. Penicillinase-resistant penicillins (e.g., flucloxacillin or methicillin) are given together with gentamicin until the results of culture are available, whereupon the treatment can be specifically tailored. Vancomycin should be given with gentamicin initially whenever the presence of penicillinase-resistant staphylococcus is likely on clinical grounds (e.g., in intravenous drug users and patients with artificial heart valves).

If emboli continue to form despite antimicrobial treatment, surgical heart valve replacement may be necessary. Anticoagulants should be withheld till at least 48 hours after the procedure, unless the infected valve is itself a previously implanted prosthesis, in which case anticoagulation should generally not be interrupted.

Mycotic aneurysms pose a special problem. Many regress spontaneously under antimicrobial therapy, but persistent aneurysms may need to be obliterated neurosurgically (722) or by endovascular treatment.

■ **Encephalitis**

■ **Whipple's Disease**

Pathological Anatomy

This is a bacterial infection of the intestinal mucosa, mesenteric lymph nodes, and reticuloendothelial system. The responsible pathogen, *Tropheryma whippelii*, generally cannot be cultured.

Clinical Features

The manifestations include arthralgias, diarrhea, intestinal malabsorption and weight loss. Some 40% of patients show neurological signs, which are the sole finding in 5%. These consist of a progressive encephalopathy with personality changes, apathy, memory impairment, and cognitive deficits that may reach the severity of dementia. Extrapyramidal signs, ataxia, ophthalmoplegia, and hypothalamic dysfunction may also be found. Oculomasticatory myorhythmia with a frequency of 1 Hz is characteristic.

Diagnosis

These clinical signs are the consequence of a perivascular nodular encephalitis that is well seen in CT and MRI. The cerebrospinal fluid may be normal, or there may be pleocytosis of up to 200 cells/μL and an elevated protein concentration of up to 2 g/L. The diagnosis rests on the demonstration of PAS-positive material in the mucosa of the small intestine or (in cases of isolated CNS disease) in the brain.

Treatment

Clinical improvement follows treatment with *trimethoprim-sulfamethoxazole* (Bactrim), which must be given for 1 year.

Focal Purulent Infections

■ **Brain Abscess**

A brain abscess is a focal purulent process in the brain parenchyma. These rarely occurring lesions are found more commonly in persons with HIV (see p. 117), bronchiectasis, hereditary hemorrhagic telangiectasia (Osler-Weber-Rendu disease), or congenital heart anomalies with a right-to-left shunt.

Pathogenesis, Sites and Responsible Organisms

Approximately one-half of brain abscesses arise by contiguous spread of infection, generally from otitis media or sinusitis; the means of spread is hematogenous in a further one-quarter of cases, and undetermined in the remainder. Dental abscesses are found in 10% of patients. Direct inoculation of pathogens into the brain is relatively rare. Abscesses are multiple in 10% to 50% of cases (the numbers in published series vary). Hematogenous abscesses are commonly found at the junction of gray and white matter in the territory of the middle cerebral artery, but may be anywhere in the brain. The source of infection is commonly the lungs, abdomen, pelvis, or bones (osteomyelitis). Temporal lobe abscesses most commonly result from otitis media, mastoiditis, and sphenoid sinusitis, and frontal lobe abscesses from frontal and ethmoidal sinusitis or dental abscess. Cerebellar abscesses are otogenic in 90% of cases. Two-thirds of the responsible organisms are aerobic, and one-third anaerobic; different flora are typically associated with each source of infection. In general, streptococci, Gram-negative bacilli, and *Staphylococcus aureus* are the most common aerobes, and *Bacteroides sp.* and streptococci the most common anaerobes. Some 30–60% of abscesses contain mixed flora (two or more species).

Pathology

An abscess develops through successive stages of early and late cerebritis followed by early and late capsule formation. At first, there is cerebritis with a necrotic focus, marked edema, and a perifocal zone of inflammation.

Table 2.**24** Differential diagnosis of ring-enhancement on CT and MRI

Primary brain tumor
Metastasis
Abscess
Granuloma
Hematoma in the process of being resorbed
Infarct
Thrombosed arteriovenous malformation
Thrombosed aneurysm
Plaque of demyelination

The focus then becomes demarcated as surrounding neovascularization and fibrosis gradually lead to the formation of a capsule. Over the course of several weeks or months, the necrotic center is replaced by granulation tissue and correspondingly shrinks in size. An abscess may also give rise to satellite abscesses or rupture into a ventricle or the subarachnoid space, causing an acute ventriculitis or meningitis.

Neuroradiology

The stages of abscess development can be followed with CT or MRI (282). CT initially shows a poorly demarcated area of hypodensity with diffuse contrast enhancement. The central hypodense zone is surrounded by edema with consequent mass effect. Later, ring-enhancement appears and the abscess capsule becomes visible in the nonenhanced views as well. On the MRI, cerebritis is T2-hyperintense and enhances diffusely with contrast. Necrosis and edema are hypointense on T1- and hyperintense on T2-weighted images, while the abscess capsule is isointense or mildly hyperintense on T1-weighted and isointense or mildly hypointense on T2-weighted images. The capsule is visible as a marked ring-enhancement (1049), which, however, is not specific for brain abscess and carries an extensive differential diagnosis (Table 2.**24**).

Clinical Features

The clinical manifestations of brain abscess include:

- general manifestations of the primary or generalized infectious process, when present,
- general signs of intracranial hypertension,
- focal signs depending on the site of the abscess in the brain (Table 2.**25**).

Fever, prostration, and shaking chills may be, but need not be present. Headache, nausea and vomiting, and papilledema indicate the presence of intracranial hypertension. Local effects of the abscess on the brain include seizures, neuropsychological abnormalities, impairment of consciousness, or focal signs such as hemiparesis, visual field defects, and cranial nerve deficits.

Laboratory Findings and Diagnosis

The blood leukocyte count, erythrocyte sedimentation rate, and C-reactive protein are usually, but by no means always, elevated. Blood cultures are positive in only about 10% of cases. The cerebrospinal fluid is normal or else shows the same picture as in chronic meningitis, usually with a normal glucose concentration. If signs of intracranial hypertension are present, lumbar puncture should not be performed, or only with a very fine needle if necessary. CT or MRI demonstrates the focal lesion. As the radiologic picture is not pathognomonic, the diagnosis must be based on the combination of clinical, laboratory, and radiologic findings.

■ Subdural Empyema and Epidural Abscess (140)

Subdural empyema is a collection of pus in the virtual space between the dura mater and the arachnoid, while epidural abscess is one in the virtual space between the dura mater and the inner table of the skull. When an epidural abscess is present, there is usually a subdural empyema as well, because the two spaces are spanned by the emissary veins. Subdural empyema can spread more or less unhindered in the subdural space; only the tentorium serves as a barrier between the supra- and infratentorial compartments. Epidural abscesses cannot spread across the cranial sutures.

Both of these types of infection usually arise as complications of *sinusitis*

Table 2.**25** Clinical manifestations of brain abscess (1031)

Manifestation	Frequency (%)
Headache	70
Triad of fever, headache, and focal neurological deficit	< 50
Fever	40–50
Focal neurological deficit	50
Seizures	22–40
Nausea/vomiting	22–50
Meningism	25
Papilledema	25

Table **2.26**   Antimicrobial therapy of brain abscess (824, 836)

Type of abscess, patient population	Probable organism	Treatment of first choice[1]	Alternative treatment
Otogenic or unknown etiology	*Streptococcus viridans*, anaerobic streptococci, *Bacteroides* sp.,, *Escherichia coli*	Penicillin G and ceftazidime[2] and metronidazole	Penicillin G, chloramphenicol
Frontal abscess and sinusitis	Anaerobic streptococci, pneumococci, *Haemophilus*	Penicillin G[3] and metronidazole	Penicillin G, chloramphenicol
Traumatic brain injury, neurosurgical procedures	*Staphylococcus aureus*, *Escherichia coli*, *Pseudomonas aeruginosa*[4]	Penicillinase-resistant penicillin and ceftriaxone[2] and rifampicin	Vancomycin and ceftriaxone[2] and rifampicin
HIV-positive	*Toxoplasma gondii*	Pyrimethamine and sulfadiazine	Pyrimethamine and trimethoprim-sulfamethoxazole

1 Unless otherwise specified, these recommendations are applicable to the most likely pathogens affecting the group of patients in question. If the responsible pathogen is known, the treatment should be correspondingly tailored. Dosages may be found in drug compendia.
2 Or other (third-generation) cephalosporin.
3 In young adults, penicillinase-resistant penicillin in place of penicillin G.
4 Often mixed flora.

Treatment

Cerebritis is treated with *antimicrobial therapy* with serial neuroradiological follow-up. If the lesion improves, the treatment should be continued; if not, a *stereotactic biopsy* should be performed for histological confirmation of the diagnosis and the obtaining of a specimen for culture.

Brain abscess is usually initially treated by stereotactic biopsy and aspiration (with or without drainage), to reduce the infectious mass and obtain material or culture. Thereafter, specific antimicrobial therapy is given (or empiric therapy until culture results are available; Table 2.**26**). If the abscess is small (< 2.5 cm in diameter), the source of infection is known, and the presumed pathogenic organism has already been identified by culture from that source, it may be possible to dispense with biopsy and proceed directly to specific antimicrobial therapy.

Parenteral antimicrobial therapy is continued for 4–6 weeks. A further 2–6 months of oral antimicrobial therapy is often given, but is of uncertain benefit.

or *otitis*, though they are sometimes the result of trauma and rarely of hematogenous spread of infection elsewhere in the body. They are most often due to a single organism, and their spectrum is comparable to that of otorhinogenic brain abscesses (streptococci, staphylococci, Gram-negative bacilli).

Clinical Features

The appearance of neurological signs and symptoms in a patient suffering from sinusitis, otitis, or mastoiditis should arouse suspicion of a subdural empyema or epidural abscess. Sometimes, however, the sinusitis or otitis may be discovered only after presentation with neurologic manifestations. The latter include fever, headache, meningism, seizures, and focal signs, usually hemiparesis (Table 2.**27**).

Diagnosis

A cerebrospinal fluid pleocytosis with 6–500 cells/µL, an elevated protein concentration, and a normal glucose concentration are found. The pathogenic organism can be identified by cerebrospinal fluid culture in only 10% of cases. The diagnosis is established by imaging studies (CT or MRI) in conjunction with the clinical findings and elevated laboratory parameters of inflammation. The images reveal a crescentic or lentiform fluid collection over a cerebral hemisphere

Table 2.**27** Clinical manifestations of subdural empyema (405)

Manifestation	Frequency (%)
Fever	88
Headache	75
Hemiparesis	75
Impairment of consciousness	74
Meningism	69
Seizures	53
Other focal neurologic deficits, such as hemianopsia or cranial nerve deficits	46
Papilledema	39
Dysphasia	22

or in the interhemispheric fissure. The adjacent gyri are inflamed and, therefore, contrast-enhancing (1010).

Course

Epidural abscess may take a relatively protracted course, but subdural empyema is a fulminant and life-threatening disease with mortality between 10% and 30%.

Spinal Epidural and Subdural Abscesses

The spinal sub- and epidural spaces, unlike the corresponding intracranial spaces, are real, rather than virtual. Infections in these areas are acute emergencies and are discussed on p. 414.

Acute Viral Infections (470)

A bewildering variety of viruses can cause acute or chronic infection of the central nervous system (see p. 104). The clinical presentation depends on which structure is predominantly involved: the meninges (meningitis), the brain (encephalitis), the spinal cord (myelitis, p. 416), or the nerve roots (radiculitis and polyradiculitis, pp. 575 ff.).

■ "Aseptic" or Lymphocytic (Serous) Meningitis

This term refers to an acute meningitis caused by a viral pathogen. The diagnosis is based on characteristic clinical and laboratory findings and on the exclusion of nonviral infectious causes. The most common pathogens are:

- enteroviruses,
- arboviruses,
- the human immunodeficiency virus (HIV), and
- herpes simplex viruses (HSV).

Rarer pathogens include:

- lymphocytic choriomeningitis virus (LCMV),
- mumps virus,
- adenoviruses,
- cytomegalovirus (CMV),
- Epstein-Barr virus (EBV),
- influenza viruses (types A and B),
- measles virus,
- parainfluenza virus,
- rubella virus, and
- varicella-zoster virus (VZV).

Clinical Features

Headache, fever, and meningeal irritation are the cardinal manifestations, usually accompanied by fatigue, prostration, anorexia, myalgias, nausea, abdominal discomfort, diarrhea, and sometimes a skin rash. The headache is usually predominantly fronto-orbital and associated with photophobia. Neck stiffness is of variable severity; sometimes passive bending of the neck induces only a local pulling sensation and mild worsening of the headache. Focal neurologic signs and impairment of consciousness are not characteristic of aseptic meningitis and point rather toward encephalitis or another diagnosis.

Diagnosis

The blood leukocyte count and erythrocyte sedimentation rate are mildly

Treatment

Both of these entities are treated by immediate intravenous antimicrobial therapy and immediate neurosurgical evacuation. The choice of antimicrobial agent follows the same principles as in the case of brain abscess.

elevated, and the differential white cell count is usually dominated by lymphocytes and monocytes. The cerebrospinal fluid is clear or mildly turbid and contains up to a few hundred mononuclear lymphocytes, though granulocytes may initially predominate. The protein and glucose concentrations are normal, or, at most, mildly elevated (see Table 2.**21**). The cerebrospinal fluid may exhibit oligoclonal bands, disruption of the blood–brain barrier, or both.

Viral infection is definitively demonstrated by serology: seroconversion usually occurs in the blood, cerebrospinal fluid, or both between the acute illness and the convalescence phase. Typically, CNS infections produce a steeper rise in antibody titers in the cerebrospinal fluid than in serum. Serologic testing is of little clinical help, however, because it enables only a retrospective diagnosis. A few viruses, including Coxsackie virus, echoviruses, LCMV and mumps virus, can be cultured or demonstrated by PCR. PCR results are sometimes falsely positive.

Differential Diagnosis

Viral lymphocytic meningitis must be differentiated from parameningeal infections, partially treated bacterial, chronic, or neoplastic meningitis, and noninfectious inflammation due to vasculitis. The possibility of HIV meningitis should be considered in individuals at risk, and evidence of seroconversion should be sought when the patient is in the convalescent phase.

Prognosis

Viral meningitis is usually a self-limited illness that passes without permanent sequelae.

Prevention

All infants and children should be routinely immunized against mumps, poliomyelitis, and measles. For prevention of HIV meningitis, see p. 119.

For prevention of HIV meningitis, see p. 119.

> ### ■ Treatment ■
>
> The treatment is symptomatic and consists of *bed rest, analgesia* against headache, and *antipyretic medication. Acyclovir* is used to treat HSV, EBV, and VZV; the latter can also be treated with *famciclovir* or *valaciclovir* (51a).

■ Viral Encephalitis (452)

In these disorders, viral infection involves either the brain exclusively (encephalitis) or both the brain and the meninges (meningoencephalitis). *The more common pathogens* are:

- arboviruses,
- enteroviruses,
- type I herpes simplex virus (HSV-I), and
- mumps virus.

Rarer pathogens include:
- CMV,
- EBV,
- HIV,
- measles virus,
- VZV,
- LCMV, and
- rabies virus.

Most of these viruses arrive in the central nervous system by hematogenous spread. Rabies virus and VZV enter the CNS by retrograde transport through peripheral nerves.

Clinical Features

Most varieties of viral encephalitis present, like meningitis, with fever, headache, and meningism. These are

Table 2.**28**   Clinical manifestations of viral encephalitis (1021)

Manifestation	Frequency (%)
Impairment of consciousness	97
Fever	87
Personality change	81
Headache	79
Dysphasia	72
Autonomic dysfunction	58
Ataxia	40
Seizures	42
• Focal (only)	21
• Generalized (only)	12
• Focal and generalized	9
Hemiparesis	35
Cranial nerve deficits	33
Visual field defects	13
Papilledema	13

practically always accompanied by impairment of consciousness, and often also by personality changes, dysphasia, autonomic dysfunction, ataxia, hemiparesis, generalized or focal seizures, cranial nerve deficits, visual field defects, and papilledema (Table 2.**28**). A history of animal bite raises the possibility of rabies; a flaccid paralysis, that of poliomyelitis or early summer meningoencephalitis (ESME). Homonymous upper quadrantanopsia is indicative of temporal lobe involvement and thus suggests HSV-I encephalitis (1021).

Diagnosis

The diagnosis is based on the cerebrospinal fluid examination and on neuroimaging studies. The findings in the cerebrospinal fluid are the same as those of viral meningitis (see above), although the pleocytosis may at first be only mild, or even absent in rare cases. In the latter situation, if pleocytosis is still not found 24 hours later, another etiology should be sought.

CT and MRI enable a differentiation between diffuse and focal encephalitis; MRI is the examination of choice because of its higher sensitivity (854). Characteristic findings are hypodensity on CT, T1-hypointensity and T2-hyperintensity on MRI.

The EEG shows generalized and sometimes also focal abnormalities.

Serologic testing may reveal antibodies against various neurotropic viruses in the blood or cerebrospinal fluid and thus indicate the presence of a specific infection, whose course can then be followed with serial titers. PCR methods are also available for the detection of some viruses.

Differential Diagnosis

Similar considerations apply as in the case of viral meningitis (1020).

■ Specific Varieties of Viral Encephalitis

■ Enteroviral Encephalitis

The group of enteroviruses includes poliovirus, Coxsackie virus, and echoviruses. All of these are transmitted by the feco-oral route and reach the central nervous system through the bloodstream. For poliomyelitis, see p. 414. Coxsackie virus and echoviruses seldom produce permanent sequelae, except in the case of perinatal infection.

■ Arboviral Encephalitis

Arboviruses (an acronym for "arthropod-borne viruses") are classified into alphaviruses, flaviviruses, and bunyaviruses and are transmitted to man by ticks and mosquitoes. Endemic and epidemic arboviral encephalitis occurs in many parts of the world, in a regional and seasonal pattern reflecting the habitat and life cycle of their specific arthropod vectors. They usually arise from early summer to fall. In the United States, *western* and *eastern equine encephalitis, St. Louis encephalitis,* and *California encephalitis* are found; in Central and South America, *Venezuelan equine encephalitis;* and, in Europe, *Russian spring-summer meningoencephalitis* and *central European tick-borne encephalitis* or *early summer meningoencephalitis (ESME)*. The latter typically appears as an encephalitis combined with a predominantly focal polyradiculitis or polyradiculomyelitis, which may severely and permanently damage the central and peripheral nervous system. Protection against ESME may be conferred by both active and (with prompt intervention) passive immunization.

■ Rabies

Rabies exclusively attacks the mammalian central nervous system and is transmitted to man by the bite of a rabid animal. Affected animals include dogs and cats (urban type), as well as wild animals such as foxes, badgers, bats, and raccoons (sylvatic type). The virus arrives in the CNS by retrograde transport through peripheral nerves and may then spread transsynaptically to the entire nervous system. After a nonspecific prodromal phase, an encephalitis appears that is initially indistinguishable from other types of viral encephalitis but then goes on to attack the brainstem, practically always causing death.

The diagnosis is suspected on the basis of a history of animal bite and confirmed by serology and by immunofluorescence staining of a specimen of skin obtained by biopsy. Active and passive immunization are feasible in persons bitten by an abnormally behaving animal. Persons at special risk, such as veterinarians, should be prophylactically actively immunized.

■ Paramyxoviruses

The paramyxoviruses include the measles, mumps, and parainfluenza viruses. Mumps may lead, 3–10 days after the parotitis, to a meningoencephalitis of generally benign course. Measles does not affect the CNS during the acute infection, but is followed in approximately one in a thousand cases by a *postinfectious autoimmune encephalomyelitis. Subacute sclerosing panencephalitis* (p. 124) appears years after the infection in approximately one child per million (468).

■ Arenaviruses

Lymphocytic choriomeningitis (LCM) and *Lassa fever* are both produced by arenaviruses. LCM usually appears in the winter months and is transmitted by rodents. The clinical illness is either a meningitis or a meningoencephalitis. Lassa fever is an often fatal hemorrhagic fever occurring in West Africa, which may lead, in survivors, to cognitive disturbances and deafness.

■ Herpes Viruses (344)

The family of herpes viruses includes:
- herpes simplex virus, types I and II (HSV-I and HSV-II),
- varicella-zoster virus (VZV),
- cytomegalovirus (CMV), and
- Epstein-Barr virus (EBV).

Herpes simplex encephalitis. Herpes simplex encephalitis is the most common sporadic form of acute focal encephalitis and is almost always caused by HSV-I (1020). It remains unclear whether this illness represents a new infection by way of the olfactory system or the reactivation of a latent infection already present. Fever, headache, confusion, bizarre behavior, lethargy, meningism, epileptic seizures (generalized or complex partial), dysphasia, focal motor and sensory deficits, and upper homonymous quadrantanopsia make up the typical clinical picture. HSV encephalitis, however, cannot be distinguished from other viral encephalitides and other illnesses in the differential diagnosis on clinical grounds alone (1021), or by the findings of the CSF examination.

CT and, especially, *MRI* help to establish the diagnosis (853). CT reveals hypodensity, and MRI reveals signal changes, in the medial temporal areas with extension to lateral portions of the basal ganglia and to the insular cortex (Fig. 2.**21**).

At the same time, there is cerebral edema with mass effect that may be severe enough to cause transtentorial herniation. The inflamed brain areas often become hemorrhagic. The brain is usually asymmetrically affected, and the differentiation from a cerebrovascular insult can be difficult. Unlike the latter, however, herpes simplex encephalitis may simultaneously affect the vascular distributions of the middle cerebral artery (insular cortex, basal ganglia) and of the posterior cerebral artery (medial temporal lobe). The *EEG* reveals periodic sharp waves every 2–3 seconds over the temporal regions on one or both sides (889). A rise in the antibody titer can be documented by serology, but occurs too late to be useful for therapeutic decision-making. The diagnosis can be established early with the use of PCR or brain biopsy (808), although the latter is seldom necessary (895).

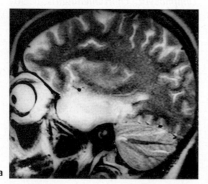 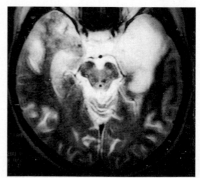

a   b

Fig. 2.**21a, b**   **Herpes simplex encephalitis.**
The T2-weighted MR images reveal extensive signal changes in the left and (to a lesser extent) right temporal lobes.
a Axial spin-echo sequence.
b Parasagittal spin-echo sequence.

The agent of choice is *acyclovir* (10 mg/kg i.v. q8h for 10 days) (886). Treatment with acyclovir reduces mortality from 60–70% to less than 30% (1019). *Foscarnet* is also effective.

HSV-II infections. HSV-II, the causative organism of genital herpes, can also lead to aseptic meningitis, zoster-like neuropathies, urinary retention (cf. Elsberg syndrome, p. 582), and, in immunocompromised patients, to a diffuse encephalitis.

Varicella-zoster virus. VZV is the cause of chickenpox (varicella) (344a). Reactivation of a childhood infection in adulthood results in *herpes zoster* (p. 739), which is more common in immunocompromised patients. Herpes zoster, in turn, can be complicated by *encephalitis* or by a granulomatous vasculitis infecting the larger arteries of the central nervous system. Small-vessel vasculitis can also occur (28a). For VZV myelitis, cf. pp. 416 and 739.

Acyclovir is the first line of therapy; *valaciclovir* and *famciclovir* are also effective.

Cytomegalovirus. CMV may produce a congenital infection, Guillain-Barré syndrome (see p. 575), or, rarely, an acquired encephalitis. In immunocompromised patients, particularly AIDS patients, CMV is a frequent cause of encephalitis, myelitis, polyradiculitis, and retinitis. The *CMV encephalitis* of AIDS mainly affects the periventricular white matter and takes a subacute course with progressive dementia, headache, cranial nerve deficits, focal and generalized weakness, and seizures. *CMV retinitis* is characterized by a painless, progressive visual loss that usually appears bilaterally and can be treated with ganciclovir and foscarnet.

Acyclovir, ganciclovir and valaciclovir are used for the prophylaxis and suppressive treatment of CMV infection in immunocompromised patients.

Epstein-Barr virus. EBV is the cause of infectious mononucleosis and, rarely, of encephalitis or myelitis.

■ **Papovaviruses**

JC virus, the causative organism of *progressive multifocal encephalopathy (PML),* belongs to the family of papovaviruses (91). PML typically affects patients whose cellular immune response is compromised (because of lymphoma, leukemia, AIDS, etc.) and is pathologically characterized by demyelination of white matter in the brain and, to a lesser extent, in the spinal cord. Its clinical manifestations include cortical blindness, dysphasia, confusion, dementia, hemi- and quadriparesis, ataxia, and other focal neurologic disturbances. The disease establishes itself rapidly and leads to death within a few months.

The cerebrospinal fluid is normal. CT reveals the foci of demyelination as hypodense areas. Altered signal intensity is always present on MRI (385) (Fig. 2.**22**). T2-hyperintensity is typical; it is at first multifocal, later confluent. The overlying gray matter is thinned but usually of normal signal intensity.

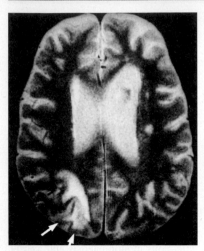

Fig. 2.22 Progressive multifocal leukoencephalopathy.
A 75-year-old man with leukemia and cortical blindness. The signal change in the white matter is typical, as are the unchanged signal intensity and thinning of the adjacent gray matter (arrows).

Chronic Meningitis (955)

Chronic meningitis is diagnosed when the clinical signs and symptoms of meningitis, including inflammatory changes of the cerebrospinal fluid, persist for at least 4 weeks. The various etiologies are summarized in Table 2.**29**. Their frequency varies highly in immune-competent and immunocompromised patients (p. 120). Relevant aspects of the patient's history include earlier illnesses, operations and malignancies, travel, tick bites, sexual behavior, and eating habits.

Clinical Features

The most prominent manifestations are headache, fever, and nuchal rigidity, but these may be very mild, and

The viral encephalitides are treated symptomatically, with the goal of preventing medical complications. Temporary hospitalization in an *intensive care unit* is often necessary, especially when respiratory dysfunction arises. If HSV encephalitis is suspected, *acyclovir* should be given (see above for dosage). Other CNS infections entering into the differential diagnosis that may require other kinds of specific treatment should be ruled out with certainty. *Cerebral edema* exerting mass effect must be treated (p. 72) whenever there is clinical or radiological evidence for its presence. Decisions whether to give anticonvulsants or ulcer prophylaxis should be made on an individual basis.

other relevant physical findings or suggestive history may be absent. Occasionally, erythema chronicum migrans will point to a diagnosis of borreliosis (Lyme disease), or the funduscopic examination will reveal signs of chorioretinitis. Rarely (e.g., in sarcoidosis), there may be signs of hypothalamic or pituitary dysfunction. Cranial nerve deficits are found more often in tuberculous, sarcoid, luetic, fungal, and neoplastic meningitis, all of which preferentially affect the basilar meninges.

Diagnosis

A complete blood count, serum enzymes, antinuclear antibodies, serology for HIV, syphilis, and cryptococcus, and a chest roentgenogram should be obtained in every patient. Cutaneous lesions may point to the correct diagnosis in borreliosis, sar-

Table 2.**29** Common etiologies and differential diagnoses of chronic meningitis (after 272)

Infectious	
• Bacterial and mycobacterial	Tuberculosis Brucellosis
• Fungal	Cryptococcosis Candidiasis Coccidioidomycosis (in North America) Histoplasmosis (in the United States)
• Spirochetal	Syphilis Borreliosis (Lyme disease)
• Parasitic	Cysticercosis Echinococcosis
• Viral	HIV
Non-infectious	Neoplastic meninigitis Sarcoidosis Granulomatous vasculitis Isolated CNS vasculitis Systemic lupus erythematosus Behçet's disease Vogt-Koyanagi-Harada syndrome
Differential diagnosis	Parameningeal inflammation—e.g., epidural abscess, osteomyelitis

coidosis, secondary syphilis, tuberculosis, or disseminated fungal infection. The cerebrospinal fluid examination should include cell count, protein, glucose, Gram and Ziehl-Neelsen stains, syphilis and *Borrelia* serologies, a touch prep for the demonstration of cryptococcus, and cytology for the detection of neoplastic cells (p. 79).

Further, the cerebrospinal fluid should be cultured for aerobic and anaerobic bacteria, fungi, and tubercle bacilli. These tests should be performed at least three times, both to increase the diagnostic yield and to assess the dynamics of the disease over time.

A CT or, preferably, MRI scan may indicate a lesion of the brain parenchyma (e.g., in cysticercosis, toxoplasmosis, and tuberculosis), and the chronically inflamed meninges enhance with intravenously administered contrast (see Fig. 2.**15**). Imaging studies are also necessary to rule out the presence of parameningeal foci of infection, hydrocephalus complicating chronic basilar meningitis, and multiple infarcts due to vasculitis. Vasculitis can be ruled out by angiography. Because chronic meningitis may be the central nervous manifestation of an infection involving other organs as well, the lymph nodes, liver, and bone marrow may need to be biopsied, and the gastric juice, sputum and urine may need to be cultured for mycobacteria and other pathogens, depending on the specific clinical

Table 2.**30**   Diagnostic questions and investigations to be considered in chronic meningitis

MRI of brain with contrast, possibly CT (parenchymal lesion, meningeal or parameningeal involvement?)
MRI of spinal cord with contrast, possibly CT (parenchymal lesion, meningeal or parameningeal involvement?)
Plain radiographs of skull and spine (bone destruction?)
Cerebrospinal fluid examination, at least 3 times (cell count, protein, isoelectric focusing, glucose, Gram stain, touch prep, Ziehl-Neelsen stain, cytology for neoplastic cells, cultures for aerobic and anaerobic bacteria, fungi, and mycobacteria, PCR studies, possibly also antibody tests)
Funduscopy with contact lens (chorioretinitis?)
Serological studies (borreliosis, syphilis, HIV, brucellosis, cryptococcosis, toxoplasmosis, cysticercosis, echinococcosis, antinuclear antibodies, etc.)
Medication history (medication-induced aseptic meningitis? intravenous immunoglobulins?)
Mycobacterial culture of sputum, gastric juice, and urine
Angiotensin-converting enzyme (sarcoidosis?)
Tuberculin test (sarcoidosis, tuberculosis?)
Chest radiograph (sarcoidosis, tuberculosis, or other specific change?)
Cerebral angiography (vasculitis?)
Tissue biopsy for histology, possibly also microbiological examination and culture (skin, liver, bone marrow)
Biopsy and possibly also microbiological examination and culture of radiologically detectable abnormalities in the meninges or brain

suspicion in each case. If the diagnosis remains unclear, the neuroradiologically visible changes in the meninges or brain should be directly investigated by biopsy and culture. The neurosurgeon should also take this opportunity to obtain ventricular fluid for culture (Table 2.**30**).

Recurrent Meningitis
The syndrome of recurrent aseptic meningitis with symptom-free intervals is known as *Mollaret's meningitis*

(622). In a recent study, PCR analysis demonstrated the presence of HSV-II in patients' cerebrospinal fluid during, but not between, the meningitic episodes; this illness is thus thought to represent an initial infection with HSV-II followed by one or more episodes of reactivation. It remains unclear whether virustatic therapy can shorten the meningitic episodes. It seems reasonable to treat frequently recurring episodes with famciclovir, 500 mg p.o. b.i.d., for 10 days.

Allergic reactions to medications, usually nonsteroidal anti-inflammatory agents, can also produce recurrent meningitis (195). Further causes include acquired or congenital dural defects, epidermoid cyst, or a parameningeal infection that repeatedly breaks into the subarachnoid space.

Treatment

When chronic meningitis is due to a known pathogenic organism, the treatment is directed at its eradication. Usually, however, the etiology is not yet known when a therapeutic decision must be taken. When borreliosis is suspected, *ceftriaxone* can be given for 3 weeks. If the patient's condition worsens despite this treatment, *tuberculostatic treatment* should be given without hesitation. In such situations, a possible fungal infection should be sought by all available diagnostic means, even while tuberculostatic treatment is in progress, and, if discovered, should be treated. If fungi are not found, and if the level of clinical suspicion for a fungal infection is not very high, then empirical antifungal therapy should not be given, in view of its high toxicity.

Fungal Meningoencephalitis

The clinical features of fungal infection cover a broad spectrum (Table 2.**31**). The immune status of the patient is a crucial variable. *Cryptococcus neoformans* is the most common pathogen in the patient with normal immune status, while *Candida sp.* and *Aspergillus sp.* are more common in the immunocompromised host. In general, fungal illness plays a greater role in arid geographic zones than

Table 2.**31** Types of fungal infection in the CNS (after Bell and McGuinness, 80)

Meningitis (acute, subacute, chronic)
Granulomatous meningoencephalitis
Abscess (solitary, multiple, microabscess)
Granuloma (microgranuloma, mass lesion)
Infarct due to arterial or venous thrombosis

in Europe. *Coccidioides immitis* is found only in the Americas, *Histoplasma capsulatum* worldwide but with a particular concentration in the Americas, and *Blastomyces dermatitidis* in North America, Africa, and the Middle East.

■ Cryptococcosis

Cryptococcus neoformans mainly affects patients with AIDS or other systemic illnesses impairing the cellular immune response (lymphoma, posttransplantation, steroid therapy), and, more rarely, patients with normal immune status (231, 1050). The primary infection occurs in the lungs. CNS infection is usually subacute or chronic and appears as a combination of meningitis and multifocal granulomatous encephalitis (the clinical signs of either of these two may predominate in individual cases). The major symptom is headache, and associated signs of encephalitis include personality changes, confusion, and focal neurological deficits. In some cases, a mild cognitive deficit is the only manifestation of disease. The cerebrospinal fluid examination usually reveals a chronically inflammatory picture (p. 84 and Table 2.**22**), which may be only mild in the presence of

Table 2.**32** Fungi causing CNS infections, in order of frequency (after Bell and McGuinness, 80)

In patients with normal immune status:
- *Cryptococcus neoformans*
- *Coccidioides immitis*
- *Histoplasma capsulatum*
- *Blastomyces dermatitidis*
- *Sporothrix schenckii*

In the immunocompromised host:
- *Candida* spp.
- *Aspergillus* spp.
- Zygomycetes (Phycomycetes)
- *Cryptococcus neoformans*
- *Histoplasma capsulatum*
- *Blastomyces dermatitidis*
- *Sporothrix schenckii*
- Others

gical procedures, intravenous catheterization, steroid treatment, intravenous drug use, and the like. It may take an acute or chronic course, with or without fever, and lead to meningitis or meningoencephalitis, with corresponding clinical features. The cerebrospinal fluid examination usually reveals a chronically inflammatory picture (see Table 2.**21**), with cell count rarely above 2000/μL. The diagnosis rests on the demonstration of spores in the cerebrospinal fluid, either directly or by culture.

Treatment

Candidiasis is treated with *amphotericin B* and *flucytosine.*

immunosuppression. The touch prep directly reveals cryptococci in more than half of all patients; when it does not, the demonstration of anticryptococcal antibodies in the serum and cerebrospinal fluid is necessary for rapid diagnosis. CSF cultures are positive by 4–6 weeks in three-quarters of all patients. Blood, sputum, urine, and stool cultures may also be helpful.

Treatment

The treatment consists of *amphotericin B* and *flucytosine.* Immunocompromised patients require long-term treatment with flucytosine for the prevention of a relapse.

■ **Candidiasis** (77)

Candidiasis is seldom restricted to the central nervous system and generally is found in the CNS as a local expression of systemic disease. It is usually a consequence of visceral sur-

Parasitic Diseases of the Brain

■ **Toxoplasmosis** (542)

Toxoplasma gondii is an intracellular parasite. Infection may be congenital, or it may be acquired at any age through the consumption of infected meat or contact with the feces of domestic animals or pets.

Congenital toxoplasmosis produces a granulomatous meningoencephalitis (p. 36).

Acquired toxoplasmosis is typically asymptomatic or else a mononucleosis-like illness with lymphadenopathy, fever, rash, myalgias, and hepatosplenomegaly. In rare cases, meningoencephalitis may be seen, with up to 500 lymphocytes per microliter of cerebrospinal fluid (948). Patients with AIDS or under pharmacological immunosuppression are at increased risk of severe toxoplasmosis infections, which may arise *de novo* or as a reactivation of latent disease.

Clinically, there may be a diffuse meningoencephalitis, or else solitary or multiple intracerebral masses (698). Gradually worsening headache, lethargy, seizures, and focal neurologic signs are typical manifestations. CT and MRI reveal solitary or multiple ring-enhancing lesions (464, 806), which may become calcified. The diagnosis is established by serology or by the direct demonstration of organisms in tissue or cerebrospinal fluid.

▋Treatment▋

The treatment of choice is a combination of *pyrimethamine* and *sulfadiazine*, together with *leucovorin* (see Table 2.**26**).

■ Amebic, Plasmodial, and Trypanosomal Infections

These protozoal illnesses affecting the brain are mainly found in Africa and the Americas.

■ Cysticercosis

Cysticercosis is endemic to Central and South America and parts of Africa, Asia, and Eastern Europe. Is caused by the pork tapeworm (cestode), *Taenia solium.* Man is the only known definitive host for the adult form of the organism (the tapeworm itself, which resides in the intestine). Man may also be infected as an intermediate host, harboring the larvae of the organism in skeletal muscle and in the brain (cerebral cysticercosis). The commonest intermediate hosts are domestic animals such as pigs, dogs, cats, and sheep. When a human being eats the flesh of an infected animal that contains larvae, an intestinal infection with the adult tapeworm results. The worm produces

eggs, which then develop into embryos; the latter penetrate the intestinal wall and spread through the bloodstream to the distant soft tissues, including the brain, where they mature further to larvae (cysticerci).

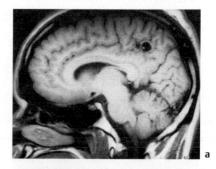

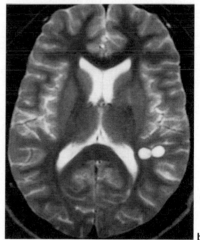

Fig. 2.**23a, b   Cerebral cysticercosis.**
a Parasagittal T1-weighted image. Two cysts are visible as hypodense areas in the parietal lobe. A larva can be seen in the larger cyst.
b Axial T2-weighted image. Two cysts can be seen as areas of increased signal lateral to the left posterior horn.

The cysticerci may be several millimeters to 2 cm in size. Their clinical manifestations are a function of their size, number, localization, and stage of development, together with the reaction of the surrounding cerebral tissue (833). They most commonly cause *epileptic seizures* (224), headache, papilledema, and vomiting, and more rarely hydrocephalus, meningitis, or spinal cord involvement.

CT and MRI are essential for the diagnosis (173) and reveal single or multiple cystic lesions, sometimes containing radiologically identifiable larvae (Fig. 2.**23**).

The dying cysticercus causes an inflammatory tissue reaction with edema and then becomes calcified. The cerebrospinal fluid may be normal or show chronic inflammation, with eosinophils. The diagnosis is established by serology or by direct demonstration of cysticerci in biopsied tissue.

■ **Treatment**

Praziquantel and *albendazole* are given in combination with corticosteroids (albendazole is more effective against neurocysticercosis than praziquantel). Cysts must occasionally be removed neurosurgically (190).

■ **Other Cestoid Infections**

The larval form of other tapeworms (cestodes) may cause infections in man, including coenurosis, sparganosis, and echinococcosis.

Echinococcosis. This disease is caused by the larvae of tapeworms for which dogs and foxes are the definitive hosts. *Echinococcus granulosus* gives rise to solitary cysts, *Echinococcus multilocularis* to locally invasive cyst agglomerates that are usually found in the liver, lungs, and skeletal muscle. The larvae may rarely stray into the brain, where they form solitary mass lesions that progress over several months and cause epilepsy, headache, papilledema, personality changes, and focal neurologic deficits. The diagnosis is made on the basis of the neuroradiologic findings and serology, which is usually, though not always, positive.

■ **Treatment**

Cysts should be *neurosurgically resected* whenever possible. If the cyst is unresectable, *albendazole* can be given.

■ **Nematoid Infections**

Trichinosis is the most common nematoid infection affecting man and is usually contracted by the consumption of undercooked pork. The ingested larvae spread through the bloodstream to the soft tissues. After an initial diarrheal phase, the disease manifests itself by fever, prostration, myalgias due to myositis, periorbital edema, and, in 10% of cases, meningitis, encephalitis, or meningoencephalitis. Eosinophilia in the peripheral blood is present, indicating a parasitic infection. The diagnosis is established by serology or muscle biopsy.

■ **Treatment**

Steroids (prednisone, 1 mg/kg, for 5 days) are effective against myositis, but antihelminthic agents are ineffective against the larvae in the soft tissues.

■ Rickettsial Infections (1034)

Rickettsiae are intracellular parasites that cause a number of illnesses including Rocky Mountain spotted fever, louse-born typhus, Q fever, and trench fever. These illnesses are transmitted by ticks, lice, and fleas. Central nervous system involvement is indicated by the presence of headache and other neurologic manifestations and may dominate the clinical picture. Serologic tests are available for most of the rickettsioses.

Treatment

Tetracycline and *chloramphenicol* are the antimicrobial agents of first choice.

Encephalopathies Caused by Immune Reaction (469)

Certain infectious diseases and immunizations rarely provoke immune reactions leading to complications in the central nervous system. An inflammatory, demyelinating encephalomyelitis typically arises days to weeks after the infection or immunization, with a monophasic course. Post-vaccinial and post-infectious encephalomyelitides are most often seen after rabies and measles immunizations or after a measles infection (p. 130), mumps, chickenpox, or rubella (360).

Cerebrospinal fluid pleocytosis is usually present, and MRI reveals multifocal signal changes (509). The differential diagnosis between one of these entities and the initial phase of multiple sclerosis may be impossible at first and become clear only after longer observation.

Spirochetal and Leptospiral Infections

■ Neurosyphilis (662, 1003)

Syphilis (lues) is a chronic, sexually transmitted infection caused by the spirochete *Treponema pallidum.* Its three phases are known as primary, secondary, and tertiary syphilis. Syphilitic meningitis may occur as early as the secondary phase, but typical *neurosyphilis* occurs in the tertiary phase. Neurosyphilis may be *meningeal, meningovascular,* or *parenchymal;* in the latter form, it is associated with the classical syndromes of *general paresis* (earlier known as "general paresis of the insane") and *tabes dorsalis.* If the patient is clinically asymptomatic and serologic tests are positive only in the blood, then one speaks of seropositive latent syphilis; if serologic tests are positive in the cerebrospinal fluid as well, one speaks of asymptomatic neurosyphilis. Cerebrospinal fluid changes appear in one-third of all syphilitic infections, usually between 12 and 18 months after the primary infection, at which time meningovascular syphilis is also most frequent. General paresis or tabes dorsalis appears years or even decades after the primary infection in 7% of all untreated syphilitics.

■ Meningeal Syphilis

Meningeal syphilis may affect the meninges of either the brain or the spinal cord and manifests itself as headache, vomiting, meningism, cranial nerve deficits, papillitis, seizures, and occasionally mental changes. It is a predominantly basal, chronic meningitis. It occasionally affects the vertex region and can lead to malresorptive hydrocephalus.

■ Cerebrovascular Syphilis (426)

Cerebrovascular syphilis produces a marked inflammation of the meninges and cerebral blood vessels, leading to infarction, usually in the distribution of middle-sized arteries. Infarction is preceded by prodromal manifestations such as headache, personality change, dizziness, sleep disturbances and other nonspecific symptoms. The vascular narrowing and parenchymal infarcts are revealed by imaging studies. The cerebrospinal fluid displays chronic inflammatory changes.

■ Tabes Dorsalis

Tabes dorsalis arises on average 8–12 years after the primary infection and is characterized by "lancinating" pain, ataxia, and bladder dysfunction. Physical examination reveals hyporeflexia and abnormal pupillary reactions (Argyll Robertson pupil, p. 665). Tabetic patients account for some 30% of patients with neurosyphilis. Men are four to seven times more commonly affected than women, in keeping with their higher rate of primary infection.

Symptoms

Pain of sudden onset, lasting several seconds or minutes, and shooting ("lancinating") into the legs or other parts of the body is a characteristic early complaint. Painful tabetic crises are often felt in the epigastrium, rectum, penis, bladder, and elsewhere. Other common phenomena include paresthesias, sensory disturbances and associated gait difficulties ("walking on cotton wool"), as well as ataxic gait. Bladder dysfunction often appears early and is usually irreversible; the bladder is typically atonic and enlarged, with a large postvoiding residual volume, but without pain. Impotence is another early manifestation.

Clinical Findings and Course

Sensory abnormalities can always be found at the time of presentation. Vibration sense and, later, position sense are either impaired or exaggerated. Sensitivity to painful stimuli is lessened in deep and visceral structures (no pain on squeezing of the testicle or Achilles tendon). Perineal pain sensation is delayed. The impairment of position sense leads to gait ataxia, which may be disabling, in about one-third of patients. Ataxia is particularly severe when the eyes are closed or in darkness, and the tandem gait and Romberg test are abnormal. Involvement of muscle afferents in the posterior roots leads to hypotonia, which may be severe, causing abnormal mobility of the joints. The deep tendon reflexes disappear in more than half of all patients, first the Achilles reflexes, and then the patellar reflexes. Pyramidal tract signs are rarely seen as well. Sooner or later, 90% of tabetics have pupillary abnormalities. The pupils are usually unequal, constricted, and misshapen and react to light weakly or not at all. All transitional states are found up to the classic Argyll Robertson abnormality, which is seen in some 20% of tabetics. About the same number of patients suffer from optic atrophy, which usually leads to blindness regardless of treatment. Oculomotor disturbances are rarer. Trophic manifestations include chronic perforating ulcer of the sole of the foot and tabetic arthropathy with severe joint destruction (Charcot joint).

Neuropathology

Thinning and sclerosis of the posterior columns of the spinal cord is appreciable on gross examination. Microscopically, a degeneration of fibers entering via the posterior horn is seen. The fibers of the posterior columns are demyelinated, with sporadic axonal degeneration, and gliosis is present.

■ General Paresis (1046)

General paresis appears 10–15 years after the primary infection, and sometimes even later. It is associated with a progressive dementia and is the clinical correlate of a parenchymal meningoencephalitis with caseating granulomatous inflammation (gumma or gummata). Men are more commonly affected than women.

Clinical Features

Progressive dementia is the most prominent manifestation and is often associated with lack of judgment, expansive features, epileptic seizures, dysarthria, pupillary dysfunction, myoclonus, and variable focal neurologic signs.

The initial symptoms are often nonspecific: headache, fatigability, and sleep disturbances. Some 10 % of patients go on to have seizures. In rare cases, there are transient focal signs, such as hemiparesis. Pupillary dysfunction, as in tabes dorsalis, is characteristic (p. 664), as is a slurred, "syllabic" form of dysarthria best brought out with certain test phrases ("around the rugged rocks the ragged rascal ran," "hopping hippopotamus," "Methodist Episcopal"). Muscular jerks known as "sheet lightning" may be seen, particularly around the mouth. The reflexes are often brisk, and a Babinski sign is often present.

Optic atrophy, posterior column dysfunction, and other signs of tabes dorsalis may be used, in which case the term "taboparalysis" is applied. Malresoptive hydrocephalus is occasionally seen (p. 39).

Mental Abnormalities

These are often more prominent than the neurologic deficits. Most common is a slowly progressive dementia with memory loss, affective disturbances, impairment of judgment, and correspondingly abnormal behavior leading to social impairment. Less frequently, the disturbance is of the hyperreactive or expansive type, in which the patient suffers from delusions of grandeur and may undertake fantastic exploits as a result. In the final, paralytic stage, dysphasia, agnosia, and apraxia complete the picture of dementia.

Neuropathology

Gross examination reveals thickening of the meninges, brain atrophy, ventricular enlargement, and granulomatous ependymitis. Microscopically, a subacute encephalitis is found, with many inflammatory cells in the perivascular spaces and in the brain parenchyma itself. Neuronal loss and glial proliferation are seen, and spirochetes can be detected with the use of special stains.

Prognosis

General paresis usually leads to death within 3 years if untreated. Spontaneous improvement is rare.

■ Other Forms of Neurosyphilis

The neurologic expression of syphilis is by no means limited to tabes dorsalis and general paresis and may take on many other forms, often mimicking other neurologic diseases. Examples include *syphilitic optic atrophy,* which leads to progressive blindness, first in one eye, and then in the other; and *syphilitic sensorineural deafness.* For congenital syphilis, see p. 37.

Diagnosis of Neurosyphilis

The diagnosis is based on serology and on the cerebrospinal fluid examination.

As for *serology,* a number of nonspecific screening tests (such as the VDRL test) and specific treponemal tests (such as FTA-ABS and TPHA) are available. The nonspecific tests are adequate for routine testing of large numbers of serum samples. Their results are expressed as a quantitative antibody titer, which provides information about the possible presence and activity of the syphilis-producing organisms. Specific tests are used to confirm the diagnosis in patients with positive nonspecific tests, or in whom there is an elevated clinical suspicion. The *cerebrospinal fluid* displays the features of chronic meningitis (see Table 2.**22**). The most pronounced CSF changes, with the highest cell counts, are found in syphilitic meningitis, the least pronounced in tabes dorsalis. The CSF protein concentration rarely exceeds 200 mg/dL and is usually below 100 mg/dL. The glucose concentration is normal or mildly low. The CSF abnormalities are very mild in some cases; rarely (usually in cases of tabes dorsalis), the cell count is normal. CSF-specific oligoclonal bands are found in ca. 50% of cases. Every patient with syphilis should also be tested for HIV, and *vice versa.*

Neuroimaging studies (CT, MRI) reveal infarcts or gummata appearing as well-demarcated contrast-enhancing masses. Cranial nerve and meningeal involvement may also be visible, particularly on MRI (92, 942).

▄▄ Treatment ▄▄▄▄▄▄▄▄▄▄▄

Patients with neurosyphilis, even if asymptomatic, should be treated with high-dose penicillin G (12–24 million units i.v. qd for 10 days), or alternatively with ceftriaxone (1 g i.v. q.i.d. for 14 days).

Successful treatment results in a decline of the VDRL antibody titer, which should be rechecked at 1, 3, 6, and 12 months after treatment. Nonspecific tests for syphilis often become negative, but the specific tests do not. The cerebrospinal fluid should be reexamined every 3–6 months for 3 years to document the expected fall in cell count and somewhat slower fall of the elevated protein concentration.

■ Borreliosis (330)

Borrelia burgdorferi, afzelii, and *garinii* are the etiological agents of the European Garin-Bujadoux-Bannwarth syndrome, and *Borrelia burgdorferi* that of North American Lyme disease (which takes its name from the town of Lyme, Connecticut). These organisms are spirochetes related to the treponemes that cause syphilis (159) and are transmitted to human beings by tick bites. The initial infection is marked by local cutaneous erythema, typically in the form of an enlarging ring *(erythema chronicum migrans),* sometimes accompanied by flu-like symptoms. *Acute disseminated borreliosis* may appear very early, but *chronic borreliosis* may not be evident until much later. The clinical picture is so varied, and the rate of seropositivity so high in the normal population (10–15%), that practically every manner of presentation of neurologic disease has been ascribed to borreliosis in at least one case report (734).

Clinical Features (595, 735)

The early stage of infection (stage I), in which the infection is still local, is characterized by erythema chronicum migrans or, less commonly, by cutaneous erythema with lymphohistiocytic infiltration. Such skin changes are seen, however, in fewer than 25% of patients with borreliosis. The disseminated infection (stage II) makes itself known with headache, fever, musculoskeletal pain, arthralgias, and sometimes a generalized lymphadenopathy. Multifocal erythema may arise in this stage. 15% of patients with disseminated borreliosis suffer from neurologic syndromes including *meningitis, cranial neuritis, radiculoneuritis, plexus neuritis, en-*

cephalitis, and *combinations* of these entities (Fig. 2.**24**).

The most common form of neurologic involvement is a lymphocytic meningitis with uni- or bilateral facial palsy or radiculoneuritis. Uni- or multifocal encephalitis or vasculitis is rarer. Radiculoneuritis is typically very painful and may dominate the clinical picture. Within weeks of presentation, cardiac involvement may become evident in the form of intracardiac conduction abnormalities or, more rarely, myopericarditis with ventricular dysfunction. In the chronic, generalized stage of infection (stage III), arthralgias (60%) and cutaneous abnormalities *(acrodermatitis chronica atrophicans)* are typical. Late-stage neurologic abnormalities include a mild, nonspecific encephalopathy with mild memory loss and mood changes, or else leukoencephalopathy with spastic paraparesis and bladder dysfunction.

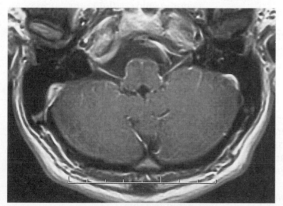

Fig. 2.**24 Cranial polyradiculitis in borreliosis,** in a 38-year-old man. This axial T1-weighted spin-echo image reveals contrast enhancement of the meninges and cranial nerves, particularly well seen in the leptomeninges around the medulla and in the hypoglossal nerves bilaterally.

Diagnosis

Acute borreliosis is associated with a cerebrospinal fluid pleocytosis of up to 100 cells/µL. The cell count is lower, or even normal, in chronic borreliosis. The diagnosis is established by serological demonstration of IgG and IgM antibodies and is most reliable when seroconversion is found to have occurred over a time span of a few weeks. IgM titers are highest a few weeks after the onset of disease, IgG titers only months or years later. The presence of intrathecal antibodies is pathognomonic of neuroborreliosis (193, 380). When interpreting positive findings, the diagnostician must remember that 10–15% of the normal population possesses IgG antibodies and will therefore have false-positive serology, that cross-reactions with other spirochetal diseases, such as syphilis, do occur, and that collagen-vascular diseases may also lead to falsely positive tests. If a test for serum antibody is positive, neuroborreliosis must be ruled in or out by lumbar puncture and cerebrospinal fluid serology.

■ **Leptospiral Infections**

The leptospiroses are acute systemic illnesses with vasculitis. The organisms are transmitted through the feces of infected animals.

Clinical Features

The leptospiroses generally present, much like a viral illness, with lymphocytic meningitis. Rare cases present with hepatic and renal failure associated with visceral hemorrhage (Weil disease due to *Leptospira icterohaemorrhagiae*).

Treatment (215)

Acute neuroborrelioses are treated parenterally with *ceftriaxone* (2 g i.v./day), *cefotaxime* (2 g i.v. t.i.d.), or *penicillin G* (20–24 million units i.v./day) for 2 weeks. Lymphocytic meningoradiculitis may also be treated with *doxycycline* 100 mg p.o. b.i.d. for 2 weeks (492). Chronic neuroborreliosis requires at least 3–4 weeks of treatment with ceftriaxone, cefotaxime, or penicillin in the above doses. Isolated facial palsy can be treated with *doxycycline* 100 mg p.o. b.i.d. or *amoxicillin* 500 mg p.o. t.i.d. for 3 weeks. Steroids are useful in the treatment of painful neuroborreliosis.

Diagnosis

The cerebrospinal fluid cell count and protein concentration tend to be higher than in viral meningitis; the glucose concentration is normal. The diagnosis can be made in the earliest phase of the illness by direct demonstration of leptospirae in the blood, cerebrospinal fluid, or urine, or 6–12 days later by serology.

Treatment

Doxycycline and *penicillin G* shorten the course of illness.

Chronic Viral Infections of the Central Nervous System

Many different viruses can produce infections of the central nervous system that persist for years or decades. The most common such diseases are listed in Table 2.**33**.

■ HIV Infection and AIDS
(290, 422, 881)

HIV-1 in North America and Europe, and HIV-2 in West Africa, are retroviruses (RNA viruses possessing the enzyme reverse transcriptase) that attack and destroy CD4+ T-lymphocytes and macrophages. They thereby produce immune deficiency leading to severe opportunistic infection, Kaposi's sarcoma, and lymphoma.

Epidemiology and History

The acquired immune deficiency syndrome (AIDS) was first described in homosexual men in 1981. It soon became clear that this was a viral illness transmitted by sexual intercourse, blood transfusion, or exchange of blood components by other means (intravenous drug use, administration of blood products to treat hemophilia, childbirth in HIV-positive mothers). Throughout the 1980s, AIDS largely remained a disease of homosexual men, intravenous drug users, and hemophiliacs. Since then, however, it has become increasingly common in the general population and has, indeed, become a worldwide pandemic. The international agency dealing with AIDS (UNAIDS) reports that the number of HIV-infected persons worldwide has increased from 13 million in 1993 to 34.3 million in 2000.

Clinical Manifestations and Definition of Disease Stages

The clinical manifestations of HIV infection run a typical course from the primary infection, through a prolonged asymptomatic period, to the advanced disease (AIDS). A standard definition of the stages of disease has been issued by the Centers for Disease Control (CDC) of the United States and was last revised in 1993 (Tables 2.**34** and 2.**35**). Staging is based on the CD4+ T-lymphocyte count and on the clinical findings. AIDS is present, by definition, in any patient in clinical category C (Table 2.**35**) or with fewer than 200 CD4+ cells per microliter, regardless of clinical condition. It is further stipulated that clinical improvement (successfully treated infections, etc.) does not entail reclassification in a better category.

In 50–70% of cases, the event by which HIV is transmitted to the patient is followed within a few weeks by a mononucleosis-like illness with fever, pharyngitis, headache and retroorbital pain, lymphadenopathy, prostration, arthralgia, and myalgia. There may also be a maculopapular rash, mucosal ulcers, acute lymphocytic meninigitis, or, more rarely, encephalitis, myelopathy, or plexus neuritis. At the time of seroconversion, most patients manifest CSF pleocytosis. This stage of primary infection is followed by an asymptomatic phase, with or without lymphadenopathy, during which the virus mul-

Table 2.**33** Chronic viral infections of the nervous system

Disease	Virus
AIDS	HIV-1, HIV-2
Tropical spastic paraparesis	HTLV-1
Progressive multifocal leukoencephalopathy	JC virus
Subacute sclerosing panencephalitis	Measles virus
Progressive rubella encephalopathy	Rubella virus

Table 2.**34**   Revised CDC classification of HIV infection

CD4+ T-lymphocyte count	Clinical stage		
	A	**B**	**C**
	Asymptomatic primary HIV infection or progressive generalized lymphadenopathy	Clinical manifestations are present, but neither A nor B symptoms	AIDS-defining clinical manifestations
> 500/μL	A1	B1	C1
200–499/μL	A2	B2	C2
< 200/μL	A3	B3	C3

Table 2.**35**   Clinical stages of HIV infection

Stage A:
- Asymptomatic HIV infection
- Progressive generalized lymphadenopathy
- Acute primary HIV infection

Stage B:
- Oropharyngeal or vulvovaginal candidiasis
- Cervical dysplasia
- Fever > 38.5 °C or diarrhea for more than 1 month
- Oral leukoplakia
- Herpes zoster
- Idiopathic thrombocytopenic purpura
- Listeriosis
- Polyneuropathy

Stage C:
- Candidiasis of the bronchi, trachea, lungs, or esophagus
- Cervical carcinoma
- Disseminated or extrapulmonary coccidioidomycosis or cryptococcosis
- Cytomegalovirus infection other than in the liver, spleen, and lymph nodes
- HIV encephalopathy
- Herpes simplex ulcers lasting longer than 1 month
- Histoplasmosis
- Kaposi's sarcoma
- Burkitt's lymphoma
- CNS lymphoma
- Mycobacterial infections
- *Pneumocystis carinii* pneumonia
- Recurrent pneumonia
- Progressive multifocal leukoencephalopathy
- Salmonella sepsis
- Cerebral toxoplasmosis
- Weight loss due to HIV infection

tiplies and the CD4+ lymphocyte count steadily falls. The first sign of the subsequent phase of symptomatic HIV infection may be herpes zoster, thrombocytopenia, oral lesions, or the regression of previous lymphadenopathy. The risk of an opportunistic infection is high if the CD4+ cell count is below 200 per microliter.

Neurologic Manifestations of HIV Infection

Neurologic manifestations are present at some time in 60–80% of patients infected with HIV. They reflect direct damage to the central and peripheral nervous system by the virus itself, as well as indirect damage through the effects of opportunistic infections, tumors, or vascular complications (Table 2.**36**).

Primary HIV Encephalopathy (AIDS Dementia) (591)

Primary HIV encephalopathy is the most frequent complication of HIV infection affecting the brain and is the AIDS-defining illness in 10% of cases. It is produced by direct viral damage to cerebral glia and macrophages. It manifests itself initially in lack of concentration, forgetfulness, and difficulty carrying out familiar but complex tasks, often given the impression of simple exhaustion or reactive depression rather than dementia. There follow a loss of inter-

Table 2.**36**   Neurologic manifestations of HIV infection

Opportunistic infections:
- Toxoplasmosis
- Cryptococcosis
- Progressive multifocal leukoencephalopathy
- Cytomegalovirus
- Syphilis
- Tuberculosis
- HTLV-1 infection

Neoplasms:
- Primary CNS lymphoma
- Kaposi's sarcoma

Direct neurologic manifestations of HIV infection:
- Aseptic meningitis
- HIV encephalopathy
- Myelopathy:
  - Vacuolar myelopathy
  - Purely sensory ataxia or paresthesiae
- Polyneuropathy:
  - Acute demyelinating polyneuropathy
  - Mononeuritis multiplex
  - Distal symmetric polyneuropathy
- Myopathy

ests, apathy, and progressive deficits of attention and memory. Later on, the behavioral and cognitive abnormalities worsen, the patient becomes disoriented, and the complete picture of subcortical dementia is produced. By the time this stage is reached, motor function is slow and ataxic. Finally, these patients lose the ability to walk, become incontinent of urine and stool, and lapse into a vegetative state.

The cerebrospinal fluid contains a mild mononuclear pleocytosis, a mildly elevated protein concentration, and oligoclonal bands. CT and MRI reveal a nonspecific brain atrophy. MRI usually reveals symmetric bilateral white matter changes (398). Unless CT or MRI is performed, AIDS dementia cannot be reliably distinguished from the effects of opportunistic infections and tumors on the brain.

Treatment

Antiretroviral therapy with *zidovudine* or *didanosine* can improve cognitive function in the short term, but AIDS dementia nevertheless remains an inexorably fatal condition.

Aseptic Meningitis

Aseptic meningitis may appear at any stage of HIV infection, but does so most commonly during the acute primary infection. It resolves spontaneously over a few weeks but may later recur or undergo a transition to chronic meningitis or meningoencephalitis. Cranial nerve deficits, particularly involving the trigeminal, facial, and vestibulocochlear nerves, are common.

The cerebrospinal fluid examination reveals lymphocytic pleocytosis, an elevated protein concentration, and a normal glucose concentration.

Myelopathy

Some 20% of AIDS patients suffer from HIV myelopathy. The most common form is a *vacuolar myelopathy,* in which a combined degeneration of the long tracts leads to spasticity, ataxia, and bladder and bowel dysfunction. Cognitive disturbances are almost always present as well. Less commonly, an isolated degeneration of the posterior columns results in sensory ataxia or in isolated paresthesiae and dysesthesiae in the lower extremities.

The differential diagnosis of HIV myelopathy includes spinal cord involvement by opportunistic infection or tumors, which may be treatable.

Treatment

Antiretroviral therapy has shown some success to date in the treatment of HIV myelopathy.

Neuropathy

Neuropathy is a common complication of HIV infection and may appear at any stage of the disease.

Acute demyelinating polyneuropathy. HIV-positive individuals who are still immune-competent may suffer from an acute demyelinating polyneuropathy with clinical features similar to those of *Guillain-Barré syndrome,* including progressive weakness, areflexia, and mild sensory changes. The cerebrospinal fluid is pleocytotic, and nerve biopsy reveals a perivascular lymphocytic infiltrate, indicating an autoimmune pathogenesis. HIV-associated acute demyelinating polyneuropathy usually resolves spontaneously.

Treatment

Plasmapheresis and *intravenous immunoglobulin,* and possibly also *steroids,* can improve and shorten the course of this condition.

CMV-associated acute polyradiculopathy. This entity is in the differential diagnosis of HIV-associated acute demyelinating polyneuropathy.

Treatment

CMV-associated acute polyradiculopathy is treated with *ganciclovir* or *foscarnet.*

Mononeuritis multiplex. Like HIV-associated acute demyelinating polyneuropathy, mononeuritis affecting one or more peripheral nerves, nerve roots, or (typically) cranial nerves tends to occur in the earlier stages of HIV infection, when the immune system is still competent, and its pathogenetic mechanism is presumably the same. The cerebrospinal fluid is usually pleocytotic.

Distal symmetric polyneuropathy/ progressive radiculopathy. In distinction to mononeuritis multiplex, distal symmetric polyneuropathy and progressive radiculopathy are both seen almost exclusively in later stages of HIV infection, in the presence of immune deficiency.

Mild sensory polyneuropathy. At least one-third of AIDS patients suffer from a mild, mainly sensory polyneuropathy that progresses over time and may cause unpleasant or painful paresthesiae, sensory loss, sensory ataxia, predominantly distal weakness, and autonomic disturbances. The cerebrospinal fluid is normal or only mildly abnormal.

Treatment

The treatment is symptomatic and consists of *tricyclic agents, anticonvulsants, analgesics,* and *combinations* of these medications.

Progressive polyradiculopathy/radiculomyelopathy. In this entity, motor disturbances are more pronounced than sensory disturbances, and the cerebrospinal fluid examination reveals pleocytosis, elevated protein concentration, and low glucose concentration.

Toxic neuropathies. The differential diagnosis of these entities specific to HIV-positive patients includes not only polyneuropathies affecting the general population, but also toxic neuropathies caused by antiretroviral agents (didanosine, zalcitabine, stavudine). These are dose-dependent and reversible if the responsible medication is discontinued early enough.

Myopathy

Myopathy may also be a complication of HIV infection. It ranges in severity from an asymptomatic elevation of creatine kinase to a marked, predominantly proximal muscle atrophy and weakness. Muscle atrophy may result from the general inanition of AIDS, from AIDS-associated inflammatory destruction of muscle fibers, or from long-term use of zidovudine.

> ██ **Treatment** ██
> *Steroids* are occasionally helpful.

Opportunistic Infections of the Central Nervous System

The intracranial lesions listed in Table 2.**37** appear in at least one-third of AIDS patients. Some 30% of patients suffer from two or more of these entities simultaneously or sequentially.

Toxoplasmosis. By far the commonest such infection is toxoplasmosis (p. 108 and Table 2.**26**), which is manifest in a CT or MRI scan of the brain as a ring-enhancing lesion.

Cryptococcosis. The next most common pathogenic organism is *Cryptococcus neoformans,* which causes meningitis or focal parenchymal infection (p. 107).

Other infections. *Candida spp., Mycobacterium tuberculosis* and atypical mycobacteria, *Listeria monocytogenes* and *Nocardia asteroides* are further pathogenic organisms causing meningitis, encephalitis, and brain abscess in AIDS patients.

Opportunistic viral infections. Meningitis, encephalitis, myelitis, and polyradiculitis can also result from an opportunistic viral infection, particularly arising from herpes viruses (HSV-I, HSV-II, CMV, VZV) and papovaviruses (JC virus, see p. 103). JC virus is the causative agent of progressive multifocal leukoencephalopathy. Retinitis is typical in CMV infection. Syphilis should be considered in the differential diagnosis.

Primary CNS Lymphoma

Primary lymphoma of the central nervous system is extremely rare in the general population (p. 71) but affects some 2% of AIDS patients. It produces subacute cognitive deficits, headache, and focal neurologic deficits (892).

Systemic Lymphoma

Systemic lymphoma generally affects the CNS by invasion of the meninges and produces a clinical picture of meningitis with cranial nerve involvement. *Kaposi's sarcoma,* a tumor typically found in AIDS patients, rarely metastasizes to the CNS.

Epileptic Seizures

Seizures are a common feature of AIDS and are seen in primary HIV encephalopathy as well as in opportunistic infections of the brain.

Diagnosis of HIV Infection

The diagnosis is made by serologic testing. HIV infection may be suspected because the patient belongs to a group at elevated risk, or because of the appearance of an infection or tumor associated with immune deficiency.

Table 2.**37** Most common causes of focal CNS lesions in AIDS

Toxoplasmosis
Cryptococcosis
Listeriosis
Herpes viral infection (HSV, CMV, VZV)
Progressive multifocal leukoencephalopathy
Primary CNS lymphoma
Syphilis

Diagnosis and Treatment of the AIDS Patient with Neurologic Manifestations

Patients with peripheral neurologic manifestations. These patients, like HIV-negative patients, are evaluated by electrophysiologic studies and cerebrospinal fluid examination. The treatment is directed toward the particular entity causing symptoms, as detailed above.

Patients with central nervous manifestations. Depending on the manner of presentation, these patients are evaluated by imaging study, cerebrospinal fluid examination, or both. If the CT or MRI scan is normal or shows nothing more than meningeal enhancement, a lumbar puncture must be performed and a treatable cause (organism) sought. If the imaging study reveals one or more mass lesions, *empirical treatment for presumed toxoplasmosis* can be given for 2–3 weeks. If the lesions become smaller, the treatment can be continued; if not, a *stereotactic biopsy* should be considered, so that tissue can be obtained for microbiological examination and culture for the determination of further therapy.

Treatment

Antiretroviral Therapy
(343a, 824)
Patients with neurologic manifestations or opportunistic infections (AIDS-defining infections), as well as HIV-positive patients with fewer than 350 CD4+ lymphocytes/μL or more than 5,000–10,000 virus particles per milliliter of plasma, should be treated with *antiretroviral medications*, as long as this is not made impossible by drug interactions, unacceptable side effects, or other contraindications. The currently available antiretroviral agents and their major side effects are listed in Table 2.**38**.

Monotherapy was preferred a few years ago, but is no longer recommended. Current therapy consists of a *protease inhibitor* combined with *two nucleoside reverse transcriptase inhibitors*. If the CD4+ lymphocyte count falls below 50/μL, *acyclovir* should also be given prophylactically.

Epileptic seizures in HIV-positive patients are treated primarily with phenytoin. Some 10% of patients develop an allergic rash and can then be treated alternatively with *phenobarbital* or *valproic acid*.

■ HTLV-I Infection (Tropical Spastic Paraparesis) (728, 978)

Tropical spastic paraparesis is rare in Europe. It takes a slowly progressive course (months) and is associated with bladder dysfunction. Sensory disturbances are mild, usually affecting only vibration sense. The causative organism is the human T-lymphotropic virus, type I (HTLV-I), which is transmitted in similar fashion to HIV. Cerebrospinal fluid examination reveals a mild lymphocytic pleocytosis ($< 50/\mu L$), a mildly elevated protein concentration, and oligoclonal bands. Demyelination and vacuolar myelopathy predominantly affecting the posterior columns may be visible on MRI. Periventricular signal changes in the brain may also be seen.

Table 2.**38**   Antiretroviral medications

Class of medication	Agent	Major adverse effects
Reverse transcriptase inhibitors-nucleoside analogues	Abacavir	Headache, hypersensitivity
	Didanosine	Pancreatitis, polyneuropathy, diarrhea
	Lamivudine	Myelosuppression, polyneuropathy
	Stavudine	Polyneuropathy
	Zalcitabine	Polyneuropathy, stomal ulcers
	Zidovudine	Anemia, headache, myopathy
Reverse transcriptase inhibitors-non-nucleoside analogues	Delavirdine	Rash, headache
	Efavirenz	Vertigo, rash
	Nevirapine	Rash
Protease inhibitors	Amprenavir	Rash, paresthesiae, depression
	Indinavir	Renal calculi, nausea
	Nelfinavir	Diarrhea
	Rifonavir	Perioral paresthesias
	Saquinavir	Diarrhea

Treatment

The occasionally beneficial effect of *steroids* is explained by a presumed direct viral and immune-mediated pathogenetic mechanism. *Zidovudine* should also be beneficial on theoretical grounds.

■ Subacute Sclerosing Panencephalitis (SSPE) (258)

This term designates a chronic measles infection of the brain that usually affects school-age children, an entity earlier known as *Dawson's inclusion body encephalitis, Pette-Döring panencephalitis,* and *van Bogaert's sclerosing panencephalitis.* The introduction of measles vaccination has lowered its incidence from 10 to one per million per year.

Pathogenesis

The pathogenesis of SSPE is not known with certainty. It has been hypothesized that incomplete viral replication results in the persistence of intracellular virus particles, which then leads to cell death.

Clinical Features

The clinical manifestations arise insidiously. At first, there are mild and then marked mental abnormalities such as irritability, intellectual deficit, lethargy, and fatigability. A few weeks later, language is affected and involuntary movements appear. External noises and other stimuli induce myoclonus and spasms, and choreoathetosis and tremor may also be seen.

Prognosis

The prognosis is poor. The characteristic manifestations progress, language function deteriorates, vegetative disturbances appear, and the patients finally become spastically rigid and then comatose. Death ensues after an average of 3 years.

Diagnosis

The diagnosis can be made by EEG, serologic testing, and cerebrospinal fluid examination.

The *EEG* reveals diffusely occurring periodic high-amplitude slow waves, usually in synchrony with myoclonus. The *cerebrospinal fluid examination* reveals a normal cell count, elevated gamma-globulin levels, and oligoclonal bands. Measles antibodies are found in elevated concentration both in the serum and in the CSF. *CT* and *MRI* reveal multiple hypodensities (areas of signal change) in the subcortical and periventricular regions, and in the basal ganglia (953).

■ Treatment

There is no known effective treatment. The effect of *isoprinosine* is debated. *Interferons* may be helpful.

■ Progressive Rubella Panencephalitis (PRPE) (1005)

This illness affects children suffering from congenital (p. 36) or acquired rubella. It is rarer than SSPE but displays a similar clinical picture, usually compounded with retinopathy and optic atrophy. Like SSPE, it leads to death within a few years.

Prion Diseases (14c, 773)

Prion diseases were long referred to as "slow-virus diseases" (Table 2.**39**). It is now known that they are caused by infectious proteins, called prions. Unlike viruses, prions contain no nucleic acids, provoke no immune response, inflammation, or interferon production, and are resistant to the usual methods of sterilization.

- The prion protein PrP^P occurs physiologically and is predominantly expressed at the neuronal cell surface.
- The abnormal ("infectious") prion protein (PrP^{SC} or PrP^{CJD}) integrates itself into normal cells, replicates within them, and has a different conformation from PrP^P.

Table 2.**39** Prion diseases of the central nervous system

Kuru
Creutzfeldt-Jakob disease
variant Creutzfeldt-Jakob disease
Gerstmann-Sträussler-Scheinker syndrome
Familial fatal insomnia
Familial progressive subcortical gliosis

PrP^{SC} can enter the neuron from outside, or arise from a new mutation occurring within and then replicate itself further. Years or decades after the initial infecting event, it leads to neuronal loss in the brain and to the formation of vacuoles and amyloid plaques, which are associated with typical patterns of neurodegenerative disease affecting both humans and other mammals. The incubation period of kuru ranges from 4.5 to 40 years (average, 12 years).

Pathological Anatomy and Clinical Manifestations

These diseases are the clinical expression of a *spongiform encephalopathy.* Once clinical manifestations appear, progression is rapid, and death usually follows within 1 year. The known prion diseases in man are:

- kuru,
- Creutzfeldt-Jakob disease,
- variant Creutzfeldt-Jakob disease,
- Gerstmann-Sträussler-Scheinker syndrome,
- familial fatal insomnia, and
- familial progressive subcortical gliosis.

The "classic" prion diseases affecting animals are mad cow disease (bovine spongiform encephalopathy, BSE) and scrapie, which affects sheep and goats.

Diagnosis

The diagnosis is established by the demonstration of abnormal prion protein (PrP^{SC}) in brain tissue homogenate, by the demonstration of a mutation in the PrP gene, or by immunohistologic characterization of cerebral amyloid plaques.

■ **Kuru** (327)

Kuru exclusively affected the Fore people of Papua New Guinea and was transmitted by ritual cannibalism. Its manifestations included cerebellar ataxia, choreoathetosis, myoclonus, tremor, and dementia. The abandonment of ritual cannibalism has led to its disappearance.

■ **Creutzfeldt-Jakob Disease** (CJD) (851)

This disease is probably the commonest of the prion diseases, with an incidence of 0.5 to 2 per million per year. It typically affects middle-aged and elderly persons, as a sporadic illness in 85% and as a familial illness in 15%.

Indirect evidence implies a link between prion diseases affecting animals, particularly mad cow disease, and CJD (see variant CJD, below). The disease may be transmitted experimentally from humans to primates, or from human to human through neurosurgical procedures (including the implantation of permanently indwelling electrodes), organ transplantation (cornea, lyophilized dura mater), and the therapeutic administration of human pituitary extract. CJD of human and bovine origin differ in the type of prion involved: human-to-human transmission involves prion type 3 exclusively, vCJD is due to prion type 4, and sporadic and familial cases are due to prion types 1–3.

Pathological Anatomy

Spongiform degeneration, with round vacuoles in the neuropil and abnormal glial proliferation, is accompanied by no more than moderate brain atrophy.

Clinical Features

Mental changes appear at first, including mood swings, depression. fatigability, sleep disturbances, and progressive forgetfulness. There follow neurologic abnormalities such as hyper- and hypotonia, pyramidal tract signs, extrapyramidal and cerebellar disturbances, fasciculations, and, typically, myoclonus, while the mental changes progress to a frank dementia. Mental and physical activity decline until a vegetative state of decortication supervenes. In one-third of patients, visual or cerebellar disturbances predominate in the initial phase of disease; cerebellar disturbances are particularly common in the iatrogenic form. The familiar form is characterized by early onset, protracted course, and (often) by a similar clinical picture among affected members of the same family.

Diagnosis

EEG usually provides the key to diagnosis (Fig. 2.**25**). There is diffuse generalized slowing at first, followed by progressively severe, bilaterally synchronous, generalized, pseudo-periodic, tri- or tetraphasic theta and delta wave activity. These pseudoperiodic waves are then gradually lost as the voltage of the EEG progressively declines. The *cerebrospinal fluid* is generally normal, although there may be a mild elevation of the cell count and protein concentration. Protein 14-S is positive. *MRI* reveals T2-hyperintensity in the basal ganglia (59).

Treatment

Unfortunately, no treatment is available. It is recommended that the body fluids, urine, and stool of patients with CJD be treated as potentially infectious, with the same precautions as in viral hepatitis.

■ Variant Creutzfeldt-Jakob Disease (vCJD) (184a, 421a)

A prion disease of cattle was first detected in the United Kingdom in 1986 and named mad cow disease (bovine spongiform encephalopathy, BSE). The responsible variety of prion turned out to be readily transmissible to other animal species, which led to the fear that human beings might also become affected by an illness similar to BSE. This fear was confirmed in 1996, when a new variant of CJD began to be recognized (1028b). The most compelling piece of evidence that BSE can cross the interspecies barrier for prion infection, is transmissible to man, and is the cause of vCJD is the finding that the prions responsible for the two illnesses are of the same type, type 4. Prion diseases are most efficiently transmitted by inoculation. Oral transmission is also possible if the dose of the infectious agent is high enough, as demonstrated by the example of kuru. Both in vCJD and in kuru, PrP^{SC} can be found in lymphoreticular tissue before the disease is clinically manifest and before it can be found in nervous tissue (421a); in the standard form of CJD, however, the abnormal prion protein is found only in nervous tissue. These findings and the current plateau in the incidence of vCJD in the United Kingdom support the hypothesis that vCJD is transmitted orally by con-

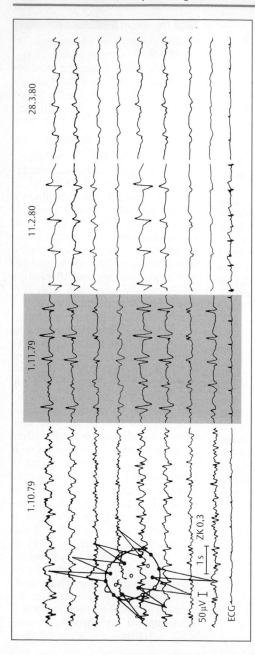

Fig. 2.25 Creutzfeldt-Jakob disease.
The course of EEG changes over time in a 57-year-old woman in whom the diagnosis of CJD was later confirmed by autopsy. Six weeks after the onset of the prodromal phase, only a hint of periodic activity is seen. It is fully developed 1 month later. The two recordings taken at later dates show a progressive decline of overall activity.

sumption of the meat of BSE-infected cattle (28c).

In addition to the dose of the infectious agent, the genetic structure of the recipient of the PrP^{SC} protein seems to play a role in determining whether that individual develops the disease. This hypothesis is supported by the observation that none of the persons who have become ill with vCJD to date were members of theoretically highly exposed groups, such as farmers or butchers; residence in the United Kingdom is the only known risk factor.

Patients with vCJD are younger, on average, than those with CJD. The youngest patient to date was a 12-year-old girl (976b). Youth is also the most important clinical feature distinguishing the two patient groups. Before the disease is fully manifest, vCJD patients complain of vague sensory abnormalities, depression, and anxiety, as do CJD patients in a comparably early phase.

Like CJD, vCJD is currently untreatable. It is also unknown at present whether a major epidemic of vCJD will strike Europe in the coming decades, now that BSE has become endemic to the continent. The most important unknown variables are the infectiousness of BSE prions and their incubation time in man. As a preventive measure, the nations of the European Union currently practice the slaughter of affected herds, while cohort slaughter is practiced in Switzerland.

■ Gerstmann-Sträussler-Scheinker (GSS) Syndrome

GSS syndrome is an autosomal dominant disorder clinically resembling CJD and mainly affecting middle-aged persons. Molecular genetic studies have consistently shown mutations of the gene for PrP (541). The clinical picture is of progressive cerebellar dysfunction and dementia, and extrapyramidal dysfunction may appear as well. Hereditary spinocerebellar degeneration should be considered in the differential diagnosis.

■ Familial Fatal Insomnia

Familial fatal insomnia, described by Lugaresi, is an autosomal dominant, heritable disorder consisting of rapidly progressive, intractable insomnia and disturbances of autonomic, endocrine, and motor function, the last including tremor, ataxia, and spasticity. Most patients experience complex hallucinations and display disturbances of attention and memory. Frank dementia is less common.

Histopathological study reveals neuronal loss and gliosis, primarily in the thalamus, where PET studies have also shown abnormally low glucose metabolism (750). As in GSS syndrome and familial CJD, a mutation of the PrP gene has been demonstrated (655).

■ Familial Progressive Subcortical Gliosis

Familial progressive subcortical gliosis is another rare prion disease. It may appear sporadically or in families, with an autosomal dominant inheritance pattern (755). It appears in the elderly and consists of slowly progressive personality changes and dementia. The clinical picture resembles that of Pick's disease (554).

Congenital Infections
(p. 36)

The organisms that most commonly cause congenital infection are:
- *Toxoplasma gondii,*
- rubella virus, and
- herpes viruses.

The most prominent clinical manifestations of congenital infection are chorioretinitis, splenomegaly, hepatomegaly, jaundice, microcephaly, and petechial rash. Toxoplasmosis commonly causes hydrocephalus, while cytomegalovirus and rubella virus often cause deafness and microcephaly.

Diseases Caused by Microbial Toxins

Microbial toxins can cause a block of synaptic transmission, as in *botulism*, or neuronal hyperexcitability, as in *tetanus* (see p. 455). Tetanus can lead to a reversible encephalopathy and to muscle atrophy.

Neurological Complications of Vaccination (297)

Paresthesias, mono- and polyneuritis and polyradiculitis, aseptic meningitis, and multiple sclerosis-like manifestations have been attributed to a number of different kinds of vaccination, sometimes with less than convincing evidence. Oral vaccination against poliomyelitis rarely leads to the development of paralytic poliomyelitis.

Infections Leading to Guillain-Barré Syndrome

HIV, herpes viruses (CMV, EBV), and *Campylobacter jejuni* are more frequently associated with Guillain-Barré syndrome than other pathogens (p. 575). It has also been suggested that vaccinations sometimes induce Guillain-Barré syndrome (297).

Chronic Fatigue Syndrome (221)

This term currently designates a symptom complex prominently involving *disabling, chronic fatigue.* Earlier designations of the same entity included neurasthenia, epidemic neuromyasthenia, myalgic encephalomyelitis, effort syndrome, chronic mononucleosis, and the like.

Clinical Features
Women are more frequently affected than men. The occasional epidemic appearance of this disorder and the mild immunological and endocrine disturbances that sometimes accompany it indicate that it is of multifactorial origin. The probable causative agents include various viral species. In addition to fatigue that does not resolve with rest and leads to a limitation of daily activities, the major clinical features include difficulty concentrating, headache, sore throat, painful lymph nodes, myalgia, arthralgia, a feeling as if febrile, sleep disturbances, and a greater than average prevalence of depression. There are no abnormal physical findings other than tenderness of the muscles or lymph nodes and a subfebrile elevation of temperature.

Diagnosis
The diagnosis mainly rests on the exclusion of other relevant somatic or psychiatric disease. There are no confirmatory laboratory tests. There is controversy over whether this disorder should be considered primarily a somatic or a psychiatric ailment.

Treatment
The most important aspect of treatment is proper psychological management of these patients, so that they feel their complaints are being taken seriously. Spontaneous improvement usually occurs within weeks. Recurrent illness lasting months or years occurs only in exceptional cases.

Disturbances of Cerebral Perfusion and Nontraumatic Intracranial Hemorrhage (6, 62, 106, 164, 936a, 999b, 1030)

Definition:
Disturbances of cerebral perfusion are due to ischemia in 80–85% of cases and to intracerebral or subarachnoid hemorrhage in the remaining 15–20%. They may present as transient ischemic attacks or as permanent neurological deficits. Two-thirds occur in the territory of the anterior circulation (the internal carotid artery and its branches), and one-third in that of the posterior circulation (the vertebral and basilar arteries). They may arise from disease of the extracranial large vessels, the intracranial large vessels, or the intracranial microvasculature, or from embolization of a thrombus formed in the heart. Each of these causes accounts for approximately 20% of disturbances of cerebral perfusion. A small percentage of strokes are due to nonatherosclerotic vascular disease, such as arterial dissection. Macroangiopathies and emboli typically cause infarction in the territory of a major vessel, while microangiopathies typically cause lacunar infarcts. Motor and sensory hemisyndromes, homonymous hemianopsia, and neuropsychological deficits are characteristic features of hemispheric strokes; lateralizing phenomena include aphasia (dominant hemisphere, usually left) and disturbances of spatial processing (right hemisphere). Vertebrobasilar disturbances produce bilateral motor and sensory deficits, cerebellar ataxia, visual field defects, diplopia, dysphagia, and other cranial nerve deficits. Stroke prophylaxis (for all patients at risk, including those who have already had a stroke) consists of the treatment or elimination of controllable risk factors, including hypertension, smoking, obesity, and hyperlipidemia; healthful diet and regular exercise; and, where indicated, the use of medications such as inhibitors of platelet aggregation and anticoagulants, statins and the surgical treatment of high-grade carotid stenosis.

Stroke is the third most common cause of death in the industrial world, after heart disease and cancer. It is the most common cause of permanent disability in young and middle-aged persons, and also the most common life-threatening neurological disease. Its incidence increases with age; in the 65–74-year-old age group, there are 600–800 strokes per 100,000 persons per year. There is geographical variation, the incidence of stroke being higher in Japan, Finland, and Scotland (for example) than in central Europe or in the white population in North America. Men are somewhat more commonly affected than women. Some 80–83% of strokes are of ischemic origin, 10–12% are due to intracerebral hemorrhage, and 7–8% are due to subarachnoid hemorrhage. The mortality of stroke is largely a function of age and of stroke etiology; it is much lower for lacunar infarction than for territorial infarction, and much higher in the elderly than in the young (122).

Diagnostic Tests in Cerebrovascular Disease

■ Computed Tomography (CT)

CT is a digital technique that produces cross-sectional anatomical images. Its physical basis, like that of conventional radiographic imaging, is the differential absorption of roentgen rays by tissues of different density. Tissue density is expressed on the Hounsfield scale, named in honor of the inventor of CT. The scale runs from –1000 to +1000 Hounsfield units. The density of water is, by definition, 0 Hounsfield units.

When CT images are acquired one section at a time, the roentgen ray tube has to be rotated through 360° for image acquisition, then back to the starting position, and the patient table must then be moved forward, in preparation for the next image. An improved technique for image acquisition, known as helical (spiral) CT, was developed in the late 1980s (402). In this technique, the roentgen ray tube continually rotates in one direction, while the patient table continually moves forward at constant speed. A helical data set results, which can then be digitally reformatted into axial or other types of sections. Current helical CT units employ multiple roentgen-ray tubes, so that multiple data sets can be acquired simultaneously. As a result, the examination time is dramatically reduced, and the images are sharper; normal and pathological anatomy are well demonstrated, and functional and dynamic CT studies can also be performed.

The use of *intravenous contrast material* enhances the visibility on CT of blood, and of tissue in which there is a disruption of the blood–brain barrier. Contrast administration thus raises the sensitivity and specificity of CT for a wide range of pathological processes. It also provides the basis for selective imaging of blood vessels (*CT angiography*): if one digitally suppresses other structures with high roentgen-ray absorption, such as bone, and then reformats the sectional images of the vasculature in three dimensions, a projectional image results, resembling the images of conventional angiography. CT angiography is a suitable technique for aneurysm screening, and for the demonstration of stenoses of the carotid artery or other vessels.

The major disadvantage of CT is the exposure of the patient to *ionizing radiation.* CT contrast substances contain iodine and may cause nausea, vomiting, and (more rarely) urticaria, bronchospasm, and kidney failure in susceptible individuals. Anaphylactic shock is extremely rare.

The indications, diagnostic capabilities, advantages, and disadvantages of CT are discussed together with those of MRI in the following sections, and throughout the book in the context of individual diseases.

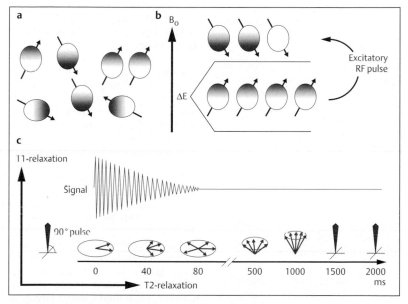

Fig. 2.**26a–c Physical principles of magnetic resonance imaging** (after Edelman and Warach).

a The magnetic axes of the protons are randomly distributed in space.

b When a magnetic field B_0 is applied, the protons align themselves parallel or antiparallel to B_0. A proton oriented parallel to B_0 is of lower energy than one oriented antiparallel to B_0. If a brief radiofrequency (RF) pulse is applied whose frequency equals the resonant (Larmor) frequency, some of the lower-energy parallel protons will "flip" to the higher-energy antiparallel position. They then fall back to the lower-energy state in a process known as "relaxation." The timing of this process is a function of two tissue-specific constants, the T1 and T2 relaxation times.

c After the 90° excitatory pulse, the protons precess in the transverse plane. Initially, they precess in phase, which results in maximal signal. Tiny inhomogeneities in the magnetic field cause the protons to precess at slightly different rates, which leads to "dephasing" and thus to loss of signal intensity. This process occurs within milliseconds and is called T2 relaxation. The MR signal is typically measured during T2 relaxation. Over a somewhat longer time period, the magnetization parallel to B_0 reestablishes itself, in a process called T1 relaxation. Various techniques, such as gradient-echo and spin-echo, are used to capture the largest possible amount of signal.

■ **Magnetic Resonance Imaging (MRI)** (43, 264, 962)

MRI is based on the theory of nuclear magnetic resonance, discovered by Bloch and Purcell in 1946. The physical entities made visible in MRI are the *protons of hydrogen nuclei,* which are, of course, richly abundant in all tissues containing water, proteins, lipids, and other biological macromolecules (Fig. 2.**26**) (266).

Magnetic field. Protons possess not only charge, but also *spin*: they rotate and precess around their own axis, and therefore possess a small magnetic field. As a result, a proton placed in an external magnetic field usually behaves like the needle of a compass, and aligns itself parallel to the field. It can also align itself antiparallel to the field, i.e., in the exactly opposite direction. This state is associated with a higher energy. In the resting state, most protons are oriented parallel to the applied field, and only a few are oriented antiparallel to it.

Larmor frequency. When protons in a magnetic field are additionally exposed to electromagnetic radiation, in the form of radio waves at a particular frequency (the resonance or Larmor frequency), they can absorb energy and "flip" from the parallel orientation to the energetically unfavorable antiparallel orientation.

Relaxation. Within a short time after this, the antiparallel protons release the absorbed energy as they return to their original, parallel state. This process is known as *relaxation*. Its time course is characterized by two tissue-specific time constants, the *T1 and T2 relaxation times.*

MR signal. During the course of relaxation, protons spinning in the transverse plane of the external magnetic field emit electromagnetic radiation, which can be detected with a radio antenna or coil. This radiation constitutes the MR signal. The T1 and T2 relaxation times are much more variable than the radiographic density of tissue; MR thus provides much better tissue contrast than conventional roentgenography or CT.

MR image. The MR image is a planar (tomographic) map of the MR signal as it varies in intensity across different types of tissue (Table 2.**40**). T1-weighted, T2-weighted, and proton density images can be obtained by suitable choice of the excitatory pulse sequence, repetition time (TR, the interval between repetitions of the pulse sequence), and echo time (TE, the interval between radiofrequency excitation and measurement of the MR signal).

Tumors and other tissues with a high free-water content appear dark on T1-weighted and bright on T2-weighted or proton density images. Cerebrospinal fluid consists largely of free water; it is thus very dark on T1-weighted images and very bright on T2-weighted and proton density images. T1-weighted images are more suitable than T2-weighted images for the demonstration of necrosis and cystic change within a tumor, or for the demonstration of subacute hemorrhage.

Gradients. The construction of an image from an MR signal is possible only because the source of the signal can be accurately localized in space. Localization is made possible by the use of *gradient fields*—i.e., small magnetic

Table 2.**40** Synopsis of signal intensities of normal and abnormal structures on MR images (after ref. 264)[1]

Tissue	T1-weighted image	T2-weighted image
Cerebrospinal fluid	Dark	Very bright
Brain:		
• White matter	Bright	Slightly dark
• Gray matter	Slightly dark	Slightly bright
• Multiple sclerosis plaque	Intermediate to dark	Bright
• Bland infarct	Dark	Bright
• Meningioma	Dark	Bright
• Abscess	Intermediate	Intermediate
• Edema	Dark	Bright
• Calcification	Intermediate or bright	Intermediate or dark
Fat	Very bright	Intermediate or dark
Cyst:		
• Mainly containing water	Dark	Very bright
• High protein content	Intermediate to bright	Very bright
• High fat content	Very bright	Intermediate to dark
Bone:		
• Cortical	Very dark	Very dark
• Yellow marrow	Very bright	Intermediate to dark
• Red marrow	Intermediate	Slightly dark
Bone metastasis:		
• Lytic	Very dark	Intermediate to bright
• Sclerotic	Dark	Dark
Cartilage:		
• Fibrous	Very dark	Very dark
• Hyaline	Intermediate	Intermediate
Intervertebral disk:		
• Normal	Intermediate	Bright
• Degenerated	Intermediate to dark	Dark
Muscle	Dark	Dark
Tendons and ligaments:		
• Normal	Very dark	Very dark
• Inflamed	Intermediate	Intermediate
• Torn	Intermediate	Bright
Tissue enhancement with Gd-DTPA:		
• Low concentration	Very bright	Bright
• High concentration	Intermediate to dark	Very dark

Table 2.**40**   Synopsis of signal intensities of normal and abnormal structures on MR images (after ref. 264)[1] *(Cont.)*

Tissue	T1-weighted image	T2-weighted image
Hematoma:		
• Hyperacute	Intermediate	Intermediate to bright
• Acute	Intermediate to dark	Dark or very dark
• Subacute	Bright rim, intermediate	Bright rim, dark center, later entirely bright
• Chronic	Dark rim, bright center, later entirely dark	Dark rim, bright center, later entirely dark

[1]   Bright means hyperintense (signal-rich), dark means hypointense (signal-poor); intermediate indicates a signal intensity resembling that of the brain.

fields whose intensity varies linearly over space, which are superimposed on the homogeneous main magnetic field. Good image quality can be obtained with a main field strength of 1.0–1.5 Tesla. The magnet strength of most MR scanners currently in use lies in this range.

Spatial resolution. The spatial resolution of MRI depends on three parameters: the size of the desired field of view (FOV, typically 25 cm for the head); the matrix (typically 256 × 256 to 512 × 512); and the slice thickness. The FOV divided by the matrix number gives the edge length of one *pixel* (picture element). This length squared (the pixel area) multiplied by the slice thickness gives the volume of one *voxel* (volume element), the three-dimensional building block of the MR image.

Time required for study. A typical MR scan of the brain employing spin-echo sequences can be obtained in 10–20 minutes. Modified sequences can be used to reduce the scanning time, and more recent developments such as *echo-planar imaging* (EPI) enable image acquisition in a fraction of a second (267, 478). EPI has opened the way to *perfusion, diffusion, and functional MR imaging* (48b, 842a).

Blood flow. The effect of blood flow on signal intensity is readily understood from theoretical considerations. In a standard spin-echo sequence, a signal is generated when the tissue is excited by two radio-wave pulses. Blood flowing rapidly through the plane of the image will encounter only the first pulse and not the second, so that no signal is generated and the blood vessel appears dark on the MR image (*flow void*). Blood flowing more slowly will be hit by both pulses, give rise to a strong signal, and appear bright on the MR image (*flow-related enhancement*). On the other hand, gradient-echo sequences use only a single excitatory pulse and produce the echo by changing the gradient. Flowing blood is always bright on gradient-echo images, while nonmoving tissue gives little signal. Flowing blood, and thus indirectly the blood vessels enclosing it, are seen in high contrast on such images.

MR angiography (MRA). Projectional algorithms can be used to stack the planar images on top of one another and thereby create a three-

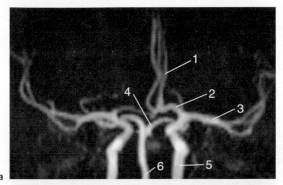

a

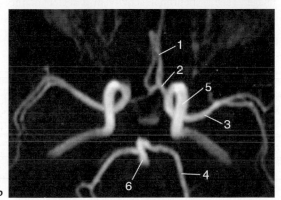

b

Fig. 2.**27a, b   MRA of the cerebral vasculature.**
This is a normal study, apart from hypoplasia of the main stem of the right anterior cerebral artery.
a Coronal view.
b Axial view.
1 Pericallosal artery
2 Anterior cerebral artery
3 Middle cerebral artery
4 Posterior cerebral artery
5 Internal carotid artery
6 Basilar artery

dimensional view of the vascular tree, known as an MR angiogram (44, 642). MRA enables visualization of the intra- and extracranial arterial and venous circulation (646) (Fig. 2.**27**). The major drawback of MRA is that it depicts flowing blood, rather than the anatomical structure of the vessel wall. Pathological abnormalities such as stenoses, where the blood flow may be slow and turbulent and give rise to little signal, may appear more severe than they are, sometimes giving the false impression of vascular occlusion; small aneurysms, on the other hand, may escape detection. Contrast-enhanced MRA is less sus-

ceptible to these difficulties, because the contrast substance rather than the blood itself is being imaged, and flow velocity and turbulence are less important as confounding factors (783b).

Perfusion MRI (48b, 842a, 961a). Gadolinium and other contrast substances shorten the T1 relaxation time and cause local inhomogeneity of the magnetic field. This leads, in turn, to loss of signal, which is most marked on gradient-echo images, especially when very long echo times (TE) are used (265). When a bolus of contrast material is injected into a brachial vein, passage of contrast through the brain can be seen on MR images within seconds. The loss of signal is proportional to the volume of contrast-containing blood flowing through the cerebral circulation. Furthermore, the transit of contrast material through the brain can be timed and expressed as the mean transit time (MTT). The degree of signal loss and the MTT provide a semiquantitative index of parenchymal blood flow, which can be represented pictorially in a perfusion MR image (see Fig. 2.**37**).

Diffusion MRI (48b, 842a). Proton spins rotate and precess about their own axes at a frequency proportional to the magnetic field strength. Spin-spin interactions and local magnetic field inhomogeneities give rise to small differences in the precession frequencies of individual spins, which, in turn, lead to loss of signal. Any proton that happens to be moving through the brain by diffusion will have a precession frequency that varies from moment to moment, because it will encounter a magnetic field that varies in each spatial dimension according to the applied gradients. This effect is intentionally enhanced with the use of diffusion-weighted sequences, which include special diffusion-gradient pulses in addition to the usual gradients. As a result, relatively little signal is lost from spins that have little or no diffusional motion, while more signal is lost from spins that do have such motion. In acute cerebral infarction, cerebral edema occurs because of a shift of water from the extra- to the intracellular compartment. This limits the ability of water molecules to diffuse, so that their signal in the

diffusion-weighted image becomes more intense (see Fig. 2.**37**). A disturbance of diffusion is noted on diffusion-weighted MRI within a few minutes of cerebral infarction. This method thus allows detection of stroke much earlier than CT, which is generally normal until several hours after the acute event.

Functional MRI. Oxyhemoglobin is diamagnetic, while deoxyhemoglobin is not. When there is an elevation of neuronal activity in a region of the brain and oxygen is extracted from the locally circulating blood, the normal physiological response is an elevation of regional cerebral blood flow that is proportionally higher than the amount of oxygen extracted. The ratio of oxy- to deoxyhemoglobin thus rises, and the gradient-echo MR signal increases by a very small amount, which is nevertheless large enough to be detected by signal averaging. This technique, known as BOLD-MRI (blood oxygen level-dependent MRI), forms the basis of functional MR imaging, which reveals regional alterations of cerebral blood flow in response to neuronal activity (Fig. 2.**28**).

Absolute contraindications to MRI. MRI is absolutely contraindicated in the presence of cardiac pacemakers, neurostimulators, cochlear implants, ferromagnetic aneurysm clips, and other ferromagnetic foreign bodies in tissues that are susceptible to injury. Most aneurysm clips in current use are MRI-compatible, but this should always be verified from the operative record before an MRI is performed. A small number of patients experience emotional stress in the MRI unit because of claustrophobia; this problem can usually be overcome, but, for ex-

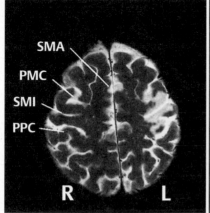 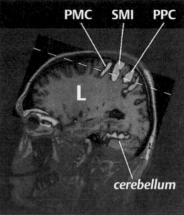

Fig. 2.**28a, b Functional MRI (fMRI) during right finger movement.**
Neural activity in the brain leads to an increase in regional cerebral blood flow and, in complex fashion, to a change in the MR signal, which can then be seen in the MR image.
a Axial image. Finger movement involves activation of the contralateral brain areas SMA, PMC, SM1, and PPC. In the ipsilateral hemisphere, SMA, PMC, and PPC are activated, but SM1 is not.
b Left parasagittal image. Cerebellar activation is predominantly ipsilateral. The image shows the side contralateral to the finger movement, with activation of SMA, PMC, SM1, and PPC, as well as of the cerebellum. Activation of the thalamus and basal ganglia is predominantly contralateral, but is not seen on this image, because these structures are out of the plane of section.
PMC: premotor cortex (= motor association cortex);
PPC: posterior parietal cortex (= secondary sensory cortex);
SM1: primary motor and sensory cortex, divided by the central sulcus;
SMA: supplementary motor area.

treme cases, open MRI units are available in some centers. Contrast reactions are negligibly rare.

■ Indications for CT and MRI Studies

CT and MRI are indicated for the diagnosis or exclusion of all diseases of the nervous system that cause structural changes in the brain, the spinal cord, the nerve roots, or the meninges.

Advantages of MRI. MRI provides better tissue contrast than CT and thus allows the diagnosis of many conditions affecting the brain parenchyma that are not usually visible on CT, including microangiopathy, axonal shear injury in head trauma, the plaques of multiple sclerosis, encephalitides, and other conditions.

Advantages of CT. CT provides better visualization of bone and of acute hemorrhage. It is also cheaper than MRI, and requires a lesser degree of patient cooperation. It should not be forgotten that each CT study (unlike MRI) delivers a dose of ionizing radiation to the patient, and that these doses are cumulative.

The decision whether to perform a CT or MRI of the brain in the individual case depends both on the clinical situation and on the availability of the scanners in question. A CT generally suffices in emergency situations, if an MRI scanner is not available. In less urgent situations, however, MRI is usually the better option, and may also be cheaper, because there will be fewer negative scans necessitating costly further work-up.

Perfusion and diffusion MRI are helpful in establishing the indication for cerebral thrombolysis in acute thrombotic stroke, but they are available on an emergency basis in relatively few centers. When there is clinical suspicion of an acute subarachnoid hemorrhage, the imaging study of choice is CT; an MRI should be performed (if at all) only when FLAIR sequences are available. For the elderly patient with focal neurological signs or confusion, a CT usually suffices to detect all potentially treatable conditions, such as hydrocephalus and chronic subdural hematoma.

For a discussion of spinal MRI, see p. 389.

■ Angiography (438)

Cerebral angiography was invented by the Portuguese neurologist and neurosurgeon Egas Moniz, who performed the first carotid angiogram in 1927. Angiography usually serves to verify or characterize in greater detail a pathologic process first revealed by CT, MRI, or cerebrovascular ultrasound.

Indications. Cerebral angiography is mainly used for the diagnosis or exclusion of the following:

- stenosis and occlusion of intra- and extracranial blood vessels,
- cerebral venous and venous sinus thrombosis,
- ruptured and unruptured cerebral aneurysms,
- specific arterial abnormalities including dissection and fibromuscular dysplasia, or irregular caliber and mycotic aneurysms in inflammatory and infectious conditions,
- arteriovenous malformations and fistulae,
- brain tumors (characterization of blood supply).
- In addition, angiography is part of the interventional treatment (by the neuroradiologist) of aneurysms, arteriovenous malformations and fistulae, and of arterial stenosis and vasospasm. It is also a part of the technique of intra-arterial thrombolysis, and of mechanical extraction of intravascular thrombi.

Technique. A catheter is introduced into the femoral artery and passed along a guide wire into the aortic trunk, thence into one of the great vessels, and finally into to the left or right internal carotid or vertebral artery, where contrast medium is injected (all four major cerebral arteries are catheterized in a complete study). Fine catheters may be passed yet more distally into the branches of the major cerebral arteries for superselective contrast injection. Images are produced by point-for-point computerized subtraction of the images obtained before and after contrast injection, so that all structures other than the injected vessels appear as very pale shadows (this method is referred to as digital subtraction angiography, DSA). The digital processing of angiographic images enables them to be superimposed exactly on images of other types, such as CT and MRI, and to be used for the planning of stereotactic neurosurgical procedures.

Interpretation of angiograms. Angiographic images of the normal cerebral vasculature are shown in Figures 2.**29** and 2.**30**, and an image of carotid ste-

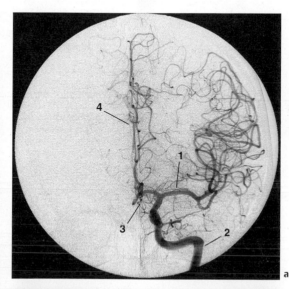

Fig. 2.**29a–c**
Normal digital subtraction angiogram of cerebral vessels in the carotid distribution.
a, b Arterial phase.
a, anteroposterior projection; **b**, lateral projection.
1 Middle cerebral artery (MCA)
2 Internal carotid artery (ICA)
3 Anterior cerebral artery (ACA)
4 Pericallosal artery

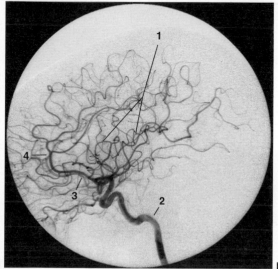

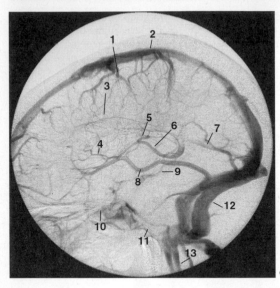

Fig. 2.29c
Venous phase, lateral projection.
1 Superior cerebral veins (of Trolard and Rolando)
2 Superior sagittal sinus
3 Inferior sagittal sinus
4 Septal vein
5 Thalamostriate vein
6 Internal cerebral vein
7 Straight sinus
8 Vein of Labbé (= inferior anastomotic vein)
9 Basal vein of Rosenthal
10 Cavernous sinus
11 Inferior petrosal sinus
12 Junction of transverse sinus (= lateral sinus) and sigmoid sinus
13 Jugular vein

c

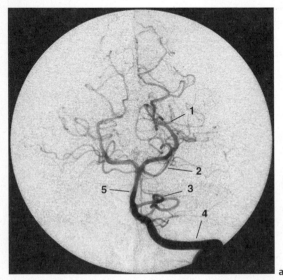

Fig. 2.30a, b
Selective angiography of the left vertebral artery.
a Anteroposterior projection.
1 Posterior cerebral artery
2 Superior cerebellar artery
3 Anterior inferior cerebellar artery (AICA)
4 Left vertebral artery
5 Basilar artery
6 Posterior inferior cerebellar artery (PICA)

a

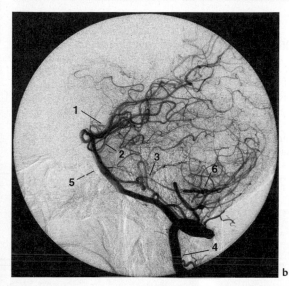

Fig. 2.**30b**
Lateral projection.
1 Posterior cerebral
 artery
2 Superior cerebellar
 artery
3 Anterior inferior cere-
 bellar artery (AICA)
4 Left vertebral artery
5 Basilar artery
6 Posterior inferior cerebellar artery (PICA)

b

nosis is shown in Figure 2.**32a**. For further abnormal cerebral angiograms, see Figures 2.**62** and 2.**65**.

Complications. Angiography is an invasive and expensive diagnostic technique. Its indications must be carefully considered in each case, because complications do rarely occur (219, 382). Femoral arterial puncture may cause a local hematoma or a vascular dissection. The angiographic catheter, in its passage into the cerebral vessels, may dislodge atherosclerotic plaques or thrombi, which can then embolize into the brain and cause a stroke. There may also be local, catheter-induced vasospasm, as well as reactions to contrast medium, including epileptic seizures, renal failure, and anaphylactic shock. Patients with atherosclerosis are more likely to suffer a complication from cerebral angiography than other patients. For spinal angiography, see p. 391.

■ Ultrasonography

Overview:
Neurologically relevant diagnostic techniques using ultrasound include Doppler and duplex ultrasonography of the intra- and extracranial arteries, and echocardiography. These are most often used in the evaluation of stroke patients, for the detection of stenosis or occlusion of the cerebral vessels and of sources of emboli in the heart and aortic arch. Transcranial Doppler ultrasonography can also be used for the noninvasive detection and serial assessment of cerebral vasospasm in the acute aftermath of aneurysmal subarachnoid hemorrhage.

■ Cerebrovascular Ultrasonography
(2, 37, 155, 489, 506, 703, 986, 1023, 1032, 1055)

Ultrasonography is used for the non-invasive diagnostic assessment of diseases of the cerebral arteries.

Indications. The most important indications for ultrasonography are the diagnosis and serial assessment of stenosis and occlusion of the intra- and extracranial arteries and their collateral circulation, of vasospasm after subarachnoid hemorrhage, of arteriovenous malformations and fistulae, of vasculitis, and of global non-perfusion of the brain (in the medicolegal ascertainment of death). Monitoring for cerebral embolization is a further application. Ultrasound lacks adequate sensitivity for the detection or exclusion of saccular aneurysms

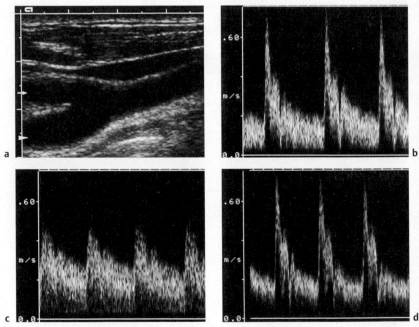

Fig. 2.**31a–d**   Doppler ultrasonography of a normal carotid bifurcation.
a   Two-dimensional sectional image (B-image) of a normal carotid bifurcation. It is rare to find the common, internal (arrowhead), and external (small arrow) carotid arteries lying in the same plane, so that they can all be seen on the same image, as here.
b–d   Doppler frequency–time spectra of the common (**b**), internal (**c**), and external (**d**) carotid arteries. The internal carotid artery, which supplies the brain, has a higher end-diastolic maximal velocity than the external carotid artery, which supplies extracranial structures and the meninges. The internal carotid artery is also less pulsatile than the external carotid artery.

and of disorders of the cerebral veins and venous sinuses, and it should not be used for these purposes (73).

Doppler ultrasonography. This technique is based on the effect first described by Christian Doppler in 1843 (268): the measured frequency of a wave emitted from a point source is shifted if the source and detector of the wave are moving relative to each other. The frequency is increased if the source is moving toward the detector, decreased if it is moving away. This fact can be exploited to measure the speed of erythrocytes in flowing blood with ultrasound waves. Waves emitted by the ultrasound device are bounced off the moving erythrocytes, and the frequency of the reflected waves is measured. The Doppler shift in frequency ("Doppler frequency") is linearly proportional to the velocity of blood flow and also depends on the angle of insonation.

Doppler signal. The Doppler signal is a composite of the Doppler frequencies of all of the individual erythrocytes in the path of the ultrasonic beam. Erythrocytes flow at different velocities depending on their position in the blood vessel (in accordance with the vessel's "flow profile" at that moment). The Doppler signal can be converted to an audio signal, or else visually represented as a *frequency-time spectrum* (Fig. 2.**31**). The latter shows the distribution of Doppler frequencies across the entire population of erythrocytes, plotted on the y-axis, against time, on the x-axis. Measured parameters relevant to the detection of stenoses include the maximal velocities in systole (V_{smax}) and diastole (V_{dmax}) and the mean maximal velocity (V_{mmax}). Resistance and pulsatility

indices can also be calculated. Cerebral vessels have a lower resistance than visceral vessels; the internal carotid artery is less pulsatile and has a softer sound than the external carotid artery (Fig. 2.**31**).

Gray scale. The detection of ultrasound waves reflected off boundaries between tissues of different acoustic resistance allows the construction of two-dimensional sectional images (Fig. 2.**31a**). The different types of reflection are depicted on a gray scale (this is the so-called B-image or B-mode, for *brightness mode*). The B-image yields morphological information: it allows the differentiation of echo-dense tissues, such as calcified atherosclerotic plaques, from echo-poor tissues, such as blood or fresh clot.

Duplex ultrasonography. The B-image is used in combination with Doppler ultrasonography for cerebrovascular diagnosis. This combination, called duplex ultrasonography, yields both morphologic and hemodynamic information.

Color duplex ultrasonography. Color duplex ultrasonography involves the color-coded representation of flow velocity and direction (information derived from Doppler ultrasound) superimposed on the B-image. The colors red and blue are usually used to represent flow in opposite directions. The color saturation represents the flow velocity (the brighter the color, the faster the flow).

Arteries that can be examined by ultrasonography. Ultrasonography can be used to examine all of the major arteries of the brain:

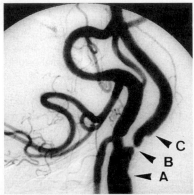

Fig. 2.**32a–c Short high-grade stenosis of the internal carotid artery.**
A, B, and C designate the prestenotic portion of the common carotid artery (A) and the stenotic (B) and post-stenotic (C) segments of the internal carotid artery. In accordance with the laws of fluid mechanics, the flow velocity in the stenotic segment increases as the square of the reduction of vascular diameter. Pulsatility is increased proximal to the stenosis and diminished distal to it.
a Angiogram.
b Ultrasonographic B-image.
c Doppler spectra.

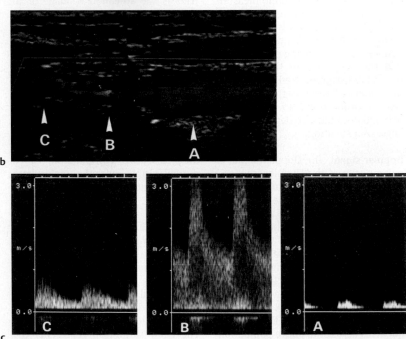

- Extracranial examination: the common, internal, and external carotid arteries, the vertebral artery, and the subclavian artery.
- Transcranial examination through the temporal bone window: the anterior, middle, and posterior cerebral arteries.
- Through the foramen magnum: the intracranial segment of the vertebral artery (V_4) and the basilar artery.

- Through the orbit: the ophthalmic artery.
- Through the carotid siphon and above the inner canthus: the supratrochlear and supraorbital arteries.

The flow velocities in all of these vessels are systematically measured, and abnormalities of the vascular walls are imaged and documented (76a). Atherosclerotic deposits are reliably seen, while dissection and arteritis are usually, but not always, detectable (844b).

Interpretation of Doppler findings. The interpretation of Doppler findings is based on hemodynamic considerations (76b). If the flow volume is held constant, the speed of flow across a stenosis increases as the inverse square of the vascular diameter. The flow velocity varies depending on position within the vessel (nearer the center, or nearer the vascular wall); for laminar flow, the flow profile is parabolic. Turbulence may occur immediately distal to a stenosis, or at points of bifurcation or curvature; turbulence is audible or visible in the

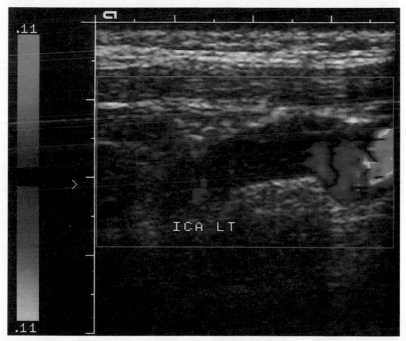

Fig. 2.**33a–c   Left internal carotid artery occlusion.**
Color-coded duplex ultrasonography of an occlusion of the left internal carotid artery 3 cm distal to the carotid bifurcation. Blood flow is seen up to the bifurcation (intense colored signal). (ICA LT = left internal carotid artery.)
a Within the internal carotid artery, only weak movement of the blood column is seen (scant red signal).

frequency-time spectrum and is characterized by the appearance of negative frequencies. Depending on the degree of stenosis, flow may be abnormal only within the stenosis, within and immediately distal to it, or within, proximal and distal to it (Fig. 2.**32**). Distal to a high-grade stenosis, the blood pressure falls so markedly that blood is supplied mainly by collateral vessels (see

Fig. 2.**41**). The demonstration of collaterals is diagnostically useful as indirect evidence of high-grade vascular stenosis or occlusion.

Vasospasm after subarachnoid hemorrhage similarly leads to an increased velocity of blood flow. The takeover of perfusion by collaterals is generally indicated by an abnormal flow profile and by reversal of the direction of flow. Arteriovenous malfor-

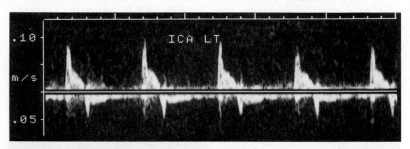

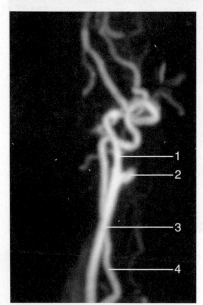

Fig. 2.**33b**
Doppler ultrasonography reveals only a brief early systolic forward flow with markedly reduced velocity, followed by backward flow already in early diastole.

Fig. 2.**33c**
The left ICA occlusion is readily seen on MRA.
1   External carotid artery
2   Stump of the occluded internal carotid artery
3   Common carotid artery
4   Vertebral artery

Table 2.**41** Classification of carotid stenoses and related ultrasonographic findings

Severity of stenosis	Grade of stenosis (%)	Finding proximal to stenosis/occlusion (in common carotid artery)	Finding at point of stenosis/occlusion	Finding distal to stenosis/occlusion (in internal carotid artery)	Collateral circulation (circle of Willis, ophthalmic artery)
Normal vessel, nonstenosing plaque	0%	Normal	Normal flow profile	Normal	None
Mild stenosis	<30%	Normal	Mild local increase in flow velocity	Normal	None
Moderate stenosis	30–70%	Normal	Significant local increase in flow velocity, spectral widening	Normal	None
High-grade stenosis	70–90%	Decreased flow velocity, increased pulsatility	Major local increase in flow velocity, spectral widening, including negative frequencies (turbulence)	Decreased flow velocity, decreased pulsatility	Usually present
Very high-grade stenosis	>90%	Markedly decreased flow velocity, increased pulsatility	Variable stenosis signal	Markedly decreased flow velocity and pulsatility	Always present
Occlusion	100%	Markedly decreased flow velocity, increased pulsatility (early systole)	No flow	No flow	Always present

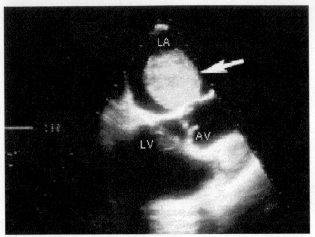

Fig. 2.34   Left atrial myxoma as a source of cardiac emboli.
Transesophageal echocardiogram.
AV: aortic valve;
LA: left atrium;
LV: left ventricle.

mations and fistulae manifest elevated flow velocity and diminished pulsatility. Cerebral nonperfusion (in death) is characterized by brief forward flow in systole, followed by backward flow in early diastole. The same profile is generally seen in internal carotid occlusion (Fig. 2.**33b**). Aneurysms are seen in color duplex sonography as zones of inflow and outflow separated by an intermediate zone without signal (73).

Microemboli appear in the frequency-time spectrum as signals of increased intensity. They can be counted as embolic events per unit time (embolic monitoring) (877, 917).

Echocardiography
Echocardiography is performed with the same duplex apparatus used for cerebrovascular ultrasonography, but with differently configured probes. It can be performed in the following ways:
- noninvasive trans-thoracic echo-cardiography (TTE), or
- minimally invasive trans-eso-phageal echocardiography (TEE) with a biplanar probe.

It is useful in the determination of stroke etiology, particularly for the detection of embolic sources in the heart and aortic arch (212) (Fig. 2.**34**). Furthermore, echocardiography after the intravenous injection of ultrasonographic contrast medium can be used to detect right-left shunts, such as through a patent foramen ovale, which may provide an anatomical pathway for paradoxical emboli.

Ischemic Stroke

■ Preliminary remarks: the physiology of cerebral perfusion

■ Cerebral Metabolism

The brain consumes glucose as its almost exclusive source of energy, at a rate of ca. 115 g daily. Some 15% of cardiac output is used to perfuse the brain, even though the brain accounts for only 2% of total body weight. Brain function is impaired when the global cerebral blood flow drops from its normal value of ca. 58 mL per 100 g of tissue per minute to values below 22 mL/100 g/min (404).

■ Autoregulatory Mechanisms

Autoregulation of cerebral blood flow enables an adequate supply of oxygen and nutrients to the brain over a wide range of hemodynamic conditions. A fall in blood pressure in the awake individual provokes a compensatory dilatation of the small cerebral arteries, so that the cerebral blood flow remains approximately constant. It starts to drop appreciably only when the systolic blood pressure falls below 70 mmHg in healthy persons, or below 70% of the initial value in hypertensive persons. Autoregulation also occurs in response to abnormal values of Pa_{CO_2}: cerebral blood flow is decreased in response to low values (hyperventilation), and increased in response to high values (hypoventilation).

■ Total (Experimental) Brain Ischemia

When the blood supply to the brain is suddenly shut off in an experimental animal, the brain is depleted of free oxygen within 2–8 seconds. Loss of consciousness occurs within 12 seconds, and EEG silence within 20–40 seconds. Histologically demonstrable, irreversible necrosis of the brain parenchyma follows within 3–4 minutes. Total brain ischemia for 9 minutes is incompatible with life, unless there is simultaneous hypothermia (Fig. 2.**35**).

■ Ischemic Thresholds and the Ischemic Penumbra (41, 65a, 404a)

Ischemic thresholds. Focal or global ischemia leads to an inadequate supply of oxygen and glucose. When cerebral blood flow falls below the *functional threshold* of 18–22 mL/100 g/min, evoked potentials are no longer obtainable, and the EEG becomes flat. If normal perfusion is then reinstated, normal function returns (both clinical and electrical). If the cerebral blood flow falls further, however, and crosses the *infarction threshold* of 8–10 mL/100 mg/min, irreversible damage occurs.

The degree of morphologic injury depends not only on whether these thresholds are crossed, but also on the duration of hypoperfusion (437). Some neurons will be irretrievably lost if the cerebral blood flow drops below the functional threshold for a long enough time, even if it always remains above the infarction threshold. Hippocampal neurons are particularly sensitive.

The ischemic penumbra. The zone of brain in which the regional cerebral blood flow lies between the two threshold values (the functional and ischemic thresholds) is called the ischemic penumbra. As a rule, a brain infarct consists of an irreversibly damaged central zone, surrounded by a penumbra whose ultimate fate depends on the timing and amount of recirculation (Fig. 2.**36**).

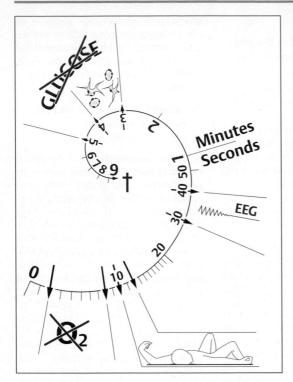

Fig. 2.**35** **Effect of ischemia on the brain.** Diagram of the effect of sudden total deprivation of blood supply to the brain on tissue metabolism, consciousness, the EEG, neuronal morphology, and tissue glucose concentration.

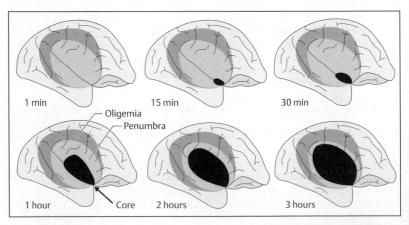

Fig. 2.**36** **Diagram of the penumbra and its development if flow is not reestablished in the occluded vessel** (adapted from J.-C. Baron).

■ **Ischemic Cerebral Edema**

Brain ischemia leads to cerebral edema. In accordance with the laws of osmosis, the intracellular macromolecules and electrolytes pull water into the cells from the extracellular space, which, because of the disabled function of the energy-dependent Na$^+$/K$^+$-ATPase, can no longer be pumped out again. The cells swell (this *cytotoxic* edema is visible on diffusion MRI). If ischemia persists, the blood–brain barrier is disrupted, and osmotically active substances escape from the plasma into the extracellular space, which then swells up with excess water as well (*vasogenic* edema).

In the early stage, consisting mainly of cytotoxic edema, CT reveals diffuse swelling and obliteration of the distinction between gray and white matter. Later, when vasogenic edema has set in, free water is seen to extend in fingerlike fashion along nerve bundles into the white matter, just like tumor-associated vasogenic edema. Extensive cerebral edema may exert mass effect and raise the local or global intracranial pressure, in turn diminishing the perfusion of the ischemic penumbra, so that the infarct is enlarged. Ultimately, upward or downward transtentorial herniation may occur (in the case of infra- and supratentorial infarcts, respectively) (213) (see Fig. 2.**67**).

■ **Preliminary Anatomical Remarks** (Figs. 2.38–2.40)

■ **Carotid Circulation**

The *common carotid artery* arises, on the right side, from the brachiocephalic trunk, and, on the left side, directly from the aorta. On either side, it bifurcates at the level of the hyoid bone into the *internal and external carotid arteries,* which supply the neurocranium and the viscerocranium, respectively. The internal carotid artery gives off its first branch at the level of the carotid siphon, namely, the *ophthalmic artery,* which supplies the eye. More distally, it gives off the *posterior communicating artery* (which joins the posterior cerebral artery) and the *anterior choroidal artery.* The latter supplies the choroid plexus of the temporal horn; through its early branches, the optic tract and (variably) the genu of the internal capsule and medial portions of the globus pallidus; through its lateral branches, the amygdala and the anterior portion of the hippocampus; and, through its medial branches, the hypothalamus, substantia nigra, red nucleus, and lateral geniculate body.

Above the carotid siphon, the internal carotid artery divides into the *middle and anterior cerebral arteries,* which together supply the entire lateral surface of the cerebral hemisphere, with the exception of the mediobasal temporal lobe and the occipital lobe. The *middle cerebral artery* supplies a major portion of the basal ganglia, as well as the internal capsule and the lateral surface of all four lobes of the hemisphere. It carries about twice as much blood per minute as the *anterior cerebral artery,* which supplies the medial surface of the hemisphere and the parasagittal region (the interface between lateral and medial surfaces). The basal portions of the middle and anterior cerebral arteries give off the striate and lenticulostriate arteries and smaller perforating vessels, which supply the basal ganglia. Other so-called perforators arise from leptomeningeal branches of the intracranial arteries and supply the cerebral cortex.

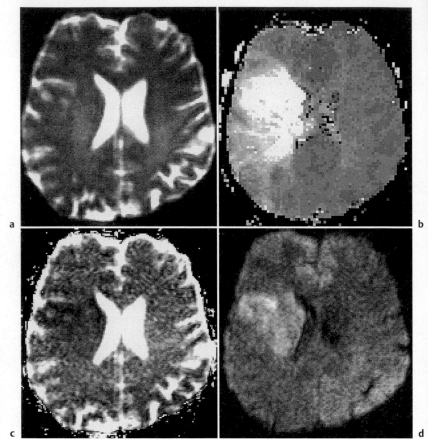

a

b

c

d

Fig. 2.**37a–d**   **Demonstration of the ischemic penumbra with perfusion and diffusion MRI in acute cerebral infarction, 2.5 hours after the onset of symptoms.**

a T2-weighted echo-planar MRI image (normal).

b Perfusion study showing the mean transit time (MTT). Blood flow is slowed and reduced in the entire distribution of the middle cerebral artery.

c, d Diffusion studies: **c** is a representation of the apparent diffusion coefficient (ADC), in which an abnormality of diffusion appears as an area of diminished signal; **d** is a diffusion-weighted image, in which the abnormality appears bright. The disturbance of diffusion occupies a triangular area that extends from the surface of the lateral ventricle to the brain surface and is significantly smaller than the hypoperfused area seen in **b**. The difference between these two areas corresponds to the ischemic penumbra.

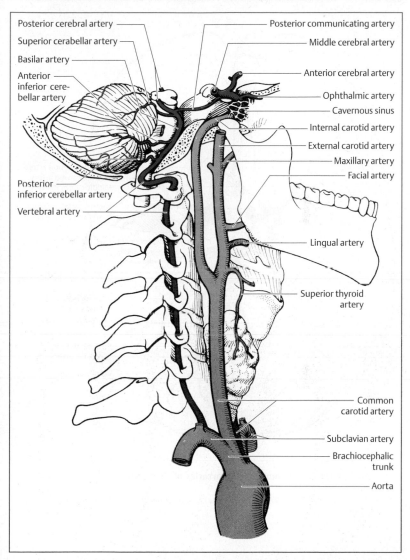

Fig. 2.**38** **Extracranial course of the major arteries supplying the brain (the carotid and vertebral arteries).** (From P. Duus, *Neurologisch-topische Diagnostik*, Stuttgart: Thieme, 1995).

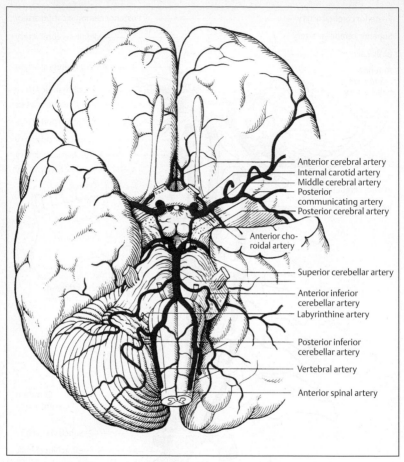

Fig. 2.**39a–f** **Intracranial course of the arteries of the brain.**
Fig. 2.**39a**
Arteries of the base of the brain. (From P. Duus, *Neurologisch-topische Diagnostik*, Stuttgart: Thieme, 1995).

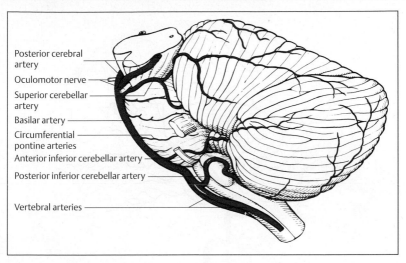

Fig. 2.**39b**   **Arteries of the posterior fossa.** (From P. Duus, *Neurologisch-topische Diagnostik*, Stuttgart: Thieme, 1995).

Key to numbered vessels in Figs. 2.**39c** and **d:**

1 Internal carotid artery
Branches of the internal carotid artery:
2 Ophthalmic artery
3 Posterior communicating artery
4 Posterior cerebral artery
   (supplied mainly by basilar artery)
5 Anterior choroidal artery
Branches of the anterior cerebral artery:
6 Pericallosal artery
7 Fronto-orbital artery
8 Common trunk of 9 and 10
9 Frontopolar artery
10 Anterior internal frontal artery
11 Middle internal frontal artery
12 Posterior internal frontal artery
13 Superior internal parietal artery
14 Inferior internal parietal artery
15 Orbitofrontal artery

Branches of the middle cerebral artery:
16 Prefrontal arteries
17 Prerolandic artery
17a Rolandic artery
18 Anterior parietal artery
19 Posterior parietal artery
20 Artery of the angular gyrus
21 Middle temporal artery
22 Posterior temporal artery
23 Temporopolar artery
24 Anterior temporal artery
25 Temporo-occipital artery

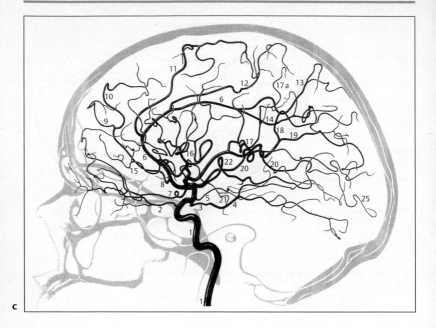

c

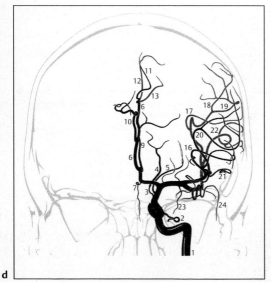

d

Figures 2.**39c, d Arteries supplying the cerebral hemispheres.** (From P. Duus, *Neurologisch-topische Diagnostik*, Stuttgart: Thieme, 1995).

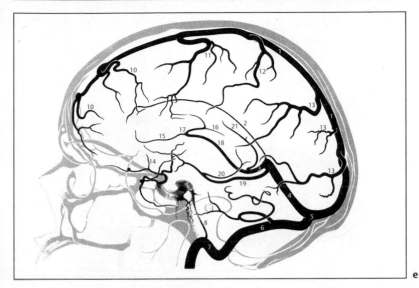

e

Figures 2.**39e, f   Cerebral veins and venous sinuses:** lateral (**e**) and Towne's (**f**) projections. (From P. Huber et al., *Cerebral angiography*, 2nd ed., New York: Thieme, 1982).

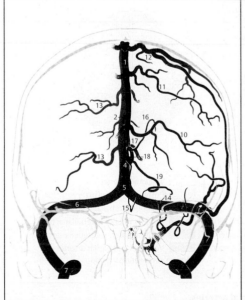

f

1 Superior sagittal sinus
2 Inferior sagittal sinus
3 Great cerebral vein (vein of Galen)
4 Straight sinus
5 Confluence of the sinuses (torcular Herophili)
6 Transverse sinus
7 Sigmoid sinus
8 Inferior petrosal sinus
9 Cavernous sinus
10 Frontal ascending veins
11 Vein of Trolard
12 Vein of Rolando
13 Parietal and occipital ascending veins
14 Veins of the Sylvian fossa
15 Septal vein
16 Thalamostriate vein
17 Venous angle
18 Internal cerebral vein
19 Basal vein of Rosenthal
20 Inferior ventricular vein
21 Dorsal vein of the corpus callosum (posterior pericallosal vein)

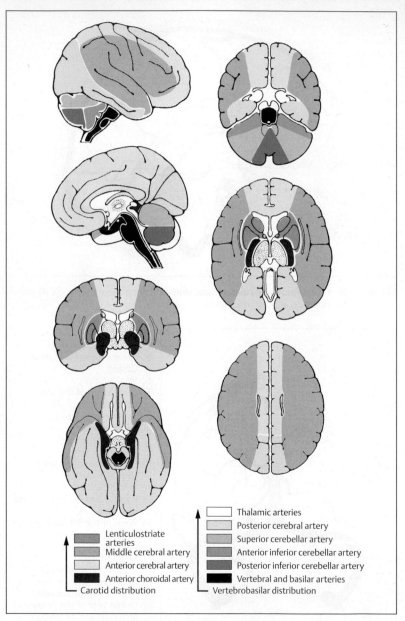

Fig. 2.**40 Territories of the cerebral arteries.**

■ Vertebrobasilar Circulation

The left and right *vertebral arteries* arise from the *subclavian arteries* and join in front of the brainstem to form the *basilar artery*. The vertebrobasilar system carries blood to the brainstem, cerebellum, and thalamus, the mediobasal portion of the temporal lobes, and the occipital lobes. Perforators and small circumferential arteries arising from the basilar artery supply the brainstem, and perforators arising more distally supply most of the diencephalon and thalamus. The vertebral artery normally gives rise to the *posterior inferior cerebellar artery (PICA),* while the basilar artery gives rise to the *anterior inferior cerebellar artery (AICA)* and superior cerebellar artery. All of these vessels supply the cerebellum (828).

The basilar artery bifurcates at the level of the midbrain to form the right and left *posterior cerebral arteries,* which supply the cerebral peduncles, the thalamus, the mediobasal portion of the temporal lobes, and the medial portion of the occipital lobes. In 7–14% of cases, the posterior cerebral artery on one or both sides arises not from the basilar artery, but from the internal carotid artery, through an enlarged posterior communicating segment *(persistent fetal origin of the posterior cerebral artery).* This less common, but by no means rare anatomical configuration may have pathophysiological significance in patients with stroke, as it explains the exceptional case in which carotid disease leads to a posterior infarct (852). Persistent fetal origin of the posterior cerebral artery may also have important implications for the planning of neurosurgical procedures, particularly the clipping of aneurysms.

■ Intra- and Extracranial Collateral Circulation

Collateral circulation is of major importance in the pathophysiology of stroke. Its variable presence or absence explains why the stenosis or occlusion of a given vessel can be asymptomatic, or cause only a small stroke, in some patients, and yet lead to extensive, or even fatal, infarction in others. The more extensive the collateral circulation, and the longer the time over which it has developed, the more likely it is that an occlusion will be well tolerated (Fig. 2.**41**). Vessels that may be recruited for the purpose of collateral circulation are found extracranially (numbers 1–4 and 9 in Fig. 2.**41**), in the arterial circle of Willis (numbers 6 and 8 in the same figure), and at the leptomeningeal level (numbers 5, 7, and 10–12). Among these sites, the circle of Willis has the greatest capacity for collateral flow.

■ Causes of Vascular Stenosis and Occlusion

Atherosclerosis. Atherosclerosis is the most common cause of arterial stenosis and occlusion (p. 189).

Further causes:

- *Dissection,* particularly of the extracranial arteries. Dissection starts from an intimal tear and progresses as the intima is peeled away from the media. A false lumen or an aneurysm may develop that may then secondarily become thrombosed, occlude the vessel, or give rise to emboli.
- *Inflammation or infection in the vicinity of the vessel* that may progress to involve the arterial wall, or intrinsic inflammation of the wall itself *(arteritis).*

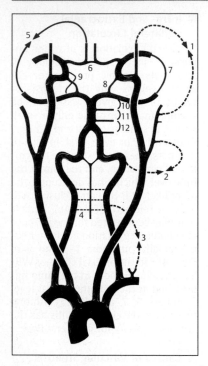

1   External carotid artery—facial artery—angular artery—ophthalmic artery—carotid siphon
2   External carotid artery—occipital artery—muscular branches—vertebral artery
3   Subclavian artery—thyrocervical trunk—occipital muscular branches—vertebral artery
4   Vertebral artery—meningeal branches—spinal arteries
5   Anterior cerebral artery—cortical branches—posterior cerebral artery
6   Right anterior cerebral artery—anterior communicating artery—left anterior cerebral artery
7A Middle cerebral artery—cortical branches—posterior cerebral artery
7B Middle cerebral artery—cortical branches—anterior cerebral artery
8   Carotid siphon—posterior communicating artery—posterior cerebral artery
9   Carotid siphon—anterior choroidal artery—posterior choroidal artery—posterior cerebral artery
10 Posterior cerebral artery—cortical branches—superior cerebellar artery
11 Superior cerebellar artery—cortical branches—AICA
12 AICA—cortical branches—PICA
    AICA: anterior inferior cerebellar artery;
    PICA: posterior inferior cerebellar artery.

Fig. 2.**41** **The most important collaterals of the cervicobrachial arteries and their branches.**

- *Cardiogenic or aortogenic embolism.* These cause about 20% of cerebral vascular occlusions (24, 476).
- *Fibrinoid and hyalinoid degeneration* and necrosis of the intima and media of small arteries and arterioles (= arteriolosclerosis) as the result of long-standing arterial hypertension (305).

■ **Basic Classification of Infarcts: Territorial, Watershed, and Lacunar Infarcts**

The patho-anatomical and neuroradiologic findings often provide a clue to the etiology of an infarct.

Territorial infarcts (Figs. 2.**42** and 2.**43**). These involve both the cerebral cortex and the subcortical white matter (790). They arise as a result of thrombotic or embolic occlusion of a single terminal branch, multiple branches, or main trunks of the major cerebral arteries. Large infarcts of the basal ganglia and thalamus may also be of this type.

Watershed infarcts. Watershed infarcts, also known as *border zone infarcts,* occur at the border between the distributions of two or more cerebral arteries, most commonly the an-

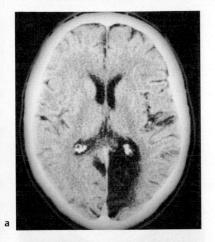

Fig. 2.**42a–e   Territorial infarcts.**
CT and MRI scans.
a   CT of a 45-year-old man with embolic
occlusion of the left posterior cerebral
artery. Note that the necrosis involves
both cortex and white matter.

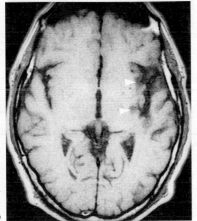

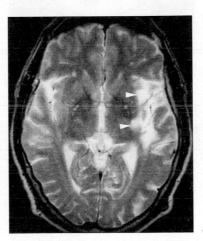

b, c T1- and T2-weighted spin-echo images of a 61-year-old man with Broca's aphasia,
which resolved within a few weeks. The sylvian fissure is wider on the left side because of
a cortical and subcortical lesion (arrowheads).

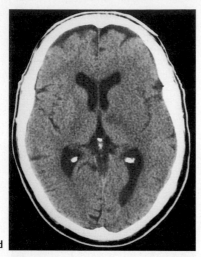

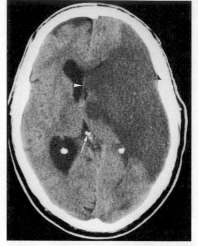

d

e

d, e CT of a 70-year-old man with a large infarct in the left middle cerebral artery distribution.

d   Six hours after the onset of symptoms. Note the mild hypodensity of the left basal ganglia, the mild effacement of the gray–white matter distinction, and the less well visualized sulci on the side of the infarct.

e   Two days later, the entire middle cerebral artery territory is hypodense. The infarct exerts mass effect, compressing the left lateral ventricle and displacing the pineal calcification (arrow) and the septum pellucidum (arrowhead) to the right.

terior and middle cerebral arteries (Fig. 2.**44**). They are of hemodynamic origin, occurring when the perfusion pressure is insufficient to bring an adequate blood supply to the periphery of the vascular territory (1052). The region of brain tissue at risk is called a watershed area, in (very loose) analogy to a mountain range separating lowlands on either side. Such infarcts generally result from stenosis or occlusion of multiple cerebral vessels, or from occlusion of a single internal carotid artery with insufficient collateral circulation. They are usually associated with a diminished vasomotor response to parenterally administered acetazolamide, or to breathing of 5 % CO_2 (789).

Lacunar infarcts. Lacunar infarcts result from inadequate blood flow in arteries less than 1.5 mm in diameter that supply the basal ganglia, thalamus, and brainstem, or that penetrate and supply the cerebral cortex. They are most commonly of *atherosclerotic* origin and, in such cases, are usually multiple. MRI reveals multiple signal changes of vascular origin in the white matter, while CT reveals multiple white matter hypodensities, typically near the frontal and occipital horns of the lateral ventricles. These radiologic findings are characteristic of subcortical arteriosclerotic encephalopathy of hypertensive origin, also known as *Binswanger disease* (Fig. 2.**45**).

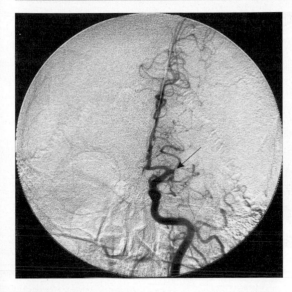

Fig. 2.**43a–c Acute right hemiplegia** in a 60-year-old man.
a The left carotid angiogram (anteroposterior view) reveals occlusion of the main stem of the middle cerebral artery at its origin (arrow). Only the anterior cerebral artery is visible.

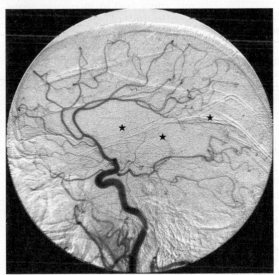

b The lateral view reveals only the pericallosal artery and its branches and the posterior cerebral artery, while the territory of the middle cerebral artery remains empty (stars). (Cf. the normal angiogram, Figs. 2.**29** on p. 141 and 2.**39c** on p. 158).

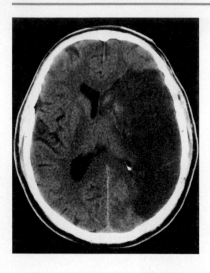

c A CT scan obtained 2 days after the onset of symptoms reveals a massive infarct in the middle cerebral artery territory, extending from the cortex to the basal ganglia.

■ Clinical Neurologic Syndromes of Cerebral Infarction
(108, 109, 636)

The goal of clinical examination is to localize the infarct to a particular area of the brain, and to determine the vessel in whose territory the infarct is located (even if, in some cases, this can be done no more specifically than to say whether the carotid or vertebrobasilar territory is involved). Accurate localization is usually possible after careful history-taking and neurological examination. Some types of infarcts, however, particularly lacunar infarcts, can be accurately localized only with the aid of ancillary neuroradiologic studies. Furthermore, certain types of middle and posterior cerebral artery territory infarcts are not distinguishable from each other on clinical grounds alone.

Ophthalmic artery. Ischemia and infarction in the territory of the ophthalmic artery lead to monocular visual disturbances, retinal infarction, and blindness. If retinoscopic examination reveals cholesterol crystals in the retinal arteries, the cause is probably atherosclerosis of the carotid artery.

Internal carotid artery. The classic clinical picture of hypoperfusion in the territory of the internal carotid artery is the oculocerebral syndrome, caused by simultaneous ischemia or infarction of the eye and the ipsilateral cerebral hemisphere. Monocular visual disturbances are accompanied by contralateral hemiparesis or hemiplegia, and by neuropsychological deficits corresponding to the involved hemisphere (dominant or nondominant) (113). The full constellation of symptoms and signs is, however, rarely seen.

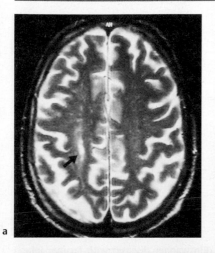

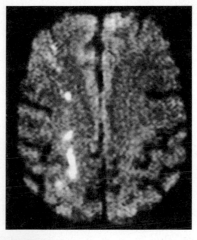

a

b

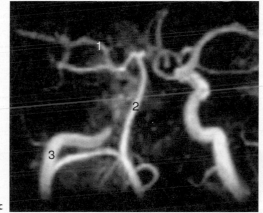

c

Fig. 2.**44a–c Watershed infarct.** A 58-year-old man with an infarct in the watershed zone between the right anterior and middle cerebral artery territories, resulting from right internal carotid artery occlusion. The territories can be seen in Fig. 2.**40** (p. 160). The infarct is seen on the T2-weighted spin-echo-image (arrow in **a**) and, even better, on the diffusion-weighted image (**b**) as a longitudinal signal abnormality in the watershed zone between the two arterial territories. The internal carotid artery is occluded below the siphon, as is seen in the MR angiogram (**c**).

1 Middle cerebral artery
2 Basilar artery
3 Right internal carotid artery

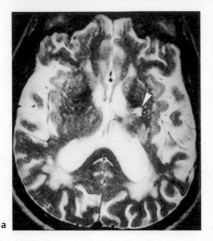 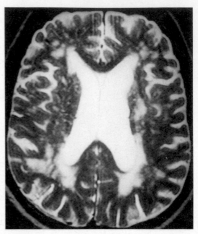

a
b

Fig. 2.45a, b Cerebral microangiopathy (Binswanger disease) with lacunar infarct (arrowhead) and severe white matter changes.
MR images in a 70-year-old man. The microangiopathic lesions are seen on the T2-weighted images as multifocal signal abnormalities in the white matter. The most severe changes are typically found in the periventricular zone abutting the frontal and occipital horns of the lateral ventricles.

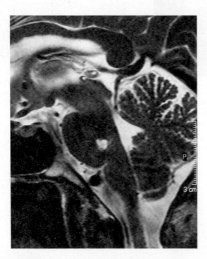

Fig. 2.46 Isolated lacunar infarct of the pons associated with atherosclerotic dolichoectasia of the basilar artery.
T2-weighted spin-echo image. Isolated lacunar infarcts have a broader differential diagnosis than multiple vascular lesions (see Fig. 2.**45**).

Middle cerebral artery (495). The symptoms and signs of hypoperfusion in the middle cerebral artery territory are variable, depending on the precise location and extent of the disturbance. The more common findings are:

- contralateral "faciobrachiocrural" hemiparesis or hemiplegia (i.e., affecting the face, arm and leg);
- hemisensory deficit;
- homonymous hemianopsia;
- contralateral gaze paresis.

Lesions of the dominant hemisphere for speech additionally cause *dysphasia* and *dyspraxia*, while lesions of the nondominant (usually right) hemisphere cause *disturbances of spatial processing* (p. 353).
Occlusion of the *superior anterior principal branch* of the middle cerebral artery produces infarction mainly involving the frontal lobe, typically manifesting as faciobrachial hemiparesis, gaze paresis, motor dysphasia and dyspraxia. Occlusion of its *inferior posterior principal branch* produces infarction mainly involving the parietal lobe, typically manifesting as a predominantly sensory hemisyndrome, often accompanied by homonymous hemianopsia, (with left-sided lesions) sensory dysphasia, or (with right-sided lesions) a disturbance of spatial processing, hemineglect, or (rarely) delirium (677). *Main stem occlusion*, if there is a high degree of collateralization through leptomeningeal anastomoses, produces infarction of the basal ganglia and internal capsule, leading to hemiparesis or hemiplegia. If there is little or no collateral circulation, then the infarct involves the entire middle cerebral artery territory, extending from the cortex to the basal ganglia.

A *thrombus or embolus that fragments and propagates distally* may cause occlusion of one or more peripheral branches of the middle cerebral artery and produce clinical signs and symptoms depending on the affected cortical area or areas.
Occlusions of the *striate and lenticulostriate arteries* and of their small branches produce small, usually lacunar infarcts in the basal ganglia and internal capsule (341). These cause sensorimotor, purely motor, or purely sensory hemisyndromes, and occasionally also extrapyramidal motor syndromes, such as hemiballism (342).
In the acute stage of hemiparesis or hemiplegia, muscle tone and intrinsic reflexes are usually diminished, and a Babinski sign is present. Spastic tone arises over the course of several days, or (in some cases) weeks. Hemispastic posture typically includes flexion at the elbow and wrist and extension at the knee and ankle. This, in turn, produces the typical hemispastic gait, with circumduction of the paretic leg and flexion of the paretic arm (Fig. 2.**47**).

Anterior choroidal artery (222). Infarcts in the territory of this artery are clinically characterized by homonymous visual field defects and by a sensory or (less commonly) motor hemisyndrome. If the optic tract is involved, retrograde axonal degeneration occurs and can be seen on examination of the retina with a slit lamp.

Anterior cerebral artery (114). The typical clinical finding of anterior cerebral artery infarction is a hemisyndrome mainly affecting the leg, though it sometimes affects the arm more than the leg and is accompa-

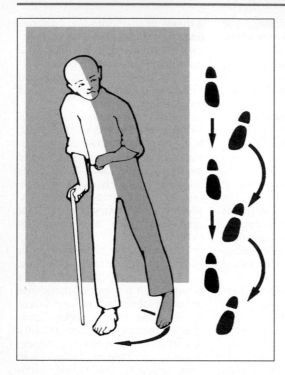

Fig. 2.**47 Typical gait disturbance of a hemiparetic patient.** Circumduction of the spastically paretic leg with predominantly extensor tone, and flexion of the spastically paretic arm at the elbow because of predominantly flexor tone (Wernicke-Mann type).

nied by ataxia. *Left-sided lesions* may produce dyspraxia of the *left* arm and leg, transcortical motor dysphasia, and behavioral disturbances such as apathy and abulia, or disinhibition and euphoria. Lesions of the paracentral lobule cause urinary incontinence. Perseveration or excessive distractibility during problem-solving are also typical. *Right-sided lesions* may cause left motor or spatial hemineglect accompanied by similar behavioral disturbances. *Bilateral anterior cerebral artery occlusion* leads to abulia or even akinetic mutism, in which the patient largely or completely lacks the motivation to act, move, or speak.

Watershed infarcts (116). These infarcts lead to motor, sensory, or combined hemisyndromes, sometimes associated with neuropsychological disturbances such as transcortical motor or sensory dysphasia, dysnomia, anosognosia, and hemineglect.

Lacunar syndromes. These are often difficult to assign to the anterior or posterior circulation on clinical grounds alone (713). They typically involve purely motor, purely sensory, or ataxic hemisyndromes, or a combination of clumsiness of one hand with dysarthria (the "clumsy hand—dysarthria syndrome") (304, 671). Lacunar infarction may also cause hemichorea, hemiballism, and an assortment of brainstem signs and symptoms.

Posterior cerebral artery (482, 752). Occlusion of the initial segment of the posterior cerebral artery proximal to the origin of the posterior communicating artery (the so-called P_1 segment) causes infarction in the cerebral peduncle, the thalamus, and the mediobasal portions of the temporal and occipital lobes. An occlusion of the next, more distal segment (the P_2 segment) spares the peduncle and thalamus. The leading symptoms and signs of P_1 occlusion may closely resemble those of middle cerebral artery occlusion, consisting of hemiparesis, hemisensory deficit, and homonymous hemianopsia. The major sign of P_2 occlusion is hemianopsia. Infarcts in the territory of the posterior cerebral artery are usually associated with neuropsychological deficits. Deficits due to *left-sided* (i.e., dominant-hemispheric) occlusion include so-called "alexia without agraphia," Gerstmann syndrome (the tetrad of agraphia, acalculia, finger agnosia, and right–left confusion), transcortical sensory dysphasia, anosmia, and color agnosia. Deficits due to *right-sided* occlusion include disorders of spatial orientation, left visual hemineglect, and prosopagnosia (see pp. 378 and 628). *Bilateral* posterior cerebral artery infarction causes altitudinal hemianopsia, cortical blindness (blindness with preservation of the pupillary light reflexes, so-called Anton syndrome), and disturbances of color perception. Severe memory impairment occurs if both sides of the thalamus or the mediobasal portions of both temporal lobes are involved.

Basilar artery. Circulatory disturbances in the basilar artery territory range in severity from occlusion of a circumferential or penetrating small artery of the brainstem to occlusion of the entire basilar trunk and all of its branches. A variable combination of brainstem, cerebellar, thalamic, temporal lobe, and occipital lobe signs and symptoms results.

Basilar artery thrombosis. Thrombosis of the basilar artery is usually preceded by prodromal symptoms and signs such as severe headache, dizziness, and seizures. These are then followed by coma and quadriplegia, or by the so-called "locked-in syndrome" (163, 298, 546). The latter consists of quadriplegia involving not only the limbs but also the cranial nerves on both sides, while consciousness is generally preserved. In typical cases, horizontal gaze (subserved by pontine centers) is paralyzed, while vertical gaze (subserved by the rostral midbrain) remains intact. The patient has no means of expression other than vertical eye movements and opening and closing of the eyelids.

The midbrain and the occipital lobes may be spared from infarction in cases of basilar artery thrombosis if they receive adequate collateral circulation from the internal carotid artery by way of the posterior communicating artery, or if the posterior cerebral artery exceptionally arises from the internal cerebral artery rather than the basilar artery (persistent fetal origin of the PCA, p. 161).

Basilar tip occlusion ("top of the basilar syndrome"). Occlusion of the rostral portion of the basilar artery causes infarction in the midbrain,

thalamus, hypothalamus, and medio-basal portions of the temporal and occipital lobes, and in combinations of these structures (546). The territory of the *superior cerebellar artery* may also be affected. The most prominent symptoms and signs are
- nuclear oculomotor paresis,
- vertical gaze palsy,
- ataxia,
- hypersomnia,
- impairments of attention and memory, of variable duration.

Thalamic infarction. The thalamus is supplied by four groups of small arteries:
- tuberothalamic (or tuberopolar) arteries,
- thalamoperforating (or paramedian) arteries,
- thalamogeniculate (or inferolateral) arteries, and
- the posterior choroidal arteries.

The first-named group arises from the posterior communicating artery and may thus depend for its adequate perfusion on either the carotid or the vertebrobasilar system, depending on the prevailing pressure relationships in the individual patient. The latter three groups all consist of branches of the posterior cerebral artery and thus belong to the posterior circulation. A vessel belonging to any of the four groups may be occluded on an embolic or microangiopathic basis. Infarcts in any of these territories are associated with a sensory hemisyndrome, usually accompanied by mild hemiparesis and by occasionally severe hemiataxia. Left-sided infarcts may produce dysphasia and memory impairment, while right-sided infarcts may produce hemineglect and disturbances of spatial orientation.

Abnormal movements (dyskinesias) are rarely present. Choroidal artery infarcts involve the lateral geniculate body and thereby produce homonymous sector- or quadrantanopsia (Dejerine-Roussy syndrome). The paramedian arteries may be represented by a single (unpaired) arterial trunk supplying the paramedian areas of both hemithalami (170). If this is the case and the trunk becomes occluded, consciousness is impaired, and (because the infarct additionally involves the midbrain) nuclear oculomotor palsy and vertical gaze palsy are also seen.

Brainstem infarctions. These are most often lacunar. Their clinical expression depends on location; a wide variety of brainstem stroke syndromes have been described, most of which carry eponymous names (Table 2.**42**). As a rule, brainstem lesions cause ipsilateral cranial nerve deficits, ipsi- or contralateral ataxia or hyperkinesias, and contralateral motor and sensory hemisyndromes. It follows that *the cranial nerve deficits and the bodily hemisyndrome are crossed.* By correlation of the clinical findings with brainstem anatomy, it is usually possible not only to localize an ischemic lesion to the midbrain, pons, or medulla, but also to give its position as medial or lateral, as well as ventral or dorsal, within the given structure.
The clinical characteristics of brainstem infarcts are described more fully below.

Midbrain infarction. Infarction in the medial portion of the midbrain is characterized by ipsilateral nuclear or fascicular oculomotor palsy and contralateral hemiparesis, hemiataxia, or coarse ("rubral") tremor. Lateral infarction causes contralateral sensory

Table 2.**42** Brainstem syndromes. (Note: descriptions of individual syndromes in the literature may be variable)

Name	Localization	Ipsilateral signs	Contralateral signs	Special features
Chiray-Foix-Nicolesco syndrome (upper red nucleus syndrome)	Midbrain, red nucleus	No oculomotor palsy	Hemiataxia (sometimes), hyperkinesia, intention tremor, hemiparesis (often without Babinski sign), sensory disturbances (sometimes)	
Benedikt syndrome (upper red nucleus syndrome)	Midbrain, red nucleus	Oculomotor palsy, sometimes gaze palsy toward the side of the lesion	Hemiataxia (sometimes), intention tremor, hemiparesis (often without Babinski sign)	Staggering gait
Claude syndrome (lower red nucleus syndrome)	Midbrain, red nucleus	Oculomotor palsy	Hemiataxia or hemi-incoordination, hemiparesis	No hyperkinesia
Weber syndrome	Midbrain, cerebral peduncle	Oculomotor palsy	Hemiparesis	
Parinaud syndrome	Region of the quadrigeminal plate			Upward gaze palsy (superior colliculi), downward gaze palsy (inferior colliculi)
Nothnagel syndrome	Region of the quadrigeminal plate	Oculomotor palsy	Hemiataxia	
Raymond-Céstan syndrome	Anterior portion of pontine tegmentum	Gaze palsy toward the side of the lesion	Hemisensory deficit (possibly including face), hemiparesis (sometimes)	

Table 2.**42**   Brainstem syndromes. (Note: descriptions of individual syndromes in the literature may be variable) (Cont.)

Name	Localization	Ipsilateral signs	Contralateral signs	Special features
Gasperini syndrome	Posterior portion of pontine tegmentum	Deficits of cranial nerves V, VI, VII, VIII	Hemisensory deficit	Nystagmus (sometimes)
Millard-Gubler syndrome	Posterior portion of pontine tegmentum	Peripheral facial palsy	Hemiparesis	
Brissaud syndrome	Posterior portion of pontine tegmentum	Facial spasm	Hemiparesis	
Foville syndrome	Posterior portion of pontine tegmentum	Abducens palsy, sometimes facial palsy	Hemiparesis	
Babinski-Nageotte syndrome	Dorsolateral portion of pontomedullary junction	Cerebellar ataxia, Horner syndrome	Hemiparesis, hemisensory deficit	Nystagmus, lateropulsion (territory of posterior inferior cerebellar artery)
Wallenberg syndrome	Dorsolateral medulla	Horner syndrome, vocal cord paresis, palatal and posterior pharyngeal paresis, trigeminal nerve deficit, hemiataxia	Dissociated sensory disturbance (body)	Nystagmus (territory of posterior inferior cerebellar artery)
Céstan-Chenalis syndrome	Lateral medulla	Horner syndrome, vocal cord paralysis, palatal and posterior pharyngeal paresis, hemiataxia	Hemiparesis, hemihypesthesia	
Avellis syndrome	Lateral medulla	Palatal and posterior pharyngeal paresis, vocal cord paralysis	Hemiparesis, hemihypesthesia	

Schmidt syndrome	Lateral medulla	Palatal and posterior pharyngeal paresis, vocal cord paralysis, sternocleidomastoid and upper trapezius paresis, hypoglossal palsy	Hemiparesis, hemihypesthesia
Tapia syndrome	Lateral medulla	Palatal and posterior pharyngeal paresis, vocal cord paralysis, hypoglossal palsy	Hemiparesis, hemihypesthesia
Vernet syndrome	Lateral medulla	Palatal and posterior pharyngeal paresis, sternocleidomastoid paresis, hemiageusia of the posterior third of the tongue, hemihypesthesia of the pharynx	Hemiparesis
Jackson syndrome	Inferior medulla	Hypoglossal palsy	Hemiparesis
Spiller syndrome	Medial medulla	Hypoglossal palsy	Hemiparesis, hemihypesthesia

and motor hemisyndromes. Rostral midbrain infarction, and infarction of the quadrigeminal plate, cause vertical gaze palsy. Patients with bilateral lesions are comatose or severely obtunded. The small arteries supplying the medial portion of the midbrain arise from the basilar artery, while those supplying the lateral regions arise from the P_1 segment of the posterior cerebral artery (Fig. 2.**48**). Mesencephalic strokes often extend rostrally into the thalamus.

Pontine infarction. Pontine infarcts usually involve only part of the pons.

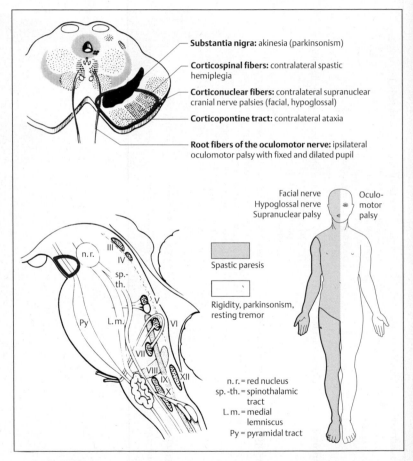

Fig. 2.**48** **Midbrain.**
Above: cross-section at the level of the oculomotor nucleus; *below:* schematic view of one half of the brainstem, cut in the midline. Weber syndrome as an example of midbrain stroke. (From P. Duus, *Neurologisch-topische Diagnostik,* Stuttgart: Thieme, 1995.)

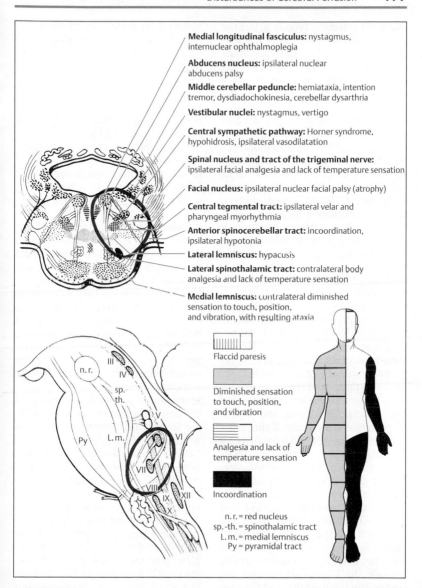

Medial longitudinal fasciculus: nystagmus, internuclear ophthalmoplegia

Abducens nucleus: ipsilateral nuclear abducens palsy

Middle cerebellar peduncle: hemiataxia, intention tremor, dysdiadochokinesia, cerebellar dysarthria

Vestibular nuclei: nystagmus, vertigo

Central sympathetic pathway: Horner syndrome, hypohidrosis, ipsilateral vasodilatation

Spinal nucleus and tract of the trigeminal nerve: ipsilateral facial analgesia and lack of temperature sensation

Facial nucleus: ipsilateral nuclear facial palsy (atrophy)

Central tegmental tract: ipsilateral velar and pharyngeal myorhythmia

Anterior spinocerebellar tract: incoordination, ipsilateral hypotonia

Lateral lemniscus: hypacusis

Lateral spinothalamic tract: contralateral body analgesia and lack of temperature sensation

Medial lemniscus: contralateral diminished sensation to touch, position, and vibration, with resulting ataxia

Flaccid paresis

Diminished sensation to touch, position, and vibration

Analgesia and lack of temperature sensation

Incoordination

n. r. = red nucleus
sp. -th. = spinothalamic tract
L. m. = medial lemniscus
Py = pyramidal tract

Fig. 2.**49** **Pons.**
Above: cross-section at the level of the facial nucleus; *below:* schematic view of one-half of the brainstem, cut in the midline. Pontine tegmental infarct as an example of pontine stroke. (From P. Duus, *Neurologisch-topische Diagnostik,* Stuttgart: Thieme, 1995.)

The most common type is a lacunar infarct in the distribution of the median, paramedian or lateral perforating arteries, most of which arise directly from the basilar trunk. As a rule, dorsal infarcts produce oculomotor disturbances, while ventral infarcts produce motor signs. Median and paramedian infarcts cause ipsilateral internuclear ophthalmoplegia, horizontal gaze palsy, one-and-a-half syndrome (see p. 649), nuclear facial palsy or contralateral hemiparesis, while lateral infarcts cause ipsilateral Horner syndrome, abducens palsy, fascicular facial palsy, hemiataxia, and contralateral sensorimotor hemisyndrome (Fig. 2.**49**).

Medullary infarction. The best known medullary infarction syndrome is that of the dorsolateral medulla, or Wallenberg syndrome (Figs. 2.**50** and 2.**51**). It is characterized by facial hypesthesia for all modalities, Horner syndrome, glossopharyngeal and vagal palsy with dysphagia and hoarseness, vertigo, spontaneous nystagmus, ipsilateral cerebellar ataxia, and contralateral hypalgesia and diminished temperature sense. If the lesion extends ventrally, there may also be a contralateral hemiparesis. Ventrolateral medullary lesions additionally involve the intramedullary fibers of the facial nerve, and caudal lesions below the pyramidal decussation produce ipsilateral bulbar palsy and ipsilateral hemiparesis. Medullary lesions can produce facial hypesthesia on either side (ipsi- or contralateral), because the trigeminal nucleus descends into the medulla, and the central trigeminal pathway crosses the midline before ascending to the thalamus. *Medial medullary syndromes* are characterized by ipsilateral hypo-

glossal (tongue) palsy and contralateral sensorimotor hemisyndrome (70a). Cardiac arrhythmia, arterial hypo- or hypertension, and apnea ("Ondine's curse") may appear, which may be acutely life-threatening, with risk of sudden death (714). Lateral medullary syndromes result from distal occlusion of the vertebral artery or proximal occlusion of the posterior inferior cerebellar artery, while medial medullary syndromes result from occlusion of paramedian branches of the anterior spinal artery.

Pseudobulbar palsy. Multiple lacunar infarcts are the usual cause of pseudobulbar palsy, while a single, larger infarct is a rarer cause. The clinical signs reflect damage to the corticobulbar pathways on both sides. Typically, the patient has a history of one or more earlier strokes, on which a new vascular event is superimposed. Only the last event produces the impressive clinical picture of acute pseudobulbar palsy. The same picture sometimes comes about in the absence of any acute event, usually on the basis of a "lacunar state" (multiple lacunar infarctions, each one of which is subclinical, but which cumulatively cause neurologic dysfunction). This syndrome may be succinctly defined as a bilateral spastic paresis of the oral and pharyngeal musculature. The patient's speech is disjointed and dysphonic (p. 384); in extreme cases, speaking is actually impossible (anarthria). Only incomplete protrusion and coarse movements of the tongue can be executed. The act of swallowing is severely impaired, so that food remains in the mouth for a long time. The masseteric and perioral reflexes are brisk. Pyramidal tract signs may also be found in

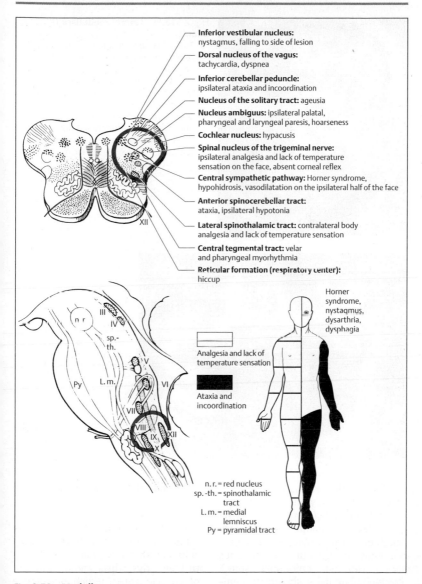

Inferior vestibular nucleus:
nystagmus, falling to side of lesion

Dorsal nucleus of the vagus:
tachycardia, dyspnea

Inferior cerebellar peduncle:
ipsilateral ataxia and incoordination

Nucleus of the solitary tract: ageusia

Nucleus ambiguus: ipsilateral palatal,
pharyngeal and laryngeal paresis, hoarseness

Cochlear nucleus: hypacusis

Spinal nucleus of the trigeminal nerve:
ipsilateral analgesia and lack of temperature
sensation on the face, absent corneal reflex

Central sympathetic pathway: Horner syndrome,
hypohidrosis, vasodilatation on the ipsilateral half of the face

Anterior spinocerebellar tract:
ataxia, ipsilateral hypotonia

Lateral spinothalamic tract: contralateral body
analgesia and lack of temperature sensation

Central tegmental tract: velar
and pharyngeal myorhythmia

Reticular formation (respiratory center):
hiccup

Horner
syndrome,
nystagmus,
dysarthria,
dysphagia

Analgesia and lack of
temperature sensation

Ataxia and
incoordination

n. r. = red nucleus
sp. -th. = spinothalamic
tract
L. m. = medial
lemniscus
Py = pyramidal tract

Fig. 2.**50**   **Medulla.**
Above: cross-section at the level of the hypoglossal nucleus; *below:* schematic view of one-half of the brainstem, cut in the midline. Dorsolateral medullary infarct causing Wallenberg syndrome, as an example of a medullary infarct. (From P. Duus, *Neurologisch-topische Diagnostik,* Stuttgart: Thieme, 1995.)

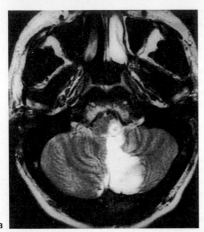

Fig. 2.51a, b   Lateral medullary (PICA) infarct.
a The T2-weighted spin-echo MR image reveals an infarct in the distribution of the posterior inferior cerebellar artery (PICA) involving the dorsolateral portion of the medulla and extending inferomedially into the cerebellum.
b The MR angiogram reveals a threadlike stenosis of the intracranial portion of the left vertebral artery, involving the location from which the PICA normally arises (arrowheads).

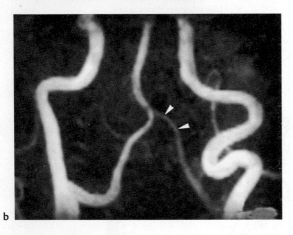

the extremities. Particularly impressive are the lability and incontinence of affect, including involuntary crying and, less commonly, involuntary laughter, in the absence of any corresponding change in the patient's mood (internal emotional state). Pseudobulbar palsy should be clinically distinguished from true bulbar palsy, brainstem processes of other than vascular etiology, lower-motor-neuron-type weakness involving the oral and pharyngeal muscles, and myasthenia gravis.

Cerebellar infarction (25). Cerebellar infarction presents with acute headache and dizziness, nausea, gait disturbance, dysarthria, and impairment of consciousness, which may range from somnolence to coma. Objective findings include truncal and gait ataxia, appendicular ataxia, a tendency to fall to the same side as the lesion (lateropulsion), dysmetria, dysarthria, and nystagmus. Practically all patients with an acute cerebellar stroke are unable to walk.

The proximal segments of the cerebellar arteries also supply portions of the brainstem; thus, proximal occlusions are often accompanied by brainstem signs, which may actually overshadow the cerebellar signs. If the cerebellum is affected in isolation, there may be no clinical signs or symptoms other than dizziness, nystagmus, and ataxia (pseudovestibular syndrome), possibly suggesting the erroneous diagnosis of an acute vestibulopathy.

Cerebellar infarcts may be accompanied by massive edema, leading to secondary brainstem compression and transtentorial and transforaminal herniation (p. 223). An acute cerebellar infarct with mass effect, threatening to compress a still-functioning brainstem, is an acute neurosurgical emergency. Open decompression by "strokectomy" is life-saving.

■ Multi-Infarct Syndrome

The most prominent clinical sign of multi-infarct syndrome is dementia, which may be combined with focal neurological signs (p. 371) (794). There is generally a history of one or more vascular risk factors. The clinical signs often progress in stepwise fashion after an initial stroke (372). Infarcts are seen on CT and MRI. Coronary artery disease and occlusive peripheral vascular disease are frequent comorbidities.

■ Temporal Classification of Cerebrovascular Events: TIA, Amaurosis Fugax, RIND, and (Completed) Stroke

Transient ischemic attack (TIA). A cerebrovascular event may be classified according to its temporal course as a transient ischemic attack (TIA), reversible ischemic neurologic deficit (RIND), or (completed) stroke (Fig. 2.**52**).

By definition, a TIA lasts for less than 24 hours, although the usual duration is 2–15 minutes. *Carotid TIAs* manifest themselves as unilateral weakness, incoordination, or sensory disturbances of the face or upper or lower limb, dysphasia, homonymous hemianopsia, or transient monocular blindness. The term "amaurosis fugax" denotes transient monocular blindness due to a carotid TIA involving the eye (i.e., the territory of the ophthalmic artery). *Vertebrobasilar TIAs*, on the other hand, characteristically present with bilateral or side-alternating weakness, incoordination, and sensory disturbances, as well as homonymous hemianopsia, total blindness, gait ataxia, dysequilibrium, and/or combinations of diplopia, dysphagia, dysarthria, and dizziness. Cases of isolated dizziness or dysequilibrium, tinnitus, scintillating scotoma, transient amnesia, and drop attacks are generally not due to TIA.

A secure diagnosis of TIA can only be made retrospectively. When a neuro-

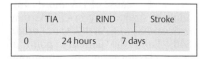

Fig. 2.**52 Definition of TIA, RIND, and stroke.**

logic deficit due to ischemia is only a few minutes old, the probability that it will revert to normal within 24 hours, and thus qualify as a TIA, is nearly 50%. Two hours later, however, the probability is only 10% (578, 1016).

Reversible ischemic neurologic deficit (RIND). By definition, the clinical manifestations of a RIND last no more than 7 days. Any longer-lasting ischemic neurologic deficit qualifies as a stroke.

Progressive stroke, stroke-in-evolution. These terms denote strokes with secondary clinical worsening at some time after the initial event (333).

Asymptomatic cerebrovascular disease. This category includes incidentally discovered stenoses and occlusions of the cerebral arteries in the absence of any corresponding neurologic deficit (or history of neurologic deficit). Stenosis or occlusion is often found in the workup of an asymptomatic carotid bruit.

Diagnostic evaluation. In the Dutch TIA Trial, CT revealed brain infarcts in 13% of cases of TIA, 34% of RIND, and 47% of small strokes. MRI was more sensitive and revealed infarcts more frequently in all of these clinical categories.
There is a broad spectrum of possible etiologies of TIA, RIND, and stroke (Tables 2.**43** and 2.**44**). Hemorrhage is very rarely a cause of TIA, more commonly of stroke. Very brief TIAs may be of cardiac (e.g., arrhythmic) origin (540). From the patient's point of view, classification by temporal course (TIA, RIND, or stroke) is less important than the establishment of

an etiology, which has implications for the prevention of further events (165). Earlier studies of stroke treatment and prevention generally classified cerebrovascular events by their temporal course. Though this had some empirical justification, a more rational, etiological classification is now commonly used (6, 936a).

■ **Etiology of Cerebral Infarction**
The etiology of stroke in the individual case can often be inferred from the history and physical examination. Further diagnostic workup should, therefore, be tailored to the clinical impression, so that "shotgun" ordering of unnecessary tests can be avoided. Figure 2.**53** provides a detailed etiological classification, which will be of greater use for younger patients, in whom atherosclerosis is less likely to be the cause.
Though needless tests should be avoided, some ancillary testing is always necessary to confirm a suspected etiologic diagnosis, and jumping to a diagnostic conclusion without such confirmation is highly per-

Table 2.**43**   Major etiologic categories of brain infarct

I	**Atherosclerosis of major intra- and extracranial vessels:** • Thrombosis • Hemodynamic insufficiency • Arterio-arterial emboli
II	**Cardiogenic and aortogenic emboli**
III	**Cerebral small vessel disease, lacunae**
IV	**Nonatherosclerotic causes:** • Vasculopathies • Coagulopathies
V	Idiopathic

ilous. Even the fundamental differentiation of cerebral *ischemia* from cerebral *hemorrhage* cannot be made reliably on clinical grounds and requires neuroradiologic confirmation.

Atherosclerosis of the extra- or intracranial portions of the major arteries supplying the brain (*macroangiopathy*) is suspected when vascular risk factors are present, when other signs of atherosclerotic involvement of the coronary or peripheral arteries are found, or when a carotid bruit is heard. Cholesterol emboli in the retinal vessels, if found, are further evidence of carotid atherosclerosis.

Hypertensive and diabetic patients are predisposed to the development of arteriolosclerosis and cerebral microangiopathy, resulting in *lacunar in-*

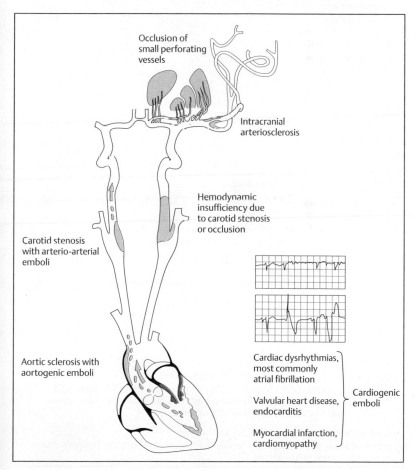

Fig. 2.**53** **The most important etiologies of stroke.**

Table 2.**44** Etiologic classification of ischemic stroke (after 636, 640)

Atherosclerosis of major intra- and extracranial arteries, including the aortic arch: thrombosis, arterioarterial emboli, hemodynamic insufficiency

Atherosclerosis of the aorta

Cerebral small vessel disease, lacunar infarction

cardiogenic emboli:

- Mural thrombus
  Myocardial infarction
  Cardiomyopathy
  Mural aneurysm
- Valvular heart disease
  Rheumatic heart disease
  Bacterial and non-bacterial endocarditis
  Mitral valve prolapse
  Prosthetic heart valve
- Dysrhythmia
  Atrial fibrillation
  Sick sinus syndrome with brady- and tachyarrhythmias
- Atrial myxoma
- Paradoxical embolism through patent foramen ovale or atrial septal defect
- Atrial septal aneurysm

Cerebral hemorrhages (see Table 2.**52**)

Hematologic diseases:

- Thrombocytopenia
  Protein C, protein S, and antithrombin III deficiencies
- Anti-phospholipid antibodies, anti-cardiolipin antibodies
- Hemoglobinopathy (sickle-cell anemia), thalassemia
- Hyperviscosity syndrome
  Erythrocytosis, thrombocytosis, leukocytosis, macroglobulinemia, myeloma
- Polycythemia vera, myeloproliferative syndromes
  Paroxysmal nocturnal hemoglobinuria

Vasculitis (see Table 2.**49**)

- Primary CNS vasculitis
  Granulomatous angiitis of the CNS
- Systemic necrotizing vasculitis with CNS involvement
  Periarteritis nodosa, Churg-Strauss syndrome, giant cell arteritis (polymyalgia rheumatica, temporal arteritis), Takayasu's arteritis, Wegener's granulomatosis, lymphomatoid vasculitis, hypersensitivity vasculitis

- Connective tissue diseases with CNS involvement
  Systemic lupus erythematosus, scleroderma, rheumatoid arthritis, Behçet's disease, mixed connective tissue disease

(Cont.) →

Table 2.**44** Etiologic classification of ischemic stroke (after 636, 640) *(Cont.)*

- Infectious vasculitis
  HIV, tuberculosis, borreliosis, neurosyphilis, fungal infection, mononucleosis, cytomegalovirus, herpes zoster,
  hepatitis B, rickettsioses, bacterial endocarditis

Medications and drugs of abuse:

- Cocaine, crack, amphetamines, LSD, heroin
- Sympathomimetic agents, ergotamines, triptans
- Intravenous immunoglobulin

Non-atherosclerotic vascular diseases:

- Dissection
  Traumatic, spontaneous, Marfan syndrome, fibromuscular dysplasia
- Traumatic thrombosis or avulsion of cerebral vessels
- Vasospasm after subarachnoid hemorrhage
- Embolism from an aneurysm
- Moyamoya disease
- Dolichoectasia
- Amyloid angiopathy

Various other etiologies:
- Homocysteinuria
- Hyperhomocysteinemia
- Fabry disease
- Fat and air embolism
- Liposculpturing
- Pseudovasculitic syndrome with cholesterol emboli
- Migraine
- Neurofibromatosis
- Pulmonary diseases
  Arteriovenous malformations, Osler's disease, pulmonary venous thrombosis
- Distal emboli from giant intracranial aneurysms
- Tumor emboli
- MELAS and other mitochondrial encephalomyopathies, CADASIL and other familial cerebral vasculopathies

Venous and venous sinus thrombosis

Stroke of indeterminate etiology (idiopathic)

Iatrogenic stroke:

- Angiography; surgery on the carotid artery, aorta, and heart
- Injection of steroid crystals, fat emboli, etc.

farction in the basal ganglia, internal capsule, thalamus, brainstem, and (rarely) cerebral cortex. Arterioslcerosis is often directly visible by retinoscopy.

Clinical examination of the *heart* and its rhythm may suggest the possibility of cardiogenic embolism. A difference in blood pressure between the two arms should arouse suspicion of an aortic aneurysm, Takayasu's arteritis, or subclavian steal syndrome.

The presence of *ecchymoses, petechiae,* and other cutaneous lesions suggests that whatever process is underlying them has affected the brain as well. *Deep venous thrombosis* in an extremity may lead to *paradoxical cerebral embolism* in the presence of an anatomical right-to-left shunt. If the physical findings yield no evidence of atherosclerosis or cardiac disease, other types of vascular disease should be considered, particularly arterial dissection. *Carotid artery dissection* should be suspected when there is a

Table 2.**45**   Initial ancillary studies for the patient with a focal neurologic deficit of acute onset

Erythrocyte sedimentation rate
Hemoglobin, hematocrit
Leukocyte count (with differential count)
Platelet count
Sodium, potassium
Glucose
BUN, creatinine
Syphilis serology
Prothrombin time
Urinalysis
Serum osmolality
ECG
Chest radiograph

history of cervical, facial, temporal, or orbital pain on one side, accompanied by ipsilateral Horner syndrome and contralateral hemiparesis or hemisensory syndrome. Carotid artery dissection may rarely cause ipsilateral cranial nerve deficits and thus misleadingly arouse suspicion of a brainstem process. Vertebral artery dissection presents with ipsilateral cervical and occipital pain and, as a rule, with brainstem symptoms and signs (p. 193). Tenderness of the temporal arteries suggests the diagnosis of *giant cell arteritis* (temporal arteritis, polymyalgia rheumatica).

■ Diagnostic Evaluation and Use of Ancillary Tests

An acute, focal neurologic deficit is usually due to a cerebrovascular event. The differential diagnostic questions discussed above are usually rapidly answered with the *ancillary tests* listed in Table 2.**45** and with a *CT or MRI scan* of the brain (cf. pp. 132, 133). An EEG is sometimes needed to distinguish TIAs from focal epileptic seizures.

In the acute phase, the *CT scan* (p. 132) may reveal early signs of infarction, such as obscuration of the gray-white matter distinction, blurring the boundaries of the cerebral cortex and of the basal ganglia. The "dense artery sign" (Fig. 2.**54**), when it is seen, indicates thrombosis of an artery (855). The *MRI scan* (p. 137) may not reveal any sign of acute ischemia unless perfusion and diffusion images are obtained (265, 998, 999). Signs of arterial dissection, venous thrombosis, or venous sinus thrombosis should always be looked for; they may be seen on either CT or MRI.

If extra- or intracranial arterial disease is considered a diagnostic possi-

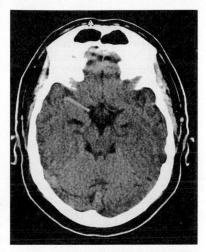

Fig. 2.**54** **Acute left hemisyndrome.** CT scan. The acute thrombus in the right middle cerebral artery is seen as a hyperdense line ("dense artery sign"). Parenchymal changes cannot yet be seen.

bility in the individual case, the next step is *cerebrovascular ultrasonography,* or else *MR or CT angiography* (p. 136). If cardiogenic embolism is suspected on the basis of the clinical history, cardiac examination, and CT or MRI, the workup should include transthoracic or, possibly, transesophageal *echocardiography* (p. 146). If cardiac dysrhythmia is suspected, *long-term ECG monitoring* (Holter monitoring) should be performed.

If the cause of a stroke remains unclear, the aortic arch should also be considered as a possible source of emboli and should be studied by transesophageal echocardiography (TEE). Further laboratory tests should be carried out, as delineated in Table 2.**46**. If these fail to provide conclusive evidence for a final diagnosis, a lumbar puncture should be considered, as this may provide a clue to

Table 2.**46** Further laboratory studies for the patient with a focal neurologic deficit of acute onset

Serum electrophoresis
Antinuclear antibodies, rheumatoid factor
Hemoglobin electrophoresis
Anti-phospholipid antibodies
Protein C, protein S, antithrombin III, and APC resistance (several weeks after the acute event)

some of the rarer causes of stroke (e.g., vasculitis, basal meningitis). *Conventional angiography* (p. 140) is performed when endovascular therapy is to be provided, or for the confirmation of an abnormal finding obtained by noninvasive means (ultrasonography, MR or CT angiography). It may also be useful as part of the primary evaluation of younger patients with stroke of unclear etiology.

■ Warning Signs and Speed of Progression

Some 25–50% of atherothrombotic strokes are preceded by TIAs; for cardioembolic and lacunar strokes, the percentage is lower. Two-thirds of all strokes progress to their full symptomatic expression within minutes, while one-third continue to progress after the patient arrives in the hospital.

■ Associated Symptoms, Temporal Course, and Complications (7)

Headache. Headache rarely accompanies ischemic stroke but may be the leading symptom in cases of venous thrombosis, giant cell arteritis, arterial dissection, and intracerebral and subarachnoid hemorrhage.

Seizures. Convulsions are common in cerebral venous thrombosis and venous sinus thrombosis. Focal seizures are seen in 2% of stroke patients overall, more commonly in acute brain hemorrhage and embolic stroke than in atherothrombotic stroke.

Disturbance of consciousness. Consciousness is impaired by midbrain and diencephalic stroke, or when a hemispheric lesion (e.g., a large intracerebral hemorrhage, or a massively edematous infarct in the distribution of the middle cerebral artery) produces mass effect leading to a dangerous elevation of intracranial pressure (p. 231).

Cerebral edema, intracranial hypertension, hydrocephalus. Particularly when a younger patient suffers a very large stroke, the associated cerebral edema may exert sufficient mass effect to elevate the intracranial pressure dangerously, perhaps leading to brain herniation (p. 222). Infratentorial strokes with mass effect may occlude the aqueduct or the pathways of CSF outflow from the fourth ventricle (foramina of Magendie and Luschka), and thereby produce hydrocephalus. Intracranial hypertension is the most common cause of death in the first few days after a stroke.

Hemorrhagic transformation, secondary hemorrhage. Ischemic strokes usually contain numerous petechial hemorrhages (302, 435), which rarely produce specific clinical signs, though they may become confluent and yield the radiologic picture of an infarct with hemorrhagic transformation. When an occluded vessel is reopened by endovascular thrombolysis, major hemorrhage may occur, leading to mass effect and clinical deterioration. Cardioembolic infarcts are more frequently hemorrhagic than atherothrombotic infarcts. As one might expect, hemorrhage is more common when anticoagulants and fibrinolytic agents are administered. The larger the infarct, the more likely that there will be an associated hemorrhage.

Respiratory disturbances. These are a feature of medullary infarction and may present a critical problem. Cheyne-Stokes respirations are also seen in patients with a large hemispheric stroke. Respiratory disturbances such as sleep apnea syndrome are both a risk factor for, and a consequence of, stroke (70c).

Dysphagia. Dysphagia in the aftermath of a stroke may lead to aspiration pneumonia.

Myocardial infarction. One of the causes of stroke is cardiogenic embolism in the setting of acute myocardial infarction. Moreover, 40–60% of stroke patients have either overt or clinically silent ischemic heart disease.

Cardiac dysrhythmia. Dysrhythmias are a frequent cause of stroke. They are also, rarely, a consequence of stroke, most commonly after medullary infarction.

ST segment changes on ECG. Such changes are found in the setting of acute stroke affecting the insular cortex. They may mimic the ECG signs of acute myocardial infarction.

Deep venous thrombosis. Not only bedridden patients, but also walking patients with a paretic limb or limbs, are at risk for deep venous thrombosis and *pulmonary embolism.*

Urinary tract infection. Urinary tract infection occurs frequently in patients with indwelling catheters.

Decubitus ulcers. Bedridden patients, particularly those with poor nutritional status, are at risk for decubitus ulcers.

Contractures, joint stiffness, reflex sympathetic dystrophy. Reduced motion across joints combined with elevated flexor tone in paretic limbs leads to joint stiffness, contractures, and trophic disturbances, such as periarthropathy of the shoulder and reflex sympathetic dystrophy.

■ Prognosis of Cerebral Infarction

The prognosis depends on the type and etiology of stroke. In general, younger patients have a better prognosis, while impairment of consciousness in the initial phase of stroke is correlated with a poorer outcome. Lacunar infarction carries a low mortality (121). Six months after cerebral infarction (of any kind), approximately 40% of patients are handicapped, and 25% are dead. The risk of recurrent stroke is 10% in the first year, and 5% in the following years (226). The risk of a cardiovascular event is also elevated (411). The clinical scales most commonly used for longitudinal study are the national Institutes of Health Stroke Scale (NIHSS) and the Modified Rankin Scale (MRS) (see Appendix, p. 940 ff.).

■ Specific Causes of Cerebrovascular Disease
■ Atherosclerosis

Frequency. Atherosclerosis is the most common disease affecting the cardiovascular system and the most common cause of death in the industrial world. It begins with microscopic intimal lesions and the accumulation of lipid-laden foam cells *(fatty streaks)*. Later, the intima thickens and contains *fibrous plaques,* consisting of cholesterol crystals enveloped in connective tissue. Fibrous plaques are found first in the aorta, later in the coronary and carotid arteries. They develop further into *complicated plaques,* containing calcification, necrosis, and ulceration, which can cause stenosis, thrombosis, em-

Table 2.**47**   Risk factors for atherosclerosis

Family history of atherosclerosis of early onset (before age 55)
Arterial hypertension*
Cigarette smoking*
Alcohol abuse*
Diabetes mellitus*
Hyperlipidemia:*   • Hypertriglyceridemia   • Low HDL-cholesterol level   • High LDL-cholesterol level
Truncal obesity*
Sleep apnea syndrome*
Oral contraceptives with high estrogen content*
Sedentary lifestyle*
Elevated fibrinogen concentration*
Elevated homocysteine concentration*
Male sex
Advanced age

* Treatable, modifiable, or preventable factors

bolism, and vascular occlusion. Patients with atherosclerosis of the arteries of the brain also have symptomatic or asymptomatic coronary artery disease in 40–60% of cases, occlusive peripheral vascular disease in 20%, and an asymptomatic abdominal aortic aneurysm in 15%.

Risk factors. The presence and severity of the risk factors listed in Table 2.**47** largely determine whether atherosclerosis will develop. Some of these factors are present at birth or constitute independent diseases (e.g., diabetes mellitus, hypothyroidism), while others are related to lifestyle (e.g., smoking, obesity, sedentary habits).

Sites of predilection. Atherosclerotic changes are most commonly found at vascular branch points and sites of curvature (Fig. 2.**55**), such as the origins and bifurcations of the major extracranial vessels (internal carotid artery, vertebral artery), the origin and bifurcation (or trifurcation) of the middle cerebral artery, and the proximal segments of the posterior cerebral artery. Involvement of the carotid siphon or of the vertebral artery at its loop around the atlas (V_3 segment) is usually found only in advanced atherosclerotic disease.

Small arteries and arterioles. Small arteries and arterioles are frequently affected by *arteriolosclerosis,* which is characterized by hyalinization, fibrous hyperplasia, and necrosis of the vascular intima and media. Arterial hypertension is the main risk factor for arteriolosclerosis.

Type of infarct. Thrombosis or arterio-arterial embolism due to atherosclerotic or arteriolosclerotic disease may produce either lacunar or territorial infarction, depending on the vessel affected.

Risk of stroke. The risk of stroke is positively correlated with the degree of vessel narrowing, as is well known in the case of the internal carotid artery. The risk becomes clinically significant once a 60–70% stenosis is

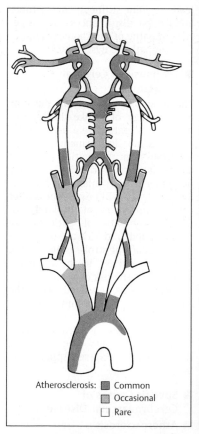

Fig. 2.**55   Localization of atherosclerosis in the cerebral arteries.**

reached, which corresponds to a residual luminal diameter of approximately 2 mm.

Identification of persons at risk. Persons at risk for stroke should be identified in young adulthood so that appropriate health counseling can be given (cf. Treatment, p. 206).

Subclavian steal syndrome. Subclavian steal syndrome is usually a manifestation of advanced atherosclerosis (412). If the subclavian artery is critically stenotic or occluded proximal to the origin of the vertebral artery, there may be a reversal of flow in the vertebral artery, so that blood is still supplied to the arm. The blood flowing in the vertebral artery is thus derived either from the contralateral vertebral artery or from the basilar artery, whence the name "subclavian steal" (187, 303). Subclavian steal is usually an incidental finding. It may manifest itself as a difference in blood pressure and in the intensity of the pulse in the two arms, or as a supraclavicular bruit. The diagnosis is established by cerebrovascular ultrasonography.

Subclavian steal occasionally causes symptoms such as weakness, pain, or sensory disturbances when the arm is used, as well as transient vertebrobasilar symptoms, such as paroxysmal dizziness, diplopia, visual impairment, or unsteadiness of gait, which arise either spontaneously, or when the arm is used. The degree of collateral flow around the circle of Willis largely determines whether symptoms will be present.

Causes of the subclavian steal syndrome other than atherosclerosis include arteritis (giant cell arteritis, Takayasu's disease) and mechanical influences leading to dissection and subsequent thrombosis of the subclavian artery (as in basketball players).

Atheromatous plaques of the aortic arch and ascending aorta. Such plaques are a possible source of arterio-arterial emboli causing stroke. They are an expression of advanced atherosclerosis, and patients in whom they are found usually have multiple other possible etiologies for stroke. Pathological studies and two different ultrasound studies have shown that such plaques are an independent risk factor for stroke, particularly when thicker than 4–5 mm (24, 476).

■ **Cardiogenic Embolism**

Cardiogenic embolism is diagnosed as the cause of stroke when a cardiac disease or dysrhythmia producing emboli is found to be present and other causes of stroke have been excluded (392). Typically, stroke due to cardiogenic embolism appears suddenly, without further progression of the deficit; the initial neurologic symptoms may be accompanied by palpitations or retrosternal pain and often reflect involvement of only a small cortical area, e.g. Wernicke's dysphasia or isolated homonymous hemianopsia. Yet even a characteristic presentation cannot be taken as conclusive evidence that cardiogenic embolism, rather than atherosclerosis, is the etiology. CT and MRI usually reveal a single, small territorial infarct, though multiple infarcts or a single lacune are sometimes seen. Hemorrhagic transformation of the infarct is more common than in the case of stroke of atherosclerotic origin. Emboli arising from infectious endocarditis or atrial myxoma may lead to the formation of cerebrovascular aneurysms, which are usually fusiform (643, 819).

The diagnosis is generally established by echocardiography and Holter-ECG monitoring, which should be performed in all stroke patients with a history of cardiac disease or an abnormality on clinical examination of the heart, and in all younger patients with stroke of undetermined cause. It has been shown that routine echocardiography and Holter monitoring in older patients with apparently normal cardiac status yield clinically relevant data in only 3% of cases, and such testing is therefore not recommended (293). Cardiac diseases associated with the production of emboli are listed in Table 2.**48**.

■ **Arterial Dissection**

Arterial dissection occurs in patients of both sexes, predominantly in early and mid-adulthood. The pathoanatomical process involves detachment of the inner (intimal) layer of the vessel wall from the tunica media. Thus, a "false lumen" between the two layers comes into being, which communicates with the true lumen through a tear in the intima. The false lumen may be a conduit for blood flow alongside the true lumen, if there is a second, distal intimal tear through which the blood can exit; it may form a saccular aneurysm; or it may become thrombosed. Thrombosis, in turn, may lead to vessel stenosis or occlusion over a long segment, distal progression of thrombus, or arterio-arterial thromboembolism and stroke. Of all cases of dissection of the cerebral arteries, 80% affect the carotid artery, 20% the vertebral artery, and 25% more than one vessel (839). Intracranial arterial dissection is rare

Table 2.**48** Cardiac conditions predisposing to cerebral emboli (after 293)

High risk:
- Atrial fibrillation
- Mitral stenosis
- Prosthetic heart valve
- Acute myocardial infarction
- Left ventricular thrombus
- Atrial myxoma
- Infectious endocarditis
- Dilated cardiomyopathy
- Nonbacterial thrombotic endocarditis
- Aneurysm of atrial septum

Low risk:
- Mitral valve prolapse
- Severe calcification of mitral annulus
- Patent foramen ovale
- Calcific aortic stenosis
- Left ventricular wall motion abnormality
- Mural aneurysm
- Spontaneous contrast on echocardiogram

in adults, but relatively common in children and adolescents (840).

Factors including trauma, hypertension, and vasculopathy (such as fibromuscular dysplasia and Marfan syndrome) predispose to arterial dissection, or are the immediate cause of it.

Carotid artery dissection presents with unilateral cervical, temporal, or orbital pain, Horner syndrome, and neurologic deficits relating to the ipsilateral cerebral hemisphere. The patient may complain of pulsatile tinnitus. The neurologic deficits are highly variable, ranging from an asymptomatic state to hemiplegia due to infarction in the territory of the middle cerebral artery. Lower cranial nerve deficits may appear, on the same side as the dissection—i.e., contralateral to the hemiparesis or other hemispheric signs. The appearance of crossed findings in the face and on the body may create the misleading impression of a brainstem syndrome.

Vertebral artery dissection causes ipsilateral cervical pain and vertebrobasilar stroke, most commonly infarction of the dorsolateral medulla (920). The manner of clinical presentation is variable, ranging from isolated pain in the neck or throat to a major brainstem stroke due to basilar artery thrombosis.

Arterial dissection can be diagnosed tentatively with ultrasound and definitively with MRI (918). Carotid artery dissection is typically seen as a stenosis or occlusion of the vessel near the skull base, in the absence of atheromatous changes of the vessel wall. In vertebral artery dissection, stenosis or occlusion is usually at the level of the loop around the atlas (V_3 segment). Spin-echo MRI may reveal a *mural thrombus* within the false lumen (Fig. 2.**56**). Residual flow in the vessel, if present, is seen as a flow void.

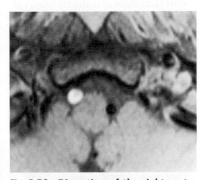

Fig. 2.**56** **Dissection of the right vertebral artery.** T1-weighted spin-echo image with fat suppression technique. The mural hematoma appears as a bright crescent surrounding the residual lumen.

■ Cerebral Infarction in Younger Patients

The annual incidence of cerebral infarction roughly doubles with each decade: it is ca. 0.4% at age 45 or 55, 0.8% at age 65, 1.8% at age 75, and 3.8% at age 85. Some 15% of all strokes affect patients under 65. The percentage of strokes due to atherosclerosis rises dramatically with age. In younger patients, the possible causes of stroke are numerous, as discussed above; the most common are cardiogenic emboli, dissection, and unknown (after a thorough diagnostic evaluation) (113, 332, 707). Practically any of the etiologies listed in Table 2.**44** may be responsible. Young adults are particularly susceptible to stroke resulting from drug and alcohol abuse (485, 576, 887) or from hypercoagulable states such as protein C, protein S, or antithrombin III deficiency, or resistance to activated protein C.

■ Venous Thrombosis and Venous Sinus Thrombosis

Thromboses of the cerebral veins and venous sinuses are somewhat more common in young women than in young men, but are still rare overall (accounting for ca. 1% of cerebral ischemic events). The more commonly involved structures are the superior sagittal and transverse sinuses, followed by the straight sinus, the cavernous sinus, and the cortical veins.

The clinical manifestations include headache, focal or generalized seizures, papilledema, and sensory and motor deficits (126). Thrombosis may be due to intracranial and systemic infection, or to a noninfectious etiology. All diseases associated with thromboembolism are possible

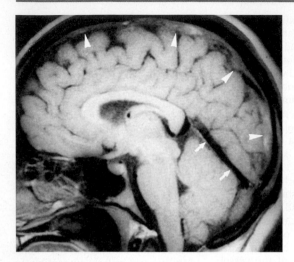

Fig. 2.**57** **Thrombosis of the superior sagittal sinus.** MRI of a 21-year-old woman. The cerebral venous sinuses usually appear dark in the spin-echo image (flow void). The sagittal T1-weighted image of this patient reveals paucity of signal in the straight sinus (arrows). The thrombosed superior sagittal sinus (arrowheads), however, is iso- or hyperintense in comparison to the brain parenchyma.

causes, in addition to gynecologic-obstetrical conditions in women and Behçet's disease in men (26). Imaging studies reveal uni- or bilateral hemorrhagic infarction. Thrombosis is usually visible by contrast-enhanced CT, or by MRI (Figs. 2.**57** and 2.**58**); MRI is the diagnostic method of choice.

■ Binswanger Disease

This disease mainly affects elderly hypertensives with multiple vascular risk factors; it may also be caused by conditions other than hypertension that cause small vessel disease, such as amyloid angiopathy or CADASIL (162) (see below). Its clinical manifestations include lacunar infarct syndromes, pseudobulbar and extrapyramidal motor syndromes, apathy, lack of interest, and cognitive deficits that progress in stepwise fashion, with stable intervals in between. The neuroradiologic and pathological findings include multiple lacunar infarcts in the basal ganglia, thalamus, pons, and white matter, as well as brain atrophy (cf. Fig. 2.**45**).

■ Amyloid Angiopathy

Cerebral amyloid angiopathy is a disease of old age (982). Rare familial forms (Icelandic and Dutch types) affect younger individuals.

Pathology

Amyloid deposits are found in small and middle-sized cerebral arteries, in the absence of systemic amyloidosis. Alzheimer-type lesions, including neuritic plaques and neurofibrillary tangles, are also seen (987).

Clinical Manifestations

Amyloid angiopathy manifests itself either as progressive dementia or as recurrent lobar hemorrhage, producing acute, focal neurologic deficits and ultimately leading to multi-infarct dementia.

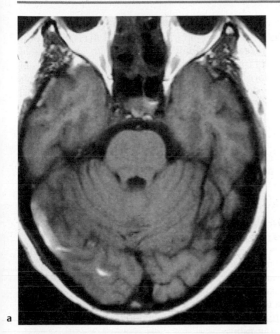

a

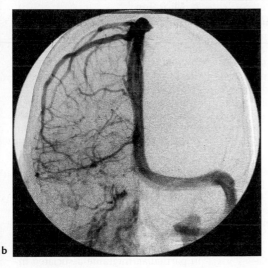

b

Fig. 2.**58a, b Thrombosis of the transverse sinus.** A 59-year-old woman with unusual right-sided headache and earache and a left homonymous visual field defect.

a The T1-weighted spin-echo image shows the thrombus in the right transverse sinus as a bright structure. A small hemorrhage in the occipital lobe is also seen.

b In the angiogram, only the left transverse sinus is seen.

Diagnostic Evaluation

The neuroradiologic findings are similar to those of Binswanger disease, often in addition to evidence of more or less recent subcortical hemorrhage (406). The diagnosis can be definitively established only by brain biopsy, but is considered highly likely in the elderly patient who has suffered 2 or more lobar hemorrhages and whose MRI reveals microangiopathic changes. There is no treatment.

■ CADASIL

Cerebral autosomal dominant arteriopathy with subcortical infarcts and leukoencephalopathy (CADASIL) is a genetic disorder of autosomal dominant inheritance that causes recurrent, usually lacunar strokes (479, 946). It has been traced to a mutation of the *notch-3* gene on chromosome 19p13.1 (478d). *De novo* mutations are rare (478c).

The pathologic findings include granular, eosinophilic deposits in the tunica media of smaller arteries in the brain, skeletal muscle, and skin. The illness often begins with complicated migraine attacks in young adulthood, later followed by clinically overt strokes. Progressive pyramidal and extrapyramidal motor signs and sensory and cognitive deficits ensue, typically leading to death by age 60 or 70. MRI reveals signal changes like those of microangiopathy of other causes; a distinct feature of CADASIL is that small vessel disease is additionally seen in the temporal poles and external capsules.

■ Fibromuscular Dysplasia (400)

Fibromuscular dysplasia is most commonly diagnosed in middle-aged women. Abnormal proliferation of the smooth muscle cells and fibrous and elastic elements of the arterial walls leads to a typical pattern of stenosis alternating with dilatation ("beads on a string"). Fibromuscular dysplasia predisposes to arterial dissection and to the formation of saccular aneurysms. It may affect the entire body and is typically most prominent in the renal arteries, visceral vessels, and extracranial and (less commonly) intracranial portions of the cerebral vasculature. It may announce its presence with a vascular bruit, pulsatile tinnitus, or TIA, or, less commonly, with a stroke, aneurysmal subarachnoid hemorrhage, or arterial dissection. Stenoses can usually be treated by endovascular dilatation.

■ Migraine

Most strokes associated with migraine affect the territory of the posterior cerebral artery (112). The following criteria must be met for the diagnosis of a migraine-associated stroke:

- history of migraine with neurologic manifestations,
- a neurologic deficit identical to that produced by previous migraine attacks,
- neuroradiologic demonstration of infarction, and
- exclusion of other possible causes.

Migraine is currently held to be a risk factor for stroke, but it is rarely the only one present in affected patients. In particular, migraine-associated infarcts must be carefully distinguished from other causes of stroke associated with headache; see also p. 805.

■ Arteritis (Vasculitis)

The vasculitides are an etiologically and morphologically heterogeneous group of conditions characterized by vascular inflammation and necrosis, which may lead to cerebral infarction. They may be either primary (i.e., idiopathic) or secondary to other illnesses (Table 2.**49**; cf. also p. 324 ff.) (383, 757).

Isolated (granulomatous) CNS angiitis. In most forms of vasculitis, the CNS manifestations are but one component of a clinical picture dominated by extracerebral involvement. In this disease, however, vascular inflammation is confined to the CNS (674) (p. 326); the peripheral nervous system, the retina, and the peripheral auditory apparatus are not involved. The major neurologic signs and symptoms include headache, cognitive impairment, and focal deficits due to usually multiple small strokes. The leukocyte count is usually elevated. Specific antibody titers may provide the key to diagnosis. CSF pleocytosis is often present, and angiography occasionally reveals inflammatory vascular changes. In some instances, the diagnosis can only be made by meningeal or brain biopsy.

CNS vasculitis. See p. 326.

Giant cell arteritis (689). See pp. 326, 816

■ Hypertensive Encephalopathy

This term designates a disturbance of brain function due to an acute, critical elevation of blood pressure, whether or not the patient previously suffered from chronic arterial hypertension. Its signs and symptoms are headache, nausea, vomiting, visual dysfunction, confusion and stupor, and (possibly)

Table 2.**49** Types of CNS vasculitis, and types of systemic vasculitis affecting the CNS (pp. 324 ff.)

Necrotizing arteritis:
- Isolated CNS vasculitis (p. 326)
- Giant-cell arteritis:
  - Cranial arteritis
  - Polymyalgia rheumatica
  - Takayasu's arteritis
- Periarteritis nodosa (p. 324)
- Wegener's granulomatosis (p. 326)
- Lymphomatoid granulomatosis
- Sarcoidosis (p. 329)

Autoimmune arteritis (p. 327):
- Systemic lupus erythematosus
- Sjögren's syndrome
- Rheumatoid arteritis
- Scleroderma
- Ulcerative colitis
- Mixed collagenosis (Sharp syndrome)

Infectious arteritis

Neoplastic arteritis

Iatrogenic arteritis due to medications

Arteritis secondary to drug abuse

Other types of arteritis:
- Sneddon syndrome
- Malignant atrophic papulosis (Köhlmeier-Degos disease)
- Behçet's disease
- Retinocochleocerebellar vasculopathy
- Cogan syndrome
- Susac syndrome
- Eales disease

focal neurologic deficits or focal or generalized epileptic seizures. The retinoscopic examination reveals retinal swelling and papilledema, as well as vasospasm of the small arteries. *Eclampsia* may be regarded as a special type of hypertensive encephalopathy arising during pregnancy.

The corresponding changes on the level of pathological anatomy include focal or diffuse cerebral edema, as well as acute or older cerebral infarcts and petechial hemorrhages, all of which are visible on MRI (177, 1009).

Treatment

Hypertensive encephalopathy is a medical emergency that must be treated by immediate pharmacologic reduction of blood pressure and the administration of anticonvulsants.

■ **"Vertebrobasilar Insufficiency"**

So-called vertebrobasilar insufficiency is a condition characterized by recurring TIAs in the vertebrobasilar distribution, over a period of months or years. In affected patients, turning the head or extending the neck often provokes such symptoms as occipital headache, diplopia, vertigo, cortical visual disturbances, drop attacks, and paresthesias and other sensory abnormalities in the face and extremities. The symptoms may be of crossed or alternating laterality; they resemble the initial symptoms of basilar artery thrombosis (298). The patients are usually elderly hypertensives with atherosclerosis, and they may also manifest a subclavian steal syndrome. The term "vertebrobasilar insufficiency" refers, not to a particular disease of unique etiology, but rather to a syndrome that may be produced by practically any type of arterial pathology in the vertebrobasilar distribution.

■ **Moyamoya**

Moyamoya is an idiopathic disease of the blood vessels of the brain that usually affects younger individuals. It presents with TIAs, ischemic stroke, cerebral hemorrhage, and epileptic seizures. It is rare in populations of European descent, and more common in Japan and elsewhere in the Far East. The major pathogenetic abnormality is slowly progressive stenosis and occlusion of the internal carotid arteries and other vessels of the circle of Willis, which induce the generation of a network of fine, abnormally fragile collateral vessels. These have the angiographic appearance of a "puff of smoke" (*moyamoya*, in Japanese) (1040).

■ **Antiphospholipid Antibody Syndrome**

The antiphospholipid antibody syndrome occurs in women and is characterized by the triad of
- recurrent spontaneous abortion,
- venous thromboses, and
- thrombocytopenia.

In this disorder, antiphospholipid antibodies cause thrombotic arterial occlusion of noninflammatory type, leading to an increased risk of ischemic stroke (294). Mitral valve abnormalities are often found on echocardiography and may lead to the formation of emboli that cause stroke.

Treatment

See Table 2.**51**, p. 204.

■ **Treatment of Stroke** (6a, 140b, 646a, 935b)

Overview:

A patient in the acute phase of ischemic stroke should be rapidly transported to a center with a fully equipped stroke treatment unit, as the chance of recovery is high if thrombolysis is performed by the intravenous route in the first 3 hours after the ictus, or by the intra-arterial route in the first 6 hours. The success of treatment depends on careful patient selection, with strict adherence to the accepted indications and contraindications. If thrombolysis cannot be performed, oral administration of aspirin is the best therapeutic alternative. Heparin is used only in specially selected cases. General medical measures for the treatment and prevention of complications of stroke are just as important as specific thrombolytic and antithrombotic therapy.

The options for the pharmacological treatment of acute ischemic stroke are listed in Table 2.50. The goal of treatment is the reopening of the arterial circulation, so that the ischemic cascade can be interrupted, and neuronal death in the ischemic penumbra prevented. Success depends on rapid intervention. Even if the vessel cannot be reopened, proper treatment may prevent the extension of a thrombus or the generation of further emboli.

Table 2.**50** Pharmacotherapy of acute ischemic stroke

First 3 hours after onset of symptoms:
• Intravenous or intra-arterial thrombolysis
• Aspirin, if thrombolysis is contraindicated
First 6 hours after onset of symptoms:
• Intra-arterial thrombolysis
• Aspirin, if thrombolysis is contraindicated
More than 6 hours after onset of symptoms:
• Aspirin
• Heparin: only in special circumstances (see Table 2.**51**)

Systemic intravenous thrombolysis:
Systemic intravenous thrombolysis with rt-PA (recombinant tissue plasmino-gen activator, 0.9 mg/kg i.v.) may be performed within 3 hours of the onset of symptoms (999a). Cerebral hemorrhage should be ruled out by CT or MRI before rt-PA is given, and neither heparin nor aspirin should be given concur-rently. Even if all of these precautions are taken, treatment may still be com-plicated by cerebral hemorrhage. It is thus advisable to adhere strictly to the NINDS guidelines for patient selection, and to have thrombolysis performed by a team of experienced neurovascular specialists (936). For every 1000 pro-cedures performed, 140 patients will be saved from permanent disability. The patients standing to benefit most are probably those with stroke of inter-mediate severity (10–30 points on the NIHSS scale). There is, however, no significant effect on mortality. The benefit of intravenous rt-PA is less after the first 3 hours and can be demonstrated, if at all, then only by post hoc analysis (179c, 373, 373b). It is therefore not recommended for use in hours 4, 5, and 6.

Selective intra-arterial thrombolysis:
Selective intra-arterial thrombolysis may be performed at any time up to 6 hours from the onset of symptoms, in a center with an interventional neu-roradiology team. It has been shown that intra-arterial application of uroki-nase can reopen occluded vessels and increase the probability of clinical re-covery (Figs. 2.**59** and 2.**60**) (352d). This was recently demonstrated in the prospective, randomized PROACT II Study, which involved the use of recom-binant pro-urokinase in patients with occlusion of the initial segment or main branches of the middle cerebral artery (322a). Treatment increased the rate of absence of disability (defined as Rankin grade 2 or lower; see mRS in the Appendix, p. 949) from 25% to 40% in absolute terms, corresponding to a 60% increase in relative terms, or to a sparing from disability in 150 of 1000 patients treated. Intra-arterial thrombolysis had no effect on stroke mortality. This technique is now increasingly combined with interventional thrombus retraction, which is expected to improve its success rate.
In cases of basilar artery thrombosis, local intra-arterial thrombolysis is gen-erally preferred to intravenous thrombolysis (373a) and can be performed more than 6 hours after the onset of symptoms, provided that the patient is not comatose. The state of consciousness before thrombolysis is an important prognostic factor.
Local intra-arterial thrombolysis with urokinase is also effective for the treat-ment of acute retinal ischemia due to occlusion of the central retinal artery (1000a).   ▶

There are no studies available at present to provide a direct comparison of the effectiveness of intravenous and intra-arterial thrombolysis. Patients with occlusion of the internal carotid artery, the initial segment or principal branches of the middle cerebral artery, or the basilar artery are probably more likely to benefit from intra-arterial than from intravenous therapy.

Treatment: Aspirin and Other Inhibitors of Platelet Aggregation

If thrombolysis is contraindicated by timing or other factors, aspirin is the best alternative for the treatment of nonembolic ischemic stroke (169a, 234a, 451a, 823). If aspirin is given in the first 48 hours, mortality is reduced by 1%, and the rate of full recovery is increased by 1%, in comparison with the natural history of the disease.

The use of other inhibitors of platelet aggregation, particularly glycoprotein IIb/IIIa antagonists, in the acute phase of stroke has so far been tested only in Phase II studies. These agents may soon become an important component of treatment.

Treatment: Nonfractionated Heparin, Low-Molecular-Weight Heparins and Heparinoids

The International Stroke Trial (823) found no therapeutic benefit of standard, nonfractionated *heparin*, given in a dose of 12,500 U s.c. b.i.d., for the treatment of acute stroke, because the excess rate of intra- and extracranial hemorrhage outweighed any possible beneficial effect. The results of this trial allow no conclusive determination of whether a lower heparin dose (5,000 U s.c. b.i.d.), given in combination with aspirin, is beneficial or detrimental. *Fractionated low-molecular-weight heparin* was of no greater benefit than standard heparin, and another study likewise showed no greater benefit from the *heparinoid* Orgaran (danaparoid). In summary, heparin or heparinoids are generally not indicated in the treatment of acute ischemic stroke, because they raise the rate of hemorrhage and thus pose a danger to the patient.

On the venous side–i.e., in cases of *cerebral venous thrombosis and venous sinus thrombosis*–two small prospective, randomized studies have shown a benefit of treatment with heparin (221c, 270). The current indications for heparin treatment are summarized in Table 2.**51**. Heparin should not be given to patients with very large infarcts of whatever etiology.

In embolic stroke due to atrial fibrillation, the risk of reinfarction in the acute phase is lower than that of heparin-induced hemorrhage. Thus aspirin, rather than heparin, is given in the first 2 weeks after the event, and then switched to oral anticoagulation. For stroke due to septic emboli in bacterial endocarditis, antibiotic therapy is the most important mode of treatment, and surgical valve replacement may be necessary. Anticoagulation should be given in cases of septic embolism only when the presence of mycotic cerebral aneurysms has been definitively ruled out (p. 192) (148).

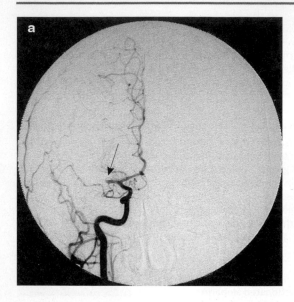

Fig. 2.**59a, b Right internal carotid artery angiogram in a patient with acute left hemiplegia, hemisensory deficit, and hemianopsia.**

a The main stem of the middle cerebral artery is occluded (arrowheads). Only the anterior cerebral artery is seen.

b After successful thrombolysis, the main stem and branches of the middle cerebral artery are well seen. The patient recovered completely and returned to work.

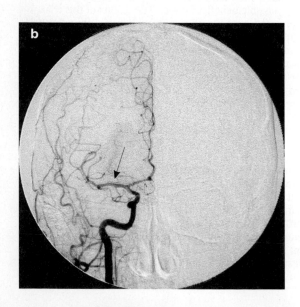

Treatment: Other Measures for Acute Ischemic Stroke; the Stroke Unit

The cerebral and extracerebral complications of stroke listed on p. 190 ff. are major contributors to stroke morbidity and mortality (7). The likelihood that they will be recognized and successfully treated is higher in a dedicated stroke unit, staffed by a specialized stroke team, than in a general medical ward (553a). Abnormalities of fluid and electrolyte balance should be corrected. An elevated hematocrit (50% or above) should be treated by hemodilution, phlebotomy, or both, epileptic seizures with anticonvulsants (phenytoin, clonazepam or others), and concomitant infections with antibiotics. No beneficial effect has been shown for the routine administration to all stroke patients of *hemodilution, calcium antagonists* and *corticosteroids,* nor have the so-called neuroprotective agents shown any benefit to date. Fever increases brain damage due to stroke and should be aggressively treated with antipyretics (374c).

Careful attention must be paid to the patient's respiratory and circulatory status, as abnormalities of either will worsen the brain damage due to stroke. The most common causes of hypoxia are partial airway obstruction, hypoventilation, aspiration pneumonia, and atelectasis. Cardiac dysrhythmias may not only cause stroke, they may also be the direct cause of death of a patient in the acute phase of stroke (714). Patients with medullary infarcts are at greatest risk. Hypertension in the acute phase of stroke should not be aggressively treated, except in cases of hypertensive encephalopathy; in general, it should be gently lowered, and only when the systolic blood pressure exceeds 200 mmHg, or the diastolic blood pressure 110 mmHg. A normal or even elevated blood pressure is necessary in the acute phase to preserve adequate circulation in the ischemic penumbra through collateral vessels.

For the same reason, *bed rest* is indicated in the first few days after stroke. In this phase, prophylactic treatment against deep venous thrombosis and pulmonary embolism must be given, including *physiotherapy, compression stockings,* and, in patients who will be bedridden for longer periods, *fractionated heparin* (822). A somewhat elevated bleeding tendency must be accepted as the inevitable price of antithrombotic therapy. If the patient remains bedridden, adequate nursing care is necessary to prevent decubitus ulcers.

Cerebral edema with mass effect may complicate larger infarcts in the carotid or middle cerebral artery territories, as well as cerebellar infarcts. Edema is of maximal severity 2–4 days after the acute event and may lead to transtentorial herniation, brainstem compression, and death, particularly in younger patients (who lack the brain atrophy associated with old age, and thus have less room in the cranial vault for an expanding mass). A *cerebellar infarct* exerting substantial mass effect should be treated by *neurosurgical decompression,* as long as a large volume of the brainstem is not infarcted as well; this would confer a poor prognosis with or without surgery. Decompression allows these patients to survive the acute phase, and often to make a good recovery, and even regain functional independence. Intracranial hypertension due to a *supratentorial infarct* with severe mass effect is treated in most centers by *eleva-*

▶

tion of the upper body and head (i.e., raising the head of the bed to 30°), the administration of *steroids* and *mannitol, intubation, pharmacologic muscle paralysis,* and *controlled, mild hyperventilation,* until the phase of maximal cerebral edema is past. The optimal treatment in this situation remains unknown. Early *decompressive craniectomy* is a rational method of providing room for the expanding, edematous brain, and thus preventing herniation and brainstem compression (315, 856c). *Hypothermia,* too, may be useful in lowering the intracranial pressure. Hypothermia has a general neuroprotective effect and may turn out to be a routine component of future therapy for acute stroke (854b).

Table 2.**51**   Indications for heparin in acute ischemic stroke

Cerebral venous thrombosis or venous sinus thrombosis[1]
Extracranial carotid or vertebral artery dissection[2]
Acute infarct associated with high-grade carotid stenosis[2]
Documented intraluminal thrombus in a cerebral artery[2]
Cardiogenic emboli with high risk of recurrence[2]
Hypercoagulable states (protein C deficiency, protein S deficiency, antithrombin III deficiency, antiphospholipid antibody syndrome)[2]

1. Recommendation based on prospective, randomized studies.
2. Recommendation based on indirect evidence.

Perfusion- and diffusion-weighted MRI 3 hours after the onset of left hemiparesis. Angiography reveals occlusion of a branch of the right middle cerebral artery. Images were obtained before (**a–c**) and after (**d–f**) local intra-arterial thrombolysis of the middle cerebral artery.

a The T2-weighted spin-echo image appears normal and fails to reveal the ischemic area.
b The diffusion-weighted image clearly reveals the ischemic area in the right central region as an area of hyperintense signal.
c In the perfusion-weighted (time-to-peak) image, the ischemic area appears bright (hyperintense), because it is less well perfused than the surrounding tissue.
d The T2-weighted image obtained after successful thrombolysis reveals a very mild signal change in the right central region.
e, f The signal abnormality has normalized almost completely on the diffusion-weighted image (**e**), and completely on the perfusion-weighted image (**f**). The latter demonstrates full reconstitution of the circulation and thus documents the successful recanalization.

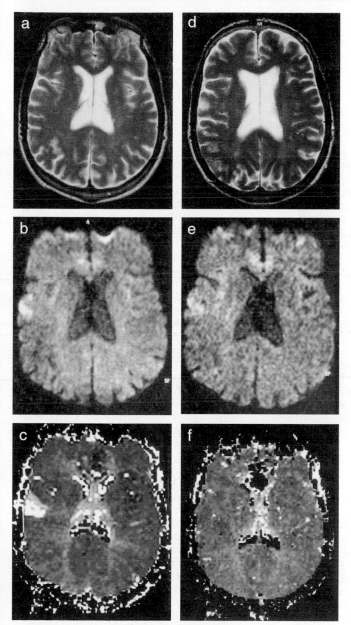

Fig. 2.**60a–f Middle cerebral artery occlusion.**

■ **Stroke Prevention** (61, 293, 352a, 637)

Definition:
Stroke prevention consists of three types of measures: the treatment or elimination of risk factors for stroke, pharmacotherapy, and surgical intervention. Endovascular techniques may soon become an important fourth modality. Modification of risk factors is the most important means of stroke prevention, whether primary or secondary (i.e., after the patient has already had a stroke or other vascular event).

Modification of Risk Factors
(see Table 2.47)
The following are treatable or eliminable risk factors for stroke:
- cigarette smoking,
- hypertension,
- diabetes mellitus,
- obesity,
- hyperlipidemia,
- sleep apnea syndrome,
- cardiac disease, especially atrial fibrillation,
- alcohol and drug abuse (34, 1004, 1033).

Furthermore, regular exercise and proper diet improve the vascular risk profile (229d, 352a, 437c, 478b, 566b) and lessen the incidence of vascular events of all types, including brain infarction.

Medical stroke prevention. The most important agents given to prevent ischemic stroke are aspirin and other *inhibitors of platelet aggregation,* and *oral anticoagulants.*
Aspirin, when used as *primary prevention* of vascular events, prevents approximately one in three nonfatal myocardial infarctions. This effect is canceled out, however, by a rise in the frequency of (presumably hemorrhagic) stroke. Aspirin thus has no effect on combined mortality due to vascular and nonvascular causes.

When used as *secondary prevention,* aspirin reduces the frequency of ischemic stroke by 23%, myocardial infarction by 36%, and death from all vascular causes by 14% (31). The reduction of relative risk for ischemic stroke was somewhat lower (13%) in a meta-analysis of the use of aspirin by patients who had already had a cerebrovascular event (but no other kind of vascular event) (17c). Thus, in patients who have already had a first stroke or TIA, aspirin may prevent between 1 in 4 and 1 in 8 further ischemic strokes. The lowest effective dose of aspirin after TIA is 30 mg p.o. qd, and after ischemic stroke 25 mg p.o. b.i.d. (935a). The optimal dose is still debated (257); we give 250 mg p.o. qd. The combination of aspirin and dipyridamole is more effective than either alone (935a). Monotherapy with clopidogrel is also more effective than aspirin; although clopidogrel is much more expensive than aspirin, its use in high-risk patients is both medically and economically justified (166a, 383a). In patients who cannot tolerate aspirin or have no therapeutic response to it, clopidogrel is the best alternative. The combination of aspirin with clopidogrel is more effective than either alone for cardiac patients, but has not been adequately tested in patients with cerebrovascular disease.

Oral anticoagulants (vitamin K antagonists) are indicated as the continuation of therapy in all stroke patients treated with heparin in the acute phase. Anticoagulants are generally given for 3–6 months on an empirical basis and then replaced with an inhibitor of platelet aggregation. For patients with venous thrombosis and venous sinus thrombosis, we usually give oral anticoagulants for 1 year; for patients with cardiogenic emboli or hypercoagulable states, we give them indefinitely. Anticoagulants may also be used for a limited time in patients who do not respond to antiplatelet agents, e.g., patients who continue to experience TIAs despite the administration of aspirin. Anticoagulants probably also protect better than aspirin against recurrent stroke in patients with stenosis of a major intracranial artery (178).

Stroke prevention is particularly important in patients with *atrial fibrillation,* a condition associated with more than 10% of all ischemic strokes (392a). Anticoagulation is the prophylactic treatment of choice in patients with symptomatic atrial fibrillation, as well as in asymptomatic patients with clinical evidence of heart failure, a history of hypertension or thromboembolism, or ultrasonographic evidence of left atrial enlargement or left ventricular dysfunction. (The optimal dose is that corresponding to an INR of 2–3 for patients with nonvalvular atrial fibrillation, and 3–4 for patients with valvular atrial fibrillation.) All other patients may be treated with aspirin, and patients under 60 years of age with isolated atrial fibrillation can be treated by clinical follow-up alone (259, 390, 392a).

Vasculitis is treated with *immunosuppressive agents* such as prednisone, cyclophosphamide, and azathioprine. *Antilipid agents* are used to treat *hypercholesterolemia* in patients with documented atherosclerosis. Lovastatin improves carotid arteriosclerosis and lowers the incidence of ischemic stroke and myocardial infarction, as well as mortality from myocardial infarction (322). In *cardiovascular* patients with high or normal cholesterol levels, simvastatin, pravastatin (1017b) or atorvastatin lowers the incidence of ischemic, but not hemorrhagic, stroke by 20 to 30% (4S, CARE, LIPID, HPS, and MIRACL studies). Studies in *cerebrovascular* patients, e.g., with atorvastatin, are in progress.

Surgical stroke prevention. Surgical prophylaxis has been shown effective in patients with *symptomatic, high-grade (> 70%) stenosis of the internal carotid artery.* A therapeutic benefit of lesser magnitude has also been demonstrated in patients with intermediate stenosis (50–70%). For these types of patients, *carotid endarterectomy* significantly reduces the risk of ischemic stroke and death from vascular causes (287, 697). Patients with asymptomatic, high-grade carotid stenosis have also been found to benefit from endarterectomy, but the risk reduction in this group is only ca. 1% per year (42).

Patients with *congenital heart defects* may benefit from surgical correction not only through the improvement in cardiac function, but also through the reduction of risk for stroke.

Endovascular therapies. Symptomatic subclavian steal syndrome may be elegantly treated by *transluminal angioplasty* of the stenotic subclavian artery (937). If the subclavian artery is occluded, a surgical external carotid–subclavian bypass may be considered. The possible benefit of angioplasty in carotid stenosis remains an open question, and is currently the subject of 4 separate studies. A *patent foramen ovale* can be closed by the endovascular route as effectively as by surgery, with a lower risk of complications (1029a). The PC Trial, now in progress, is intended to determine whether cerebrovascular events can be prevented by this technique.

The importance of treatment. It is clear that physicians in ambulatory practice and in smaller community hospitals have fewer resources at their disposal for the diagnosis and treatment of stroke than their counterparts in major university centers. Nonetheless, stroke being the third most common cause of death in our society, we strongly advise that its occurrence should not simply be accepted fatalistically, but that a major professional effort, as well as material resources, should be directed toward its prevention and treatment. The physician must decide in each case how intensively the available diagnostic and therapeutic modalities are to be used.

■ **Rehabilitation after Stroke**

Rehabilitation after a stroke is tailored to the neurologic deficit(s) of the individual patient, and includes physical and occupational therapy, speech therapy, and other directed neuropsychological exercises, as well as psychological support. The goals of rehabilitation are the prevention of complications of immobility (pneumonia, decubitus ulcers, deep venous thrombosis and pulmonary embolism); the promotion of independence, including, if possible, return to work; and the psychological support of the patient and his or her family, including encouragement of the patient as he or she learns to live with neurological disability.

Intracerebral Hemorrhage of Nontraumatic Origin (493, 630)

Definition:

Intracerebral hemorrhage accounts for 10–12% of all cases of stroke. Its hallmark is a rapidly progressive neurologic deficit; large hemorrhages often present with coma. The nature and severity of the deficit are directly related to the location and magnitude of the hemorrhage. Persons with long-standing, untreated arterial hypertension are at greatest risk. Other causes include amyloid angiopathy, tumors, coagulopathies and anticoagulant medications, aneurysms, arteriovenous malformations, cavernomas, drug abuse, trauma, and secondary hemorrhage into an infarct. The diagnosis is established by CT or MRI, and further diagnostic studies are indicated depending on the findings. Neurosurgical clot evacuation is indicated as a potentially life-saving measure in patients with lobar supratentorial or cerebellar hemorrhages that are large enough to impair consciousness.

Table 2.**52**   Causes of cerebral hemorrhage

Chronic arterial hypertension	**Head trauma:**
Aneurysm	• Primary hemorrhagic contusion
Vascular malformation:	• Shear injury
• Arteriovenous malformation	• Vascular avulsion
• Cavernoma	• Secondary (Duret) hemorrhage
• Capillary telangiectasis	**Hemorrhage into preexisting lesions:**
• Venous angioma	• Primary brain tumors
Abnormally fragile vessels:	• Metastases
• Amyloid angiopathy	• Granulomas
• Vasculitis	**Hemorrhagic infarct, secondary hemorrhage into infarct**
• Sickle-cell anemia	**Other, rare causes:**
Bleeding diatheses:	• Migraine
• Use of anticoagulants (vitamin K antagonists, heparin, inhibitors of platelet aggregation)	• Acute hypertension in eclampsia, pheochromocytoma, glomerulonephritis
• Use of fibrinolytic agents	• Vasopressor medications
• Thrombocytopenia	• After carotid endarterectomy
• Hemophilia	• After surgery for an arteriovenous malformation
• Leukemia	• Extreme physical exertion
Drug abuse	• Severe, acute pain
Venous thrombosis, venous sinus thrombosis	• Acute cold exposure
	• Fat embolism
Infectious endocarditis, septic embolism	• Supratentorial hemorrhage after surgery in the posterior fossa

Patients with spontaneous (nontraumatic) intracerebral hemorrhage are 10 years younger, on average, than patients with ischemic stroke. Intracerebral hemorrhage accounts for 10–12 % of all cases of stroke.

There are many possible causes, and the etiologic spectrum varies with age. In children, the more common causes are vascular malformations, aneurysms, and hematologic conditions such as thrombocytopenia, leukemia, and hemophilia. The causes in young adults include all of these, as well as arterial hypertension, alcohol intoxication, and drug abuse (943). In middle-aged and elderly patients,

most intracerebral hemorrhages are caused by arterial hypertension, amyloid angiopathy, tumors, vascular malformations, and aneurysms, and, occasionally, vasculitis (Table 2.**52**) (630). A low serum cholesterol level confers a mildly *elevated* risk of intracerebral hemorrhage, though it lowers the risk of ischemic stroke, as discussed above.

Clinical Manifestations

Spontaneous intracerebral hemorrhage occurs more commonly in waking hours than during sleep (307). The typical presentation is the sudden appearance and rapid progression of a neurologic deficit, whose nature is determined by the site of the hemorrhage (494, 796). Nearly half of all patients have intense headache, as opposed to only 5–15% of those with ischemic stroke. Nine percent have epileptic seizures. One-third of patients vomit, often when blood enters the cerebral ventricles or when the intracranial pressure rises as the result of a large intraparenchymal hematoma. Reflex elevation of blood pressure usually occurs in the acute phase of intracerebral hemorrhage and may be interpreted as a homeostatic response to maintain cerebral perfusion. High blood pressure on admission is thus not indicative of prior chronic hypertension, which can, however, be suspected if hypertensive retinopathy is found on retinoscopic examination, or if the left ventricle is enlarged.

Etiological Differential Diagnosis

The history and imaging studies provide clues to the etiology of hemorrhage in the individual case. Abnormalities of the brain parenchyma should be sought. The site of the hemorrhage may make some etiologies more likely and others less, although, in principle, any type of hemorrhage may occur at any site. Multiple hemorrhages have a different etiologic spectrum than single hemorrhages; they may be due to a bleeding diathesis, metastases, vasculitis, sepsis, amyloid angiopathy, or thrombosis of the cerebral veins and venous sinuses.

■ Etiology and Site of Hemorrhage

Hypertensive hemorrhage. The more common sites of hypertensive hemorrhage are the basal ganglia, thalamus, pons, and cerebellum (Fig. 2.**61**). Bleeding arises from tiny, miliary protuberances (Charcot-Bouchard aneurysms) of small arteries affected by lipohyalinosis, a type of pathological change caused by chronic arterial hypertension. Sensory and motor hemisyndromes, hemianopsia, and (in cerebellar hemorrhage) ataxia are typical clinical findings. Hemorrhages larger than 3 cm in diameter confer a worse prognosis.

Lobar hemorrhage. These are defined as hemorrhages in the cerebral hemispheres not involving the basal ganglia and thalamus. They may be of any of the following types:

- *Aneurysmal hemorrhage:* aneurysms of the anterior communicating artery, or of the bi- or trifurcation of the middle cerebral artery, may rupture into the parenchyma of the frontal lobe (preseptal area) or the temporal lobe, respectively. Subarachnoid hemorrhage usually occurs simultaneously.
- *Amyloid angiopathy:* see p. 194.
- *Bleeding diathesis:* Vitamin K antagonists, heparin, fibrinolytic agents, thrombocytopenia, leukopenia, sepsis, and hepatic disease predispose to intracerebral hemorrhage. In patients with these conditions, headaches that are unusual in quality or intensity should prompt suspicion of an intracerebral hemorrhage (312, 635).
- *Drug abuse:* The use of various illegal drugs may be complicated by intracerebral hemorrhage, particularly "crack" cocaine and amphetamines. Hemorrhage is presumably due to a sudden elevation of blood pressure, or to drug-induced vasculitis. Persons who abuse heroin in-

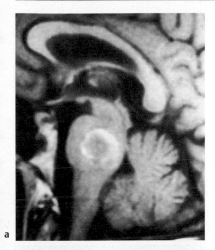

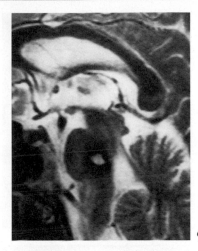

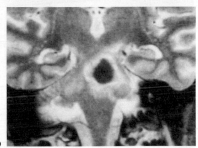

Fig. 2.**61a–c Pontine hemorrhage, probably due to cavernoma.**
a Sagittal T1-weighted spin-echo image after onset of symptoms. Signal hyperintensity at the periphery of the hematoma is due to methemoglobin.
b T2-weighted image in the acute phase. The hematoma still appears hypointense and is surrounded by a ring of edema (hyperintensity).
c T2-weighted image 2 months after hemorrhage. There is central hyperintensity, due to methemoglobin, and peripheral hypointensity, due to hemosiderin.

travenously may develop endocarditis complicated by septic embolism, mycotic cerebral aneurysms, and subarachnoid hemorrhage.

• *Tumors:* Hemorrhage associated with brain tumors is often multiple. It occurs mainly in cases of metastatic disease, particularly bronchial carcinoma, melanoma, choriocarcinoma, renal cell carcinoma, and thyroid carcinoma. Marked edema is usually seen in the area surrounding the hemorrhage. For hemorrhagic infarction and secondary hemorrhage into an infarct, see p. 188.

• *Cavernoma:* See Fig. 2.**12**, p. 70.

Arteriovenous malformation. An arteriovenous malformation (AVM; Fig. 2.**62**) (646b, 933a) is a congenital anomaly consisting of abnormally dilated arteries and veins on either side of a cluster of capillaries (nidus) containing numerous direct arteriovenous anastomoses. 10% of AVMs have one or more saccular aneurysms on their feeding arteries. The lesion is

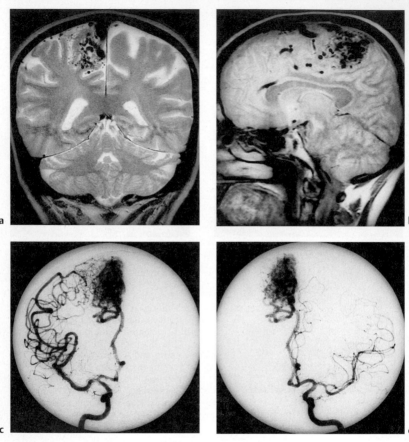

Fig. 2.**62a–d Arteriovenous malformation** (unruptured).

a Coronal, T2-weighted spin-echo image. The feeding and draining vessels, and part of the nidus, appear as zones of decreased signal (flow voids).

b Parasagittal, proton-density image of the same lesion.

c Right carotid arteriography. The malformation is fed by the right middle cerebral and pericallosal arteries.

d Left carotid angiography. The left pericallosal artery also contributes to the arterial supply of the lesion, which lies in the right hemisphere.

surrounded by gliotic tissue. Most AVMs lie on the cortical surface. The most important characteristics affecting the planning of treatment for an individual AVM are: the size of the ni-

dus, the number of feeding vessels, the type of venous drainage (superficial or deep), and the functional importance of the brain area in which it is located (555, 898). AVMs are often incidentally discovered on CT or MRI studies ordered for other purposes. Ultrasonography reveals increased flow velocity and decreased pulsatility of the feeding vessels as compared to normal cortical arteries (75).

Clinical Presentation

Seventy percent of symptomatic AVMs present with intracerebral and subarachnoid hemorrhage. Some 30–65% cause focal and generalized epileptic seizures in the absence of prior hemorrhage (188c). Other manifestations include migraine-like headache, focal neurologic deficits depending on the location of the AVM, pulsatile tinnitus, and intracranial hypertension.

Natural History

The annual risk of hemorrhage is 1–2% for an unruptured AVM and 2–4% for one that has already ruptured at least once. The mortality of the first hemorrhage is ca. 10%, and that of subsequent hemorrhages ca. 20% each; the risk of permanent disability from each hemorrhage is ca. 25% (144, 194, 725). The incidence of epilepsy (i.e., the risk of newly developed epilepsy) is ca. 1% per year.

Treatment

The goal of treatment is the elimination of the AVM. The feasibility and attendant risks of neurosurgical resection, of endovascular occlusion by the interventional neuroradiologist, and of radiosurgical obliteration by means of a gamma knife, linear accelerator, or proton beam must be assessed individually in every case. A combined technique, consisting of endovascular occlusion followed by resection or radiosurgery, has been found useful. Epilepsy is treated symptomatically with anticonvulsants. In view of the high cumulative risk of hemorrhage from an untreated AVM, as well as the demonstrated beneficial effect of treatment on AVM-associated epilepsy, a neurosurgical or interventional-endovascular treatment is considered advisable, whenever the risk is not prohibitive. Stereotactic radiosurgery has a lower immediate risk than surgery or endovascular treatment but, unlike them, does not result in immediate elimination of the AVM, because the effect of radiation therapy takes place over time. Hemorrhage may still occur at any time until the AVM is completely obliterated, which may be 2 or 3 years after radiosurgical treatment.

Special types of AVM. *Intraventricular AVMs* may present with spontaneous ventricular hemorrhage. *Orbital AVMs* may present with unilateral exophthalmos, worsening on lowering of the head or performance of the Valsalva maneuver. *Carotid–cavernous fistulae* are often of traumatic origin and are thus not true AVMs in the histological sense. They present with painful, pulsatile exophthalmos, tense dilatation of retinal and conjunctival veins, disturbances of ocular motility and vision, and a both subjectively and objectively audible vascular bruit over the orbit or the zygoma. Purely *dural AVMs* ("dural arteriovenous fistulae") are mostly located in the posterior fossa and usually present with pulsatile tinnitus. They may cause intracerebral hemorrhage if the elevation of venous pressure is transmitted in retrograde fashion to nearby cerebral veins.

Venous angioma. This term refers to an unusually dilated vein at an anatomically anomalous location in the deep white matter. Venous angiomas are generally of no clinical consequence. Similar-looking anomalous veins sometimes represent the venous side of an arteriovenous fistula and thus contain abnormally high blood flow under elevated (arterial) pressure. Venous angiomas are occasionally seen in association with cavernomas or other malformations. In such cases, it is the cavernoma, rather than the venous angioma, that poses a risk of hemorrhage (788).

Intracerebral hemorrhage of undetermined etiology. It is not always possible to establish the etiology of an intracerebral hemorrhage. Patients in this situation should undergo follow-up imaging a few months after the hemorrhage, because certain tumors or vascular anomalies (AVMs) may escape detection in the acute phase.

Traumatic intracerebral hemorrhage (335). See p. 50.

Brainstem hemorrhage. Pontine hemorrhage is usually due to hypertension, while midbrain and medullary hemorrhages are often due to a cavernoma. The clinical features of brainstem hemorrhage depend on its location. Major pontine hemorrhages of hypertensive origin often produce locked-in syndrome and are usually fatal.

Cerebellar hemorrhage (Fig. 2.63). Cerebellar hemorrhage is most commonly caused by hypertension, followed by anticoagulation, arteriovenous malformations, and embolic stroke. It presents with a disturbance of limb coordination and gait. Larger hemorrhages cause brainstem compression, leading to impairment of consciousness, coma, or death.

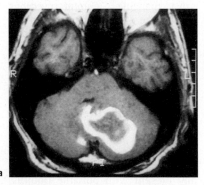

a

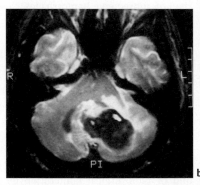

b

Fig. 2.**63a, b Cerebellar hemorrhage due to cavernoma.** MRI in subacute phase, a few days after the hemorrhage.

a T1-weighted spin-echo image. The periphery of the hematoma is bright because of its high methemoglobin content. Observe the mass effect with displacement and compression of the fourth ventricle.

b T2-weighted spin-echo image. At this early phase, deoxyhemoglobin and methemoglobin are still contained in intact erythrocytes. The hematoma appears dark and is surrounded by a thin, brighter rim of cerebral edema.

■ Diagnostic Evaluation of Intracerebral Hemorrhage

Intracerebral hemorrhage is diagnosed by imaging. CT is the modality of choice. In many centers, only a CT scan is available for acute neuroradiologic study, but CT may fail to detect relevant changes of the brain parenchyma, particularly cavernomas, the abnormal vessels of an AVM, or traumatic shear injuries. Thus, whenever the etiology of an intracerebral hemorrhage remains unclear after a CT scan, an MRI scan should be obtained. If the MRI is not sufficiently informative, an *angiogram* should be performed in all younger patients; angiography may be dispensed with for older patients, in whom hypertension or amyloid angiopathy are presumed to be the most likely etiologies. CT has the disadvantage, compared to MRI, that an initially hyperdense hematoma becomes isodense to the surrounding brain within a few weeks, and hypodense afterward, so that, in later stages, it is no longer recognizable as a hematoma (p. 132). Cerebrospinal fluid examination is rarely helpful in the diagnostic evaluation of intracerebral hemorrhage. If a tumor is suspected, follow-up imaging or a biopsy may be required.

▌Treatment and Prognosis▐

Impaired consciousness, a large hematoma, midline shift, and intraventricular rupture are all negative prognostic factors (956). If a hematoma is large enough to impair consciousness, *emergency neurosurgical evacuation* may be life-saving (721). Patients with brain hemorrhages (particularly in the cerebellum) should be kept for at least 48 hours in a center where immediate neurosurgical intervention can be performed if necessary. Clot evacuation does not, however, reduce neurologic disability. It is thus not warranted in awake patients, in patients with hypertensive hemorrhages with mass effect, or in patients with hemorrhages due to amyloid angiopathy. If the hemorrhage is due to coagulopathy or anticoagulation, blood clotting should be normalized by the *intravenous infusion of fresh frozen plasma or clotting factors*. Approximately 25% of surviving patients have a neurologic deficit 1 year after hemorrhage (299).

Subarachnoid Hemorrhage (268a, 538, 647, 972, 860b)

Definition:

Nontraumatic subarachnoid hemorrhage (SAH)—i.e., hemorrhage into the subarachnoid space—is usually due to rupture of a saccular aneurysm and usually presents with sudden, intense headache and meningism. Focal neurologic deficits are often absent; when present, they are mostly due to vasospasm, or to bleeding directly into the brain parenchyma. If untreated, aneurysmal subarachnoid hemorrhage confers a high mortality. The goal of treatment is the elimination of the source of bleeding as soon as possible. Neurosurgical treatment is usually required.

Nontraumatic SAH accounts for ca. 7% of all cerebrovascular accidents ("strokes," in the widest sense of the term). More than half of all cases of nontraumatic SAH are due to the rupture of saccular aneurysms; cigarette smoking, hypertension, and alcohol abuse are risk factors for aneurysmal SAH. Nontraumatic SAH may also arise from arteriovenous malformations, tumors, vasculitides, amyloid angiopathy and coagulopathies (791). The source of bleeding cannot be determined in up to 20% of cases of SAH; benign perimesencephalic SAH is a subgroup of cases of this type (971).

Saccular aneurysms are rarely familial. Predisposing conditions include polycystic kidney disease, Ehlers-Danlos syndrome, Marfan syndrome, and fibromuscular dysplasia (141). Aneurysmal SAH is somewhat more common in women. The average age at the time of hemorrhage is 50 years. The source of bleeding is occasionally at the spinal level; in such cases, the initial pain is often in the back or neck, rather than the head. Aneurysms develop preferentially at bifurcations of the major arteries of the base of the brain, where the internal elastic layer of the vessel wall is at its weakest (Fig. 2.**64**). Aneurysms are

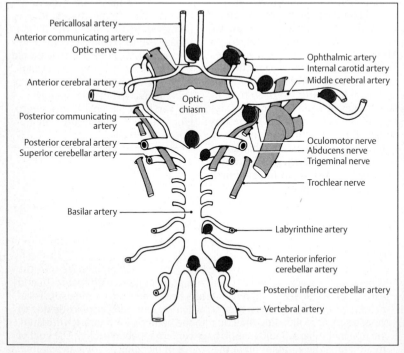

Fig. 2.**64 Common locations of saccular aneurysms, and their relations to some of the cranial nerves.** Aneurysms are typically found at vascular bifurcations.

sometimes multiple, though an acute aneurysmal SAH is generally due to rupture of a single aneurysm, even when multiple aneurysms are present.

General Clinical Features

The characteristic presenting symptom of SAH is a sudden, intense headache which is unusual for the patient in both intensity and quality, even if he or she has previously suffered from headache. The headache of SAH is usually diffusely localized, but may be predominantly occipital. The appearance of headache may be accompanied by a brief loss of consciousness, nausea, and vomiting, as well as focal neurologic deficits, including cranial nerve deficits. More than a few cases are preceded, in the days or weeks before the overt hemorrhage,

by minor symptoms that are usually traced to the aneurysm only in retrospect (the so-called "warning leak") (561). Meningism usually develops gradually, though it may be present immediately after the acute event in some cases, or absent in small hemorrhages. Preretinal vitreous hemorrhage is found in one out of 10 patients (Terson syndrome) (1011).

The clinical severity of SAH is assessed on two different scales (Table 2.53). The Hunt and Hess scale is older, and more familiar in neurosurgical practice, while the WFNS scale has largely replaced it in published reports.

Special clinical features, depending on type and location of aneurysm. Aneurysms of the *anterior communicating artery* may bleed into the un-

Table 2.**53a**   Hunt and Hess grading scale for subarachnoid hemorrhage (446)

Hunt and Hess grade	Clinical features
I	Headache, mild meningeal signs
II	Severe headache and severe meningeal signs
III	Somnolent, disoriented, possible mild focal neurologic deficit
IV	Unresponsive, severe focal neurologic deficit
V	Comatose, possibly with signs of transtentorial herniation

Table 2.**53b**   WFNS grading scale for subarachnoid hemorrhage (860b)

WFNS grade	Glasgow Coma Scale	Focal neurologic deficit
I	15	Absent
II	13–14	Absent
III	13–14	Present
IV	7–12	Present or absent
V	3–6	Present or absent

WFNS: World Federation of Neurological Societies.

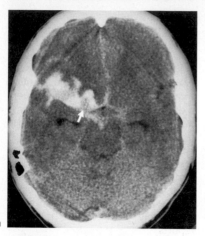

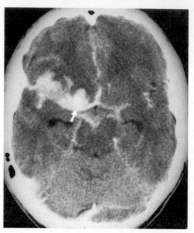

Fig. 2.**65a–c Subarachnoid hemorrhage.** Ruptured saccular aneurysm at the bifurcation of the internal carotid artery to form the anterior and middle cerebral arteries.

a The non-enhanced CT reveals blood in the subarachnoid space, particularly along the course of the middle cerebral artery.

b The lumen of the aneurysm, dark in **a**, turns bright after the administration of intravascular contrast (arrows in **a** and **b**).

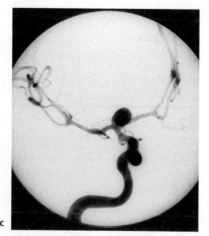

c Carotid angiography demonstrates the aneurysm.

dersurface of the frontal lobe, causing marked abulia. Aneurysms of the *internal carotid artery* lie in the subarachnoid space if their point of origin is above the level of the anterior clinoid process, but parasellar carotid aneurysms lie within the cavernous sinus, and infraclinoid aneurysms are extradural. Rupture of the latter two types of carotid aneurysm leads not to SAH, but rather to sudden, painful ophthalmoplegia, often with involvement of the optic nerve and chiasm, as well as sensory loss in the ophthalmic distribution (pp. 656–670). Ruptured aneurysms of the extracranial portion of the internal carotid artery may cause cranial nerve deficits mimicking the signs of a posterior fossa lesion. Aneurysms of the *poste-*

rior communicating artery often lie adjacent to the oculomotor nerve and may cause a painful oculomotor nerve palsy, affecting both the pupil and the extraocular muscles, even before aneurysmal rupture. A rapidly progressive oculomotor nerve palsy, in an otherwise asymptomatic patient, may be a vital warning sign of impending subarachnoid hemorrhage and should provoke an immediate diagnostic evaluation for an aneurysm. Ruptured aneurysms of the middle cerebral artery may cause contralateral hemiparesis, dysphasia, focal epilepsy, and other focal neurologic signs. Aneurysms of the vertebral and basilar arteries, whether ruptured or unruptured, may cause neurologic deficits related to the brainstem, cerebellum, or lower cranial nerves. Giant aneurysms are defined as those with diameter greater than or equal to 25 mm and may produce neurologic signs and symptoms by mass effect on the brain. Thrombus may form in the lumen of an aneurysm; it may then break off and be carried distally by the bloodstream as an arterio-arterial embolus, producing corresponding ischemic deficits.

Course

Twenty-five percent of patients with aneurysmal subarachnoid hemorrhage die within 24 hours of the event; many die before they reach the hospital. If the patient survives the initial event, the risk of rebleeding is 3–4% in the first 24 hours thereafter, 1–2% per day in the ensuing month, and 3% per year after 3 months. The only way to prevent rebleeding is to obliterate the aneurysm, either surgically or by endovascular occlusion. 40% of untreated patients are dead at 3 months (8).

Arterial vasospasm may occur at any time from 3 to 14 days after the hemorrhage, particularly in vessels that are in extensive contact with blood in the subarachnoid space. Vasospasm often presents clinically with new neurologic deficits and impairment of consciousness. It subsides spontaneously in 3–4 weeks but may, in the meantime, cause neurologic complications, including TIA and ischemic stroke.

Clinical deterioration after aneurysmal SAH may also be due to acute hydrocephalus, resulting from the blockage of CSF flow by blood clot. Finally, acute hyponatremia may arise, due either to abnormal natriuresis, or to abnormal free water retention (syndrome of inappropriate antidiuretic hormone secretion, SIADH) (1025).

Diagnostic Evaluation

SAH is a neurological emergency requiring prompt diagnosis and treatment. The preferred initial diagnostic study is CT (Fig. 2.**65**); MRI with FLAIR sequences may also be used. A negative scan, however, does not rule out the diagnosis of SAH, because a small quantity of blood in the subarachnoid space may escape detection in this way. Thus, if the CT or MRI scan is negative, or if these imaging modalities are unavailable, a lumbar puncture should be performed. SAH is revealed by the presence of blood (or xanthochromia, see p. 79) in the CSF. Once the diagnosis is established, cerebral angiography should be performed as soon as possible to reveal the source of bleeding, which is usually a saccular aneurysm. MR and CT angiography are currently less sensitive than conventional angiography and should not be used in its stead, though they may be valuable complementary studies. *Transcranial Doppler or duplex ultrasonography* is used to detect cerebral vasospasm and follow its course.

Treatment

The goal of treatment is to exclude the aneurysm from the bloodstream rapidly and completely, and thereby prevent further bleeding. *Neurosurgical clipping* is generally performed in the first 12–72 hours after SAH, in patients in Hunt and Hess grades I–III. *Endovascular occlusion* of the aneurysm with intraluminal coils (performed by an interventional neuroradiologist) is mainly reserved for patients in poor condition, those with basilar tip aneurysms, and those at elevated surgical risk. Coiling may be performed as an adjunct to later clipping.

Vasospasm, and the neurologic deficits it causes, can be prevented to some extent with the calcium antagonist *nimodipine*, which is given routinely to all patients with aneurysmal SAH. Once vasospasm occurs, it is generally treated by administering fluids and raising the arterial blood pressure, with systemic pressors if necessary (so-called *"triple-H therapy"*: hypertension, hypervolemia, hemodilution). If clinical signs of vasospasm persist, *endovascular arteriodilatation* is performed in some centers (either by angioplasty, or by the direct intraluminal injection of a vasodilator substance).

Hydrocephalus can be treated by *external ventricular drainage.* The risks of external ventricular drainage include aneurysmal rebleeding (because lowering the intracranial pressure increases the pressure gradient across the aneurysm wall) and catheter infection. *Serial lumbar puncture* is an alternative (394). If hydrocephalus fails to subside once the acute hemorrhage has been cleared from the CSF, permanent *ventriculoperitoneal shunting* may be necessary. Hyponatremia associated with hypovolemia is treated by the administration of isotonic fluids, while SIADH is treated with fluid restriction.

Seizures increase the risk of rebleeding, and the prophylactic administration of *anticonvulsants* is therefore recommended in the acute phase of aneurysmal SAH; it need not be continued afterward. *Steroids* are usually given in addition, as they may reduce the frequency of early and late complications, such as malresorptive hydrocephalus.

Unruptured aneurysms. The widespread use of neuroimaging has led to the incidental discovery of a large number of otherwise unsuspected, unruptured aneurysms. These have an annual rate of rupture of approximately 1 % if their diameter exceeds 5–7 mm. The findings of a recent prospective study have been interpreted to imply that unruptured aneurysms should be clipped only if their diameter exceeds 10 mm, but this runs contrary to studies published earlier, and to the experience of many neurosurgeons. In most centers, young and middle-aged patients with unruptured aneurysms measuring 5–7 mm or more are advised to undergo prophylactic clipping or coiling (451b, 482a).

The Comatose Patient (306, 764)

Overview:
Consciousness and wakefulness require normal functioning of the cerebral cortex, as well as of the midbrain reticular formation and its ascending projections. Bilateral structural lesions or functional disturbances of these brain areas can impair consciousness and produce coma. The bodily posture and brainstem reflexes of the comatose patient provide clues as to whether the lesion lies in the brainstem or in the cerebral hemispheres. Brainstem reflexes are usually preserved in coma due to bilateral hemispheric dysfunction, including metabolic, anoxic, and toxic coma. Ancillary tests are used to answer specific diagnostic questions. The treatment of coma depends on its etiology.

■ Consciousness, Wakefulness, Coma

Consciousness is a biological phenomenon arising in the cerebral cortex (72). It may be defined as awareness of oneself and one's environment. Coma is the absence of consciousness–i.e., *lack of awareness of oneself and one's environment,* including lack of awareness of external stimuli (764). Consciousness requires normal functioning of the midbrain arousal system (see below) and of the cerebral cortex. Any diminution of consciousness is pathological, except sleep. The cerebral metabolic rate is slowed in coma, but normal during sleep.

The scale of consciousness ranges from *wakefulness,* through *somnolence* (synonym: lethargy) and *stupor,* to coma (p. 225). Somnolence and stupor are imprecisely defined. A somnolent patient is relatively easy to awaken and, once awake, speaks and acts slowly, but otherwise normally. A patient in stupor can be no more than partially awakened, even with intense stimulation, and falls back into stupor as soon as the stimulus is removed. Such a patient may produce unintelligible sounds, but cannot communicate. If a patient cannot be awakened by any kind of stimulus and keeps his or her eyes closed at all times, he or she is said to be in coma.

■ Anatomical and Pathophysiological Considerations

The anatomical substrate for normal arousal is composed of the *ascending reticular activating system (ARAS)* and its projections to the cerebral cortex (Fig. 2.**66**).

The most important component of the ARAS is the reticular formation, which lies in the periaqueductal region and extends from the pontine tegmentum to the hypothalamus. Its dorsal projections travel by way of the intralaminar nuclei of the thalamus to the cerebral cortex, while its ventral projections travel directly to the basal forebrain (477). Bilateral dysfunction of these structures impairs consciousness, whether it is due to permanent structural lesions or to transient functional disturbances. A lesion or disturbance will be sufficient to impair consciousness if it affects the periaqueductal region of the midbrain, or if it bilaterally involves the pontine tegmentum, the thalamus, the deep white matter of the cerebral hemispheres, or the cerebral cortex.

■ Brain Shift and Herniation (261, 764)

Supra- and infratentorial mass lesions of sufficient size cause displacement ("shift") of adjacent and distant structures. Unilateral supratentorial masses such as tumor, hemorrhage, edema, or abscess push the brain to the opposite side. This is most easily detected on radiologic images as lateral shift of midline structures such as the septum pellucidum or the pineal calcification. A significant degree of midline shift is associated with impairment of consciousness (797); 3–5 mm of pineal shift is typically associated with somnolence, 5–8 mm

with stupor, and > 8 mm with coma. As the mass effect increases, the cingulate gyrus is displaced under the falx cerebri toward the opposite side (*subfalcine herniation*, Figs. 2.67 and 2.**68**), and the mediobasal portion of the temporal lobe is displaced medially and downward across the tentorial notch. The uncus of the hippocampal gyrus is wedged between the tentorium and the brainstem. Excessive pressure on structures crossing the tentorial notch causes damage to the uncus, the cerebral peduncle, and the oculomotor nerve (*uncal transtentorial herniation*). The clinical signs include impairment of consciousness, ipsilateral pupillary dilatation, and ipsilateral oculomotor nerve palsy.

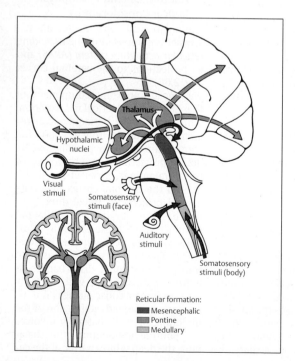

Fig. 2.**66 The ascending reticular activating system (ARAS): the neural substrate of arousal and wakefulness.** The ARAS is susceptible to excitation by exogenous stimuli. Bilateral structural lesions or functional disturbances of the rostral brainstem, thalami, or cerebral hemispheres (cortical or subcortical regions) lead to coma.

Thalamus

Hypothalamic nuclei

Visual stimuli

Somatosensory stimuli (face)

Auditory stimuli

Somatosensory stimuli (body)

Reticular formation:
■ Mesencephalic
■ Pontine
■ Medullary

Bilateral supratentorial masses cause downward displacement of the diencephalon and midbrain through the tentorial notch *(central transtentorial herniation)*. Infratentorial masses (e.g., cerebellar hemorrhage) compress the brainstem, including its reticular formation, directly, and also cause upward displacement of brain tissue through the tentorial notch *(upward transtentorial herniation)* and downward displacement of the cerebellar tonsils through the foramen magnum and into the spinal canal *(tonsillar herniation)*. Brain herniation may cause secondary hemorrhage in the midbrain (Duret hemorrhage) (493). Furthermore, a major

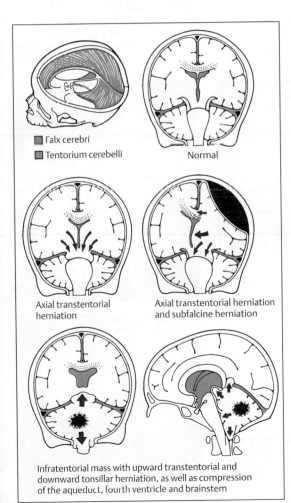

Fig. 2.**67** **Diagram of subfalcine herniation, uncal transtentorial herniation, and infratentorial mass with both upward (transtentorial) and downward (tonsillar) herniation.**

Falx cerebri
Tentorium cerebelli

Normal

Axial transtentorial herniation

Axial transtentorial herniation and subfalcine herniation

Infratentorial mass with upward transtentorial and downward tonsillar herniation, as well as compression of the aqueduct, fourth ventricle and brainstem

blood vessel may be occluded by brain herniation, so that a stroke results. Most commonly affected are the anterior cerebral artery and its branches (in subfalcine herniation) and the posterior cerebral artery (in transtentorial herniation).

■ Intracranial Hypertension

A small intracranial mass has little effect on the intracranial pressure because of compensatory shifting of cerebrospinal fluid out of the intracranial compartment and into the spinal canal. Depending on the age of the patient, a maximum of 40–80 mL of cerebrospinal fluid may be shifted in this way. If the mass is larger than the displaceable fluid volume, the intracranial pressure rises rapidly. The cerebral perfusion pressure (defined as intracranial pressure minus mean arterial blood pressure) is lowered, the cerebral blood flow is impaired, and loss of consciousness may result (1). Prolonged critical impairment of cerebral blood flow results in complete brain failure, which may be followed

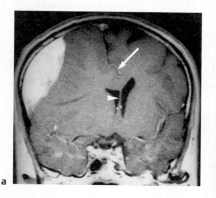

a

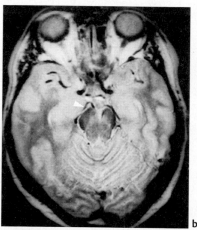

b

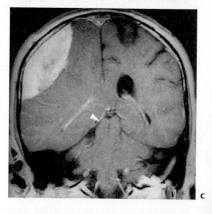

c

Fig. 2.**68a–c Incipient transtentorial herniation due to acute, right-sided subdural hematoma:**
magnetic resonance images.
a Coronal T1-weighted spin-echo image. The midline (arrowhead) and the lateral ventricles are displaced to the left, and the cingulate gyrus (arrow) is herniated under the falx cerebri to the left.
b Axial proton-density-weighted spin-echo image. The uncus is displaced toward the midline (arrowhead).
c Coronal T1-weighted spin-echo image in a plane passing through the cerebral peduncles. The brainstem is slightly displaced to the opposite side by pressure from the medially displaced temporal lobe. The lateral ventricle on the side of the hematoma is compressed.

at a shorter or longer interval by systemic circulatory collapse (396). Transient intracranial hypertension leading to reduction of cerebral blood flow is the pathogenetic mechanism of cough syncope (644).

■ Examination of the Comatose Patient

The immediate first step in the care of the comatose patient is the securing of breathing and circulation. Intubation and artificial ventilation are usually required. In the comatose trauma patient, a cervical spine radiograph should be obtained and an intra-abdominal hemorrhage should be ruled out by peritoneal lavage, if necessary. If the cause of coma is unclear from the available history and preliminary physical examination, and if the blood glucose concentration cannot be measured immediately, an intravenous bolus of 50–100 mL of 50% dextrose should be administered before further examination is carried out. If Wernicke's encephalopathy is suspected, thiamine should also be given. Suspected opioid or benzodiazepine intoxication should be treated by administration of the corresponding antagonist (naloxone or flumazenil, respectively).

The Glasgow Coma Scale. The *Glasgow Coma Scale* (932) is in use all over the world as a simple, reproducible means of grading impairment of consciousness of whatever etiology, whether traumatic or nontraumatic (Table 2.**54**). A fully oriented patient receives the maximum of 15 points, while a deeply comatose patient with no reaction whatever receives the minimum of 3 points. For the definition of some descriptive terms referring to impairment of consciousness

Table 2.**54** The Glasgow coma scale. The patient's overall score is the sum of the scores in the three categories

Category	Points
Best verbal response:	
• None	1
• Unintelligible sounds	2
• Inappropriate words	3
• Disoriented	4
• Oriented	5
Eye opening:	
• None	1
• To painful stimuli	2
• To auditory stimuli	3
• Spontaneous	4
Best motor response:	
• None	1
• Abnormal extension	2
• Abnormal flexion	3
• Withdraws (pulls away from pain)	4
• Localizes (fends off painful stimulus)	5
• Follows commands	6

of varying degrees of severity, the reader is referred to a table in a later chapter (Table 7.**21**).

Focal and global brain dysfunction. The next step in the diagnostic process is to determine whether the disturbance of brain function is focal or global, and, if focal, to localize it as precisely as possible. The most important elements of diagnostic assessment are discussed in this section, and below on p. 233 (Fig. 2.**69**).

• *Pupillary size and reactivity* (p. 664): Normal size and reactivity of the pupils indicate integrity of the visual afferent pathway and of the sympathetic and parasympathetic efferent pathways. A diencephalic

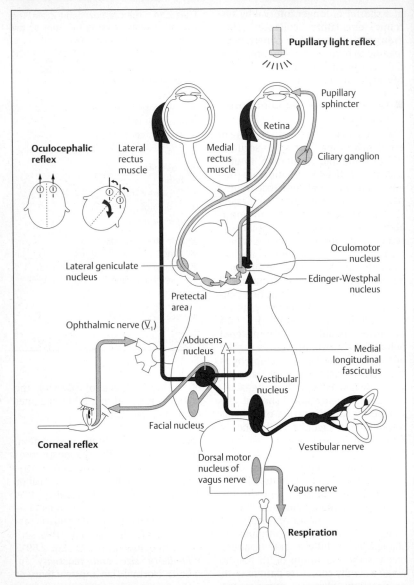

Fig. 2.**69**   **Brainstem reflexes to be examined in the comatose patient.** Midbrain function is tested with the pupillary light reflex, and pontine function with the corneal, vestibulo-ocular and oculocephalic reflexes. Respiration is subserved by the medulla.

lesion produces small and reactive pupils, a pontine lesion even smaller and reactive pupils. Midbrain processes may lead to nonreactivity of one or both pupils; if both pupils do not react, they may be unequal in size. (Definition: *anisocoria* = inequality of the pupils, from Greek *koré*, pupil. It is thus redundant to state, "The pupils are anisocoric.") A single fixed (i.e., nonreactive) and dilated pupil indicates the presence of a process affecting the midbrain or the oculomotor nerve, often as the secondary effect of a supratentorial mass causing uncal transtentorial herniation. In general, lesions above the thalamus or below the pons affect the pupils only indirectly, by mass effect on the midbrain and oculomotor nerve, in the herniation syndromes described in the section above. The *ciliospinal reflex* consists of pupillary dilatation in response to painful pinching of the trapezius muscle and, if intact, indicates an intact central sympathetic pathway. The use of mydriatic agents for ophthalmologic examination should be avoided in comatose patients, as it renders the neurologic examination of the pupils misleading or impossible. Likewise, before examining the pupils, the neurologist should make sure that no such agents have been given.

• *Corneal reflexes* (p. 726): The corneal reflexes are subserved by the trigeminal afferent pathway and

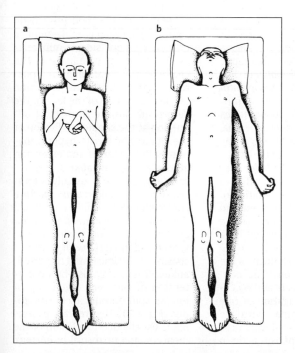

Fig. 2.**70a, b Decorticate (a) and decerebrate (b) posturing.**
(From M. Mumenthaler, *Synkopen und Sturzanfälle*, Stuttgart: Thieme, 1984.)

the facial efferent pathway. The absence of one or both reflexes in the comatose patient indicates the presence of a lesion in the brainstem or cerebral hemispheres.

- *Ocular motility* (571) (p. 634): *Abnormal position of the eyes at rest* indicates a lesion of the cranial nerves subserving oculomotor function (III, IV, and VI), of their respective brainstem nuclei, or of their supranuclear connections. *Conjugate deviation* indicates a contralateral brainstem lesion or an ipsilateral hemispheric lesion (or, in status epilepticus, an epileptogenic focus in the *contralateral* hemisphere). *Nystagmus* may be caused by an irritative lesion at brainstem or supratentorial levels, or by seizure activity. *Ocular bobbing* (rapid downward movement of the eyes, followed by slow return to the primary position) is seen in intrinsic lesions of the pons, and in anoxic, ischemic or metabolic coma. *Inverse ocular bobbing* has also been described. *Oculopalatal myoclonus* indicates an infratentorial lesion (p. 652). As spontaneous eye movement is absent in coma, only reflex eye movements can be examined; of interest are the *oculocephalic and oculovestibular reflexes.* The oculocephalic reflex is elicited by rapid, passive rotation of the head in the supine patient and consists of initial movement of the eyes with the head, followed by a prompt return of the eyes to the vertical position (also known as the *doll's-eyes phenomenon*). The oculovestibular reflex is elicited by caloric stimulation. Irrigation of one external auditory canal with ice water causes a slow, conjugate drift of the eyes to the opposite side in

comatose patients; irrigation with warm water causes a drift toward the side of irrigation. Awake patients subjected to the same test respond with nystagmus, representing the drift seen in comatose patients followed by a rapid, "corrective" phase back into primary position. If the oculovestibular response cannot be obtained by irrigation of one or both ears, then a brainstem or labyrinthine lesion on the corresponding side(s) is present. A disjugate reflex drift implies a lesion of the oculomotor system, either in cranial nerves III, IV, and VI or in their central nuclei and connections. Failure of adduction of one eye represents *internuclear ophthalmoplegia* (see discussion, p. 649).

- *Bodily posture and motor function:* A bodily posture resembling that of normal sleep is a good prognostic sign. If spontaneous movement is only seen on one side, hemiparesis or hemiplegia may be present. The characteristic pathological postures, if present, may provide a clue to the localization of the lesion. *The decorticate posture* consists of adduction at the shoulders, flexion at the elbows and wrists, hyperpronation of the forearms and extension at the knees and ankles; the responsible lesion is usually supratentorial. *The decerebrate posture* consists of adduction and internal rotation at the shoulders, extension at the elbows, and flexion at the wrists and fingers, with extensor spasms of the knees and (inverted) ankles. There may also be overextension of the neck and thoracolumbar spine, producing opisthotonus (Fig. 2.**70**). Decerebrate posturing is usually due to a lesion of the diencephalon or rostral brainstem.

Either type of abnormal posture may be present spontaneously in the comatose patient, or only in response to noxious stimuli. Decorticate posturing has the better prognosis of the two; a deliberate defensive response, which usually requires abduction of the limb, confers a still better prognosis. Unilateral posturing of either type may indicate a focal lesion and is often seen in combination with asymmetries of tendon reflexes and muscular tone. The *Babinski sign* (extensor response to plantar stimulation) may be present in any form of coma and disappears when the patient awakens. Absence of a plantar response confers a worse prognosis than an extensor response. *Myoclonic jerks* are most often seen in hypoxic and metabolic coma.

- *Respiration:* Respiratory abnormalities in coma are listed in Table 2.**55**.
- *Meningism:* Meningism is commonly associated with meningitis, subarachnoid hemorrhage, an infratentorial mass with tonsillar herniation, and spinal trauma. It may be absent, however, in early meningitis or in the first few hours after subarachnoid hemorrhage, or in deep coma.
- *General physical examination:* The following are relevant to the diagnosis of coma: measurement of body temperature (fever or hypothermia?), retinoscopy, otoscopy, and examination of the oral cavity (bitten tongue?), skin (needle tracks or bruises?), heart, lungs, abdomen, and peripheral circulation.
- *History:* An effort should be made to find an informant, preferably an eyewitness, who can relate the circumstances and manner in which the patient's coma came about. The

past medical and surgical history should be obtained from the patient's relatives. Personal effects such as the patient's briefcase and wallet can sometimes yield crucial information, such as a previous diagnosis, a list of medications, or the address of a treating physician.

■ Conditions That Can be Mistaken for Coma

Delirium (p. 362) and the conditions listed below are not the same as coma, but are occasionally mistaken for it:

Locked-in syndrome (712). This syndrome, already mentioned above (p. 171), is most often the result of basilar artery thrombosis, with consequent infarction of the caudal portion of the pons. Other etiologies include pontine tumors and hemorrhages, central pontine myelinolysis, and traumatic brain injury. Locked-in patients are awake and aware of their surroundings, but they cannot move, as they suffer from quadriplegia combined with bilateral cranial nerve deficits. Typically, horizontal gaze is paralyzed, and the patient can only communicate by *vertical gaze and eyelid movements.* A similar or identical clinical picture may be produced by neuromuscular blocking agents, cranial polyradiculitis, or a severe crisis of myasthenia gravis.

Persistent vegetative state (463). Patients in a persistent vegetative state have normal brainstem functions, such as respiration, autonomic regulation of the circulatory system, and sleep–wake cycles, but lack cognitive or volitional motor function (685). *Apallic syndrome* and the French term *coma vigil* are synonyms. These patients have predominantly *neocortical*

Table 2.**55** Respiratory abnormalities in coma

Type of respiration	Definition	Site of responsible lesion	Remarks
Cheyne-Stokes respiration (periodic respiration)	Oscillatory alternation of hyperpnea and apnea	Cerebral hemispheres (diffuse dysfunction) or diencephalon	
Central hyperventilation	Persistent hyperventilation	Brainstem reticular formation; intracranial hypertension	Central hyperventilation is much less common than reflex hyperventilation in response to metabolic acidosis.
Apneustic respiration	Brief respiratory pause at full inspiration (variant: brief pauses during inspiration)	Mid- or caudal pons; dorsal tegmentum	Seen e.g. in massive infarction due to basilar artery occlusion
Atactic respiration (Biot respiration)	Irregular alternation of superficial and deep breathing, with irregular pauses	Dorsomedial medulla	Usually due to posterior fossa processes or meningitis
Temporary loss of automatic respiration ("Ondine's curse")	Normal breathing while awake, but cessation of breathing during sleep or when distracted	Reticulospinal projections of medullary respiratory center	A sign of acute medullary dysfunction, differential diagnosis: sleep apnea syndrome

brain damage. They have little or no spontaneous movement and lie in bed with open eyes. They mostly fail to withdraw from a painful stimulus, and, when put into an artificial, uncomfortable posture by the examiner, will not change it. In the initial stage, extensor spasms and mass movements are often seen. Later, rigidity and extrapyramidal hyperkinesia may develop. Primitive reflexes become prominent; spontaneous chewing, yawning, and grasping of visually or tactilely presented objects may arise. The persistent vegetative state is usually caused by traumatic brain injury or anoxic–ischemic injury (cardiac arrest, near-drowning, carbon monoxide poisoning), more rarely by metabolic disorders, degenerative disorders, and congenital anomalies of the nervous system. The vegetative state is considered to be persistent 1 year after traumatic brain injury and 3 months after anoxic injury (798).

Akinetic mutism (p. 386) (160). Patients in this state appear to be awake, fix and follow with their eyes, but do not speak or move spontaneously. They can be brought to speak or move only through massive stimulation. This condition is usually accompanied by major cognitive impairment, hypersomnia, and urinary and fecal incontinence, but only mild rigidity or spasticity, if any. "Abulia" is a synonym for "akinetic mutism." The responsible lesion affects the *fronto-orbital cortex* on both sides, or the frontally projecting fibers of the *ascending reticular activating system.* Because of the anatomical relationships of these structures, large areas of the *limbic system* are practically always affected as well, which accounts for the cognitive impairment. The more common etiologies of akinetic mutism are bilateral infarction in the territory of the anterior cerebral artery, vasospasm after rupture of an aneurysm of the anterior communicating artery, bilateral basal ganglionic or thalamic infarcts, traumatic brain injury, tumors of the third ventricle, hydrocephalus, and anoxic brain injury (110). A continuum of pathological conditions exists that ranges from akinetic mutism to the persistent vegetative state; the nomenclature of transitional states is not precisely defined.

Catatonia or akinetic crisis in Parkinson's disease. These conditions, too, must be distinguished from coma.

Psychogenic (pseudo-)coma. For a discussion of this entity, see p. 562.

■ The Causes of Coma

If the clinical examination yields evidence of a focal lesion, then structural brain injury is more likely than a metabolic, toxic, or anoxic–ischemic condition. The latter types of disorder generally lead to global hemispheric dysfunction but largely spare brainstem function, except in very severe cases with very deep coma. Structural lesions affecting both hemispheres in an approximately symmetrical fashion may yield a clinical picture resembling that of a nonstructural lesion; examples include multiple brain abscesses or bilateral large infarcts in the territory of the middle cerebral artery. On the other hand, a metabolic, toxic, or anoxic–ischemic disorder may produce focal clinical signs, particularly in elderly patients, and thus mimic a structural lesion. As a rule, however, abnormalities of pupil-

lary size and reactivity, corneal reflexes, ocular motility, and bodily
posture and movement are due to a
structural lesion, unless neuroimaging studies demonstrate the contrary.

Such studies should always be performed when focal clinical findings
are present. The causes of coma are
listed in Table 2.**56**.

Table 2.**56**   Causes of coma

Symmetric, nonstructural:
- Toxic (medications, alcohol, drugs of abuse, other substances)
- Metabolic:
  - Ischemia
  - Hypoxia
  - Hypercapnia
  - Hyper- or hyponatremia
  - Hypoglycemia
  - Hyperglycemia, with or without ketoacidosis
  - Lactic acidosis
  - Hyper- or hypocalcemia
  - Hypophosphatemia
  - Hypermagnesemia
  - Hyper- or hypothermia
  - Wernicke's encephalopathy
  - Uremic encephalopathy
  - Hepatic encephalopathy
  - Porphyria
  - Hypothyroidism
  - Addisonian crisis
  - Panhypopituitarism
- Infectious:
  - Meningitis
  - Encephalitis
  - Sepsis
  - Malaria
- Psychiatric:
  - Catatonia
  - Psychogenic (pseudo-)coma
- Postictal state
- Basilar migraine
- Malignant neuroleptic syndrome
- Reye's syndrome

Symmetric, structural:[1]
- Bilateral infarction in the territory of the internal carotid artery
- Bilateral infarction in the territory of the anterior cerebral artery
- Bilateral infarction in the territory of the middle cerebral artery
- Brainstem infarction or hemorrhage
- Subarachnoid hemorrhage
- Thalamic hemorrhage
- Concussion, traumatic brain injury
- Hydrocephalus
- Brain tumor (infratentorial or midline supratentorial)
- Fat embolism
- Hypertensive encephalopathy

Asymmetric, structural:[1]
- Unilateral hemispheric mass with midline shift or herniation
- Large or bilateral ischemic strokes
- Cerebral venous sinus thrombosis
- Sub- or epidural hematoma
- Subdural empyema or epidural abscess
- Endocarditis
- Cerebral vasculitis
- Thrombocytopenic purpura
- Disseminated intravascular coagulation
- Acute disseminated encephalomyelitis, multiple sclerosis
- Progressive multifocal leukoencephalopathy
- Creutzfeldt-Jakob disease
- Marchiafava-Bignami disease
- Adrenoleukodystrophy and other leukodystrophies
- Gliomatosis cerebri
- Carcinomatous meningitis

1) The clinical presentation, too, may be symmetrical or asymmetrical.

■ Diagnostic and Therapeutic Approach

Once the immediate life-saving measures have been taken and the clinical examination has been performed, directed ancillary tests and therapeutic interventions are performed depending on the cause of coma; for example, if status epilepticus is suspected, an EEG is performed, and anticonvulsants are given. Ancillary tests to be considered when the diagnosis is unclear are listed in Table 2.**57**.

Any metabolic disorder revealed by laboratory testing should be corrected. The more common types are hypoglycemia, hypoxia, hypo- or hyperthermia, hypercapnia, metabolic alkalosis or acidosis, and fluid and electrolyte disorders.

CT and MRI. The definitive demonstration of a structural lesion of the brain or of an intracranial mass requires a CT or MRI scan (see pp. 132 and 134) (335). One should remember that the diagnosis of a metabolic disorder does not rule out the presence of a structural brain lesion, and vice versa; metabolic disorders often arise as an indirect consequence of structural lesions, e.g., hypernatremia when a mass lesion impairs the normal mechanism of drinking in response to thirst.

Electroencephalography. The EEG may be very helpful in the diagnostic evaluation of comatose patients. It occasionally reveals a specific disease as the cause of coma, such as epilepsy, herpes simplex encephalitis, or Creutzfeldt-Jakob disease. Nonconvulsive status epilepticus can be diagnosed, and differentiated from a toxic or metabolic disorder, only by EEG. Furthermore, EEG is useful in assess-

Table 2.**57** Ancillary diagnostic tests in the comatose patient

Head CT or MRI
Electroencephalography
Lumbar puncture
Laboratory tests:

- Electrolytes
  - Sodium
  - Potassium
  - Calcium
  - Magnesium
  - Phosphate
- Glucose
- Serum osmolality
- Blood urea nitrogen, creatinine
- Hemoglobin, hematocrit
- Leukocyte count with differential
- Platelet count
- Prothrombin and partial thromboplastin times
- Hepatic enzymes, ammonia
- TSH, fT_3, fT_4, cortisol
- Creatine phosphokinase
- Arterial blood gases
- Toxicology screen and specific toxicological testing
- Blood culture

ing the severity and prognosis of toxic and metabolic encephalopathies and traumatic brain injuries (69, 368).

The alpha rhythm of the EEG is normally reactive in the locked-in state and in psychogenic pseudocoma (397). A nonreactive alpha rhythm is characteristic of "alpha coma," a prognostically unfavorable state due to a high pontine or diffuse cortical lesion (47).

Evoked potentials. *Somatosensory and auditory evoked potentials* are used to test specific sensory pathways in the peripheral and central nervous system. Sedatives suppress them to a lesser extent than the EEG. They are thus suitable for monitoring and prognostic prediction in pharmacologically paralyzed and sedated coma patients (e.g., after head trauma or anoxic injury) (369, 994, 995). In the locked-in syndrome, *motor evoked potentials* may indicate the potential for recovery (70).

Prognosis. Prognostication in coma is very difficult because of the extreme heterogeneity of etiology and underlying pathology. This remains true even when electrophysiologic studies are performed. As a rule, the longer the coma persists, the less favorable the prognosis. The absence of brainstem reflexes is also a poor prognostic sign (68, 179, 462, 570).

■ Death

Death is the complete and irreversible cessation of function of all parts of the brain, including the brainstem. Irreversible cardiac or respiratory arrest causes death by depriving the brain of its necessary supply of oxygen. Death may also occur through primary brain failure. (The term "brain death" is synonymous with "death" and, therefore, both unnecessary and potentially misleading.)

The clinical determination of death is an important issue in intensive care medicine and organ transplantation. The precise guidelines to be followed have been established by law and vary slightly among jurisdictions, but the major clinical aspects are, nonetheless, constant (672, 716a, 738, 857, 908, 1027):

- *Death by irreversible cardiac arrest* is diagnosed when, despite adequate measures of cardiopulmonary resuscitation that have been continued for a defined period of time, the patient remains without pulse, respirations, or any motor response (with the possible exception of spinal reflexes).
- *Death by primary brain failure* is diagnosed, regardless of whether the heart is beating, when the following criteria are met:
  - bilaterally fixed and dilated pupils,
  - absence of reflex eye movements,
  - absence of corneal reflexes,
  - absence of response to noxious stimuli,
  - absence of coughing and swallowing reflexes,
  - absence of spontaneous respiration.

Spinal reflexes are sometimes still present in dead individuals; this is more commonly seen in children. If death occurs by primary brain failure and the heart is still beating, then its pulse is invariable (without response to, e.g., atropine), and the maintenance of an adequate blood pressure for extracerebral organ perfusion will likely require the administration of pressors. Diabetes insipidus is often present.

At least two clinical death examinations should be performed, with a defined interval between them. Six hours is sufficient if the nature of the brain lesion is evident, and no reversible metabolic disorders or intoxications are present that might invalidate the findings of the examination. If an intoxication cannot be definitively ruled out, the interval between examinations should be at least 24 hours, and at least 48 in some cases. Absence of spontaneous respiration is demonstrated by an apnea test (90). Further diagnostic studies are not legally required in most countries, but may nonetheless yield valuable information. The EEG is flat, evoked potentials are unobtainable, and such methods as cerebral angiography (conventional, MR, or CT), transcranial Doppler ultrasonography (396), perfusion-weighted MRI, and radioisotope angiography reveal the absence of cerebral perfusion.

Extrapyramidal Syndromes

Definition:
The extrapyramidal system, like the cerebellum, plays an important role in motor function. It enables rapid and harmonious execution of movement and optimal performance of complex motor sequences. Extrapyramidal disorders may produce either an abnormal decrease of muscle tone (hypotonia) or an abnormal increase (rigidity). In like fashion, they may bring about either an overall paucity of movement (hypokinesia) or superfluous movement of various types, including tremor, chorea, athetosis, and other involuntary movements.

Anatomy

The functional unit known as the extrapyramidal system comprises the caudate nucleus, putamen, globus pallidus, subthalamic nucleus, substantia nigra, and red nucleus on both sides.

The traditional nomenclature in this area is potentially confusing, and thus merits a brief exposition here. The corpus striatum, or striatum for short, consists of the caudate nucleus and putamen. The lentiform nucleus consists of the putamen and globus pallidus. The globus pallidus is sometimes referred to as the pallidum, and the subthalamic nucleus as the corpus Luysii.

These nuclei are connected not only with each other, but also with the midbrain, thalamus, and cerebral cortex through ascending and descending fiber tracts. The major connections of importance for the pathophysiology of Parkinson's disease, the most common extrapyramidal disorder, are illustrated in Fig. 2.**71**.

Pathophysiology

The gray-matter nuclei of the extrapyramidal system are interconnected in complex regulatory circuits that enable the execution of automatic and semi-automatic motor programs, the modulation of muscle tone, and the harmonization of movement. If one or more of these regulatory circuits should be interrupted through the loss or dysfunction of a component structure, there may result either a net removal of inhibition, leading to excessive movement (e.g., tremor, dystonia), or a net decrease in motor activation, leading to impaired movement (e.g., rigidity, akinesia).

Neurochemistry

The biochemistry of neurotransmission is basic to a pathophysiological understanding of extrapyramidal disease. Dopamine is the neurotransmitter used by the nigrostriatal neurons, which exert an inhibitory influence on the cholinergic interneurons of the striatum. Gamma-aminobutyric acid

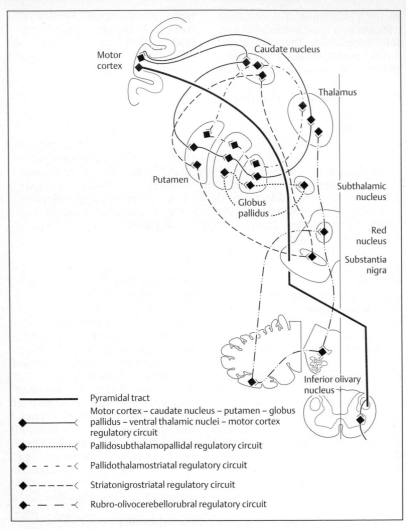

Fig. 2.**71**   **Neural pathways in Parkinson's disease.**

(GABA) is the neurotransmitter of the inhibitory striatopallidal and striatonigral pathways, among others. The pars compacta of the substantia nigra contains about 80% of the total dopamine content of the brain in healthy individuals, but is severely depleted of dopamine in patients with Parkinson's disease (see p. 246).

■ Classification of the Extrapyramidal Disorders

The extrapyramidal syndromes may be broadly classified into two categories, as in Table 2.**58**.

■ The Parkinsonian Syndrome (14a, 603, 723a)

Epidemiology

It is estimated that 0.1–0.2% of the population suffer from some form of parkinsonism, and as much as 1% of the population over 60 years of age. The incidence is said to be 0.1 cases per 1000 persons per year overall, and two cases per 1000 persons over 65. The Rotterdam Study (277a) yielded prevalence figures of 1.2% for men and 1.5% for women over 55. The prevalence rises rapidly with age: it is 0.3% from 55 to 64 years, 3.1% from 75 to 84, and as high as 5% in women aged 95 to 99.

Clinical Features

The major clinical manifestations of the parkinsonian syndrome ("parkinsonism") are listed in Table 2.**60** and will be individually discussed in this section. The diagnosis is based on a characteristic constellation of findings, though no single finding is essential for the diagnosis (not even tremor).

Impairment of primary automatic movement is the most impressive manifestation and sooner or later becomes prominent in all parkinsonian patients. At first, there is a generalized reduction of spontaneous movement, called *hypokinesia* or, more commonly but less accurately, *akinesia*. The characteristic mask-like facies is a result of akinesia. Blinking is less frequent than normal, the head is turned "en bloc" with the neck and trunk, and all movements are slow and viscous. The patients may thus take on a wooden appearance. Paucity of movement causes reduction in size of the patient's handwriting (micrographia), which may be simultaneously impaired by tremor. The *paucity of accessory movements* is easily observed as a lack of arm swing while the patient is walking.

Pro- and retropulsion are the inability of the patient to regain his or her balance when briskly pushed forward (or backward) by the examiner. The steps needed to recover from the disturbance are too small, too slow, or absent, and the patient stumbles, or even falls, in the direction of the shove. The same difficulty may arise spontaneously if the patient should trip while walking, or, for example, when the patient opens a door that

Table 2.**58** Broad classification of extrapyramidal syndromes

Group	Clinical features	Examples (see also Table 2.59)
Akinetic-rigid syndromes	Paucity of spontaneous movement and accessory movements, increased tone (rigidity), sometimes also involuntary movements	Parkinson's disease, progressive supranuclear palsy
Hyperkinetic-hypotonic syndromes	Irregular (nonrhythmic) involuntary movements, often at varying sites in a single patient; diminished muscle tone at rest	Chorea, athetosis, ballism, dystonias

Table 2.**59** The most common extrapyramidal syndromes

Syndrome	Clinical features	Pathological correlate	Causes
Parkinsonism	Akinesia, rigidity, (sometimes) rest tremor at 4–8 Hz	Loss of neurons in the substantia nigra and other melanin-containing nuclei, in the globus pallidus, and in the striatum	Usually idiopathic (Parkinson's disease); may also be genetic, toxic (iatrogenic), vascular, or postinfectious (postencephalitic)
Progressive supranuclear palsy (Steele-Richardson-Olszewski disease)	Downward gaze palsy, rigidity, pyramidal signs, retraction of the head, subcortical dementia	Loss of neurons in the lentiform nucleus, thalamus, midbrain	Idiopathic (a degenerative disease classed among the multisystem atrophies)
Chorea	Irregular, rapid, asymmetric, brief, mainly distal involuntary movements	Loss of small striatal neurons	Genetic, infectious, post-stroke
Athetosis	Irregular, slow, mainly distal involuntary movements at varying sites, with joint hyperflexion and hyperextension	Loss of neurons in the striatum and external pallidal segment	Birth injury, esp. kernicterus; genetic, brain tumors, post-stroke
(Hemi-)ballism	Irregular, sudden, large-amplitude, ballistic involuntary movements of an entire limb or limbs	Loss of neurons in the subthalamic nucleus	Infarct, tumor
Dystonic syndromes: • Spasmodic torticollis • Torsion dystonia • Localized dystonias	Involuntary tonic contractions of shorter or longer duration affecting individual muscles or muscle groups (against the resistance of antagonist muscles)	Loss of neurons in the putamen and thalamus	Birth injury, esp. kernicterus; genetic, idiopathic

Cont. →

Table 2.**59** (Cont.)

Syndrome	Clinical features	Pathological correlate	Causes
Hepatolenticular degeneration (Wilson's disease) (p. 296)	Progressive, "wing-beating" tremor, rigidity, dysarthria, mental changes, hepatic dysfunction, corneal Kayser-Fleischer ring	Loss of neurons in the putamen	A genetic disorder of copper metabolism
Myorhythmia	Involuntary, rhythmic twitching of a single muscle group at 1–3 Hz	Degeneration of the central tegmental tract (in the case of so-called palatal nystagmus)	Birth injury, vascular, encephalitis
Myoclonus	Involuntary, irregular, rapid, brief twitches of individual muscles or muscle groups	Loss of neurons in the dentate nucleus, inferior olive, red nucleus, possibly also in the peripheral nervous system	Birth injury, vascular, diffuse hypoxic injury, toxic

Table 2.**60** Clinical features of parkinsonism

Impairment of primary automatic movement:
- Akinesia
- Diminished accessory movements
- Pro- and retropulsion

Hypertonia of extrapyramidal type:
- Rigidity
- Increased postural tone
- Increased antagonist tone
- Cogwheel phenomenon
- Postural abnormalities

Tremor

Other somatic symptoms and signs:
- Micrographia
- Dysarthria
- Breathing disturbances
- Motor "weakness"
- Accentuated nasopalpebral reflex
- Autonomic signs (seborrhea, drooling, sweating attacks)
- Oculogyric crises and other oculomotor disturbances
- Dystonia

Mental abnormalities:
- Cognitive slowing
- Mood lability
- Affect disturbances
- Dementia

Late and iatrogenic manifestations:
- On–off phenomenon
- L-dopa dyskinesia
- Drug-induced hallucinations and psychosis

Hypertonia of extrapyramidal type manifests itself mainly as *parkinsonian rigidity,* an exaggerated, viscous, waxy resistance to passive movement that can be felt by the examiner during the entire movement. In Fig. 2.**72**, parkinsonian rigidity is compared with (pyramidal) spasticity, in which resistance is felt mainly at the beginning of passive movement.

Rigidity is best felt on irregular passive flexion and extension at the elbow. Rigidity at the wrist can be demonstrated by shaking the forearm and watching the movement of the unsupported hand.

In addition to rigidity, hypertonia is also manifest as *increased postural tone.* In the parkinsonian patient, passive movement tends to be followed by abnormally strong tensing of the muscles that fix the limb in the new

suddenly and unexpectedly gives way. When a patient with Parkinson's disease develops this problem and becomes conscious of it, the prognosis for disease progression and for the effect of treatment has taken a turn for the worse.

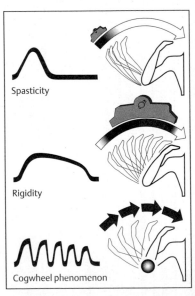

Spasticity

Rigidity

Cogwheel phenomenon

Fig. 2.**72a–c Abnormalities of tone and the cogwheel phenomenon.**

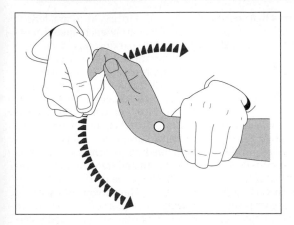

Fig. 2.**73** **Testing for the cogwheel phenomenon in the wrist.**

position. Thus, when one passively dorsiflexes the patient's foot, there follows a strong, active contraction of the tibialis anterior muscle (fixation reflex). *Increased antagonist tone* can be demonstrated by suddenly removing resistance against which the patient has been exerting force (e.g., pressure from the examiner's arm); the giving-way that follows is briskly checked by action of the abnormally strongly tensed antagonist muscles. This phenomenon is the opposite of the "positive rebound" seen in cerebellar disorders, and can also be strikingly brought out by the so-called "head dropping test": if the examiner gently lifts the patient's head off of the pillow and then suddenly removes the supporting hand, the head does not immediately fall back, but rather slowly sinks to rest, or else it is actively held in the air for some time. In fact, parkinsonian patients sometimes lie supine without any support under the head, which seems to float on an invisible cushion ("l'oreiller psychique"–the psychic pillow).

Testing of muscle tone often reveals the so-called *cogwheel phenomenon*:

the examiner, applying passive movement across a joint, feels a varying resistance, as if the two opposing joint surfaces were composed of cogwheels repeatedly engaging and disengaging with each other (Fig. 2.**72**). This phenomenon may be especially pronounced at the wrist (Fig. 2.**73**). It may be evident even if the patient has no visible tremor.

Tremor is perhaps the most impressive, though by no means an obligatory involuntary movement in Parkinson's disease (it is minimal or absent in the so-called akinesia-dominant variant of the disease). Parkinsonian tremor is practically always most prominent at rest and is a regular, rhythmic, mainly distal tremor, with a frequency of 4–8 Hz and variable intensity, that abates or disappears on voluntary movement. Characteristic "pill-rolling" or "coin-counting" movements of the fingers may be seen. The tremor is increased by strong emotion and abolished in sleep. It is reduced during active muscle contraction and when the limbs are placed in extreme positions.

The characteristic parkinsonian *posture*, with mild forward stooping, lowered head, and moderately flexed knees, hips and elbows, is evident when the patient stands or walks. The accessory movements of walking, particularly arm swing, are reduced (Fig. 2.**74**.)

Other somatic symptoms and signs of parkinsonism are mostly consequences of the abnormalities just described. The loss of postural reflexes leads to *frequent falling* (usually forwards), occasionally as an early sign of disease. The patient's *speech* is soft, monotonous and poorly articulated.

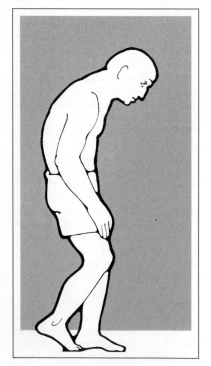

Fig. 2.**74**   **Posture of a patient with Parkinson's disease.**

Saccadic dysarthria is characteristic of the now rarely encountered post-encephalitic parkinsonian syndrome, as are iterations and palilalia (the involuntary repetition of sentences and sentence fragments, at increasing speed), and, sometimes, true (akinetic) mutism, in which the patient speaks only when under emotional stress. Parkinsonism in general is accompanied by an irregular variation in the depth and frequency of *breathing*, which can be detected with special testing. The patient may seem to be truly weak (paretic) but can move with full, normal strength under certain circumstances. The impression of *motor weakness* was, incidentally, what led James Parkinson, in 1817, to name the disease he described *"the shaking palsy."* The intrinsic muscle reflexes are unaltered, and pyramidal tract signs are usually absent in parkinsonism, though there are many exceptions to this rule. If present, pyramidal tract signs may be a sign of cervical myelopathy, which is more frequently seen in parkinsonian patients (336b), or of a form of multisystem atrophy with parkinsonian features (p. 250). *Accentuated nasopalpebral reflexes* and other intrinsic reflexes of the facial musculature are a constant feature. *Pain* is often present in the form of generalized tenderness of the muscles and bones, or as painful dystonia secondary to L-dopa therapy. *Sensory function* is intact except for diminished position sense in the great toe, which is common (1047a). Patients often report a disturbance of smell. The *autonomic signs* of parkinsonism (profuse sweating, hot flashes, seborrhea) are particularly prominent in post-encephalitic cases. *Drooling* is a manifestation, not of increased salivation, but of hypokinesia: patients swallow less frequently, and saliva escapes from the corner of the mouth (844c). A bloated feeling, obstipation, and orthostatic hypotension are also common. Bowel and bladder disturbances are not infrequent; the latter consist of urinary urgency, frequent urination and occasional incontinence, usually at night. Most such problems are due to a "hyperactive bladder," of a type responsive to apomorphine injections (33). Two-thirds of male patients suffer from erectile dysfunction (882b). *Oculogyric crises* are seen only in post-encephalitic parkinsonism and in phenothiazine-induced dyskinesia: the patient's gaze is rigidly fixed upwards for a period of minutes to hours, while the head is (sometimes) tilted backwards. Attacks of *blepharospasm* are likewise seen in post-encephalitic cases and may last for a variable time. Disturbances of convergence and accommodation, and gaze pareses, are seen in some forms of parkinsonism (for progressive supranuclear palsy, see p. 252). Dystonia may accompany parkinsonism. *Parkinsonian crises* consist of severe akinesia and rigidity, high fever (due to impaired temperature regulation), and profuse sweating; they are a rare occurrence, seen occasionally in association with L-dopa use.

Mental abnormalities are almost always present, but of highly variable severity. Mood lability and irritability are common. Above all, cognitive processes are slowed, just as motor processes are; patients must, as it were, force themselves to think. Both reactive and primary depression are common. Memory is impaired, particularly for verbal and pictorial information (780). Even aside from patients with the inherited Parkinson-dementia complex (see below), almost one-third of patients with Parkinson's disease suffer from more or less severe psycho-organic abnormalities, particularly cognitive deficits (249a). Hallucinations were occasionally described in parkinsonian patients before the introduction of dopaminergic agents, but have become increasingly common under this form of treatment and are now seen in some 40% of patients (295a, 1033b). Hallucinations are more common in patients with cognitive deficits. They are treated by reduction of the dose of antiparkinsonian medications and, if necessary, by administration of a so-called atypical neuroleptic agent such as clozapine, quetiapine, or olanzapine (317b, 319a, 930b, 1033b). The prevalence of dementia is positively correlated with male sex, advanced age, and the duration and severity of other parkinsonian manifestations (443b). Demented patients derive less benefit from L-dopa treatment.

The individual parkinsonian syndromes can be analyzed separately and rated quantitatively according to well-defined scales. This makes it possible to assess the course of the disease over time and to document the response to therapy. The Webster scale, introduced in 1968, and the Unified Parkinson's Disease Rating Scale (UPDRS) are reproduced in the Appendix (pp. 935 and 945).

Specific Etiologies

The manifestations of parkinsonism are similar regardless of etiology, though some etiological forms have specific, distinguishing clinical features (see below). The more common etiologies of parkinsonism are listed in Table 2.**61**.

Table 2.**61**   Causes of parkinsonism

Idiopathic Parkinson's disease (paralysis agitans)
Hereditary disorders: • Hereditary form of idiopathic Parkinson's disease • Parkinson–dementia complex of Guam
Other degenerative (hereditary) disorders
Post-encephalitic
Atherosclerotic
Rarer causes: • Trauma (multiple, e.g., pugilistic parkinsonism; controversial for single trauma) • Carbon monoxide poisoning • Manganese poisoning • Other intoxications • Drugs (neuroleptics, antiemetics) • MPTP • Brain tumor • Polycythemia vera • Wilson's disease

MPTP, 1-methyl-4-phenyl-1,2,3,6-tetrahydropyridine.

Familial Parkinson's disease. Idiopathic Parkinson's disease (paralysis agitans) is rarely found in a familial pattern with autosomal dominant inheritance. A prospective study revealed that 23% of patients with Parkinson's disease had one or more affected relatives, although there was only one in most cases. The age of onset of illness was not significantly different in familial cases, so defined, than in isolated cases. Yet, when the affected relative was a child of the patient, the age of onset was earlier than in the parent–a phenomenon known as "anticipation" (142b). It is thus clear that genetic factors play a role in Parkinson's disease (965a), even though direct genetic transmission can be shown only in very rare cases (350c). In a small number of affected families, the autosomal dominant form of the disease has been found to be associated with a mutation of the *PARK1* gene, which encodes α-synuclein, a protein found in Lewy bodies. An autosomal-recessive form of juvenile Parkinson's disease is associated with a mutation of the *PARK2* gene, which is located on chromosome 6 near the gene for ubiquitin (626a). A further locus (*PARK3*) has been found on chromosome 2p13.

The *Parkinson–dementia complex* is linked to chromosome 4p, mainly affects men, and usually arises in the sixth decade of life. It is of highly variable penetrance; only about 60% of persons with the mutation develop signs of the disease, typically akinesia, a fine tremor, and dementia. This disorder is classed among the multisystem atrophies (p. 250).

The island of *Guam* in the Marianas is home to a particular familial form of *parkinsonism with dementia,* in which some of the affected individuals also suffer from amyotrophic lateral sclerosis. Men are more frequently affected than women, and the onset of the disease is between the ages of 30 and 65. Rigidity and akinesia dominate the clinical picture; there is little or no tremor. A more or less severe dementia is invariably present.

Post-encephalitic parkinsonism. This post-infectious condition can arise during a bout of encephalitis or not till months or as many as 30 years later. The best-known cases were those resulting from the epidemic of encephalitis lethargica (von Economo's encephalitis) in the 1920s. New cases of parkinsonism continue to appear in the aftermath of isolated cases of encephalitis, not of the von Economo type. Pronounced autonomic abnormalities are typical of post-encephalitic parkinsonism. Oculogyric crises, dystonia, palilalia, and iterations (see above) are striking features of the disease.

Drug-induced and toxic parkinsonism. Parkinsonism may arise as a result of treatment with neuroleptic agents, particularly phenothiazines and butyrophenones, or with antiemetics such as metoclopramide. Drug-induced parkinsonism typically presents with marked akinesia and rigidity, and relatively less severe tremor. (For other side effects of chlorpromazine, see p. 300.) Amiodarone can cause a Parkinson-like tremor (1017). Certain pesticides and herbicides may also predispose to the appearance of a parkinsonian syndrome (684b, 860a, 974b). Smoking is considered a risk factor for Parkinson's disease by some authors (974b), but not by others (860a).

MPTP-induced parkinsonism. MPTP (1-methyl-4-phenyl-1,2,3,6-tetrahydropyridine) came to attention as a cause of parkinsonism in the early 1980s, when it was produced as a contaminant by underground chemists trying to synthesize an illegal street analogue of the opiate drug meperidine. It causes parkinsonism when ingested orally or by inhalation or injection (51). It causes a highly selective loss of melanin-containing neurons in the pars compacta of the substantia nigra. MPTP-induced parkinsonism in nonhuman primates is an important animal model for the study of Parkinson's disease. It is not yet clear whether neuronal loss is limited to the time of exposure to MPTP or continues to progress afterward.

Arteriosclerotic parkinsonism. This etiologic attribution, once commonly made, is probably incorrect in most, if not all, cases.

Idiopathic Parkinson's disease. Most cases of parkinsonism without a known etiology represent idiopathic Parkinson's disease. The manifestations usually appear on one side and then progress to involve both. Men are more commonly affected than women; the age of onset is usually between 50 and 60 years. Any putative role of heredity in these cases is hard to define. Children of affected parents have a 19% chance of suffering from the disease, which seems to rule out a simple dominant or recessive pattern. A multifactorial etiology is assumed.

Rare causes of parkinsonism:

- *Post-traumatic parkinsonism* (567a) should only be diagnosed in strict adherence to published criteria: a single traumatic event (severe concussion or brain contusion), causing demonstrable, permanent structural injury, is followed by the emergence of parkinsonian manifestations, either immediately or after an interval of a few days to weeks, during which time transitional signs may be present (457b, 974b). Parkinsonism has also been described after trauma not involving the head (166c, 852a).
- *Pugilistic parkinsonism* results from the cumulative effect of the numerous concussions, of greater and

lesser severity, to which boxers are subject, and is associated with dementia ("punch-drunk state," "dementia pugilistica").

- *Carbon monoxide poisoning* may be followed, within a few weeks, by the development of bilateral parkinsonism.
- *Chronic manganese poisoning,* an occupational hazard of miners and workers in various industries, causes parkinsonism that usually becomes manifest only after many years of exposure.
- *Other toxic etiologies* have been described in small numbers of cases, including intoxications with methanol, certain hypnotic drugs, carbon disulfide, sulfur dioxide, and thallium. Intoxication with organic phosphates, such as pesticides, may lead to transient, severe parkinsonian manifestations (684b).
- *Taurine deficiency* has been demonstrated in the serum, CSF, and brain (at autopsy) of patients suffering from an autosomally inherited disease manifested by depression arising in old age, followed by sleep disturbance and, finally, by parkinsonism.
- *Case reports* document the rare emergence of parkinsonism after electrical trauma, chronic subdural hematoma, brain tumors (particularly meningioma), and polycythemia vera.

Pathology

Loss of melanin-containing neurons in the substantia nigra with glial proliferation is the pathological *sine qua non* of Parkinson's disease. Other melanin-containing nuclei in the globus pallidus, the striatum, the reticular formation of the brainstem, the dentate nucleus and the thalamus are less constantly affected. Still-alive but diseased neurons in the affected nuclei may contain round, hyaline, tyrosine-rich inclusion bodies called *Lewy bodies.* Specific etiological causes of parkinsonism other than idiopathic Parkinson's disease have their own characteristic pathological features; for example, neurofibrillary tangles resembling those of Alzheimer's disease are found in postencephalitic parkinsonism and in the Parkinson-dementia complex. In parkinsonism of any etiology, a diminished concentration of dopamine in the substantia nigra and striatum can be demonstrated with immunofluorescence.

Pathophysiology and Biochemistry

Parkinsonism is caused by the anatomical or functional disturbance of certain portions of the complex system of regulatory circuits depicted above in Fig. 2.**71**. The cause of "idiopathic" Parkinson's disease is at least partly genetic (965a) and may also involve (auto-)immune processes (176b).

A low dopamine concentration is found in normally dopamine-rich structures such as the caudate nucleus, putamen, and substantia nigra. This leads to a preponderance of *cholinergic* over *dopaminergic* neurotransmission in the extrapyramidal motor system.

Treatment

Initiation of Treatment:
There are differing views as to when medical treatment should be initiated in patients diagnosed as having Parkinson's disease. We tend to do so when the patient, subjectively assessing his own impairment, feels it is necessary.

Pharmacotherapy:
The initial treatment of idiopathic Parkinson's disease is always with medications (457a) and varies according to the stage of disease and the age of the patient. Milder forms may be treated with parasympathetic antagonists and amantadine, which have few side effects. Beta-blockers were once thought effective against tremor in Parkinson's disease, but this was subsequently not confirmed. Clozapine has significant effectiveness against tremor (458). Selegiline, at a dose of 10 mg/day, is thought to have a neuroprotective effect.

The mainstay of medical treatment for Parkinson's disease is levodopa (combined with a decarboxylase inhibitor) and/or dopaminergic agonists (bromocriptine, pergolide, ropinirole, cabergoline, pramipexole, lisuride). Levodopa remains the most effective antiparkinsonian medication, but its prolonged use may lead to late adverse effects (dyskinesia, motor fluctuations), and a long-term neurotoxic effect, though not proven, is theoretically possible. It is thus advisable, particularly in patients under 60 years of age, to defer levodopa treatment as long as possible, and to keep the dose low whenever possible. The dopaminergic agents seem not to have these long-term adverse effects, but their practical management is more difficult. A further temporizing measure to defer the introduction of levodopa is the use of adjuvant agents, singly or in combination, such as amantadine (initially 100 mg/day, then increasing to a target dose of 100 mg b.i.d. or t.i.d.), and selegiline (5 mg qd or b.i.d.), and anticholinergic agents to treat tremor, such as biperiden or trihexyphenidyl (these should be used cautiously in elderly and confused patients). Patients under 60 years of age are usually initially treated with a dopaminergic agonist (765a) such as pergolide, bromocriptine, pramipexole, cabergoline, or ropinirole (863b). These drugs should be introduced in very slowly increasing doses, in order to prevent the sudden appearance of side effects that may necessitate discontinuation of therapy, such as nausea, vomiting, or changes of blood pressure. If these side effects should arise, they may be treated temporarily with domperidone. The initial dose is usually 0.05 mg/day for pergolide, 1.25 mg/day for bromocriptine, 0.375 mg/day for pramipexole, or 0.25 mg/day for ropinirole; the dose is increased over several weeks till a satisfactory effect is obtained. Patients initially treated with ropinirole are less likely to suffer from dyskinesia 5 years later than those initially treated with levodopa (780c), and the same holds for patients initially treated with cabergoline (791a). Sudden falling asleep during the day has been reported as an adverse effect of pramipexole and ropinirole (321a, 424b) but probably occurs with all other dopaminergic agonists as well (498b), and is, in any case, a frequent occurrence in Parkinson's disease, with

▶

a reported prevalence of 27% (930a) to 50% (287e). Approximately one-third of patients treated with dopaminergic agonists develop orthostatic hypotension (547b). Most dopaminergic agonists, except pramipexole and ropinirole, are ergot derivatives that can (rarely) cause retroperitoneal fibrosis.

Patients over 60 years of age should be treated initially with levodopa at an initial dose of 50 mg in the morning, increasing over several weeks to 300–1000 mg/day, in 3 to 5 divided doses. If a satisfactory result cannot be obtained, or is first obtained and then lost, the next step may be the potentiation of levodopa by the addition of a COMT inhibitor, such as tolcapone or entacapone (777b). The use of tolcapone requires very careful monitoring of hepatic function, as severe hepatotoxicity has been described. Tolcapone treatment is begun at a dose of 100 mg t.i.d., while the dose of levodopa is simultaneously reduced by a third, to prevent an excessive effect.

Entacapone is given initially at 200 mg with each levodopa dose, while the total dose of levodopa is reduced by 20% to 30%. The levodopa dose is cautiously brought back to its original level in a second step, until a satisfactory effect is obtained.

Advanced Parkinson's disease is characterized by adverse effects and complications of medical therapy: dyskinesia, motor fluctuations, and akinetic crises (so-called "on-off phenomena") of variable severity become prominent. Levodopa may be given in fractionated doses or in timed-release format to lessen variation in blood levels over the course of the day; when this is done, the early-morning dose must still be high enough to achieve a therapeutic level in the morning. Timed-release preparations are helpful overnight. Amantadine reduces dystonia (890b, 976a). The dose of dopaminergic agonists may also be cautiously increased: pergolide up to 1 mg q.i.d., bromocriptine up to 20 mg/day, ropinirole up to 5 mg q.i.d. (15, 723). Refractory "off periods" may be treated with a rapidly absorbable or liquid form of levodopa, if necessary. Crises can sometimes be managed when they occur with subcutaneous injection of apomorphine (1–3 mg/dose) (731).

If the measures described above are no longer sufficient, triple therapy with levodopa, a dopaminergic agonist, and a COMT inhibitor may be necessary. As the disease progresses, the therapeutic window narrows.

Dyskinesia and hallucinations can sometimes be treated with an atypical neuroleptic agent, such as clozapine in an initial dose of 12.5 mg, increasing (if necessary) up to 25 mg b.i.d., with regular monitoring of the complete blood count because of the risk of agranulocytosis, or olanzapine. In older patients with advanced disease, however, a reduction and simplification of the dose schedule may be necessary, particularly if cognitive disturbances or confusion should arise.

Neurosurgical treatment:
Stereotactic operations for the treatment of Parkinson's disease were introduced in the 1950s, fell into disuse after the introduction of levodopa in the late 1960s, and have experienced a major revival in the last 15 years. The ma-

▶

jor reasons for this are, on the one hand, the emergence of a population of patients with intractable parkinsonism despite exhaustion of medical treatment options, and, on the other hand, the vast improvements in neurosurgical technique made possible by recent technical advances, particularly CT and MRI.

Until recently, the neurosurgical treatment of Parkinson's disease necessarily involved the placement of a lesion in the brain, usually either in the internal pallidal segment (pallidotomy, for the treatment of rigor and akinesia) or in the ventral lateral nucleus of the thalamus (thalamotomy, for the treatment of tremor) (65b, 465b). The lesions were made by many different means in the early years, including cryosurgery and mechanical and chemical tissue destruction, but, at present, lesions are usually made thermally, with a radiofrequency current applied through a stereotactically placed probe. An important limitation of lesion-making in the brain is that bilateral lesions may have severe undesired side effects. Bilateral pallidotomy, for example, may produce severe emotional and behavioral disturbances, as well as corticobulbar dysfunction (340b). Lesions can be made without open surgery by means of so-called stereotactic radiosurgery, using a linear accelerator or gamma knife device (709c); the drawback of this technique is the inability to check the target site intraoperatively, with electrophysiologic testing, before making the lesion.

The latest major development in stereotactic neurosurgery for Parkinson's disease has been the introduction of deep brain stimulation. Instead of making a lesion at the target site, the neurosurgeon implants an electrode connected by a subcutaneous extension cable to a small impulse-generating device ("neuropacemaker"), which is implanted subcutaneously below the clavicle.

High-frequency current delivered through the electrode causes a physiological inactivation of the target site, which lasts as long as the current is turned on. Stimulation thus mimics the physiological effect of a lesion, but has the advantage of reversibility. It is also adaptable, in that its electrical parameters (amplitude, frequency, pulse width) can be adjusted for optimal therapeutic effect. When electrodes are implanted bilaterally for the control of bilateral symptoms, the parameters can usually be adjusted to eliminate the side effects that would occur with bilateral lesion-making. The feasibility of bilateral treatment is thus another major advantage of deep brain stimulation. The impulse generator must be changed surgically every 3–5 years, when its battery runs out.

The targets for deep brain stimulation are essentially the same as those of stereotactic lesion-making for Parkinson's disease. In patients with tremor-dominant disease (as well as patients with tremor of nonparkinsonian origin, such as essential tremor), thalamic stimulation has been found to be at least as beneficial as thalamotomy (718a, 856a). Patients with akinetic-dominant disease benefit from pallidal stimulation (982a); like pallidotomy, this treatment is particularly effective against levodopa-induced dyskinesia. In the last few years, stimulation of the subthalamic nucleus has been shown to counteract both tremor and akinesia in Parkinson's disease (586d). ▶

Neural transplantation for Parkinson's disease, in the hope of reconstituting the deficient dopaminergic pathway, has been an object of research for decades but remains an experimental technique at present. The implantation of fetal mesencephalic cells or autologous adrenal medullary cells into the caudate nucleus was found to delay progression of the disease in a minority of patients so treated (1015). The results were less than spectacular, the procedure was not devoid of risk, and psychiatric problems sometimes developed postoperatively (232). Transplantation of fetal nigral cells into the putamen yielded encouraging results in another study involving 4 patients (317), and PET studies have shown increased fluorodopa uptake after transplantation (396a).

A randomized, controlled, double-blinded study of the transplantation of fetal mesencephalic cells to treat Parkinson's disease has been published very recently (317c). Sham surgery was used in control patients to preserve blinding, and a subjective rating of symptoms was chosen as the primary endpoint. The result was negative overall, in that the 20 treated patients had no significant benefit compared to the sham-surgery group. Yet the subgroup of treated patients less than 60 years old did appear to benefit from the transplant. Three of the treated patients developed intractable dyskinesia. Although this was a negative study, the results seem to offer hope that further technical refinements will make neural transplantation a real option for the treatment of Parkinson's disease.

Prognosis

All of the parkinsonian syndromes described above are, by definition, progressive illnesses, with the exception of drug-induced syndromes, which are, to some extent, reversible. Most lead to invalidism within a few years. Levodopa therapy, though it is usually highly effective at first, can merely delay rather than prevent the severe disability of Parkinson's disease, which, as must be realized, is an irreversible neuropathological process rather than a simple chemical deficiency in the brain.

According to an earlier Japanese study, the mean duration of Parkinson's disease until death is 7.4 years; this figure seems extremely low to us and may reflect not only an earlier era of treatment, but also cultural differences regarding the time of presentation. The more common causes of death in that study, at a median age of 70 years, were heart disease and pneumonia. A recent American study (599a) revealed a two- to fivefold elevation of mortality in persons with Parkinson's disease compared to age-matched controls. Mortality was found to be correlated with the severity of hypokinesia.

■ Multisystem Atrophies

A number of other, rare illnesses are associated with symptoms and signs whose differential diagnosis includes idiopathic Parkinson's disease (84a, 592a). Among these are the so-called multisystem atrophies (MSA), which are listed with their major features in Table 2.**62**.

Mixed and transitional forms of MSA are not uncommon, and the diagnos-

Table 2.**62**   Major features of the multisystem atrophies

Disorder	Major manifestations	Ocular findings	Parkinsonism	Dementia
Shy-Drager syndrome	Orthostatic hypotension without reflex tachycardia, resulting in (pre-)syncope; sweating, impotence, incontinence; fasciculations and muscular atrophy	Extraocular pa sy, iris atrophy	Rigidity, tremor, akinesia	No
Striatonigral degeneration	Initial parkinsonism followed by autonomic dysfunction; hypotonia, syncope, incontinence		Often initial, poorly responsive to levodopa	
Olivopontocerebellar atrophy	Sporadic or familial; initial cerebellar manifestations (tremor, ataxia); later parkinsonism (often mild) and autonomic failure		Late, often mild	Yes
Progressive supranuclear palsy	Usually in males, often starts with akinesia; predominantly truncal rigidity; falls; dysarthria	Vertical gaze palsy, slowing of downward vertical saccades	Akinesia is the most prominent parkinsonian feature; truncal rigidity	Yes (subcortical dementia)
Corticobasal degeneration	Rapidly progressive akinetic–rigid parkinsonian syndrome; asymmetrical; cortical neuropsychological deficits; alien limb syndrome; severe gait ataxia		Asymmetric, akinetic-rigid	
Lewy body dementia	Prominent dementia; progressive cognitive impairment; abnormal response to neuroleptics		Yes, with gait impairment and falls	Prominent

tic classification of individual cases is often difficult, particularly early in the course of disease (14a, 84a, 84b, 592a, 833a, 980a). All forms of MSA first appear in the fourth decade of life or later. Their parkinsonian manifestations respond poorly to levodopa. Pain is prominent in MSA, being present in approximately half of all patients, beginning a mean of 3 years after disease onset (942c). The administration of clonidine may lead to an elevation of serum growth hormone concentration in Parkinson's disease, but does not in the multisystem atrophies (517b).

■ Shy-Drager Syndrome
Pathology
Loss of neurons is found most prominently in the basal ganglia, substantia nigra, other brainstem nuclei, and the gray matter of the spinal cord, as well as in the cerebral and cerebellar cortices. Some 60–80% of the neurons of the intermediolateral cell columns of the spinal cord are lost.

Clinical Features
The illness begins in middle or advanced age and is more than twice as common in men as in women. The initial symptoms are usually exclusively those of orthostatic hypotension—i.e., dizziness, weakness, visual disturbance, and possible loss of consciousness on standing up. In contrast to idiopathic orthostatic circulatory collapse, these symptoms are not accompanied by reflex acceleration of the pulse, yawning, or sweating.

Months or years usually elapse before other neurological disturbances appear (though they may, in some cases, appear before orthostatic hypotension). These include loss of sweating, impotence, incontinence, pyramidal tract signs, and most prominently rigidity, akinesia,

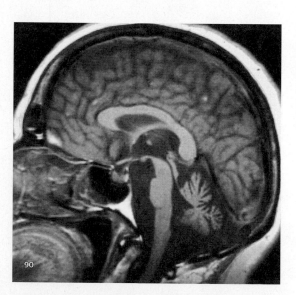

Fig. 2.75 Sporadic cerebellar atrophy/olivopontocerebellar atrophy.
Sagittal T1-weighted spin-echo image in a 64-year-old woman. The cerebellum and pons are markedly atrophic.

90

tremor, muscle atrophy, fasciculations, extraocular muscle weakness and atrophy of the iris. These disturbances progress even if the orthostatic drop in blood pressure is pharmacologically stabilized (see below). Shy-Drager syndrome may cause death in as little as 1 year or as long as several years. Dementia is not a part of this syndrome.

Treatment

Fludrocortisone, indomethacin, and sympathomimetic agents may lessen the orthostatic drop in brood pressure, but they do not influence the progression of the underlying pathogenetic process. Orthostatic hypotension may also be treated with a pressure suit (similar to the G-suit of the air force pilot).

■ Striatonigral Degeneration

Striatonigral degeneration is a disease of adults, with onset generally later than age 30. It is characterized by parkinsonian manifestations that are resistant to dopamine substitution and, as the disease progresses, by severe autonomic dysfunction (orthostatic hypotension, syncope, urinary incontinence, impotence), cerebellar dysfunction, and pyramidal tract signs.

■ Olivopontocerebellar Atrophy

This disease appears in familial and sporadic forms with roughly equal frequency (185, 185d, 345a, 748). The autosomal dominant inherited form is due to an abnormality involving polymorphic CAG repeats on the short arm of chromosome 6 (800a). Cerebellar manifestations are prominent at first, while the parkinsonian manifestations remain relatively mild (345a). Autonomic dysfunction and pyramidal tract signs appear later. The disease generally begins in middle age, but occasionally earlier, and leads to death within 1–4 years (Fig. 2.**75**).

■ Progressive Supranuclear Palsy

Definition:

This disease, often initially misdiagnosed as Parkinson's disease, is also known as Steele-Richardson-Olszewski syndrome, in honor of its describers, and in the French literature as "dystonie oculo-facio-cervicale" (563, 684, 824a, 829b, 904). By definition, it is characterized by hypokinetic parkinsonian manifestations and gaze palsy. With a prevalence of ca. five per 100,000 persons, it accounts for roughly 4% of all patients suffering from parkinsonian syndromes. It occurs sporadically, and only exceptionally in families. A τ-gene mutation has been postulated as a pathogenetic factor, but this hypothesis is not uniformly supported by research to date (424a).

Clinical Features

This disorder usually strikes men aged 50–70. Poverty of movement progresses gradually and turns into severe akinesia over the course of 1 year or several years. The patients have a parkinsonian appearance but are distinct from patients with Parkinson's disease in that the head is not inclined forward, but rather extended backward, because of hypertonia of the nuchal muscles. Rigidity is more pronounced in the trunk than in the extremities. Dysphagia and pyramidal tract signs are common. The disturbance of ocular motility, which is of diagnostic importance, is often not noticed by the patient at first, but often progresses to a practically complete external ophthalmoplegia. Voluntary eye movement and ocular pursuit are almost entirely abolished, but the doll's-eyes reflex (p. 228) can still be evoked and Bell's phenomenon is preserved; these findings on examination serve to exclude a nuclear or subnuclear lesion. Downward vertical saccades are slowed most severely, horizontal saccades somewhat less so (791b).

When the patient is tested by provocation of vertical optokinetic nystagmus, the fast component is typically lost, while the slow component is preserved. There is usually also a slowly progressive dementia, which is said to be of the "subcortical" type, though its manifestations would be equally compatible with bilateral frontal lobe dysfunction: forgetfulness, cognitive slowing, apathy, occasional irritability, and difficulty applying acquired knowledge.

Dementia may be the presenting sign, and ocular motility may be disturbed only late in the course of disease, or not at all. Pyramidal tract signs are found in half of all patients, cerebellar signs less frequently. The occasional disturbance of micturition has been shown to be due to loss of neurons in Onuf's nucleus in the sacral spinal cord (829b).

Treatment

Cerebrospinal fluid shunting may temporarily improve cognition and walking, but not the vertical gaze palsy or parkinsonism. The latter is better treated with *dopamine agonists* than with *levodopa*. *Methysergide* also appears to be beneficial.

Prognosis

The prognosis is poor, and death usually ensues within a few years. Occasional patients with similar clinical manifestations will turn out to meet the clinical and radiological criteria for malresorptive hydrocephalus (p. 39).

■ Corticobasal Degeneration

This disorder is characterized by a rapidly progressive akinetic-rigid parkinsonian syndrome, which often begins on one side (534a, 592a, 1015b). Gait ataxia and dysarthria are prominent, as is disturbed cortical function, manifesting as aphasia, astereognosis, and pyramidal tract signs. A markedly delayed onset of horizontal saccades is characteristic and establishes the differential diagnosis from other syndromes with parkinsonian features (791b). Further findings include dystonia, action and postural tremor, myoclonus, and the so-called alien hand syndrome, in which an extremity is not recognized as part of oneself. A supranuclear disturbance of ocular motility may also be found.

■ Chorea

Clinical Features

Chorea is a hyperkinetic-hypotonic form of extrapyramidal dysfunction, of varied etiology, characterized by irregular, asymmetric, sudden, brief, shooting *involuntary movements,* which are usually more pronounced in distal segments of the extremities. If mild, these movements may be misinterpreted as "fidgeting," and their organic, pathological nature is thus often not realized at first. When severe, however, they may be of very high amplitude, randomly directed, and extremely disturbing. Grimacing and lip-smacking may be prominent. These involuntary movements interfere with the carrying out of normal voluntary movements, endanger the patient, and afford no rest, often leading to complete exhaustion. Sometimes they are less evident during sleep. Chorea is often seen in combination with athetosis (p. 260); it may be generalized, or only on one side of

the body (hemichorea). Senile hemichorea is depicted in Fig. 2.**76a–e** (still images from a film recording).

The *neurological examination* often reveals, beside the involuntary movements described, nothing more than a generalized decrease in muscle tone. Occasionally, if the knee-jerk reflex is tested while the patient is seated with legs hanging, the leg may return to its original position more slowly than normal (Gordon phenomenon) or make an additional extensor movement after the reflex jerk. Both of these phenomena reflect an involuntary movement interfering with the reflex process. Occasionally, the abdominal wall may be abnormally sucked in during inspiration, as in phrenic nerve palsy.

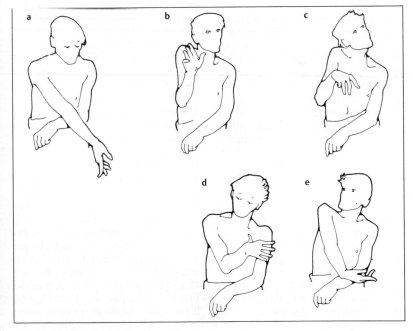

Fig. 2.**76** **Senile hemichorea.**

Etiologies

Table 2.**63** provides an overview of the hyperkinetic extrapyramidal syndromes, including chorea, with their various etiologies. These will be discussed individually in the following section.

Chorea minor (Sydenham's chorea). This most common form of chorea, also known as chorea rheumatica and chorea infectiosa, was described by Sydenham in 1686. It most commonly affects school-aged girls and is predominantly seen between the ages of 6 and 13, though it is occasionally seen as late as age 40. It is usually associated with childhood infectious diseases, primarily rheumatic fever. Some two-thirds of cases arise a few weeks after a bout of streptococcal pharyngitis or rheumatic arthritis or endocarditis. The known increased prevalence of chorea and other neurological disorders in patients' relatives indicates that there is also a genetic predisposition. *Nonspecific symptoms* such as fatigue, emotional lability and irritability develop a few days to weeks after the initial infectious illness and are later followed by specific, *objective findings,* primarily the involuntary movements, which may be mild at first, resembling "fidgeting," but progress to frank chorea in a matter of weeks. Only rarely does the chorea begin or remain on one side of the body. Fever is present only during the acute infectious illness. The diagnosis may be supported by a positive throat culture or an elevated anti-streptolysin antibody titer. The cerebrospinal fluid is almost always normal. Mental disturbances may be evident, sometimes as severe as a frank psychosis.

Chorea mollis ("soft" chorea) is said to be present when hypotonia and muscle weakness are the major findings and the involuntary movements are minimal or absent. Its prognosis is good, in that the findings generally regress after a few weeks or months, but there is a tendency to relapse, and about one-third of patients have residual abnormalities (jitteriness when under stress, anxiety, tics).

Treatment

The treatment is mainly that of the underlying infectious illness and consists of *salicylates, antihistamines, cortisone, pyridoxine,* and prolonged administration of *penicillin.*

Chorea gravidarum. This form of chorea usually arises between the third and fifth month of a first pregnancy and resembles chorea minor in its symptoms, associated findings, and prognosis. There is often a prior history of chorea minor in childhood. The use of inhibitors of ovulation is also associated with chorea, which is reversible once the drug is discontinued.

Huntington's disease. This serious disease is of autosomal dominant inheritance (1051a) and is due to an expanded CAG repeat (a so-called unstable trinucleotide sequence) on the short arm of chromosome 4. The expanded CAG repeat tends to be longer in paternally inherited cases, which therefore tend to have an earlier age of onset, in some cases as early as the first decade of life. Onset after age 50 is more than twice as common when the patient's mother, rather than father, was the affected parent. The rate of spontaneous mutation is ca. 3% (351). The visual evoked potentials (VEP) are abnormal in patients with Huntington's disease, the more so with greater severity and longer duration of illness, but are always normal in their asymptomatic children and thus cannot be used as a predictive test. *Clinically evident disease* usually arises between the ages of 30 and 50. *Hyperkinesia* develops gradually, more slowly than in chorea minor, and with a greater admixture of athetotic movements. Gait is often severely impaired. Mental disturbances are typically found, but their severity need not parallel that of the involuntary movements; they may arise years earlier or later. These include disturbances of affect and drive, delusions, paranoid-hallucinatory psychoses, and, finally, dementia. The rare cases of childhood onset usually present with generalized rigidity and spasticity with pyramidal tract signs, epileptic seizures, and rapidly progressive dementia. The choreiform movements appear later, and then progress very rapidly. The *Westphal variant* of Huntington's disease involves the onset, during childhood, of hypokinesia and rigidity. Presymptomatic diagnosis by genetic testing (562) is currently possible (899). The *prognosis* of Huntington's disease is very poor; death usually ensues 10–15 years after the diagnosis.

Treatment

There is no etiologic treatment; for the symptomatic management of chorea, see below.

Benign familial chorea. A further autosomal dominant form of chorea is of benign prognosis and is not associated with dementia. The responsible gene is on chromosome 14q (229b). This form of chorea begins in childhood but, in many families, does not progress further.

Rarer etiologies of chorea. *Chorea-acanthocytosis* also runs in families and seems to be of autosomal recessive inheritance. It begins between the ages of 20 and 30 with orofacial dyskinesia and tongue-biting and then progresses, with the development of mild choreiform movements of the extremities. The reflexes are diminished or absent, the CPK is elevated, and acanthocytosis with a normal beta-lipoprotein level is found. Dementia is not a component of this disease. *McLeod syndrome* is due to a deletion and point mutation on the X chromosome, causing a lack of Kx protein. The affected men suffer from chorea, neurogenic muscle atrophy with areflexia, cardiac anomalies, epileptic seizures, and mental disturbances, occasionally psychosis. The onset of disease is between the ages of 20 and 50. Female carriers may suffer from cognitive impairment and other mental abnormalities. The serum CPK is elevated, and MRI reveals atrophy of the caudate nucleus and putamen. *Postapoplectic hemichorea* is rare even among patients who have sustained a putaminal stroke. Chorea arising after hemiplegia is often accompanied by hemiballism. A number of other rare etiologies are listed in Table 2.**64**. Hemichorea due to *cerebral arteriovenous malformation* deserves mention, as does *Hunt's progressive pallidal atrophy,* a sporadically occurring, hereditary illness characterized by choreoathetotic and dystonic involuntary movements, with progressive devel-

Table 2.**63** Differential diagnosis of hyperkinetic extrapyramidal syndromes

Syndrome	Features	Etiology	Remarks
Chorea:			
• Chorea minor	Sudden, usually rapid, distal, brief, irregular involuntary movements; hypotonia	Autoimmune; streptococcal infection	Often a sequela of streptococcal pharyngitis, most commonly in girls aged 6–13 years
• Chorea mollis		Autoimmune; streptococcal infection	Hypotonia is prominent
• Chorea gravidarum		3rd–5th month of pregnancy	Usually during first pregnancy, often with prior history of chorea minor
• Chorea due to inhibitors of ovulation			Rare, reversible with drug discontinuation
• Huntington's disease		Autosomal dominant	Onset usually ages 30–50; associated with progressive dementia
• Benign familial chorea		Autosomal dominant	Onset in childhood, no further progression, no dementia
• Chorea-acanthocytosis		Autosomal recessive	Mainly orofacial, tongue-biting, elevated CPK, hyporeflexia, acanthocytosis
• Postapoplectic chorea		Vascular (prior stroke)	Sudden hemichorea and hemiparesis, often combined with hemiballism
• Senile chorea		Vascular and degenerative	Occasional presenile onset, often more severe on one side, occasionally with dementia
• Rarer forms			See Table 2.**64**
Athetosis			
• Status marmoratus	Slow, exaggerated movements against resistance of antagonist muscles, predominantly distal, appear uncomfortable and cramped	Perinatal hypoxia	Soon after birth, increasingly severe athetotic hyperkinesia, often cognitive impairment, sometimes also spasticity

• Status dysmyelinisatus		Kernicterus of the newborn	Begins in the neonate, often with other signs of perinatal brain damage; later progressive
• Pantothene kinase-associated neurodegeneration (formerly Hallervorden-Spatz disease)	Joint hyperflexion/hyperextension (see Fig. 2.77)	Autosomal-recessive disorder of pigment metabolism	Choreoathetotic movements beginning at age 5–15 years, rigidity, dementia, and retinitis pigmentosa in one-third of all cases; progressive, death by age 30
• Hemiathetosis		Focal lesion of pallidum and striatum	Unilateral, may come about some time after the causative lesion
Ballism/hemiballism	Unilateral, lightning-like, high-amplitude flinging movements involving multiple limb segments	Ischemic or neoplastic lesion of the subthalamic nucleus	Sudden onset, usually in the setting of preexisting hemiparesis
Dystonic syndromes:			
• Torsion dystonia	Slow, tonic contractions of muscles or muscle groups, shorter- or longer-lasting, usually against the resistance of antagonist muscles	Familial syndrome	Families often of Jewish ancestry, onset 1st–2nd decade of life with focal dystonia, later rotating movements of head, trunk and extremities, as well as athetotic finger movements
	As a secondary manifestation of other diseases	E.g., in Wilson's disease, Huntington's disease, pantothene kinase-associated neurodegeneration	
• Spasmodic torticollis	Slow contraction of cervical and nuchal musculature against antagonist resistance, with turning movement of the head	Idiopathic, occasionally after neck trauma and a variety of other causes	One-third recover spontaneously, one-third remain unchanged, one-third develop torsion dystonia
• Localized dystonia	See p. 266		E.g. writer's cramp, faciobuccolingual dystonia, oromandibular dystonia

opment over the years of accompanying tremor, rigidity, and akinesia. The disease usually appears between the ages of 5 and 15 and progresses until middle age. For *paroxysmal choreoathetosis*, see p. 557.

Pathology

Chorea is typically associated with loss of smaller neurons in the striatum (i.e., the caudate nucleus and putamen). Coronal sections of the brain, and coronal MRI images, correspondingly reveal flattening of the bulge of the caudate nucleus into the lateral ventricle. A focal lesion, such as a metastatic tumor, is very rarely the cause of chorea, which seems to develop only when the striatum is diffusely damaged.

Pathophysiology

The substantia nigra receives afferent input from the premotor fields and sends its output to the anterior horn cells of the spinal cord. The activity of the substantia nigra is regulated by the striatum, which projects to it by way of the striatonigral fasciculus. When this influence is lost, the substantia nigra can no longer normally control accessory movements and muscle tone. Meanwhile, the striatal projection to the external pallidal segment is also lost, which causes not only a loss of inhibitory activity in pallidoreticular fibers, but also disinhibition extending over multiple synapses, from the internal pallidal segment, to the ventral thalamic nuclei, to the premotor cortical fields 6A-alpha and 4S. The latter structures, bereft of their normal, modulating inhibitory influence, in turn act abnormally upon the reticular inhibition system, the substantia nigra, and the anterior horn apparatus.

▬ Treatment ▬

Choreiform movements may be treated symptomatically with *perphenazine*, at an initial dose of 4 mg, increasing till the desired effect is obtained, or with *haloperidol, thioridazine*, or *tiapride*, or, in severe cases, *tetrabenazine*. The common and occasionally serious side effects of these medications must be carefully weighed against their therapeutic benefit.

■ Athetosis

Clinical Features

Athetosis consists of slow, irregular, exaggerated, uncomfortable- and cramped-appearing *involuntary movements* that are more pronounced in distal portions of the extremities. It often involves hyperflexion or hyperextension of the joints. Strong contraction of antagonist muscles is always observed. This results in bizarre, cramped *postures* in which the limbs may be frozen for several seconds at a time (particularly the hands, Fig. 2.**77**) and which may even lead, over time, to subluxation of the interphalangeal joints ("bayonet finger").

Voluntary and automatic movements (e.g., walking) are impaired by abnormally strong accessory innervation. Athetosis is not uncommonly accompanied by chorea. In many cases, the *neurological examination* reveals no other abnormality. The intrinsic muscle reflexes are normal. Dystonic dorsiflexion of the great toe may produce a "pseudo-Babinski" sign. The Strümpell phenomenon may be observed, consisting of dorsiflexion and supination of the foot and toes when the patient tries to flex the knee and hip against the examiner's resistance. Other findings in individual cases

Table 2.**64**   Rarer etiologies of chorea

Etiology	Features	Remarks
Chorea-acanthocytosis	Autosomal recessive inheritance, onset in the 2nd and 3rd decades of life, begins in the orofacial area, no dementia	Acanthocytosis with normal beta-lipoprotein
Postapoplectic hemichorea	Combined with hemiparesis, often with ballistic component	Putaminal stroke (visible in MRI)
Hemichorea due to tumor	Other tumor-related signs	Rare
Senile chorea	Usually accompanied by senile dementia, rarely isolated	Not hereditary
Toxic chorea		CO, manganese, carbon disulfide, phenytoin, chlorpromazine
Systemic lupus erythematosus		
After acute rash		
Pantothene kinase-associated neurodegeneration (formerly Hallervorden–Spatz disease)		
Wilson's disease		
Ataxia telangiectasia		
Creutzfeldt-Jakob disease		
Thyrotoxicosis		
Polycythemia vera		
Hypernatremia		
Hyperparathyroidism		
Disorders of purine metabolism	Marked elevation of serum uric acid concentration, lack of tissue hypoxanthine-guanidine phosphoribosyl transferase	Torsion dystonia and self-mutilation (Lesch-Nyhan syndrome)
Kernicterus		Usually accompanied by athetosis and other manifestations of cerebral palsy

Cont. →

Table 2.**64**   *(Cont.)*

Etiology	Features	Remarks
Perinatal hypoxia	First years of life	With spasticity and cognitive deficit
Portocaval encephalopathy		
Glutaric acidemia		
Progressive pallidal atrophy	Hereditary, onset age 5–15 years	With athetosis, later tremor
Paroxysmal choreoathetosis	Familial as well as symptomatic forms, e.g. phenytoin intoxication, multiple sclerosis, hyperparathyroidism	See p. 557

may reflect an underlying neurological disease.

Etiologies

Status marmoratus. Status marmoratus is the most common cause of "double athetosis" and is usually a sequela of perinatal asphyxia, leading to loss of small neurons in the putamen and caudate nucleus, with foci of hypermyelination. The movement disorder begins shortly after birth or in the first few years of life, rarely later. Bilateral athetotic hyperkinesia, mainly in the arms, is accompanied by mental deficiency in half of all cases. Other clinical signs of brain damage, such as spastic paraparesis or pyramidal tract signs, are rare. The clinical manifestations progress until a plateau is reached, and remain stable thereafter.

Status dysmyelinisatus (Vogt). Status dysmyelinisatus is characterized by demyelination of the intrinsic fibers of the globus pallidus and by loss of the intrinsic fibers of the subthalamic nucleus. There is extensive loss of pallidal cells, resulting in shrinkage of both pallidal segments. This clinical and pathological entity may be due to any of a number of etiologies, including birth trauma, perinatal asphyxia, and kernicterus (p. 38). Athetosis begins immediately after birth or in the first year of life and is often accompanied by other signs of brain damage.

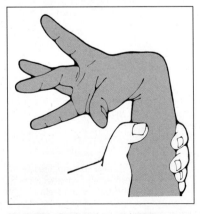

Fig. 2.**77**   **The hand in athetosis.**

Pantothene kinase-associated neurodegeneration (formerly Hallervorden-Spatz disease). This is a familial disorder, probably of autosomal recessive inheritance, that generally becomes clinically manifest before age 15, rarely in adulthood. Patients suffer from progressive rigidity, mainly in the legs, and choreoathetotic movements, often accompanied by progressive dementia and epileptic seizures. One-third also suffer from retinitis pigmentosa. Progression is relatively rapid; most patients die by age 30.

Note: As this book goes to press, a laudable movement is underway to rename this disease. It was originally named after its describers, Hallervorden and Spatz, two academic neuropathologists who were personally involved in the mass murder of mentally ill children and adults in Nazi Germany. It is widely felt that their memory should no longer be honored.

Focal processes. Focal processes may cause hemiathetosis in both childhood and adulthood. Focal hemorrhage or infarction causes "postapoplectic" hemiathetosis, most commonly in adults, but also in children (as a result of birth trauma, encephalitis, etc.). There may be an interval of weeks to months between the cerebrovascular event and the onset of hemiathetosis, but, when the hemiathetosis does appear, spastic hemiparesis is almost always still present. *Paroxysmal choreoathetosis* and other *paroxysmal dyskinesias* are discussed on p. 557.

Differential Diagnosis

Chorea and athetosis must be distinguished from psychogenic tics and from the pseudochoreoathetosis caused by severe impairment of proprioception (866).

Pathology

Athetosis is due to lesions of the striatum and globus pallidus, more rarely to lesions of the thalamus and red nucleus.

Pathophysiology

Loss of neural input from the internal pallidal segment to the thalamic nuclei leads to disordered regulation of neural activity in a cascade leading from the thalamus, to the premotor extrapyramidal cortical fields, to deeper centers, and thence to the spinal cord. The reticular system, too, loses its normal pallidal regulatory input, and also receives disordered excitatory input from the premotor cortical fields.

> **■ Treatment**
>
> See under dystonic syndromes, pp. 264 ff.

■ Hemiballism and Ballism

Clinical Features

These disorders are characterized by lightning-like, high-amplitude, flinging ("ballistic") movements simultaneously involving multiple segments of a limb. This creates the impression of a coordinated, but excessive movement that vastly overshoots its target. Hemiballism is unilateral by definition, while ballism is bilateral. The excursion of the involved limb(s) is very wide, so that it may be forcefully thrown against a wall or other obstacle, or indeed pull the rest of the body along. Injuries are not uncommon. This form of hyperkinesia is not present during sleep, but it may continue almost without interruption during waking hours, particularly in newly developed cases, and is worsened by external stimuli and by emotion. *Neurological examination* usually reveals an accompanying hemiparesis.

Etiologies

The most common cause is a *cerebrovascular event*, most characteristically a stroke involving the subthalamic nucleus, which produces the sudden onset of contralateral hemiballism. The onset may also be sudden, however, in cases due to *focal space-occupying lesions*. Bilateral heredodegenerative ballism is rare.

Pathology

There is usually a primary lesion of the contralateral subthalamic nucleus, less commonly a secondary involvement of this structure due to damage of the striatum and globus pallidus.

Pathophysiology

Loss of regulatory input from the subthalamic nucleus to the magnocellular portion of the red nucleus leads, by way of the rubrospinal tract, to disordered firing of the anterior horn cells of the spinal cord.

Treatment

Reserpine and neuroleptic agents are sometimes helpful, but hemiballism usually resolves spontaneously in a matter of weeks.

■ **Dystonic Syndromes** (605)

Clinical Features

Dystonia is the involuntary tonic contraction of muscles or muscle groups. It may be of shorter or longer duration. It is characterized by a mismatch between the relative degrees of contraction of agonist and antagonist muscles. Dystonia may be:

- either focal, affecting only a single muscle group, as in spasmodic torticollis or writer's cramp,
- or generalized, as in torsion dystonia (see also Table 2.**65**).

Physical Examination

Neurological examination usually reveals no abnormality other than the involuntary muscle contraction, though sometimes additional signs of an underlying illness are present. The types of dystonia are listed in Table 2.**65** and will be discussed individually in the following sections.

Note that the present system of classification is only partly based on etiologic criteria. The pathogenesis of dystonia is poorly understood. It may be due to a reorganization of inhibitory mechanisms in the spinal cord after peripheral nerve injury, as has been demonstrated, for example, in musicians with dystonic disorders (345c).

■ **Torsion Dystonia**

Clinical Features

Generalized torsion dystonia is characterized by slow, forceful, mostly rotatory movements of the head and trunk, accompanied by variable movements of the extremities, most often athetotic finger movements. The involved muscles seem to struggle continually against the contraction of their antagonist muscles, so that the patients appear to be in discomfort. A stationary posture, once reached, tends to be maintained for a long time, no matter how unusual or uncomfortable it may be. Torsion may be induced by voluntary movement or by emotion and is absent during

Table 2.**65** Symptomatic forms of torsion dystonia

Early Wilson's disease
Early Huntington's disease
Pantothene kinase-associated neuro-degeneration (formerly Hallervorden-Spatz disease)
Brain tumor
Postencephalitic
After cerebral venous thrombosis
G_{M2} gangliosidosis

sleep. Tone in the remaining muscles is often diminished, and the joints may be hyperextensible. Patients gradually fall into a permanent dystonic posture, involving, for example, hyperlordosis of the lumbar spine with flexion of the hips and internal rotation of the arms and legs. Torsion dystonia is said to be *myostatic* when a severe elevation of muscle tone produces an abnormal dystonic posture, but hyperkinesia is absent or no longer present.

Etiologic Forms

Hereditary idiopathic torsion dystonia. This disorder is of autosomal recessive inheritance and is usually found in Jewish families; large non-Jewish affected families have also been described, in some of which the inheritance pattern is autosomal dominant. There are *two major forms*, which differ in the age of onset and other clinical features: early onset is associated with a lesion on chromosome 9q34, later onset with a lesion on chromosome 8q or 18p. The *onset of illness* is usually in the first or second decade of life (before age 15 in two-thirds of all cases). Often, only

mild focal motor disturbances are present at first (resembling spasmodic torticollis or writer's cramp), and the full picture of torsion dystonia develops later. Gait disturbance is usually the first sign when the disease manifests itself in childhood, and its diagnostic significance is often, at first, unclear. In three-quarters of patients, the disease then progresses within 5–10 years to generalized dystonia, which is frequently severe. In contrast, if the disease first manifests itself in young adulthood, the initial signs are often in the trunk and upper extremities, and severe generalized dystonia develops in only one-third of such patients. Neuropathological study reveals loss of mainly the larger neurons in the putamen and other deep nuclei.

Treatment

This disorder is difficult to treat. *Diphenhydramine* (952) and other medications used to treat localized dystonia and chorea are recommended (see pp. 254 and 266).

DOPA-responsive dystonia. This disorder, which is often but not always hereditary (57b, 161, 860, 393), was earlier known as progressive dystonia with severe daily fluctuations (Segawa's disease) and presents in childhood with dystonia in varying locations, or, occasionally, with tremor. It is due to a mutation of the GTP cyclohydrolase I gene on chromosome 14q 22.3 (322a, 450b) and is inherited in an autosomal dominant pattern with low penetrance (448a). The dystonic movements vary considerably in severity over the course of each day, but become increasingly severe over the years as the disease progresses.

■ **Treatment**

As the name says, this disorder responds well to levodopa treatment. The designation "DOPA-responsive dystonia" is also given to other, rare types of dystonia that respond to levodopa, but are not associated with daily fluctuations (161, 393). This disorder may be difficult to differentiate from juvenile-onset Parkinson's disease with dystonic features (161).

■ **Localized Dystonias**

By definition, localized dystonia is confined to a particular part of the body. A single muscle group, or a small number of nearby muscle groups, tend to undergo involuntary tonic contraction, which hampers voluntary movement and produces an abnormal posture whenever certain types of voluntary movement are attempted. Many different areas of the body may be affected, most commonly the shoulders, feet, or legs (in walking) or the hands (in certain manual activities). Genetic studies have shown that ca. 25% percent of affected patients have relatives with dystonia. Autosomal dominant transmission with low penetrance is therefore assumed (991). Rare progressive cases may be the result of a brain lesion, and may first become apparent only after a long latency period (857a).

Many localized forms of dystonia are the product of excessive demand on the coordination of rapid movements; musicians' dystonia is a good example. The mechanism by which this occurs is, in most cases, unclear.

■ **Spasmodic Torticollis**

Clinical Features

This most common form of dystonia is limited to the cervical and nuchal musculature. Patients suffer from protracted, cramp-like, uncomfortable involuntary muscle contractions, which usually pull the head strongly to one side in a few seconds' time, while simultaneously tilting the head to the same, or opposite, side. Agonist and antagonist muscles contract simultaneously, creating the vivid impression that two forces are struggling with each other until the stronger one slowly prevails, as in an arm-wrestling match. The most commonly involved muscles are those innervated by the spinal accessory nerve – i.e., the sternocleidomastoid and the upper portion of the trapezius – though other cervical and nuchal muscles may also take part. Spasmodic torticollis is equally common in men and women and may appear at any age, but most often in middle age. When the abnormal muscle contractions are symmetrical, the head is strongly pulled straight backward (retrocollis). Mobile spasmodic torticollis is the more common type, but a more or less permanent dystonic posture, known as fixed torticollis, can also occur. The involuntary contractions may be provoked by voluntary movement or by emotional influences, and cease during sleep. Certain minor hand movements, such as gently supporting the chin with the hand, may suppress the dystonia ("geste antagoniste"). Torticollis is often accompanied by personality disorders. It is associated with blepharospasm and contraction of the facial musculature in Meige syndrome (see description, below).

Etiologic Forms

Spasmodic torticollis is not a unitary disease in the etiologic sense. Some cases are familial, while others are associated with an encephalitis in the patient's remote history, often years before. It may be the expression of incipient torsion dystonia, of Wilson's disease, or of Huntington's disease. It occurs with appreciable frequency in the aftermath of traumatic brain injury or cervical spine trauma.

Pathology

A heterogeneous collection of striatal lesions are associated with spasmodic torticollis.

Course

Approximately one-fifth of all patients with spasmodic torticollis undergo spontaneous remission, usually within 5 years. In a further one-third, dystonia progresses to involve other areas of the body (457).

Differential Diagnosis

Spasmodic torticollis must be distinguished from *psychogenic tics*, for which it is all too frequently mistaken. Furthermore, this disorder, particularly its fixed form, must be differentiated from other causes of a fixed *wry neck*, including the following:

- congenital anomalies of the cervical spine,
- muscular wry neck due to scarring of the sternocleidomastoid muscle secondary to birth trauma (caput obstipum musculare),
- compensatory tilting of the head away from the side of a trochlear nerve palsy,
- head tilt due to syringomyelia or high spinal cord tumor,
- acute torticollis in cervical intervertebral disc disease.

▌Treatment▐

Neurosurgical treatment with multiple upper cervical rhizotomy (the classic Dandy-McKenzie operation and more recent, selective variants, cf. ref. 540a) has lately been largely supplanted by local injection of botulinum A toxin into the affected muscles under electromyographic control (285); for details, see p. 268.

■ Writer's Cramp

This localized form of dystonia occurs almost exclusively with writing by hand, and only exceptionally with writing at the typewriter or computer console. Recently, it has been argued that writer's cramp may be due to a chronic lesion of the median nerve at the point where it crosses under the pronator teres muscle. Cases have also been described among patients with hereditary neuropathy, who have a tendency to develop pressure palsies (913a). Functional brain imaging has revealed that moving the index finger of the dominant hand is associated with less activation of the contralateral cerebral cortex in patients with writer's cramp than in normal controls (227a).

Treatment

Local injection of botulinum toxin is occasionally effective.

■ Blepharospasm (356, 374d, 619)

Nearly all cases of blepharospasm are first misdiagnosed as a psychogenic tic (833b). The disorder is generally seen in older adults, more often women than men, and consists of recurrent, spasmodic contraction of the orbicularis oculi muscles, of variable frequency and duration. During the phase of eye closure, which is of variable length, the patient can see nothing and is, therefore, helpless. A subgroup of patients are unable to open their flaccid, closed eyelids; this type of blepharospasm is also known as *lid opening apraxia.* The treatment consists of botulinum toxin injections (see below) and, occasionally, myectomy. Secondary forms of blepharospasm occur in Brueghel syndrome (see below), postencephalitic Parkinson's disease, Wilson's disease, Huntington's disease, and basal ganglionic infarction.

■ Dystonic Movements of the Mouth, Tongue, and Face

Faciobuccolingual dystonia generally arises as an adverse effect of medication, as discussed on p. 299. Phenothiazine derivatives, such as are found in antipsychotic, antivertiginous, and antiemetic medications, are most often responsible. Dystonic movements may also arise acutely and dramatically after a single dose of medication, just as oculogyric crises can. Faciobuccolingual dystonia also occurs in the absence of provoking medication, usually in the elderly, and presumably because of a midline cerebellar lesion, in most cases. The combination of blepharospasm with an *oromandibular dystonic syndrome* (dystonic jaw and lip movements with forced opening or closure of the mouth, accompanied by tongue movements) is known as *Meige syndrome* or *Brueghel syndrome;* some cases are familial. Cervical dystonia is frequently a further component of this disorder, which usually affects elderly patients and may progress to a generalized torsion dystonia. Buccofacial dystonia is occasionally seen

as a consequence of dental malocclusion; such cases respond well to reconstruction of the patient's bite by a dentist. *Spasmus nutans,* to be discussed below, should be considered in the differential diagnosis. Infants suffering from dystonic posture, or simply from wry neck, may concomitantly suffer from gastroesophageal reflux in the so-called *Sandifer syndrome.*

■ Other Dystonic Syndromes at a Wide Variety of Sites

The rare dystonic syndrome known as *"the yips"* affects golfers primarily during putting (648). *Musicians* may be affected by nonprogressive, but professionally disabling dystonias affecting many different types of movement, depending on the instrument played (704). *Paroxysmal stridor* and *spastic dysphonia* (p. 386) are focal dystonias of the laryngeal musculature (615, 1022). *Dystonia secondary to the use of neuroleptic medication* is described on p. 306. *Status dystonicus* has been described as arising in patients with primary localized dystonia, often in the absence of a known provoking factor (611a). These increasingly frequent and generalized dystonias may be quite dramatic in their clinical expression and cause the patient considerable impairment and physical danger. The rare, familial, exercise-induced *paroxysmal dystonia* is described on p. 557.

■ Treatment

The mainstay of current therapy is the *local injection of botulinum A toxin* into the affected muscles (as mentioned above under torticollis), in a dose of e.g. 10–40 ng. This ▶

treatment is relatively free of adverse effects, and its systemic effect is negligible. The injections must be repeated every few weeks at first, later much less frequently, and are particularly helpful in cases of spasmodic torticollis, blepharospasm, and writer's cramp (1031a). *Pharmacotherapy* is of secondary importance; the most effective agents are those that are also known, in another context, as causes of medication-induced parkinsonism, e.g. *haloperidol* (3–5 mg/d) or *reserpine* (0.5–3 mg t.i.d.). Buccolingual dystonia responds to *tetrabenazine*, 25–200 mg/d. *Levodopa* treatment is particularly recommended for patients with fixed, myostatic dystonia. Dystonia may also respond to *diazepam* or to high doses of bromocriptine. Blepharospasm may occasionally be alleviated by *clonazepam* (if the effect of botulinum toxin injections is inadequate). Deconditioning exercises may also be tried, for example in musicians.

■ Other Extrapyramidal Disorders

■ Tremor

Tremor may be classified according to its etiology or its clinical features; in Table 2.**66**, we have done the latter. Some of the varieties of tremor listed will be discussed in greater detail in this section.

Epidemiology

Tremor is said to be familial in anywhere from 17% to 100% of cases, according to a critical review of the literature (599b). Estimates of its prevalence range from 0.3% to 1.7%.

Clinical Features

Essential tremor is phenotypically no different from autosomal dominant *familial tremor*, but its onset is somewhat later on average. The age of onset has two peaks, one in the 2nd and another in the 6th decade of life (599). Tremor of the hands is always present and is often accompanied by tremor of the head, occasionally by leg tremor, and sometimes by leg pain, dyskinesia, or ataxia. Such combined forms, particularly when progressive, must, of course, prompt a search for another etiology, such as hepatolenticular degeneration (p. 297) or hyperthyroidism. A tremor with a frequency of 5–9 Hz is present in the hands at rest and worsens with emotional stress and on the attempt to maintain a fixed posture, e.g., to hold a glass of water in the air. Drinking alcohol alleviates the tremor in nearly half of all patients. Rarely, it may be unilateral. Histopathological study reveals loss of the small neurons of the striatum. Klinefelter's syndrome is associated with a type of tremor that is similar to essential tremor. Children who later develop overt familial tremor may, in infancy, suffer from *shivering attacks*, lasting several seconds, that may recur at brief intervals, but generally disappear during the first decade of life. The literature generally does not support the hypothesis that such children are more likely than others to develop Parkinson's disease later in life (532). Yet, in a large clinical series of patients with essential tremor, nearly half had associated dystonic findings, and 20% had associated parkinsonism (599).

A familial, nonprogressive *intention tremor*, without other signs of disease, occurs less commonly, and

Table 2.**66**   The most common types of tremor

Type of tremor	Features	Examples	Remarks
Physiological tremor	Very fine, only detectable with electrophysiologic techniques; 8–12 Hz; also present during sleep		
Rest tremor	Present when the limb is resting on a table or other support, without active muscle contraction; often diminishes or disappears with voluntary movement	Parkinson's disease	
Intention tremor	Present during voluntary movement; amplitude increases as the movement approaches its target	Polyneuropathy (sometimes), toxic conditions, multiple sclerosis (often)	Lesion of the dentate nucleus or its efferent tracts
Postural tremor	Present when a given position is actively maintained against gravity by voluntary muscle contraction	Essential and familial tremor	
Kinetic tremor (= action tremor)	Present during any type of active movement		E.g., during writing
Orthostatic tremor (= standing tremor)	Present in leg muscles when the patient stands, only detectable with electrophysiologic techniques, causes mild difficulty standing		
Action-specific tremor	Present exclusively during a specific kind of movement, usually one that requires a high degree of skill and coordination		
Isometric tremor	Present during active isometric muscle contraction – i.e., contraction against nonyielding resistance		
Functional tremor	Variable frequency, irregular intensity, assumes the frequency of passive movement of another limb		

Cont. →

Table 2.**66** *(Cont.)*

Type of tremor	Features	Examples	Remarks
Rubral tremor	Present at rest, becomes more intense with actively maintained posture, and even more intense with movement	"Flapping tremor" of Wilson's disease	Midbrain lesion
Cerebellar tremor	Highly variable: slow tremor in proximal joints of arms and legs, also of head or trunk when the patient stands	Lesion of the superior cerebellar peduncle	Often associated with other cerebellar signs

tremor secondary to peripheral trauma is a rarity (166c, 457b).

Orthostatic tremor, with a frequency of ca. 16 Hz, appears in the legs when the affected individual is standing (139, 623b, 1028). Patients complain of difficulty walking and sometimes even dizziness or falls, particularly in the dark. Orthostatic tremor is often invisible to the naked eye and can only be detected by electromyography. It responds to primidone, levodopa (1028c), and clonazepam.

Hypomagnesemia in the neonatal period may present with paroxysmal tremor and epileptic seizures.

Senile tremor has a frequency of 4–5 Hz, appears at rest, and affects not only the hands, but often also the head and mandible. *Geniospasm* is an isolated tremor of the chin inherited in an autosomal dominant pattern (211). It appears in childhood and is aggravated by emotional stress. Its differential diagnosis includes facial myoclonus and essential tremor affecting the head.

Differential Diagnosis

These forms of tremor must be differentiated from the distal, rhythmic tremor of Parkinson's disease, toxic tremor (e.g., in alcoholism, p. 307, and other addictions), the fine tremor of hyperthyroidism, and "flapping tremor," otherwise known as asterixis – an irregular, coarse tremor of the hands when the arms are outstretched.

The last-mentioned entity, which may be described as the inability to maintain a given posture, is usually symmetrical in cases of portocaval shunt and other hepatic diseases, as well as in uremic encephalopathy (p. 331), but may rarely be unilateral when caused by contralateral focal lesions at various sites in the brain (930c), particularly the thalamus (930d).

Treatment

Many of the forms of tremor mentioned above, particularly essential and familial tremor (but with the exception of orthostatic tremor), respond well to treatment with beta-blockers (623b). *Propranolol*, at an initial dose of 40 mg/day and gradually increasing as tolerated to as much as 240 mg/day, is the treatment of choice for essential ▶

and familial tremor. So-called *cardioselective beta-blockers*, such as *atenolol*, are also effective.

When beta-blockers are contraindicated (e.g. by asthma, atrioventricular block, or diabetes), cause intolerable side effects, or fail to relieve tremor, *primidone* may be used, at an initial dose of 62.5 mg h.s., slowly increasing to no more than 750 mg/day (given over the course of the day, in divided doses). Patients must be advised of the fatigue and somnolence that this drug induces when it is first taken and must temporarily refrain from driving.

Stereotactic operations in the thalamus, involving the creation of lesions or the implantation of electrodes for chronic *deep brain stimulation* (718a, 856a, 865a, 1048a), are an established, effective form of treatment for medically intractable tremor of any etiology, and may be performed in patients of any age, including the elderly.

■ Organic Tics

Tic disorders with complex psychomotor features are of organic etiology. One such disorder is *Gilles de la Tourette syndrome*, which the recent literature more simply, but less accurately, calls "Tourette syndrome" (38a, 345, 567). Affected patients suffer from involuntary twitching in the throat and face, as well as compulsive behaviors including the forced vocalization of obscenities (*coprolalia*); left-handedness and asymmetry of motor function are commonly associated findings. The disorder is genetically based, with what has been called a "semidominant" inheritance pattern. There is evidence for genetic imprinting, i.e., a differential effect of the abnormal allele depending on whether it was paternally or maternally inherited (583). A similar syndrome has also been observed as a transient manifestation of neuroleptic withdrawal. Gilles de la Tourette syndrome can be treated not only with neuroleptics, such as haloperidol, but also with plasmapheresis and immunoglobulins (684a, 751a) and with the atypical neuroleptic agent olanzapine (725a).

A similar, but different inherited disorder is that of the so-called "jumping Frenchmen of Maine" (a small, formerly genetically closed, Francophone population residing near the U.S.–Canadian border). Affected persons respond to an unexpected stimulus of any kind with a high-amplitude jump, and manifest compulsive repetition of words (*echolalia*) and command automatisms.

Hyperekplexia, an autosomal dominant disorder, also belongs to this group of familial tic disorders. It has been alternatively called *startle disease*, but must not be confused with the noninherited childhood disorder of the same name (p. 559). Affected individuals respond to an unexpected stimulus with a convulsive twitch, or sometimes by falling (942a). There is no loss of consciousness. The so-called "jerking stiff-man syndrome" may be related.

Somatosensory evoked potentials reveal a strong C response 60–75 ms after a peripheral nerve stimulus. Other electrophysiologic tests of brainstem reflexes also reveal an organically based tendency toward an excessively high amplitude of brainstem reflexes (627).

Jactatio capitis nocturna (nocturnal head banging or rocking) is a rhythmic movement of the head that occurs when the patient lies supine, during the transition between wakefulness and sleep. It is usually seen in children, less commonly in adults. It often resolves spontaneously with time. It is sometimes treated with psychotherapy.

■ Myoclonus
Nonrhythmic twitching of an entire muscle or several muscles is called myoclonus (as opposed to clonus, which affects an entire body part or, indeed, the entire body, and is rhythmic). Its origin is not necessarily in the extrapyramidal system. It appears preferentially during the transition from sleep to wakefulness, and also while the individual is falling asleep; the nonpathological *hypnagogic myoclonus* ("sleeping jerks") is well known. *Action myoclonus* occasionally occurs during voluntary movement in patients who have sustained anoxic brain damage (Lance–Adams syndrome), usually with associated cerebellar signs (550) (p. 341). Myoclonus is a nonspecific manifestation of many different disorders affecting the brainstem, including toxic and medication-induced encephalopathy, anoxic brain damage (740a), metabolic disorders, certain epilepsy syndromes, paraneoplastic syndromes, and Creutzfeldt-Jakob disease.

■ Treatment
Nitrazepam, valproic acid, clonazepam, and *piracetam* are beneficial. Very severe myoclonus may require a combination of two or more of these drugs (718).

■ Myorhythmia
Myorhythmia is persistent, rhythmic twitching in a single muscle group at a frequency of 1–4 Hz; it most commonly occurs in the face (platysma, orbicularis oculi) and in the swallowing apparatus (rhythmic protrusion of the tongue). It is generally due to a lesion in the brainstem or cerebellum and may appear with a latency varying from days to years. Persistent, intractable hiccupping (myorhythmia of the diaphragm) may be very troublesome, earning the French designation "hoquet diabolique"; this situation may arise in the setting of encephalitis, after general anesthesia, in multiple sclerosis, or without any known cause. For palatal myorhythmia ("palatal nystagmus"), see p. 652. Oculomasticatory myorhythmia is seen in Whipple's disease, along with other oculomotor and neurologic abnormalities (856d) (p. 93).

■ Treatment
Myorhythmia may be treated with an intravenous bolus of *methylphenidate (Ritalin)*, 20 mg, or of *isometheptene (Octinum)*, 100–200 mg (slow i.v. bolus).

■ Other Forms
Myokymia. This term refers to repetitive waves of contraction of individual fibers of a particular muscle or muscle group (e.g. facial myokymia, cf. p. 679), sometimes induced by pharmacotherapy with gold or with phenytoin, among other causes.

■ Treatment
It has been reported that a hereditary form of myokymia, associated with paroxysmal ataxia, responds well to *acetazolamide* (599e).

Paramyoclonus multiplex. This term refers to persistent (years), spontaneous, irregular twitching of the shoulder muscles.

Myoclonic epilepsy and myoclonus epilepsy. See p. 516.

Myoclonus multiplex fibrillaris (Morvan's fibrillary chorea). This disorder is characterized by irregularly distributed, partial muscle twitches accompanied by pain, autonomic dysfunction, mental changes including hallucinations, refractory insomnia, and sometimes sweating. It is usually toxic, due to mercurial salts, but has also been described as a paraneoplastic syndrome (566a).

Infantile polymyoclonus. This disorder begins in childhood with irregular, "dancing" eye movements, myoclonus, ataxia, and irritability. It takes a protracted, stepwise course. Laboratory findings include quantitative serum IgG abnormalities and cerebrospinal fluid plasmocytosis.

Serotonin syndrome. This condition may be caused by serotoninergic medications, particularly antidepressants, used alone or in combination with monoamine oxidase inhibitors. It is characterized by myoclonus and other involuntary movements as well as hyperreflexia, rigidity, orthostatic hypertension, confusion, and agitation.

Cerebellar Syndromes

Definition:
Like the extrapyramidal system, the cerebellum, too, plays an important role in motor processes. It receives sensory input from the periphery and integrates this information into the neural substrate of voluntary movement. It regulates muscle tone and orchestrates the coordinated functioning of muscle groups. Cerebellar dysfunction causes a diminution of muscle tone as well as an impairment of the coordination, modulation, and effectiveness of motor processes. Hypotonia, ataxia, and dysequilibrium are the clinical correlates of cerebellar dysfunction.

Functions of the Cerebellum
The cerebellum coordinates the activity of agonist, accessory, and antagonist muscles to assure fluid, precise, and efficient execution of movement. The *anatomical and physiological prerequisites* for this task are:
• The *neural input* to the cerebellum must continuously convey, not only instructions about movement from higher centers, but also instantaneously updated information from the periphery about the position and movement of all body parts.

• The integrated result of cerebellar processing, based on all of these inputs, determines its *neural output*, which, in turn, travels to other components of the motor system and ultimately affects the impulses arriving at muscles throughout the body.

The cerebellum should thus be regarded as a stabilizing regulatory system, which:
• is notified of all impending movements,

- continuously compares the desired movement with afferent feedback data about the actual course of movement, and
- makes all of the necessary adjustments and corrections.

Afferent tracts: The cerebellum receives input concerning the position of the limbs and the activity of the muscles through the restiform body of the inferior cerebellar peduncle and, in small part, through the superior cerebellar peduncle. Vestibulocerebellar fibers enter the cerebellum through the juxtarestiform body of the inferior cerebellar peduncle. Impulses from the cerebral cortex arrive first at the precerebellar nuclei of the pons, from which they are relayed to the cerebellum through the middle cerebellar peduncle.

Efferent tracts: The neural output arises from the deep cerebellar nuclei and exits the cerebellum through the superior cerebellar peduncle (brachium conjunctivum). Most fibers of the superior cerebellar peduncle terminate in the contralateral ventrolateral nucleus of the thalamus. Others terminate in the red nucleus, which in turn projects both to the thalamus and, by way of the rubrospinal tract, to the brainstem and spinal cord.

General Clinical Features of Cerebellar Dysfunction

The speed, fluidity, and automatic coordination of movement are disturbed, resulting in the following major findings:

Dyssynergy. Lack of coordination of the individual muscles and muscle groups participating in a given movement. Examples include: backward bending of the trunk without concomitant knee flexion, resulting in loss of balance; walking on all fours without precise alternation of contralateral arm and leg.

Dysmetria. Incorrect amplitude or velocity of a planned movement. The patient may open the fingers excessively while grasping a small object, or raise the leg too high while attempting to plant the foot on a chair with the eyes closed.

Ataxia. Failure of harmonious cooperation of muscle groups in the performance of a motor task. The finger-nose and heel-knee-shin tests may be performed with deviations to one or both sides of the optimal path of movement.

Intention tremor. Oscillating deviation from the optimal path of movement that increases in amplitude as the target is approached, generally due to lesions of the dentate nucleus or its efferent tract (the superior cerebellar peduncle). It is easily detected with the finger–nose (Fig. 2.**78**) and heel–knee–shin tests.

Pathological rebound phenomenon. Antagonist muscles are not contracted in time to brake an excessive movement. To test this phenomenon, the examiner asks the patient to contract a muscle against resistance, then suddenly removes the resistance. Figure 2.**79** shows how this phenomenon is elicited at the elbow. The examiner can also ask the patient to push apart his outstretched arms against resistance.

Dysdiadochokinesia. Impaired performance of rapid alternating movements, due to inadequately rapid and

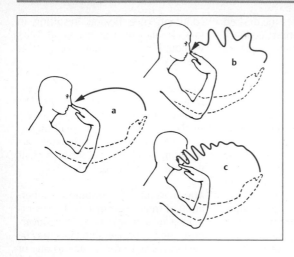

Fig. 2.**78a–c**   **Finger-nose test.**
a Normal.
b Ataxia.
c Intention tremor.

fluid alternation of agonist and antagonist contraction. One may test this with rapid alternating pronation and supination of the forearm (Fig. 2.**80**) or rapid alternating striking of the thigh with the dorsal and volar surfaces of the hand.

Hypotonia. Diminished muscle tone on passive movement. If the patient is rapidly shaken backwards and forwards, or rotationally about the vertical axis, the arms make a larger than normal excursion.

Sinking of the arm on positional testing. Tonic muscle contraction is no longer maintained with adequate constancy. When the patient raises his arms in front with eyes closed, the arm on the side of the lesion tends to sink.

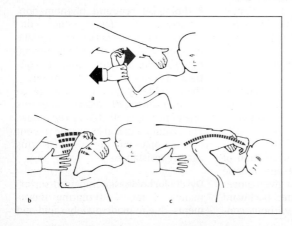

Fig. 2.**79a–c**   **Elicitation of the rebound phenomenon in cerebellar dysfunction.**
a Technique. **b** Normal finding: prompt braking of movement.
c Pathological rebound phenomenon with insufficient braking due to an ipsilateral cerebellar lesion.

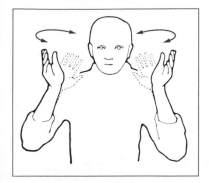

Fig. 2.**80 Testing of diadochokinesia.** Rapidly alternating pronation and supination of the hand.

Past-pointing in the Bárány pointing test. The patient is asked to point at an object and then close his eyes; the arm on the side of the lesion slowly drifts downward and to the side.

Unstable stance (in the Romberg test).

Truncal ataxia on sitting.

Unstable, broad-based gait. Patients may complain of "dizziness" in the absence of true vertigo.

Nystagmus. Coarse nystagmus with fast phase toward the side of the lesion, increasing in amplitude on lateral gaze toward the side of the lesion, and decreasing in amplitude when the eyes are closed.

Pathological nystagmus suppression test. See p. 643 and Fig. 9.**9**.

Cerebellar ("scanning") dysarthria. Chopped, explosive speech with separate, effortful pronunciation of each syllable.

Localizing Significance of Findings
Lesions affecting the caudal portion of the vermis. Truncal ataxia and dysequilibrium, particularly on sitting.

Lesions affecting the rostral portion of the vermis. Incoordination of stance and gait.

Lesions affecting the cerebellar hemispheres. Incoordination of fine movements of the ipsilateral extremities. N.b.: If the clinical findings suggest localized cerebellar dysfunction, a neuroimaging study should be performed. Focal lesions of the cerebellum are more readily detected by MRI than by CT.

Clinical Features of Various Cerebellar Disorders
The clinician can often infer the etiology of a cerebellar disorder from the temporal course of presentation, the nature of the cerebellar signs, and the accompanying neurologic deficits. Table 2.**67** has been constructed to reflect the logical sequence of the diagnostic process. The more important cerebellar disorders are discussed in this section; other disorders appearing in Table 2.**67** will be presented elsewhere.

■ Acute Cerebellar Ataxia of Childhood (186)
Acute cerebellar ataxia sometimes arises a few days or weeks after a bout of chickenpox, but more frequently follows a nonspecific illness. It usually affects children in the 2nd to 5th year of life. There is usually a subacute onset of progressively unsteady gait, tremor, oculomotor disturbances, and nystagmus. These abnormalities resolve fully and sponta-

Table 2.**67** Diseases predominantly affecting the cerebellum

Time to development of full disorder	Disease	Age	Features
Hours	Psychogenic ataxia	Adolescents and young adults	Varying manifestations depending on the test situation, normal eye movements, no nystagmus
Hours	Acute cerebellar hemorrhage or infarction	Any age	Usually in hypertensive individuals; intense headache, increasing confusion and signs of intracranial hypertension
Days	Acute cerebellar ataxia of childhood	First decade of life	After nonspecific premonitory illness; prognosis usually good
Days	Fisher syndrome	Any age	Usually young adults, mainly male; oculomotor disturbance, ataxia, and areflexia; prognosis always good
Days	Multiple sclerosis	Young adults	Ataxia is rarely the first sign of multiple sclerosis; tends to persist
Days	Intoxications	Any age	E.g., DDT, diphenylhydantoin, organic mercurial salts, piperazine, 5-fluorouracil, lithium
Hours–days (intermittent)	Hartnup disease, pyruvate dehydrogenase deficiency	Early childhood	Autosomal recessive, also choreoathetotic involuntary movements
Hours–days (intermittent)	Familial episodic ataxia	Any age	Usually autosomal dominant; ataxia, dysarthria, nystagmus; responds to acetazolamide
Hours–days (intermittent)	Multiple sclerosis	Young adults	Ictal form with dysarthria and tonic brainstem attacks; responds to carbamazepine

Months	Symptomatic, progressive cerebellar atrophy	Any age	E.g., paraneoplastic, due to alcohol abuse
Months	Myxedema	Any age	Always accompanied by other signs of severe hypothyroidism
Weeks	Cerebellar tumor	Mainly children	Rapid development of signs of intracranial hypertension
Weeks	Infantile myoclonic encephalopathy	Early childhood	Rapidly progressive ataxia with myoclonus and opsoclonus; seen in association with neuroblastoma; remission possible
Months to years	Cerebellar heredoataxia	Any age	Family history, slow progression, often other progressive deficits such as nystagmus, spasticity, optic atrophy
Months to years	Late cortical cerebellar atrophy (Marie-Foix-Alajouanine syndrome)	4th and 5th decades	Progressively unsteady gait, less commonly nystagmus; predominantly truncal ataxia; not hereditary
Months to years	Olivopontocerebellar atrophy	3rd to 5th decades	Ataxia, tremor, parkinsonism, urinary incontinence, occasionally dementia; a form of multisystem atrophy; half of all cases are familial

neously in some two-thirds of cases, but the remaining patients may suffer from residual gait imbalance, impaired learning ability, and ataxia even years later. The cause is presumably a bland encephalitis.

■ Cerebellar Encephalitis in Adulthood

Adults, too, may suffer from acute cerebellar ataxia similar to the childhood type just discussed. A serologically detectable viral illness precedes the encephalitis in only a minority of cases. The cerebellar signs generally resolve spontaneously, but may persist, particularly in older patients (522, 534).

■ Transient Ataxia in Fisher Syndrome

See p. 278.

■ Toxic Causes of Cerebellar Dysfunction

Certain substances cause cerebellar dysfunction that arises within days of ingestion and generally resolves completely thereafter. These include the following:

- DDT,
- organic mercury,
- piperazine,
- the mitotic inhibitor 5-fluorouracil,
- lithium, and
- diphenylhydantoin (in toxic doses).

The last-mentioned agent may, however, cause persistent cerebellar dysfunction even after its withdrawal, particularly in women and in patients with a preexisting brain lesion (p. 305).

■ Hereditary Cerebellar Ataxias of Known Pathogenetic Mechanism (251)

A number of systemic illnesses primarily involve the cerebellum. Some of these have a known pathogenetic mechanism, including:

- abetalipoproteinemia (Bassen-Kornzweig disease, cf. p. 296),
- hexosaminidase deficiency,
- pyruvate dehydrogenase deficiency, and
- glutamate dehydrogenase deficiency.

A rare disorder has also been described involving autoantibodies to glutaric acid decarboxylase (816a).

Xeroderma pigmentosum, whose manifestations are predominantly cerebellar, *and Cockayne syndrome,* of which deafness is often a prominent feature, are both due to abnormalities of DNA synthesis.

Ataxia telangiectasia (Louis-Bar syndrome) is an autosomal-recessive disorder in which cerebellar ataxia begins in infancy and gradually progresses, so that the affected patients become disabled before reaching adolescence. Choreoathetotic movements are often present, and eye movements are notably slow. Telangiectasias appear later, first on the conjunctiva, then on the skin, particularly at the bends of the elbows and knees. Pneumonia and upper respiratory tract infections are frequent. This disorder belongs to a group of disorders characterized by chromosomal fragility and predisposition to the development of neoplasms. The responsible gene, called ATM, has recently been identified (827). The gene product appears to possess regulatory functions for many different cellular processes and thus probably plays a role not only in ataxia telangiectasia, but also in carcinogenesis.

Rett syndrome is a progressive ataxia affecting only girls and associated with autism, dementia, and incoordination of the hands. Certain individuals with *gluten hypersensitivity* may develop ataxia, predominantly affecting gait, even in the absence of other manifestations of celiac disease. Many such patients also suffer from polyneuropathy; the combination has been termed *gluten ataxia* (373c).

A number of hereditary forms of cerebellar ataxia with a known pathogenetic mechanism are characterized by *intermittent ataxia*; these include:

• Hartnup disease (p. 292),
• pyruvate dehydroxygenase deficiency, and others.

There is also a *familial periodic paroxysmal ataxia* of autosomal dominant inheritance, due to an abnormal gene on chromosome 19p (965). Even though all patients have the same underlying genetic abnormality, the clinical expression of the disorder is highly variable (57a). Attacks of ataxia, dysarthria, nystagmus, and vertigo begin in early childhood, last for hours to days, and occur at intervals of approximately one week. Cerebellar dysfunction is no more than mild in between attacks. Acetazolamide has a beneficial effect.

■ Hereditary Cerebellar Ataxias of Unknown Pathogenetic Mechanism

Most disorders in this group are thought to be due to an inborn error of amino acid metabolism. The individual disorders listed below do not, for the most part, possess a unitary clinical picture, as the signs and symptoms of each may vary from one affected family to another. In general, ataxia with onset in the 1st and 2nd decades of life is transmitted in an autosomal recessive pattern, while ataxia of later onset is usually autosomal dominant.

Ataxia is the major finding in all of these disorders. Additional neurologic signs may develop later, including hypertonia, paralysis, muscle atrophy, pyramidal tract signs, disturbances of ocular motility, nystagmus, optic atrophy, and dementia. The ataxia and other abnormalities progress slowly, perhaps even over several decades. Histopathological study reveals cell loss in various cerebellar nuclei and in the cerebellar cortex, as well as atrophy of the long tracts of the spinal cord.

Menzel type. This autosomal dominant form of hereditary cerebellar ataxia first appears at a mean age of 35 years (range, 14–73) and lasts for a mean of 12.5 years until death (range, 4–23). Additional abnormalities, such as chorea, retinopathy, and optic atrophy, are occasionally found.

Dejerine–Thomas type. This disorder appears sporadically or in families, with an autosomal-dominant inheritance pattern. The mean age of onset is 50 years (range, 17–65), and the mean duration of illness is 6.5 years (range, 1–18). In addition to ataxia, further abnormalities include disturbances of autonomic regulation, orthostatic hypotension, impotence, and supranuclear oculomotor disturbances.

Cerebello-olivary atrophy of Holmes. This disorder is usually of autosomal dominant inheritance, begins at a mean age of 46 years (range, 10–70), and lasts for a mean of 17 years until death. Ataxia may be accompanied by spasticity, dementia, and urinary incontinence.

Dyssynergia cerebellaris progressiva (Ramsay Hunt syndrome). There is some controversy over whether this entity, also known as *progressive myoclonic ataxia* (618), is an independent disorder, as some cases may be difficult to distinguish from myoclonus epilepsy (p. 516). It is characterized by myoclonus, appearing particularly during voluntary movement, cerebellar signs (mostly of hemispheric type), and occasionally cerebellospinal signs such as ataxia, as well as epileptic seizures. Dementia is not a component of this disorder, as distinct from myoclonus epilepsy. It progresses over several years and occurs frequently in families. The histopathological findings are heterogeneous.

Marinesco-Sjögren syndrome. This disorder is characterized by cerebellar ataxia, congenital cataracts, and oligophrenia.

■ Nonhereditary Cerebellar Disorders

Late cortical cerebellar atrophy. This disorder, also known as Marie-Foix-Alajouanine syndrome after the French neurologists who described it, is associated with a symmetrical pathologic process predominantly involving the paleocerebellum, in which the vermis is more severely affected than the hemispheres. There is a severe loss of Purkinje cells, and a somewhat less severe loss of granule cells. The primary degenerative form of this disorder has its clinical onset at a mean age of 47 years; it generally begins relatively suddenly and then progresses slowly thereafter. The initial findings include gait instability, truncal ataxia affecting stance and gait, and then incoordination of the hands. Nystagmus, hypotonia, and pyramidal tract signs are rarely seen. Cognitive function usually remains normal, and the life expectancy is not diminished. The primary degenerative form may be considered a type of premature aging occurring locally in the cerebellum.

Diffuse cerebellar atrophies. These are a group of disorders of heterogeneous etiology and course. Their clinical expression may at first resemble that of late cortical cerebellar degeneration. Only the further course provides an indication of the specific etiology.

Late cerebellar atrophy in chronic alcoholism (p. 310).

Subacute cerebellar cortical atrophy as a paraneoplastic process (p. 321).

Infantile myoclonic encephalopathy (of Kinsbourne). About half of all cases of this syndrome are a paraneoplastic manifestation of childhood neuroblastoma, and the remaining cases are idiopathic. Acute or subacute cerebellar signs arise at the age of a few months to years, accompanied by variable myoclonic twitching of the skeletal muscles and an irregular dyskinesia of the eyes (opsoclonus, p. 652). The affected children are often irritable, and they later become mentally retarded. The EEG reveals no epileptiform activity. The signs of this illness tend to resolve in large measure after treatment of the neuroblastoma or, in children without tumors, after ACTH therapy.

Kuru. This prion disease was formerly seen in New Guinea, predominantly in young women, and was transmitted by ritual cannibalism (p. 125). It was characterized by unsteady gait, tremor, and the later development of other cerebellar signs and led inexorably to death in a few months to years.

A classification scheme for degenerative disorders of the cerebellum with ataxia is given in Table 2.**68**.

Table 2.**68**   Classification of degenerative cerebellar disorders causing ataxia (after 523)

Hereditary ataxias
- Autosomal recessive ataxias:
- Friedreich's ataxia (FRDA)
- Abetalipoproteinemia (Bassen–Kornzweig syndrome)
- Refsum's disease
- Ataxia telangiectasia (Louis-Bar syndrome)
- Ataxia of vitamin E deficiency
- Early-onset cerebellar ataxia (EOCA) with preserved intrinsic muscle reflexes (Fickler–Winkler)
- Other types of EOCA, with individual distinguishing characteristics
  Autosomal dominant cerebellar ataxia (ADCA):
- With additional extracerebellar signs (ADCA-I) (Nonne, Marie, Menzel):
  – Spinocerebellar atrophy (SCA1)
  – SCA2
  – SCA3 (Machado–Joseph disease)
  – SCA4
  – Other types
- With retinitis pigmentosa (ADCA-II) (Nonne, Marie, Menzel), SCA7
- With purely cerebellar signs (ADCA-III) (Nonne, Marie):
  – SCA5, SCA6
  – Other types

Non-hereditary ataxias
Idiopathic cerebellar ataxias (IDCA):
- With purely cerebellar signs (IDA-C) (Marie-Foix-Alajouanine)
- With additional extracerebellar signs in the setting of multisystem atrophy (IDCA-P, MSA) (Dejerine, Thomas)
  Symptomatic ataxias:
- Ataxia due to alcohol abuse
- Ataxia due to other intoxications
- Ataxia due to hypothyroidism
- Ataxia due to malabsorption syndrome
- Paraneoplastic ataxia
- Ataxia of physical (non-cerebellar) origin

■ Other Cerebellar Syndromes

Infectious mononucleosis and *Mycoplasma pneumoniae* infection (79a) may both cause a transient cerebellar syndrome. *Macroglobulinemia* may cause not only a polyneuropathy (p. 606) but also a progressive cerebellar ataxia, which regresses when the underlying disorder is treated. *Myxedema* may be associated with cerebellar and other neurological signs. *Sprue* in adults, in addition to the commonly encountered polyneuropathy and long spinal tract degeneration (p. 441), may also produce cerebellar signs, including palatal nystagmus, sometimes before the appearance of gastrointestinal symptoms. *Heatstroke* may cause lasting cerebellar damage with permanent deficits. A number of *medications* are known to cause cerebellar dysfunction, which may persist, among them anticonvulsants, lithium salts, and haloperidol (344b). For a discussion of cerebellar tumors, see pp. 62 f.

■ Ataxias of Extracerebellar Origin That May Mimic a Cerebellar Disorder

The motor incoordination sometimes appearing after prolonged hospitalization, so-called *"bed ataxia,"* should not be confused with a cerebellar disorder. *"Optical ataxia"* is the extreme incoordination of grasping and manipulation of objects that is seen in patients with bilateral disconnection of the visual cortex from the motor tracts. Severe *deafferentation* – e.g., in polyneuropathy or pathological processes affecting the posterior columns – also produces ataxia, particularly of gait, which must be differentiated from cerebellar ataxia. Gait ataxia is also seen in the rare syndrome of bilateral vestibular dysfunction.

Treatment

Etiological treatment of a cerebellar disorder as such is only possible when there is an underlying, correctable toxic or metabolic disturbance. In most cases, only symptomatic treatment can be provided. Medications that have been found beneficial against ataxia to a limited extent include *neostigmine* (38b), the 5-HT$_3$ antagonist *ondansetron* (785a), and *amantadine hydrochloride* (124a).

Metabolic Disorders with Cerebral Or Other Neurologic Involvement (807a)

Overview:
Familial disorders of brain metabolism are most often of autosomal recessive inheritance. They commonly cause mental retardation, ataxia, spasticity, epileptic seizures, myopathy, and progressive dementia. The clinical signs are usually symmetric and generalized. The neuropathological and neuroradiological findings are also usually symmetric; depending on the disorder, they may be localized in the gray or white matter, the basal ganglia, the cerebellum, the optic nerves, or the spinal cord. Most of the metabolic disorders to be discussed are due to a known enzyme deficiency, and the underlying genetic defect is also known for many of them. The identification of abnormal metabolic products in the urine, serum, or tissue or the determination of a specific histological abnormality is often helpful in diagnosis. The definitive diagnosis is provided by the demonstration of the causative enzyme deficiency or genetic defect. Effective treatment is available for some of these disorders. Accurate diagnosis even of untreatable disorders is important, as it provides the basis for genetic counseling.

Advances in biochemistry and molecular biology have enabled identification of the molecular defects underlying many of the metabolic disorders affecting the nervous system. These are usually enzyme deficiencies of autosomal or X-linked recessive inheritance (9). They first manifest themselves in infancy or childhood, or, in exceptional cases, in adolescence or adulthood. "Dead-end" metabolic intermediates often accumulate in the nervous system or other parts of the body. Broadly simplifying, one may say that phospholipids and gangliosides are mainly stored in nerve cell bodies and synapses. The resulting *neuronal disorders* present with dementia, seizures, and visual disturbances and later progress to ataxia and dementia. On the other hand, disturbances of sulfatide and cerebroside metabolism most often cause *myelin sheath disorders*, in which pyramidal tract signs, spasticity, and ataxia are present from the beginning, while dementia and seizures come only later (Table 2.**69**).

An increasing number of adult-onset cerebral metabolic disorders are be-

Table 2.**69** Neurological signs of metabolic disorders

Spasticity and other pyramidal tract signs
Ataxia
Motor and cognitive developmental delay
Dementia
Epileptic seizures
Visual disturbances
Polyneuropathy and myopathic syndromes

ing recognized which present with, for example, dementia or muscle atrophy (184). The more than 500 types of enzyme deficiency known to date may be classified according to the age of onset of overt disease or the type of metabolic or genetic abnormality (621, 651). Some are amenable to etiologic or symptomatic treatment; in such cases, proper treatment can give the patients a new lease on life. Even if the disorder turns out to be untreatable, it is still important to provide an accurate diagnosis for purposes of genetic counseling, the identification of carriers, and prenatal diagnosis.

When a Metabolic Disorder Should Be Suspected

Any of the following should arouse suspicion of a metabolic disorder (660):

- similar neurologic disturbances in siblings or near relatives;
- repeated impairment of consciousness or unexplained vomiting in an infant or small child;
- repeated episodes of unexplained ataxia or spasticity;
- progressive CNS degeneration;
- mental retardation in siblings or near relatives;
- mental retardation without evidence of a congenital structural anomaly or perinatal injury.

Many metabolic disorders are associated with specific somatic abnormalities of the skin or hair, coarse facial features, a characteristic smell of the urine or body odor, or ocular abnormalities such as cataract, corneal opacity, or macular cherry-red spot. A metabolic disorder is less likely if congenital malformations are present in association with mental retardation or focal neurologic deficits.

Practical Diagnostic Evaluation

The following steps are recommended (660):

Laboratory examination of the urine: Amino acid screening reveals the commoner disorders of amino acid and carbohydrate metabolism.

Serum ammonia, fasting blood sugar, lactate, pyruvate, and blood gas analysis: Urea cycle disorders are associated with hyperammonemia in the fasting state or when the patient consumes a protein-rich diet. Recurrent hypoglycemia or intermittent acidosis with elevation of either the lactate or the pyruvate concentration is associated with a range of conditions, including disorders of the pyruvate dehydrogenase complex, of glucose metabolism or gluconeogenesis; carboxylase defects or organic acidurias; and also many acquired disorders.

Serum levels of amino and other organic acids: These studies should be performed whenever the lactate or pyruvate level is elevated. The demonstration of long-chain fatty acids is characteristic of adrenoleukodystrophy.

Radiographs of the skull, spine, and long bones: These studies may aid in the diagnosis of the mucopolysaccharidoses, Gaucher's disease, Niemann–Pick disease, and the G_{M1} gangliosidoses.

Screening for lysosomal enzymes: As a minimum, this should include beta-galactosidase, arylsulfatase, and hexosaminidase.

Tissue biopsy: The definitive diagnosis of a metabolic disorder (particularly the lipidoses and leukodystrophies) is based not only on the specific clinical presentation, but also on histologic and biochemical study of tissue specimens. Depending on the disorder, the tissue to be examined may be peripheral nerve, skin, conjunctiva, muscle, lymphocytes, bone marrow, or brain.

Molecular analysis: In an increasing number of disorders, DNA analysis can be used to reveal the specific genetic defect, while biochemical analysis reveals the defective gene product.

Neuroimaging (60, 507, 566, 729)

A metabolic disorder is suspected if the MRI reveals symmetric involve-

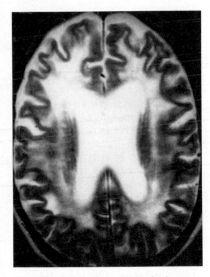

Fig. 2.**81 Adult form of polyglucosan body disease.** This 43-year-old man had been suffering from progressive spasticity, mild ataxia and fasciculations for 3 years, and had recently become demented. The T2-weighted image reveals symmetric signal abnormalities in the white matter of both hemispheres, as well as atrophy of both the white and the gray matter. The patient died 2 years after this scan was taken. An adult form of polyglucosan body disease was diagnosed at autopsy.

ment of the gray matter, white matter, or both, or of the basal ganglia (Fig. 2.**81**). The likelihood of a metabolic disorder is lower if the CT or MRI reveals structural anomalies or focal or asymmetric signal abnormalities. MRI is useful in distinguishing disorders predominantly affecting the white or gray matter (Table 2.**70**). It should be borne in mind that the state of cerebral myelination undergoes rapid changes over the course of normal development in the first few years of life. A child's brain does not resemble that of an adult on MRI until about the age of 18 months (158).

Lysosomal and Other Storage Diseases (471, 700)

If a specific catabolic enzyme is deficient, intracellular deposition of lipids or saccharides will result, thus producing a storage disease. If the lesion involves a lysosomal enzyme, a lysosomal storage disease results. Most of these diseases are transmitted in an autosomal recessive inheritance pattern, while a few are X-linked. The more important diseases in this group are listed in Table 2.**71**. Of these, only Gaucher's disease is treatable.

■ Lipidoses

Lipidoses are storage diseases involving neutral lipids, glycolipids, phospholipids, or gangliosides.

The G_{M2} gangliosidoses (472). These disorders are due to a genetically based deficiency of the enzyme hexosaminidase. The best known is *Tay-Sachs disease*, an autosomal recessive disorder that is most common among Jews of Ashkenazi (eastern European) origin. Affected infants develop my-

Table 2.**70**   MRI findings of metabolic disorders and some neurodegenerative disorders (729)

Disorders mainly affecting the white matter of the brain (leukodystrophies):

- Disorders of amino acid metabolism
- Lysosomal disorders and other storage diseases:
  - Metachromatic leukodystrophy
  - Alexander disease
  - Krabbe's globoid cell leukodystrophy
  - Degenerative diffuse sclerosis of neutral lipid type
  - Pelizaeus-Merzbacher disease
  - Batten-Kufs disease
  - Adrenoleukodystrophy
  - Diffuse cerebral sclerosis (Schilder's disease, encephalitis periaxialis diffusa)
- Spongiform degeneration of the nervous system (Canavan's disease)

Disorders mainly affecting the gray matter of the brain:

- Tay-Sachs disease and other lipidoses
- Hurler syndrome and other mucopolysaccharidoses (325)
- Mucolipidoses and fuscinoses
- Glycogen storage diseases

Disorders affecting both white and gray matter:

- Leigh syndrome
- Mitochondrial encephalomyopathies (p. 902)
- Zellweger syndrome and other peroxisomal disorders

Disorders mainly affecting the basal ganglia (423):

- Wilson's disease
- Fahr's disease
- Pantothene kinase-associated neurodegeneration (formerly Hallervorden-Spatz disease) (30, 829)
- Huntington's disease

Table 2.**71**   Lysosomal and other storage diseases affecting the nervous system

Lipidoses:
G_{M2} gangliosidoses
G_{M1} gangliosidoses
Fabry's disease (angiokeratoma corporis diffusum)
Gaucher's disease
Niemann-Pick disease
Farber's lipogranulomatosis
Wolman's disease
Refsum's disease
Cerebrotendinous xanthomatosis
Neuronal ceroid lipofuscinosis

Leukodystrophies:
Metachromatic leukodystrophy
Krabbe's globoid cell leukodystrophy

Mucopolysaccharidoses

Mucolipidoses

oclonus and generalized seizures in the first few months of life, followed by blindness, decorticate posturing, and death at 3–5 years. The diagnosis is made either by enzyme assay or by direct DNA analysis (the preferred method). In both Tay-Sachs disease and *Sandhoff disease*, a clinically similar disorder affecting non-Jewish infants, a characteristic cherry-red spot is seen on the macula of the retina. Adult forms of hexosaminidase deficiency lead to dementia, spasticity, ataxia, and muscular atrophy, or else to motor neuron disease, as seen in the Kugelberg-Welander and Aran-Duchenne syndromes. MRI reveals T2 hyperintensity of the basal ganglia and cerebellar cortical atrophy (913, 1042).

The G_{M1} gangliosidoses. These disorders are due to a deficiency of galactosidase. They clinically resemble

Tay-Sachs disease (1041) and, like it, may be diagnosed by enzyme assay or by direct DNA analysis.

Fabry disease (angiokeratoma corporis diffusum) (500). This X-linked disorder affects the skin, kidneys, and blood vessels as well as the peripheral and autonomic nervous system. A deficiency of alpha-galactosidase causes intracellular deposition of trihexosylceramide. The symptoms and signs arise either because of the primary cellular involvement or because of vascular compromise. The initial manifestations usually appear in childhood or adolescence and consist of burning pains in the extremities, which are particularly severe in warm weather, but respond to diphenylhydantoin. Sweating is lost soon afterward. Maculopapular, reddish-purple skin lesions appear, and, in the third or fourth decade of life, kidney failure occurs. Stroke and acute vestibular dysfunction are also common. A mild form of the disease may occur in female carriers of the gene.

Gaucher's disease. This autosomal recessive disorder is due to glucocerebrosidase deficiency, which results in accumulation of glucocerebroside. It occurs in juvenile and adult neuronal forms, as well as an adult nonneuronal form. In the juvenile form, developmental delay is evident in the first few months of life, and affected children die before their second birthday. The adult neuronal form causes psychosis, dementia, myoclonus, generalized seizures, akathisia, supranuclear gaze palsy, bulbar signs, spasticity, and polyneuropathy, while the nonneuronal form causes splenomegaly, thrombocytopenia, bone erosion, and bone pain. Characteristic foam cells ("Gaucher cells") are found in the bone marrow, and the enzyme deficiency can be detected in the leukocytes. Enzyme replacement (intravenous infusion of recombinant or human placental glucocerebrosidase) is an effective, though expensive form of treatment (67).

Niemann-Pick disease. A deficiency of *acid sphingomyelinase* (ASM) underlies both Type A and Type B Niemann-Pick disease. These two disorders represent opposite ends of a spectrum of disease, in which patients with lower levels of ASM activity become ill earlier, have more severe neurologic involvement, and die at an earlier age. The inheritance pattern is autosomal recessive, and the responsible genetic defect lies on chromosome 18 (169). In Type A disease, progressive encephalopathy is manifest as dementia, spasticity, ataxia, and generalized seizures, and results in death by the age of 2 years. Accompanying findings include a cherry-red spot on the retinal macula (in some cases) and hepatosplenomegaly. In Type B disease, organomegaly and respiratory disturbances are the most prominent clinical features, and patients may survive into adolescence or adulthood.

Adult-onset Niemann-Pick disease (Types C, D, and E according to the current nomenclature) is a different disease, due to a defect of cholesterol metabolism; ASM activity may be secondarily impaired. Hepatosplenomegaly is a prominent feature, and foam cells are found in the bone marrow and liver, as in Gaucher's disease. A schizophrenia-like psychosis may be the presenting sign (250).

Type A or B disease may be diagnosed by measurement of ASM activity in leukocytes, or by DNA analysis. Type C disease is generally diagnosed by specialized biochemical testing of fibroblasts obtained by skin biopsy.

Refsum's disease (heredopathia atactica polyneuritiformis) (783). Refsum's disease is unusual in that it involves storage of a substance derived from the diet. A deficiency of *phytanic acid alpha-dehydrogenase* leads to accumulation of phytanic acid in the tissues of the body, particularly the liver and kidneys. The first signs of illness may appear in childhood or as late as middle age. The most prominent neurologic abnormalities are night blindness secondary to retinitis pigmentosa, sensorineural deafness, polyneuropathy, and ataxia (both axial and appendicular). Psychiatric manifestations may also be seen. The serum phytanic acid level is elevated, and the enzyme defect may be demonstrated in fibroblasts. The patients' condition improves on provision of a low-phytanic-acid diet, and plasmapheresis can also be helpful (445, 907).

Cerebrotendinous xanthomatosis (cholestanol storage disease) (76). This autosomal recessive disorder is due to an anomaly of bile acid synthesis which results in the accumulation of cholestanol in the plasma and brain, as well as the formation of xanthomata of tendon sheaths (typically on the Achilles tendon) and lungs. Although the xanthomata contain cholesterol, the serum cholesterol level is usually not elevated. Mental retardation may begin early, but the characteristic clinical picture, with xanthomata, cataracts, progressive spasticity, and ataxia, does not develop until adolescence or later. Polyneuropathy

and muscle atrophy may also be seen. Dementia may develop in adulthood, and severe pseudobulbar signs may appear in the preterminal phase; death usually ensues at some time between the ages of 30 and 60. Molecular genetic diagnosis is possible even in the presymptomatic phase, and treatment with bile acids (chenodeoxycholic acid) can mitigate the disease manifestations and delay their progression (93, 658).

Other lipidoses. *Farber's lipogranulomatosis* and *Wolman's disease* both cause death a few months after birth. Patients with *neuronal ceroid lipofuscinosis (Batten-Kufs disease)* often die in infancy or early childhood (subforms known, respectively, as Haltia-Santavuori disease and Jansky-Bielschowsky disease), but some survive into adolescence (Spielmeyer-Vogt disease) or even adulthood (Kufs disease) (94, 168). Ataxia, myoclonus, and intractable epilepsy are characteristic. Adolescents suffer progressive loss of vision. Patients with the adult form of the disease do not become blind, but do suffer from progressive dementia (243).

■ Leukodystrophies

The leukodystrophies are disorders of myelin metabolism.

Metachromatic leukodystrophy. In this autosomal recessive disease, a deficiency of arylsulfatase A leads to an accumulation of sulfatide in the brain, peripheral nerve tissue, and other tissues, including the kidneys. The disease usually becomes manifest in *late infancy*. Spasticity appears first, typically in the second year of life, followed by deterioration of mental function, disappearance of the intrinsic muscle reflexes, and development of bulbar and pseudobulbar signs, including dysarthria. Optic atrophy and blindness ensue, and, finally, quadriplegia and a persistent vegetative state. The *juvenile form* appears between the 3rd and 10th years of life and is usually associated with a gait disorder, sometimes also with emotional disturbances and dementia (864). The adult form becomes manifest around age 30 with psychiatric abnormalities or dementia, spasticity, and ataxia. T2-weighted MR images reveal confluent hyperintensity of the cerebral and cerebellar white matter. The cortex is atrophic (566) and the ventricles are dilated. The subcortical U-fibers are spared at first, but are later involved as the disease progresses. Biochemical analysis of leukocytes and of urine reveals the deficiency of arylsulfatase A. The progression of the disease may be slowed or halted by bone marrow transplantation (543, 864).

Krabbe's globoid cell leukodystrophy (488). *Galactocerebrosidase* is the missing enzyme in this disease, whose most prominent signs are spasticity, optic atrophy, and diminished nerve conduction velocity. When the disease arises in *infancy*, it is fatal in the first 2 years of life. *Childhood and adult forms* have also been described, with clinical features resembling those of metachromatic leukodystrophy (976).

■ **Mucopolysaccharidoses** (859)
The abnormalities of facial appearance that are specific to this group of diseases have been termed "gargoylism" (see under Hurler's disease, below). Each of these conditions is due to a deficiency of a specific enzyme

(hydrolase), resulting in accumulation of acid mucopolysaccharides in the tissues.

Hurler's disease. This classic and most severe type of mucopolysaccharidosis begins in infancy and usually leads to death by age 10. A lumbar gibbus deformity and corneal opacity are already evident in the first year of life. The joints become stiff and swollen, the chest deformed; the hands and feet remain small and chubby, and stunted growth and mental retardation are evident by age 2 or 3 years. The facial features are coarse, typified by a projecting forehead, bushy eyebrows, saddle nose, hypertelorism, and a lumpy tongue. The meninges may be thickened, and there may be hydrocephalus or spinal cord compression leading to quadriparesis. Cardiac involvement is not infrequently the cause of death. *Scheie's disease* is a variant of Hurler's disease with onset in childhood.

Other mucopolysaccharidoses. These include *Hunter's, Sanfilippo's, Morquio's,* and *Maroteaux-Lamy* diseases. Hunter's disease is X-linked recessive. Sanfilippo's disease mainly affects the brain, while the two last-named diseases mainly affect the skeleton.

■ **Mucolipidoses** (859)
These diseases, clinically similar to the mucopolysaccharidoses, are diagnosed by the finding of elevated oligosaccharide and glycopeptide levels in the urine. The sialidoses are a subclass.

Disorders of Amino Acid and Uric Acid Metabolism

Phenylketonuria. Phenylalanine hydroxylase deficiency, though rare, is the most common disorder of amino acid and protein metabolism. It is transmitted in an autosomal recessive inheritance pattern. In untreated children, *failure of hydroxylation of phenylalanine to tyrosine* impairs cerebral myelination and causes mental retardation and epilepsy. Spasticity and (often) tremor appear as the disease progresses. The affected children are often blond and blue-eyed, because tyrosine is a precursor of melanin. The clinical neurologic findings are nonspecific. T2-weighted MRI reveals hyperintensity of the white matter (747). Since the 1960s, all newborns have undergone diagnostic screening for this disorder by measurement of the serum phenylalanine concentration. A phenylalanine-restricted diet enables phenylketonurics to undergo normal motor and mental development (682).

Maple syrup urine disease. This disorder is an autosomal recessive enzyme deficiency leading to impaired metabolism of the branched-chain amino acids valine, leucine, and isoleucine. Like phenylketonuria, it is associated with mental retardation. The urine has a characteristic sweet smell like that of maple syrup. The neuroradiologic findings are nonspecific (T2-hyperintensity of white matter) (138).

Hartnup disease (286). This autosomal recessive disorder is due to a defect in the intestinal and renal tubular transport of the neutral amino acids tryptophan, alanine, and histidine. Characteristic findings include a progressive, photosensitive, pellagra-like dermatitis, ataxia, nystagmus, impaired gait, spasticity, and dementia. (Hartnup was the surname of the family in which the disease was originally described.)

Homocystinuria. This disorder of methionine metabolism leads to arterial and venous thromboembolism, ectopia lentis, and mental retardation. Heterozygous carriers are at increased risk for stroke and occlusive peripheral vascular disease.

Reye's syndrome. This disease is characterized by encephalopathy and fatty infiltration of the viscera. It is discussed further below (p. 296).

Disorders of Carbohydrate Metabolism

Glycogen storage diseases (235). Table 2.**72** provides an overview of inherited enzyme deficiencies that impair the metabolism of glucose and glycogen. Most are inherited in an autosomal recessive pattern; only type IX and the hepatic form of type VIII are X-linked recessive. Glucose-6-phosphatase deficiency and glycogen synthetase deficiency are characterized by recurrent hypoglycemic crises, presenting with somnolence, stupor, or coma and generalized seizures, which may cause lasting neurologic damage (p. 898). The generalized forms (types II, III, IV, and IX) cause intraneuronal glycogen storage, and thus mental retardation. Skeletal muscle involvement leads to exercise intolerance, or to a myopathy resembling that of muscular dystrophy (p. 895). In type IX glycogen storage disease, severe hemolytic anemia may be the major clinical finding.

Table 2.72 Glycogen storage diseases

Type	Eponym	Deficient enzyme	Involved organs and tissues	Clinical features	Other remarks
I	von Gierke	Glucose-6-phosphatase	Liver, kidney	Hypoglycemic crises, hepatomegaly	
II	Pompe	Acid maltase	Generalized	Cardiomegaly, weakness, hypotonia, death by 1 year	Infantile form
		Acid maltase	Generalized	Muscular dystrophy, respiratory insufficiency	Childhood form
		Acid maltase	Generalized	Proximal myopathy, respiratory insufficiency	Adult form
III	Cori, Forbes	Debranching enzyme	Generalized	Hepatomegaly, hypoglycemia, progressive weakness	
IV	Andersen	Branching enzyme	Generalized	Hepatosplenomegaly, cirrhosis, hepatic failure	
V	McArdle	Myophosphorylase	Skeletal muscle	Exercise-induced weakness, myalgia, contractures, myoglobinuria	
VI	Hers	Hepatic phosphorylase	Liver, skeletal muscle, erythrocytes	Mild hypoglycemia, hepatomegaly	
VII	Tarui	Muscle phosphofructokinase	Skeletal muscle, erythrocytes	Exercise-induced weakness, myalgia, contractures, myoglobinuria	

Cont. →

Table **2.72**   (Cont.)

VIII	Phosphorylase kinase	Liver	Asymptomatic hepatomegaly	X-linked
	Phosphorylase kinase	Liver, skeletal muscle	Hepatomegaly, short stature, hypotonia	
	Phosphorylase kinase	Skeletal muscle	Exercise intolerance, myoglobinuria	
	Phosphorylase kinase	Heart	Lethal infantile cardiomyopathy	
IX	Phosphoglycerate kinase	Generalized	Hemolytic anemia, mental retardation, exercise intolerance, myoglobinuria	X-linked
X	Muscle phosphoglycerate mutase	Skeletal muscle	Exercise-induced weakness, myalgia, contractures, myoglobinuria	
XI	Muscle lactate dehydrogenase	Skeletal muscle	Exercise-induced weakness, myalgia, contractures, myoglobinuria	
Fanconi-Bickel	Muscle lactate dehydrogenase	Liver	Hypoglycemic crises, hepatomegaly	

Myoclonus epilepsy (497) (p. 512). Generalized epilepsy, myoclonus, and dementia are the characteristic features of this autosomal recessive disease. Its clinical signs include ataxia, spasticity, rigidity, and dysarthria. The disease usually appears in adolescence and then progresses inexorably to death in early adulthood. Autopsy reveals intraneuronal Lafora bodies containing polyglucosans.

Polyglucosan body disease (Fig. 2.**81**). This is a further disease in which polyglucosans accumulate. Patients generally present in the fifth or sixth decade of life with spasticity, weakness due to involvement of the spinal anterior horn cells, sphincter disturbances, sensory disturbances, and, later, dementia (97d). This disease may be confused at first with amyotrophic lateral sclerosis (p 434).

Disorders producing hypoglycemia. As discussed below, intermittent disturbances of carbohydrate metabolism lead to systemic hypoglycemia and its consequences for the brain (p. 113). Disorders of glucose transport from the plasma across the blood-brain barrier into the neurons are much rarer. They are characterized by intractable epileptic seizures that first appear in early childhood and take different forms depending on the age of the patient (229a). Cognitive and motor development are slowed. Low CSF concentrations of glucose and lactate are essential to the diagnosis.

Treatment
A *ketogenic diet* can control the seizures, but unfortunately does not improve cognitive and motor development.

Disorders of Glycosylation

Carbohydrate-deficient glycoprotein syndrome (CDG syndrome) comprises a group of multisystemic disorders due to congenital defects of protein glycosylation, resulting in the formation of functionally deficent glycoproteins. The most common type is phosphomannomutase deficiency (CDG-Ia), an autosomal recessive disorder characterized initially by poor feeding and failure to thrive, and later by psychomotor retardation, pronounced axial hypotonia, muscle weakness, and cerebellar ataxia. Seizures may also occur, and abnormalities of the glycoproteins involved in hemostasis may cause both hemorrhagic and ischemic strokes and cerebral veous thrombosis. Neuropathological examination reveals olivopontocerebellar atrophy. Patients surviving into adolescence and adulthood sometimes achieve some degree of social funtioning, but not independence.

Diseases Whose Pathogenesis is Incompletely Understood

Alexander disease (124). This illness appears in early childhood and is characterized by macrocephaly, spasticity, seizures, and dementia, progressing within a few years to a vegetative state and death. It rarely arises in adulthood, in which case it presents with dementia. The histological findings include Rosenthal fibers and diffuse demyelination.

Schilder's diffuse cerebral sclerosis (encephalitis periaxialis diffusa). This is a progressive leukoencephalopathy manifesting as progressive dementia, psychosis, corticospinal signs, and blindness, which may be the result either of optic neuritis or of cortical lesions. It is considered a variant of multiple sclerosis (p. 484 ff.) (766) and its cause is unknown.

Pelizaeus-Merzbacher   disease (chronic infantile cerebral sclerosis). This disease, one of the sudanophilic leukodystrophies, is inherited in an autosomal recessive pattern and presents in the first few months or years of life. Its major features are tremor, cerebellar ataxia, nystagmus, and, later, paraparesis and dementia. MRI shows T2-hyperintensity of the white matter (878).

Adrenoleukodystrophy (679). This X-linked recessive heritable disorder is due to a deficiency of *lignoceroyl CoA synthetase*, an enzyme that is necessary for the beta-oxidation of long-chain fatty acids. Boys are affected in the first or second decade of life, at first with mental changes, gait disturbance, visual impairment, and dysarthria, and later with progressive quadriparesis. In adult patients, adrenal insufficiency rather than spasticity may dominate the clinical picture. Adrenomyeloneuropathy is a form of the disorder in which there is also a polyneuropathy. A diagnostic finding is an elevation of the serum concentration of very-long-chain fatty acids. The progression of neurologic impairment may be slowed by a diet low in fatty acids and by bone marrow transplantation. The hope of therapeutic benefit from "Lorenzo's oil," which inspired a popular film of the same name, has, unfortunately, not been fulfilled (679).

Canavan's disease. This autosomal recessive disorder becomes clinically apparent in the first few months of life. A deficiency of enoyl CoA hydratase impairs myelination and thus causes developmental delay with blindness, hypotonia, spasticity, and macrocephaly.

Reye's syndrome. In 1963, Reye et al. described a *childhood encephalopathy with fatty infiltration of the viscera* (784). The syndrome is probably mediated by mitochondrial dysfunction of multifactorial cause (967). It appears a few days after a viral infection and consists of persistent vomiting, somnolence, delirium, and coma. There is a statistically significant association with the use of aspirin. The CSF is normal. Imaging studies show cerebral edema, and the EEG reveals evidence of encephalopathy (slowing and triphasic waves). There is no specific diagnostic test. In the first few years after its original description, Reye's syndrome was usually fatal; with current intensive-care methods, its mortality has been reduced to 30%.

Leigh syndrome. This neurodegenerative disease was described in 1951 (569). It may already be manifest as lactic acidosis in the neonate, or it may appear later with ataxia, flaccid weakness, hyporeflexia, ophthalmoplegia, optic atrophy, and delayed growth and development. MRI reveals symmetrical lesions resembling infarcts in the basal ganglia, thalamus, and brainstem. The serum and CSF concentrations of pyruvate and lactate are elevated (825). Point mutations of mitochondrial DNA have been found in a few patients; thus, at least some patients with Leigh syndrome suffer from a mitochondrial encephalomyopathy (p. 899) (235, 825).

Alipoproteinemias

Lipoproteins are needed for lipid transport in the blood. *Abetalipopro-*

teinemia (Bassen-Kornzweig disease) results from a disorder of apolipoprotein B synthesis. The serum cholesterol and triglyceride concentrations are very low, and there is a deficiency of lipophilic vitamins, particularly vitamin E. Just as in Friedreich's ataxia, this leads to a fat malabsorption syndrome, retinitis pigmentosa, progressive ataxia, nystagmus, ophthalmoplegia, polyneuropathy, and acanthocytosis.

Hypobetalipoproteinemia can also be associated with an ataxic syndrome and signs of polyneuropathy, but without acanthocytosis (14). *Acanthocytosis with normal serum betalipoprotein concentration* is seen in an autosomal recessive disorder characterized by glossal atrophy, polyneuropathy, chorea, and elevated serum creatine kinase concentration. A similar constellation of findings, termed *chorea-acanthocytosis* and *neuroacanthocytosis* (817), is typically inherited in an autosomal dominant pattern and is only rarely seen in isolated cases; the genetic defect lies on chromosome 9q21. In *Tangier disease*, the serum cholesterol concentration is low, but the serum triglyceride concentration is normal. The major findings are massive enlargement of the tonsils, hepatosplenomegaly, a fluctuating, asymmetric polyneuropathy, and, frequently, eyelid ptosis and ophthalmoplegia.

Disorders of Copper Metabolism

■ **Hepatolenticular Degeneration (Wilson's Disease, Westphal-Strümpell Pseudosclerosis)**
(669, 719, 834a, 902)

Pathogenesis
The prevalence of this autosomal-recessive disorder of copper metabolism is ca. one in 30,000, corresponding to a frequency of the causative allele of ca. one in 140-200. The affected gene, on chromosome 13q14.3, encodes a copper-transporting ATPase. The defect causes an abnormally low plasma concentration of the copper-transport protein ceruloplasmin, which, in turn, results in an increase in urinary copper excretion and toxic accumulation of copper in the liver, brain, and other organs. Unbound ("free") copper is present in the plasma in an elevated concentration.

Clinical Features
The major clinical features of hepatolenticular degeneration are:
- liver failure,
- hemolytic anemia,
- and neurologic or psychiatric abnormalities.

Any of these may be the predominant or even sole manifestation of the disease.

In cases of childhood onset, the initial manifestation is usually either *liver failure* or *hemolytic anemia*, while cases arising during adolescence or early adulthood more commonly present with neurologic or psychiatric abnormalities.

Neurologic and psychiatric abnormalities, if present, are always accompanied by copper deposition in Descemet's membrane, externally visible as a brown discoloration of the edge of the cornea, the so-called Kayser-Fleischer ring (300), which is sometimes detectable only by slit-lamp examination. The neurologic abnormality is usually a movement disorder, of which the more common manifestations are *dysarthria, dysphagia, dystonia*, and *rigidity* (of extrapyramidal type). Less commonly, tremor may affect the head, trunk, or limbs and is typically a coarse postural and intention tremor, often called "flapping" or "rubral" tremor. (The older term "pseudosclerosis" for hepatolenticular degeneration refers to the possible misdiagnosis of the tremor as a manifestation of multiple sclerosis.) Spasticity is rare, and sensory disturbances practically nonexistent. Epileptic seizures are seen in occasional cases.

The psychiatric manifestations of hepatolenticular disease include emotional lability, personality changes, depression, and psychosis.

Diagnostic Evaluation

MRI reveals signal abnormalities in the basal ganglia. CT and MRI are usually normal in the presymptomatic stage of the disease, and thus cannot be used as a screening test.

Hepatolenticular degeneration should be suspected in any child or adolescent with liver failure, hemolytic anemia, a movement disorder, or a mental disturbance. The diagnosis is established by the measurement of a serum ceruloplasmin concentration below 200 mg/L and the observation of a Kayser-Fleischer ring. Most patients, whether symptomatic or presymptomatic, will also be found to have an excessive elimination of copper in the urine (more than 100 µg per day) and an elevation of the free serum copper concentration. In doubtful cases, the diagnosis can be established by liver biopsy for histopathologic examination, including determination of copper content. Asymptomatic relatives of patients suffering from the disease should be screened for it by measurement of the serum ceruloplasmin concentra-

tion and urinary copper elimination, so that early treatment can be provided and the development of overt disease prevented.

Treatment

The goal of treatment is the removal of the accumulated, toxic copper deposits from the tissues of the body. In the first 6–24 months of treatment, this is done by administration of the copper chelator d-*penicillamine* at a dose of 1 g/day, or, in children under 10 years of age, 0.5 g/day. Patients must concurrently take *pyridoxine* (vitamin B_6), at a dose of 25 mg/day, to counteract the anti-pyridoxine effect of d-penicillamine. A hypersensitivity reaction consisting of fever, lymphadenopathy, rash, leukopenia, and thrombocytopenia, may appear just after the onset of treatment. Such reactions should not be mistaken for the leukopenia and thrombocytopenia that are sometimes a component of the disease itself.

d-penicillamine may also induce a lupus-like syndrome or a myasthenic syndrome. Such cases are treated with a *combination of triethylenetetramine and tetrathiomolybdate*, two other chelating agents that promote elimination of copper in the urine (834).

Zinc sulfate and *potassium sulfide* counteract the absorption of copper in the intestine (431). Zinc sulfate is currently the standard agent both for maintenance treatment and for treatment in the presymptomatic phase. Treatment must be continued for the life of the patient, and its discontinuation confers a high risk of death.

■ Menkes' Kinky Hair Syndrome

This X-linked recessive disturbance of copper metabolism causes abnormally low concentrations of ceruloplasmin in the plasma and of copper in the tissues, and an impairment of intestinal copper absorption (660). Seizures, cognitive impairment, blindness, hyperthermia, and disturbances of bone appear in the first few months of life. Kinky hair is a characteristic associated finding.

Mitochondrial Encephalomyopathies (235, 467)

Disorders of mitochondrial function that cause both encephalopathy and myopathy are discussed below on p. 902.

Symmetrical Calcification of the Basal Ganglia (Fahr Syndrome)

Calcification of the basal ganglia, usually clinically irrelevant and of unknown cause, is a common incidental finding on CT and MRI. In this familial disorder, however, calcification of the basal ganglia and dentate nucleus of the cerebellum are associated with progressive parkinsonism, dystonia, or chorea leading to premature death. Other diseases associated with basal ganglionic calcification include various forms of mitochondrial encephalomyopathy (p. 902), and pseudohypoperparathyroidism (p. 318). Calcification anywhere in the brain is always hyperdense on CT, and, in most cases, hypointense on T1- or T2-weighted MR images. Basal ganglionic calcification is an exception to the latter rule: it tends to be hyperintense on T1-weighted images, and hypo- or hyperintense on T2-weighted images (48).

Systemic Diseases Affecting the Nervous System (27)

Overview

Neurologic signs and symptoms may be the most prominent or sole manifestations of systemic disease. Their recognition may provide the key to accurate diagnosis and effective treatment. This section concerns systemic diseases with major neurologic manifestations.

Toxic and Iatrogenic Conditions (623, 741, 768, 785)

Introduction

Toxic substances (especially medications) and medical procedures may produce neurologic abnormalities resembling those of primary neurologic disease and distinguishable from them only by the history of the causative event. Such abnormalities may be either subjective (e.g., headache) or objective (cognitive impairment, cerebellar ataxia, extrapyramidal movement disorders, etc.) and are usually reversible, unless they reflect an underlying anatomic injury. Thus, permanent damage is rare after drug-induced seizures, but common after drug-induced (or other iatrogenic) hemorrhage or ischemic stroke.

The multifarious neurologic signs and symptoms of intoxication may closely resemble those of primary neurologic disease, but a physician alert to the possibility of intoxication can usually make the diagnosis from a pertinent history. Neurologic conditions that may be caused by intoxications of various types are listed in Table 2.**73**. This list is, necessarily, incomplete.

Table 2.**73** Neurologic manifestations of toxic or iatrogenic origin

Manifestation	Cause
Headache	Nearly all headache preparations; withdrawal of caffeine, ergotamine, or amphetamine; oral contraceptives and other hormone preparations (pseudotumor cerebri); nitrates, aminophylline, tetracycline, sympathomimetics, i.v. immunoglobulins, tamoxifen, H_2-antagonists, dipyridamole, interferon
Ischemic stroke	Oral contraceptives and other hormone preparations (413), antihypertensive agents, ergotamine, amphetamine, cocaine, sympathomimetics, i.v. immunoglobulins, intra-arterial methotrexate, angiography, interventional intra-arterial procedures, cardiovascular surgery, radiotherapy, fat injection ("liposculpturing") (269), steroid injections into the nasal mucosa (269), chiropractic manipulation
Hemorrhage (intra-cerebral, extracerebral, spinal) (312,635, 638)	Anticoagulants, fibrinolytic agents, inhibitors of platelet aggregation, amphetamine, cocaine, sympathomimetics; femoral nerve palsy due to psoas hematoma
Seizures (664)	Antibiotics (penicillin, isoniazid), general and local anesthetics (e.g., lidocaine), insulin, radiological contrast media, withdrawal of benzodiazepines or other sedatives, anticonvulsant withdrawal, phenytoin overdose, antidepressants, aminophylline and theophylline, phenothiazines, pentazocine, tripelennamine, cocaine, meperidine, cyclosporine, antineoplastic agents, other
Coma (pp. 221 ff.)	Insulin, barbiturates, benzodiazepines and other sedatives, analgesics, other
Neurasthenic symptoms, acute and chronic encephalopathy	Heavy metals, lithium, aluminum, heroin pyrolysate, cyclosporine, anticholinergics, dopamine agonists, benzodiazepines and other sedatives, antihistamines, antibiotics, anticonvulsants, corticosteroids, H_2-antagonists, disulfiram, methotrexate, organic solvents, hallucinogens, radiotherapy, dehydration, water intoxication, dialysis encephalopathy, other
Extrapyramidal movement disorders (acute dystonia, dyskinesia, akathisia, drug-induced parkinsonism, tardive dyskinesia)	Neuroleptics (phenothiazines, thioxanthenes, butyrophenones, dibenzepins), antiemetics containing metoclopramide or phenothiazines, dopamine agonists, levodopa, antihypertensive agents (e.g., reserpine, captopril), flunarizine, cinnarizine, MPTP

(Cont.) →

Table 2.**73** *(Cont.)*

Manifestation	Cause
Cerebellar ataxia	Phenytoin, carbamazepine, barbiturates, lithium, organic solvents, heavy metals, acrylamide, 5-fluorouracil, cytosine arabinoside, procarbazine, hexamethylmelamine, vincristine, cyclosporine, ciguatera poisoning
Central pontine myelinolysis	Too rapid correction of hyponatremia (p. 335)
Malignant neuroleptic syndrome	Neuroleptics
Malignant hyperthermia	Succinylcholine, halothane, other general anesthetics (p. 900)
Polyneuropathy	See p. 582
Optic neuropathy	Tobacco, ethanol, methanol, ethambutol (p. 582)
Deafness	See Table 9.**12**
Disorders of neuromuscular transmission	Penicillamine, muscle relaxants, procainamide, magnesium, quinine, aminoglycosides, interferon-alpha (p. 911)
Myopathy and rhabdomyolysis	Ethanol, cocaine, heroin and other opiates, pentazocine, benzene, corticosteroids, thyroxine, antimalarial agents, colchicine, antilipid agents (fibrates and statins), zidovudine, cyclosporine, diuretics (via hypocalcemia), ipecac

Physicians confronted with a case that may be of this type should consult the current version of a reference work or web site that is regularly updated for this purpose.

■ Acute and Chronic Encephalopathies

Encephalopathy caused by medications, drugs of abuse, or toxic industrial products usually manifests itself in delirium, tremor, myoclonus, asterixis, ataxia, seizures, or a combination of these. In exceptional cases, an extrapyramidal movement disorder or cerebellar ataxia may be the most prominent finding.

Before these overt neurologic signs develop, most patients go through a "neurasthenic phase" characterized by impaired psychomotor performance, deficits of attention and concentration, headache, fatigue, insomnia, vivid dreams and nightmares, dys- or euphoria, restlessness, irritability, photo- and phonophobia, dizziness, paresthesiae, and loss of sexual interest.

The elderly, in particular, may react to medications usually thought harmless with behavioral and cognitive disturbances, including perceptual illusions and hallucinations.

■ Heavy Metal Intoxication (559)

Mercury. Chronic exposure to mercury vapor or to mercury contained in organic compounds, e.g. in pesticides or industrial waste products, causes both *gastrointestinal* and *neurologic* disturbances (620, 990). The former include gingivitis, stomatitis, excessive salivation, anorexia, and abdominal pain. The latter include a fine tremor (beginning in the hands, tongue, and perioral region, later spreading to the head and legs), dysarthria, dysphagia, and sometimes ataxia, combined with a neurasthenic syndrome (anxiety, irritability) and, rarely, psychotic manifestations, paresthesiae around the mouth and in the extremities, and paresis. Muscle atrophy, fasciculations, and pyramidal tract signs are occasionally present (4).

Treatment

Penicillamine, which promotes the renal excretion of urine, may be used to treat chronic mercury intoxication.

The clinical features of mercury intoxication are summarized in Table 2.**74**.

Lead. Lead poisoning has many causes, such as the use (formerly) of lead-containing ceramic dishes, or chronic exposure in the lead-processing industry. It causes an encephalopathy with cerebral edema, as well as a polyneuropathy mainly affecting extensor muscles, which may

be misdiagnosed as an isolated radial nerve palsy (174). The symptoms and signs of lead-induced encephalopathy include headache, vomiting, seizures, papilledema, abducens palsy, optic atrophy, delirium, and coma. Florid encephalopathy may be preceded by general signs and symptoms such as irritability, headache, tremulousness, nausea, vomiting, and colic due to lead-induced porphyria.

On examination, the characteristic gingival lead line may be seen. Lumbar puncture reveals an elevation of the CSF pressure and of the CSF protein concentration. There is basophilic spotting of the erythrocytes, the serum lead level exceeds 0.5 µg/L, the concentrations of hemoglobin precursors such as delta-aminolevulinic acid are elevated in serum and urine (> 20 mg/dL), and the urinary coproporphyrin excretion is elevated (> 150 mg/24 h). The clinical features of lead intoxication are summarized in Table 2.**75**.

Treatment

Lead intoxication is treated with chelators such as *dimercaprol* (BAL), *ethylene diamine tetra-acetic acid* (EDTA), *penicillamine*, and (in children) *succimer* (678).

Table 2.**74** Manifestations of mercury poisoning

Tremor
Dysarthria
Stomatitis, gingivitis
Neurasthenic symptoms
Paresthesia (sometimes)
ALS-like or other motor abnormalities (sometimes)

Table 2.**75** Manifestations of lead poisoning

Signs of intracranial hypertension
Optic atrophy
Seizures
Delirium
Polyneuropathy, esp. hand drop
Colic
Lead ring

Bismuth salts. Bismuth salts are used to treat various gastrointestinal disturbances (481). Bismuth intoxication is manifest as a neurasthenic prodrome consisting of impaired psychomotor performance, deficits of attention and concentration, headache, insomnia, and anxiety, followed by muscle twitching and an impairment of balance and coordination. If the intoxication is not promptly diagnosed and treated in this phase, it progresses to acute encephalopathy, with delirium, myoclonus, severe ataxia, and variable impairment of consciousness, ranging from mild confusion to coma (631). Abdominal radiographs reveal bismuth in the intestine. The diagnosis is confirmed by the demonstration of bismuth in the urine, serum, or cerebrospinal fluid. The clinical features of bismuth intoxication are summarized in Table 2.**76**.

Table 2.**76** Manifestations of bismuth poisoning

Neurasthenic prodrome
Delirium
Gait ataxia, limb ataxia
Dysarthria
Myoclonus

Treatment
Dimercaprol (BAL) is beneficial, and the long-term prognosis is good once bismuth salts have been discontinued.

Other heavy metals. Arsenic, thallium, manganese, and zinc cause clinically similar forms of encephalopathy; arsenic and thallium also cause polyneuropathy (p. 610). Thallium sometimes causes subacute myelopathy and optic neuropathy (p. 625) (79). Manganese poisoning is typically manifest as parkinsonism, more rarely as chorea (pp. 245 and 261).

■ Intoxication with Organic Solvents and Other Industrial Products

The most important organic solvents are carbon disulfide, n-hexane, meth-ylbutylketone, perchlorethylene, trichloroethylene, and toluene. These highly lipid-soluble agents, widely used in the home, in the hobbyist's workshop, and in industry as solvents, diluents, and cleaning and defatting agents, pose a danger to the central and peripheral nervous systems. They are highly volatile and their vapors are easily inhaled, either accidentally or intentionally (glue sniffing). They generally have nonspecific sedative or anesthetic effects.

Acute exposure. Acute exposure to organic solvents leads to encephalopathy, manifesting itself through cognitive impairment, confusion, dysequilibrium, tinnitus, paresthesiae, ataxia, weakness, headache, nausea, and vomiting, and, in more severe cases, impaired consciousness ranging to coma. Once the exposure is terminated, recovery in minutes to hours is the rule, though headache may persist thereafter for a few hours or even days.

Chronic exposure. Depending on its severity and duration, chronic exposure to organic solvents causes either a neurasthenic syndrome or toxic encephalopathy with cognitive impairment, insomnia, delirium, and a movement disorder. Nystagmus and ataxia are the most consistent, objective neurologic signs. There is, however, some controversy as to whether a chronic encephalopathy with cognitive deficits exists in some occupational groups, e.g., painters. Longstanding, repeated exposure to certain types of organic solvents, such as trichloroethylene, n-hexane, and other hexacarbons, may cause axonal polyneuropathy (p. 612).

Toluene. Toluene causes psychoorganic changes of variable severity, up to overt dementia, as well as cerebellar, brainstem, and pyramidal tract signs and cranial nerve deficits (482). These disturbances tend to be severe in persons who sniff toluene deliberately for its intoxicating effect, in whom MRI may reveal brain atrophy and white matter changes (434).

Methanol. Methanol, when accidentally or intentionally drunk in place of ethanol, causes a frequently lethal metabolic acidosis with acute encephalopathy and optic neuropathy (873). *Methyl acetate*, which is metabolized to methanol, and *methyl formate* can also cause optic neuropathy.

Nitrous oxide. Nitrous oxide abuse can cause myeloneuropathy with spastic paraparesis, sensory ataxia, and sphincter disturbances (102, 558).

Carbon monoxide. Acute carbon monoxide poisoning causes hypoxic injury to the central nervous system, potentially resulting in coma or death. Autopsy reveals diffuse neuron loss in the cerebral cortex and bilateral necrosis of the globus pallidus. Survivors may have severe cognitive

deficits, spasticity, and parkinsonism (p. 245).

Other industrial products. In principle, nearly any gas that is present in sufficiently high concentration can cause acute encephalopathy and hypoxic brain damage. *Ethylene oxide*, used to sterilize surgical instruments, can cause central nervous system damage and polyneuropathy (197). *Acrylamide* causes acute encephalopathy, as well as polyneuropathy after chronic exposure.

■ Organophosphate (Pesticide) Intoxication (863)

Organophosphates are used as insecticide and rodent poison, and as a weapon in chemical warfare; one particular kind, *triorthocresyl phosphate*, is used as an additive to industrial oils. They inhibit acetylcholinesterase in the central nervous system and the "neuropathy target esterase" in the peripheral nervous system, causing synaptic depolarization block.

Intoxication causes bronchospasm, excessive salivation, diarrhea, miosis, impaired pupillary accommodation, fasciculations, behavioral disturbances, anxiety, agitation, delirium, seizures, and paralysis. Respiratory paralysis may be lethal, and atropine is life-saving (432). Surviving patients develop polyneuropathy 1–3 weeks later, followed by spasticity and ataxia (for a further discussion of triorthocresyl phosphate and triaryl phosphate poisoning, see p. 611).

Chronic exposure may also impair memory (487). If organophosphate rodent poison is eaten, perhaps with suicidal intent, coma ensues, with opsoclonus, myoclonus, and flaccid paresis, which later converts, if the patient survives, to spasticity.

■ Medications

Various medications may cause encephalopathy with cognitive impairment, delirium, extrapyramidal or cerebellar movement disorders, or seizures, usually on a dose-dependent basis. These include anticonvulsants, corticosteroids, dopaminergic agonists, cimetidine, isoniazid, monoamine oxidase inhibitors, pentazocine, propoxyphene, cyclosporine, interferon, methotrexate, vincristine, and other cytostatic agents. Water-soluble contrast agents used in myelography, such as *metrizamide*, may cause acute encephalopathy and seizures. Hypoglycemia caused by an overdose of *insulin* can produce encephalopathy, as can iatrogenic SIADH with hyponatremia (see p. 334 f.). *Penicillin* rarely causes an encephalopathy that manifests itself through myoclonus, seizures, and impairment of consciousness.

■ Cerebellar Ataxia Caused By Medications and Other Substances

Anticonvulsant overdoses (e.g., of phenytoin, carbamazepine, or barbiturates) can cause an encephalopathy mainly affecting the cerebellum, characterized subjectively by dizziness and imbalance, and objectively by end-gaze nystagmus, dysarthria,

ataxia, and gait impairment ranging to astasia-abasia. Prompt recognition of *phenytoin intoxication* is important, because, if unchecked, it may lead to irreversible ataxia (862). Phenytoin also causes gingival hypertrophy and polyneuropathy, though the latter is usually subclinical (767) (Table 2.**77**). The ordering physician should be aware that the pharmacokinetics of phenytoin predispose to overdose: the serum concentration of the drug rises exponentially in relation to the dosage.

Lithium intoxication, too, causes a primarily cerebellar encephalopathy. Two-thirds of patients receiving lithium at therapeutic doses develop mild tremor and cog-wheel rigidity, and diabetes insipidus and weight gain are also common. Severe, acute encephalopathy (ataxia, rigidity, hypokinesia, mutism, seizures, coma) and polyneuropathy are rare (240, 739).

Ataxia may also result from treatment with *cytostatic agents* including 5-fluorouracil, cytosine arabinoside, procarbazine, hexamethylmelamine, and vincristine, and the immunosuppressive agent *cyclosporine* (768). Ataxia may also be the most prominent sign of encephalopathy caused by organic solvent, heavy metal, or acrylamide poisoning. Ciguatera fish poisoning is characterized by acute ataxia and paresthesiae.

■ Medication-Induced Extrapyramidal Disorders (337)

Medications may be the cause of several different kinds of extrapyramidal disorder (Table 2.**78**).

Acute dystonia and dyskinesia. Neuroleptics such as phenothiazines,

Table 2.**77** Manifestations of phenytoin intoxication

End-gaze nystagmus
Ataxia Gait disturbance
Dysarthria
Gingival hypertrophy

Table 2.**78** Medication-induced movement disorders

Akathisia
Tardive dyskinesia (incl. orofacial dyskinesia)
Tardive dystonia
Medication-induced parkinsonism
Malignant neuroleptic syndrome
Tremor
Tics
Myoclonus

butyrophenones, and the antiemetic metoclopramide may induce acute dystonia and dyskinesia, usually limited to the muscles of the head and neck and consisting of grimacing, trismus, abnormal movements of the tongue, dysphonia, orofacial dyskinesia, oculogyric crises, or torticollis and retrocollis. Generalized forms affecting the muscles of the trunk and limbs are less common. Physicians unaware of the possibility of acute iatrogenic dystonia and dyskinesia may misdiagnose them as hysteria. Intravenously administered anticholinergics (e.g., 10–20 mg of biperiden) usually bring immediate relief.

Akathisia. This term refers to a state of motor unrest (literally, the inability to sit still) (50, 553), which is to be distinguished from restless legs syndrome (p. 845). Affected patients feel an irresistible inner urge to move. Akathisia may be a side effect of antipsychotics (phenothiazines and butyrophenones), antiemetics, and dopaminergic agonists.

Medication-induced parkinsonism. Antipsychotic medications, antihypertensives (e.g. reserpine, captopril), flunarizine and cinnarizine, MPTP, and other substances may induce parkinsonism that is distinguishable from idiopathic Parkinson's disease only by history (p. 245). It usually regresses after a few weeks or months and may be treated in the meantime with antiparkinsonian medication, if necessary.

Other movement disorders. The prolonged use of antipsychotic dopaminergic antagonists may induce *late ("tardive") dyskinesia and dystonia* (153, 945), which appear either during the course of drug treatment or immediately after discontinuation or reduction of the dose. Their pathophysiology is not entirely clear; it is assumed that long-term use of antidopamine agents causes either denervation hypersensitivity of the striatal dopamine receptors or a loss of GABA-mediated thalamocortical inhibition. (Involuntary movements also frequently complicate the long-term use of levodopa in patients with Parkinson's disease; cf. p. 247). Tardive movement disorders may be of practically any kind. The most common variety is the *buccolinguomasticatory syndrome*, with stereotypic chewing, licking, and smacking movements, resembling those seen in Meige syndrome (p. 268). Dyskinesia and dystonia may also affect the extremities, however, e.g. as dystonia of the toes or as an appendicular tremor, tardive myoclonus, tic disorder, or even iatrogenic pseudo-Gilles de la Tourette syndrome (519, 901; cf. p. 272). *Pisa syndrome*, involving lateral inclination and torsion of the trunk, neck, and head, is most commonly seen in elderly patients after chronic neuro-leptic use (548). (The odd, and per-haps inappropriate, name is an allu-sion to the Leaning Tower of Pisa.) Most patients with tardive movement disorders are unaware or barely aware of them, but some find them profoundly disturbing (605).

Treatment of Tardive Movement Disorders

The first step is the *removal of the causative agent*. If the movement disorder worsens, treatment should then be begun with an *anti-cholinergic* medication or a *benzo-diazepine*. Bothersome focal dyski-nesias, such as blepharospasm, can be treated with *botulinum toxin*. Only if such measures fail should a *dopamine antagonist* be tried, e.g. tiapride, tetrabenazine, or reser-pine. These medications should not be given indefinitely, but rather slowly tapered, and then discontin-ued.

Once the causative agent is re-moved, it may take months or even years for the tardive movement disorder to remit (520). *Neuroleptic medications* should therefore be prescribed sparingly and for no longer than clinically necessary in each case. If antipsychotic treat-ment must be continued in the face of a potential, or actual, movement disorder, then an agent with fewer extrapyramidal side effects is pref-erable (e.g. clozapine).

Malignant neuroleptic syndrome (371, 539, 763). The initial adminis-tration of a neuroleptic agent, or an increase in its dose, may cause sweat-ing, tachycardia, and fluctuations of blood pressure, followed by rigidity,

dystonia, and fever. The serum con-centration of creatine kinase is dra-matically elevated. Malignant neuro-leptic syndrome is often life-threatening; without treatment, its mortality is ca. 25%.

Treatment

The neuroleptic agent is discontin-ued at once, fluid and electrolyte substitution is given, and any med-ical complications, such as pulmo-nary embolus or pneumonia, are treated. *Levodopa, dopaminergic agonists*, and *spasmolytics* such as dantrolene may shorten the dura-tion of the syndrome (see also ma-lignant hyperthermia, p. 900).

■ Alcohol and the Nervous System

Table 2.79 provides an overview of the effects of ethanol (ethyl alcohol, colloquially "alcohol") on the nervous system (176, 979). The most common long-term complication of alcohol overuse is polyneuropathy. Genetic, metabolic, and environmental factors account for the variable predisposi-tion to alcoholism among individuals, as well as the multifarious forms this addiction can take.

■ Acute Alcohol Intoxication

Drunkenness expresses itself as eu-phoria or dysphoria, complaisance or aggressiveness, diminished concen-tration, prolonged reaction times, and loss of interpersonal distance, includ-ing loss of sexual inhibition. Further signs include slurred speech, ataxic gait, diplopia, nausea, dizziness, tachycardia, sudden outbursts of rage, and antisocial behavior, and, with very high blood alcohol concentra-

Table 2.**79** Alcohol and the nervous system

Alcohol intoxication:
- Euphoria or dysphoria
- Loss of inhibition
- Ataxia
- Somnolence
- Stupor
- Coma
- Respiratory suppression

Alcohol withdrawal:
- "Hangover"
- Tremor
- Hallucinations
- Partial or generalized seizures
- Delirium tremens

Dementia:
- Pellagra
- Marchiafava–Bignami syndrome
- Hepatocerebral degeneration
- Hepatic encephalopathy (portocaval encephalopathy)
- Alcoholic dementia

Wernicke's encephalopathy

Korsakoff syndrome

Alcoholic cerebellar degeneration

Central pontine myelinolysis

Tobacco-alcohol amblyopia

Alcoholic polyneuropathy

Alcoholic myopathy
- Acute necrotizing myopathy
- Chronic myopathy, occasionally cardiomyopathy

Alcohol and stroke

Pachymeningeosis hemorrhagica interna

Fetal alcohol syndrome

Special features of alcoholism
- Dipsomania
- Alcohol-induced hypoglycemia
- Accidental intoxications with other substances: optic neuropathy due to methanol consumption, lead encephalopathy in moonshine drinkers, etc.

tions, somnolence, stupor, coma, respiratory suppression, and death.

■ Alcohol Withdrawal, Alcoholic Hallucinosis, Alcoholic Seizures

Alcohol withdrawal. The declining concentration of alcohol in the blood after a single binge is accompanied by a "hangover" consisting of headache, dysphoria, tremulousness, and sweating. Morning tremulousness improving with alcohol consumption, nervousness, timidity, facial and conjunctival erythema, sweating, anorexia, nausea, tachycardia, tachypnea, and hypertension are signs of longer-term overuse of alcohol (for at least several days); they regress after a few days of abstinence.

Alcoholic hallucinosis. Severe alcohol abuse causes perceptual disturbances including nightmares, *illusions*, and *hallucinations*. Illusions and hallucinations may be visual, auditory, tactile, or olfactory, and often involve (imaginary) animals or insects. If they last for more than a few minutes, a true *alcoholic hallucinosis* with paranoid psychotic features, or a *pre-delirium*, may develop.

Alcoholic seizures. Alcoholic seizures ("rum fits") may appear in the presence or absence of alcoholic hallucinosis and are usually generalized, but sometimes focal. Alcohol may be the factor that induces the first seizure in a patient with another underlying cause of seizures; thus, seizures occurring during alcohol use or alcohol withdrawal still require diagnostic evaluation.

■ Delirium Tremens

Delirium tremens is heralded by an epileptic seizure in 10% of cases, typically 2–3 days after the cessation of alcohol consumption. Patients with delirium tremens are disoriented, sleepless, anxious, and agitated, fumble with the bedclothes, and suffer from perceptual illusions and hallucinations, usually involving animals (particularly rodents) or insects. They often experience these illusions and hallucinations as threatening, and may make violent efforts to "defend themselves." They are highly suggestible and may, for example, start reading from a blank sheet of paper. Tremor, sweating, and tachycardia are characteristic findings.

Seizures, if they occur, should always prompt suspicion of another underlying cause besides alcohol withdrawal, e.g. meningitis. It is also not uncommon for delirium tremens itself (with or without seizures) to be induced by an intercurrent illness in an alcoholic. The prevention and treatment of alcoholic delirium are detailed in Table 2.**80** (418, 531, 820). Mild withdrawal phenomena can be treated on an ambulatory basis if home circumstances allow, but all patients with fever, seizures, or hallucinations should be hospitalized. Delirium tremens is fatal in 15% of cases if untreated.

■ Dementia in Various Conditions Due to Alcohol Abuse

Alcoholic dementia. Chronic alcohol abuse causes cognitive deficits that are largely reversible with abstinence. Histopathological study may reveal neuronal loss and brain atrophy.

Table 2.**80** Treatment of alcohol withdrawal and alcoholic delirium

- *Thiamine* 100 mg i.m. or i.v., and *multivitamin preparation*

- *Diazepam (Valium)* 10–40 mg p.o. or i.v., or *chlordiazepoxide (Librium)* 25–200 mg p.o. or i.v., or

  Clomethiazole (Distraneurin) 0.6–1.2 g p.o. or 0.8% solution i.v., initially 24–60 mg/min, then 4–8 mg/min; the initial dose should be high enough to produce sedation. Repeat every 1–4 hours, reduce dose by 25% daily. (Note: not available in USA)

- *Fluid replacement* with sufficient glucose, potassium, calcium, magnesium, phosphate

- Treatment of seizures due to alcohol withdrawal with *phenytoin*, initially 500–1000 mg i.v., then 300 mg/d for 1–3 weeks (should not be given indefinitely)

- Treatment of any *accompanying illnesses* (meningitis, subdural hematoma, variceal bleeding, pancreatitis, etc.)

Korsakoff's amnestic syndrome and Wernicke's encephalopathy (388, 979). Both of these conditions are due to thiamine deficiency and are sometimes caused by poor nutrition in nonalcoholics, e.g. in patients with anorexia nervosa. *Korsakoff's syndrome* (p. 388) consists of acute anterograde and retrograde amnesia, with confabulation. *Wernicke's encephalopathy* is characterized by oculomotor disturbances and ataxia in addition to the signs of Korsakoff's syndrome. The oculomotor disturbances are bilateral and asymmetrical and may consist of abducens palsy, horizontal or rotatory nystagmus, and conjugate gaze palsy or even total external ophthalmoplegia. The pupillary reflexes may be slowed. Dysarthria, appendicular ataxia, and (most prominently) truncal ataxia are usually present; the patient may be unable to stand or walk. EEG usually reveals slowing of the background rhythm. T2-weighted MR images show abnormal signal intensity, and sometimes contrast enhancement, in the periaqueductal region and adjacent to the third ventricle (329), corresponding to the histopathological findings of neuron and axon loss, demyelination, and small foci of hemorrhage.

> **Treatment**
>
> *Thiamine* (100 mg/d i.v. or i.m.), *multivitamins* (particularly including the vitamin B complex), and *glucose-electrolyte solutions* are given acutely. Glucose, however, should be given only after thiamine has been given, as it may otherwise induce acute worsening of Wernicke's encephalopathy.
>
> The syndrome regresses after treatment, but there are often residual oculomotor disturbances, ataxia, and memory impairment.

Alcoholic cerebellar degeneration (see Table 2.**79**). Prolonged alcohol abuse (years) can lead to *cerebellar atrophy*, mainly affecting the vermis. Its major clinical manifestation is ataxia of the limbs (mainly the legs), as opposed to the truncal ataxia seen in Wernicke's encephalopathy.

■ Marchiafava-Bignami Syndrome (66, 336, 979)

This syndrome, closely related to central pontine myelinolysis, is seen in alcoholism or malnutrition of other origin and is characterized by highly symmetrical demyelination in the corpus callosum, the centrum semiovale, and other white matter areas. It is clinically expressed by acute confusion, seizures, and impairment of consciousness. Surviving patients are usually permanently abulic and demented. Before the advent of MRI, this condition could only be reliably diagnosed at autopsy.

Hepatocerebral degeneration and pellagra. *Hepatocerebral degeneration* and *pellagra* are further causes of dementia in alcoholics. The former is a consequence of long-standing, chronic portocaval encephalopathy (p. 342), the latter of niacin or tryptophan deficiency. Pellagra is characterized by glossitis, diarrhea, anemia, erythematous changes in exposed areas of the skin, and encephalopathy leading to dementia. In industrialized countries, this condition is rare even among alcoholics, because the enrichment of grain with niacin is mandated by law.

■ Other Conditions Due to Alcohol Abuse (see Table 2.79)

Alcoholic hypoglycemia (p. 313) is due to an alcohol-induced disturbance of gluconeogenesis. *Dipsomania* is an unquenchable craving for alcohol that usually arises episodically and is associated with phases of unusually high alcohol consumption, which may cause lasting somatic damage. Alcoholics are also at elevated risk of ischemic and hemorrhagic *stroke* (p. 210). Finally, grievous harm may result if *methanol* (p. 304), *ethylene glycol*, or *other neurotoxic substances* are consumed by accident instead of ethanol.

■ Drugs of Abuse and the Nervous System (149)

Drug abuse may lead to physical and psychological *dependence* and *addiction* (see Table 2.81 for a list of the more commonly abused drugs).

Table 2.81 The most commonly abused drugs

Opioids:
• Heroin
• Morphine
• Methadone
• Codeine
• Propoxyphene, etc.
Stimulants:
• Cocaine
• Amphetamine
• Methylphenidate
• Phenylpropanolamine
• Ephedrine
Sedatives and hypnotics:
• Barbiturates
• Diazepam and other benzodiazepines
• Methaqualone
Cannabis (marijuana)
Hallucinogens:
• LSD
• "Ecstasy" (= 3,4-methylenedioxymethamphetamine, MDMA)
• Psilocybin
Inhaled ("sniffed") substances: Solvents, gasoline; glue or paint containing toluene, n-hexane, aliphatic hydrocarbons, nitrous oxide, trichloroethylene, etc.
Phencyclidine ("angel dust")
Anticholinergics
Ethanol
Tobacco

Withdrawal may produce an extreme craving for the drug and somatic effects such as nervousness, tremor, sweating, and tachycardia.

Effects on the nervous system. Most drugs of abuse cause a pleasant state of altered consciousness with disinhibition, euphoria, or depersonalization, which may, however, rapidly convert into a state involving undesired illusions, hallucinations, paranoid psychosis, or depression. Motor hyperactivity normally accompanies this state altered of consciousness when some of these drugs are used. A *drug overdose* can cause nystagmus, ataxia, myoclonus, hypothermia, analgesia, hypertension, orthostatic hypotension, respiratory depression, and impaired consciousness ranging to coma. Drug withdrawal usually causes nausea, vomiting, abdominal cramps, loss of appetite, headache, sweating, skin erythema, tremor, tachycardia, cardiac dysrhythmia, fever, seizures, or "flashbacks" (intense reliving of past experiences).

Bodily harm directly or indirectly due to drug abuse. Drug abusers are prone to bodily harm of many different kinds. *Accidents*, e.g. those caused by drunk or otherwise intoxicated drivers, and *suicide* are major risks associated with drug abuse. Intravenous drug abuse predisposes to *infections* of many different kinds (local infections, hepatitis, AIDS, endocarditis, tetanus, mycotic cerebral aneurysms). *Ischemic and hemorrhagic stroke* are devastating complications seen in abusers of alcohol, tobacco, heroin, cocaine, pentazocine, tripelennamine, amphetamine, LSD, phencyclidine, and ecstasy. Drug-induced coma with respiratory depression may lead to permanent *anoxic injury* to the brain and other organs (485, 576, 887). *Rhabdomyolysis* and consequent *renal failure* are known complications of heroin, amphetamine, cocaine, and phencyclidine abuse. *Dementia* may be the ultimate result of long-term alcohol abuse or a consequence of addiction-related malnutrition, head trauma, ischemic and hemorrhagic strokes, and brain infections. Various substances, particularly solvents, can cause *polyneuropathy.* Heroin injection by addicts has been reported to cause lumbar and *brachial plexopathy* as well as *Guillain-Barré syndrome*, presumably through an autoimmune mechanism. *Pressure neuropathies and plexopathies* often result from the lack of shifting movements during drug-induced stupor and coma, in distinction to normal sleep (e.g., the well-known "Saturday night palsy" of the radial nerve). Finally, MPTP (p. 245) causes *parkinsonism*, and the smoking of heroin pyrolysate causes *leukoencephalopathy* (444).

▌Treatment▐

Acute opioid or benzodiazepine intoxication can be treated with the respective receptor antagonists, *naloxone (Narcan)* and *flumazenil (Romazicon).* General supportive care is given to maintain fluid and electrolyte homeostasis and prevent complicating conditions (see above discussion). Such conditions, if already present, will require specific treatment.

Endocrine Disorders with Neurologic Manifestations

Overview:
Endocrine disorders cause metabolic derangements that, in turn, give rise to metabolic encephalopathy, which may manifest itself in an impairment of cognitive function, alteration of consciousness, or both. They can also cause myopathy and peripheral neuropathy of various types.

■ Hypoglycemia (313,610)

Glucose is, for all practical purposes, the exclusive energy source for cerebral metabolism. If the plasma glucose concentration falls below a critical level, the CNS and autonomic nervous system can no longer function normally. The more important causes of hypoglycemia are listed in Table 2.**82**. Hypoglycemia can arise postprandially as well as after a prolonged fast.

Clinical Features

The manifestations of hypoglycemia (Table 2.**83**) are independent of its etiology. They may last only a few minutes, or for hours or longer. Autonomic disturbances usually appear first, followed by central nervous disturbances. The autonomic manifestations include dizziness, sweating, nausea, pallor, palpitations, a precordial pressure-like sensation, abdominal pain, hunger, anxiety, and headache; the central nervous manifestations include seizures, impairment of consciousness, and focal neurologic deficits.

Thus, the initial stage of hypoglycemia usually consists of paresthesiae, cloudy or double vision, tremor, and abnormal behavior; focal neurologic deficits and seizures follow, with impairment of consciousness. The neurologic deficits may be of any conceivable type; acute hemiparesis is the most common. Seizures may be

simple partial, complex partial, or generalized, and consciousness may be impaired to any extent from somnolence to deep coma.

Table 2.**82** Causes of hypoglycemia

Postprandial (reactive) hypoglycemia:
- Alimentary hyperinsulinism
- Fructose intolerance
- Other causes

Hormone deficiency:
- Hypopituitarism
- Hypoadrenalism
- Catecholamine deficiency
- Glucagon deficiency

Disorders of carbohydrate metabolism:
- Glycogenoses (cf. Table 2.**72**)

Substrate deficiency

Hepatopathy

Medications and drugs of abuse:
- Alcohol
- Beta-blockers
- Salicylates

Hyperinsulinism:
- Insulinoma
- Exogenous insulin
- Sulfonylurea

Accelerated glucose metabolism:
- Extrapancreatic tumors
- Systemic carnitine deficiency
- Lipid oxidation disorders
- Cachexia with fat depletion

Table 2.**83**   Clinical manifestations of hypoglycemia

Autonomic manifestations:
- Dizziness
- Sweating
- Nausea
- Palpitations
- Precordial pressure sensation
- Abdominal pain
- Hunger
- Anxiety
- Headache

Central nervous manifestations:
- Paresthesiae, clouded vision, diplopia, tremor, unusual or abnormal behavior
- Seizures (simple partial, complex partial, generalized)
- Impairment of consciousness ranging form somnolence to coma
- Focal neurologic deficits – e.g., hemiparesis, hemianopsia, aphasia, apraxia

Permanent neurologic injury:
- Cognitive deficits, dementia
- Specific cognitive deficits, focal neurologic deficits
- Predominantly distal muscle atrophy (damage of the anterior horn cells and their axons)

Diagnostic Evaluation

The nonspecific *EEG changes* include diffuse and focal slowing and triphasic waves.

The diagnosis is based on a low serum glucose concentration (< 2.5 mmol/L) measured during the clinical event. Repeated postprandial hypoglycemia can be diagnosed with the aid of a *glucose tolerance test*, fasting hypoglycemia with a *fasting test* or elevated insulin concentration.

Permanent Neurological Injury from Recurrent Hypoglycemia

Hypoglycemia is a deficiency of the key metabolic substrate of the neuron and thus leads to neuronal injury. Recurrent hypoglycemia causes a decline in cognitive ability that may be severe enough to qualify as dementia; it may also cause lasting focal neurologic disturbances such as aphasia, apraxia, hemianopsia, or hemiparesis, which may be more readily apparent than the cognitive impairment. Insulinomas that cause recurrent, prolonged episodes of hypoglycemia sometimes produce a so-called hypoglycemic neuropathy, which presumably reflects injury to the anterior horn cells and their axons. It clinically resembles a predominantly distal form of spinal muscular atrophy (459).

■ Hyperglycemia

Clinical Features

Hyperglycemia is almost always due to diabetes mellitus. It can produce a metabolic encephalopathy of variable severity, ranging to coma. There are two forms of hyperglycemic coma:
- ketoacidotic coma and
- hyperosmolar diabetic coma.

Diabetic ketoacidosis. This syndrome is encountered in insulin-dependent diabetics and is characterized by an impairment of consciousness with *Kussmaul respiration.* The extracellular volume deficit is less than that of hyperosmolar coma.

Hyperosmolar, nonketotic diabetic coma. This syndrome is typically seen in non-insulin-dependent diabetics in whom a hyperglycemic diuresis has led to extracellular volume loss. If the patient does not drink enough fluid to compensate for this, a severe volume deficiency with hyperosmolarity results (p. 336).

Diagnostic Evaluation

The diagnosis is based on the demonstration of glucose and ketones in the urine, and of hyperglycemia, metabolic acidosis, and an anion gap in the serum. Lactic acidosis, uremia, alcoholic ketoacidosis, and a number of intoxications may produce a similar picture.

Treatment
The treatment of diabetic ketoacidosis consists of *insulin administration and fluid replacement* (usually 3–5 liters), *potassium,* and *bicarbonate.* In hyperosmolar, nonketotic coma, the serum glucose concentration is usually higher than in diabetic ketoacidosis, and the acidosis is usually only mild. The treatment requires larger volumes of fluid (as much as 10 liters), as well as insulin, potassium, and (if acidosis is present) bicarbonate.

■ Hypothyroidism (927)

Clinical Features

A deficiency of thyroid hormone *in utero* or during infancy leads to *cretinism;* childhood hypothyroidism causes *stunted growth* and *mental retardation.* Hypothyroid adolescents and adults suffer from a wide variety of disturbances affecting the CNS, PNS, and muscles. The neurologic manifestations are largely independent of the etiology of hypothyroidism.

General manifestations. Hypothyroidism is characterized by slowly progressive lethargy, fatigue, constipation, and cold intolerance.

Neurologic manifestations. The neurologic manifestations of hypothyroidism include (Table 2.**84**):

* Headache, rarely pseudotumor cerebri.
* An axonal polyneuropathy (657) (p. 614) is seen in 80% of chronically hypothyroid individuals, presenting with marked paresthesiae and a sensory deficit along with a tendency toward compression neuropathies such as carpal tunnel syndrome.
* Cranial nerve deficits rarely caused by hypothyroidism include tinnitus, hearing loss, vertigo, ptosis, hoarseness (due to infiltration of the vocal folds with mucopolysaccharides), and facial pain.
* Myopathy (p. 914) (830, 929, 975, 1029) is common in hypothyroidism, typically presenting with myalgia and a feeling of stiffness. Some 30–40% of patients develop myopathic weakness, which usually involves the pelvic muscles and the proximal muscles of the lower

limbs, less often the proximal muscles of the upper limbs and the distal muscles of all the limbs. Hyporeflexia is most easily observed at the ankles. Tapping a muscle may produce a visible bump (myoedema). Disturbances of neuromuscular transmission, muscle hypertrophy, and myotonia are also encountered.

- Cerebellar dysfunction is occasionally clinically prominent, manifesting as dysequilibrium, ataxia, impaired coordination, dysarthria, and nystagmus (378).
- Mental abnormalities include apathy, impairment of attention, concentration, and memory, dementia, depression, hallucinations, and psychotic delirium, sometimes leading to coma.
- Seizures are a further feature of hypothyroidism.

Diagnostic Evaluation

CSF examination may reveal an elevated protein concentration. The *EEG* is diffusely slowed and low in amplitude. The serum concentration of the *thyroid hormones* fT$_3$ and fT$_4$ is low, while that of TSH is elevated (except in the rare case of a primary deficiency of hypothalamic TSH secretion).

Treatment

The treatment of hypothyroidism generally requires *lifelong thyroid hormone supplementation*.

■ Hashimoto's Thyroiditis

Encephalopathy with a high antithyroid antibody titer in the setting of Hashimoto's thyroiditis (869, 539a) is a clinical entity distinct from the usual form of hypothyroid encephalopathy. It presents with confusion, impairment of consciousness, delirium, and focal and generalized seizures.

Treatment

The clinical manifestations improve with corticosteroids.

Table 2.**84** Clinical manifestations of hypothyroidism

Infancy:
- Cretinism

Childhood:
- Stunted growth, mental retardation

Adulthood:
- General manifestations including lethargy, fatigue, constipation, cold intolerance
- Headache
- Polyneuropathy (mainly sensory), carpal tunnel syndrome, cranial nerve deficits (rare)
- Myopathy, delayed relaxation of intrinsic muscle reflexes, myxedema
- Ataxia and other cerebellar signs
- Behavioral and neuropsychological abnormalities, apathy, dementia, depression, psychotic delirium, coma
- Seizures

Treatment:
- Hormone supplementation brings clinical improvement
- Corticosteroids in Hashimoto's thyroiditis

■ Thyrotoxicosis (927)

Definition:
Thyrotoxicosis (an abnormal elevation of the serum concentration of thyroid hormone) may be due to *hyperthyroidism* (overproduction of hormone by the thyroid gland) or to other causes.

Clinical Features
Thyrotoxicosis has similar manifestations whatever its etiology. In Graves' disease, hyperthyroidism is accompanied by endocrine ophthalmopathy.

General manifestations. The general manifestations of thyrotoxicosis include nervousness, insomnia, tremor, diaphoresis, tachycardia, diarrhea, and heat intolerance.

Neurologic manifestations. The neurologic manifestations of thyrotoxicosis include (Table 2.**85**):
- *Myopathy* (465) predominantly causes weakness of the pelvic and proximal limb muscles, making it difficult for the patient to rise from a chair or raise the arms. It may be accompanied by myasthenia gravis that worsens during a thyrotoxic crisis, by an acute oculofaciobulbar myopathy with dysarthria, dysphagia, and ocular ptosis, or by thyrotoxic periodic paralysis (p. 914). As in familial hypokalemic paralysis, there are attacks of focal or generalized weakness that may last for minutes, hours, or days. Polyneuropathy is very rare.
- *CNS manifestations:* the behavioral abnormalities range from mild irritability to psychosis (rare). Tremor is practically always present; it may be very fine, like a catecholamine-induced tremor, or – particularly in older patients – coarse and of lower frequency, like

Table 2.**85** Clinical manifestations of thyrotoxicosis

General manifestations:
- Nervousness
- Insomnia
- Tremor
- Diaphoresis
- Tachycardia
- Diarrhea
- Heat intolerance

Muscle manifestations:
- Thyrotoxic myopathy with mainly proximal weakness
- Myasthenia gravis
- Thyrotoxic periodic paralysis
- Polyneuropathy (very rare)

Cerebral manifestations:
- Irritability
- Psychosis
- Tremor
- Choreoathetosis
- Spasticity with pyramidal tract signs

Ocular manifestations:
- Decreased frequency of blinking
- Lid retraction (Graefe's sign)
- Impaired convergence (Möbius's sign)
- Exophthalmos
- Diplopia
- Ophthalmoplegia
- Optic neuropathy

Partial and generalized seizures

Therapeutic alternatives:
- Thyrostatic agents
- Thyroidectomy
- Radiotherapy

an essential tremor (p. 270). Chore-oathetosis, spasticity, and pyramidal tract signs are rarely encountered (230, 869). Partial and generalized seizures may occur (454).

• *Ocular manifestations* include diminished frequency of blinking (Stellwag's sign), lid retraction (Graefe's sign), and impaired convergence (Möbius's sign), as well as uni- or bilateral exophthalmos. The latter reflects an endocrine ophthalmopathy, which may also cause diplopia, ophthalmoplegia, and optic neuropathy (p. 661).

Diagnostic Evaluation

The diagnosis is made by the demonstration of an elevated serum concentration of the *free thyroid hormones* fT$_3$ and fT$_4$. The TSH concentration is low, except in the rare case of primary hypothalamic hypersecretion of TSH.

Treatment

The options for treatment include *thyrostatic drugs, thyroidectomy*, and *radiotherapy*. The neurologic manifestations usually resolve once the serum thyroid hormone concentration has been normalized.

■ Hypoparathyroidism and Hypocalcemia (436, 770, 894)

Clinical Features

Hypoparathyroidism is a disturbance of calcium and phosphate homeostasis due to a hereditary or acquired (often post-surgical) deficiency of parathyroid hormone. The identical clinical picture is produced when parathyroid hormone is present at normal concentration, but fails to

interact normally with parathyroid hormone receptors on the surface of the effector cells; this is the case in both *pseudohypoparathyroidism and pseudo-pseudohypoparathyroidism.*

The characteristic laboratory findings are
• hypocalcemia,
• hypomagnesemia, and
• hyperphosphatemia.

General manifestations. These disease states often produce abdominal pain, nausea, and vomiting.

Neurologic manifestations. The neurologic manifestations, largely due to hypocalcemia, include:
• *Tetany* is characterized by a feeling that the extremities are "falling asleep," carpopedal spasm (with the classic "obstetrician's hand" posture), and stridor (p. 554). Objective findings include brisk reflexes and positive Chvostek, Lust, and Trousseau signs.
• *Seizures* are usually generalized and poorly responsive to anticonvulsants.
• *Headache and papilledema* are seen in hypoparathyroid states, as in pseudotumor cerebri.
• *Basal ganglionic dysfunction* manifests itself in a variety of hypo- and hyperkinetic movement disorders, e.g., choreoathetosis.
• *Behavioral and neurasthenic manifestations* include abnormal fatigability, apathy, confusion, hallucinations, and psychosis.

Other manifestations. *Cataracts* and *myopathy* with an elevated creatine kinase concentration have been described (361). *Intracranial calcifications*, with a predilection for the basal ganglia, are common (p. 299).

Diagnostic Evaluation

The serum concentration of *parathyroid hormone* is low in hypoparathyroidism. The *EEG changes* are nonspecific. Hypocalcemia with a normal parathyroid hormone concentration is seen in chronic renal failure, vitamin D deficiency, and (transiently) in severe disease states of many different kinds.

Treatment
Hypoparathyroidism is treated with *vitamin D* and *calcium*. Normalization of the serum calcium and phosphate concentrations results in clinical improvement.

■ Hyperparathyroidism and Hypercalcemia (609, 744, 770)

Clinical Features

Hyperparathyroidism is usually due to a hypersecretory parathyroid tumor; the classic clinical triad of hyperparathyroidism consists of kidney stones (calcium oxalate or phosphate), ostitis fibrosa cystica, and duodenal ulcer. Its neurologic manifestations (see below) are caused by hypercalcemia.

Neurologic manifestations. The neurologic manifestations of hyperparathyroidism are those of hypercalcemia:

- Emotional lability, fatigability, apathy, agitation, insomnia, depression, nausea, vomiting, anorexia, confusion, psychosis, progressive lethargy, coma.
- Memory impairment and dementia.
- Neuromuscular manifestations with weakness and atrophy predominantly affecting the muscles of the shoulder and pelvic girdles (958). The reflexes usually remain brisk. The EMG reveals myopathic changes (100). Fasciculations, sensory deficits, paresthesiae, and hyporeflexia are occasionally encountered.
- Ataxia, oculomotor dysfunction, spasticity, dysarthria, dysphagia.
- Seizures.

Diagnostic Evaluation and Differential Diagnosis

The diagnosis is based on the demonstration of elevated serum concentrations of calcium and parathyroid hormone. If a parathyroid-hormone-secreting adenoma is found, further testing should be performed to determine whether it has arisen in the context of a multiple endocrine neoplasia syndrome (type I or II). The differential diagnosis of hypercalcemia in the setting of a normal or low parathyroid hormone concentration includes cancer (of the breast, lung, kidney, or hematopoietic system), renal failure, hypervitaminosis D, sarcoidosis, and diseases causing accelerated metabolism of bone.

Treatment
Surgical resection of a parathyroid adenoma (if present) is curative. Hypercalcemia of other causes is treated etiologically, symptomatically, or both. Treatment is usually by *hydration with forced diuresis* and the administration of *bisphosphonates* and *calcitonin*.

Paraneoplastic Syndromes Affecting the Nervous System
(414, 362a, 768)

> **Definition:**
> Cancer can affect the nervous system not only by primary and metastatic involvement and the predisposition to opportunistic infection, metabolic derangement, and ischemic and hemorrhagic stroke, but also by humorally mediated, long-distance mechanisms. The specific, causative anti-neuronal antibodies have been identified for a number of these so-called paraneoplastic syndromes.

■ Paraneoplastic Neurologic Syndromes

This term designates the long-distance effects of cancer on the central and peripheral nervous system that are not due to metastasis, infection, or cancer-related coagulopathy (Table 2.**86**).

General Aspects

As a rule, paraneoplastic syndromes become clinically evident before the underlying tumor itself does, or when the tumor is in remission, or when it is still so small as to be curable. The syndromes designated as "paraneoplastic" are not exclusively seen in connection with a tumor; they are seen, with variable frequency, in nonneoplastic autoimmune diseases, too. The likelihood that there is an underlying tumor is so high as to merit an intensive search for it in all cases of subacute cerebellar degeneration, opsoclonus-myoclonus syndrome in children, and Lambert-Eaton myasthenic syndrome. An intensive search for a primary tumor is less urgently indicated in other paraneoplastic syndromes.

Pathogenesis

An autoimmune pathogenesis is presumed for most of these syndromes. In a number of them, the responsible autoantibody has already been identified – an antibody directed against the tumor, which keeps its growth in check, but which also reacts with neurons or with an opportunistic virus in the nervous system.

Diagnostic Assessment

"Paraneoplastic syndrome" is essentially a diagnosis of exclusion at present, though a number of *specific antibodies* have been determined whose detection can support the diagnosis of particular syndromes (Table 2.**87**) and can also facilitate the search for a primary tumor. In many cases of paraneoplastic syndrome, CSF examination reveals an inflammatory picture, with pleocytosis, elevated protein concentration, and oligoclonal bands.

> **Treatment**
> Most paraneoplastic neurologic syndromes respond poorly, or not at all, to treatment and ultimately produce marked functional impairment. It is nonetheless worthwhile to attempt treatment with *immune suppressants, plasmapheresis*, or *intravenous immunoglobulins* (IvIG). Plasmapheresis is generally successful in cases of Lambert-Eaton myasthenic syndrome, and IvIG is

effective against cerebellar degeneration, at least when it occurs in childhood (191).

■ Paraneoplastic Cerebellar Atrophy (= Subacute Cerebellar Cortical Atrophy)

Clinical Features
Paraneoplastic cerebellar atrophy is the most common paraneoplastic neurologic syndrome and is seen mainly in association with small-cell lung cancer, ovarian cancer, and Hodgkin's lymphoma. The neurologic manifestations appear several months or (rarely) years before the primary tumor becomes symptomatic. The initial presentation is usually with a mild impairment of coordination, which progresses within a few weeks or months to a symmetrical, disabling truncal and appendicu-

Table 2.**86**   Paraneoplastic syndromes of the nervous system (768)

Brain and cranial nerves:
- Subacute cerebellar degeneration
- Opsoclonus-myoclonus syndrome
- Limbic encephalitis and other dementias
- Brainstem encephalitis
- Optic neuritis
- Photoreceptor degeneration (= paraneoplastic retinopathy)

Spinal cord and spinal ganglia:
- Necrotizing myelopathy
- Anterior horn cell disorders, amyotrophic lateral sclerosis
- Myelitis
- Denny-Brown's sensory polyneuropathy (227)

Peripheral nerves:
- Subacute and chronic sensorimotor polyneuropathy
- Acute polyradiculoneuropathy (Guillain-Barré syndrome)
- Mononeuritis multiplex, plexus neuritis
- Autonomic neuropathy
- Paraprotein-associated polyneuropathy

Neuromuscular junction and muscle:
- Lambert-Eaton myasthenic syndrome
- Myasthenia gravis
- Dermatomyositis, polymyositis
- Acute necrotizing myopathy
- Carcinoid myopathy
- Myotonia
- Myopathy of cachexia

Miscellaneous:
- Encephalomyelitis
- Neuromyotonia
- Stiff man syndrome

Table 2.**87**   Autoantibodies associated with paraneoplastic neurologic syndromes (207, 575, 768)

Antibody	Syndrome	Tumor
Anti-Yo = PCA-1	Cerebellar degeneration	Ovarian carcinoma, breast cancer, (rarely) lymphoma or lung cancer
Anti-Hu = ANNA-1	Encephalomyelitis, limbic encephalitis, opsoclonus-myoclonus syndrome (415), sensory polyneuropathy	Small-cell lung cancer, neuroblastoma, prostate cancer, seminoma
Anti-Ri = ANNA-2	Opsoclonus-myoclonus syndrome	Neuroblastoma, breast cancer, small-cell lung cancer
Anti-Retina	Paraneoplastic retinopathy	Small-cell lung cancer
Anti-NMJ	Lambert-Eaton myasthenic syndrome (Ab against calcium channel)	Small-cell lung cancer
Anti-NMJ	Myasthenia gravis (Ab against acetylcholine receptor)	Thymoma
Hodgkin-Ab	Cerebellar degeneration	Hodgkin's lymphoma

ANNA: antineuronal nuclear antibody;
NMJ: neuromuscular junction;
PCA: Purkinje-cell antibody.

lar ataxia with dysarthria, dysphagia, nystagmus, oscillopsia, and vertigo. These cerebellar manifestations are often accompanied by diplopia, hearing loss, pyramidal tract signs, posterior column signs, polyneuropathy, or dementia. Most patients lose the ability to walk.

Diagnostic Evaluation
CT and *MRI* reveal cerebellar atrophy. *CSF examination* usually initially reveals inflammatory changes, which later resolve. *Antibodies* that react with Purkinje cells and other types of neurons (some of them outside the cerebellum) are often found in both the serum and the CSF (Table 2.**87**). Histological examination reveals a loss of the Purkinje cells of the cerebellar cortex. If a primary tumor is found, it is usually still in the localized stage. Anti-Yo antibodies appear only in association with gynecological tumors; their detection should therefore prompt a search for such a tumor. Cerebellar degeneration in association with Hodgkin's disease is more common in men. Plasmapheresis or intravenous immunoglobulins can bring clinical improvement in some cases.

■ **Limbic Encephalitis** (206, 954)

Clinical Features
This term refers to a form of paraneoplastic encephalitis that mainly affects the structures of the limbic system and is most commonly seen in association with small-cell lung cancer, though it may also accompany

tumors of other kinds. Over the course of a few weeks, patients develop a severe deficit of explicit memory, along with personality changes, affective disturbances, confusion, and sometimes agitation, hallucinations, and both partial and generalized seizures.

Diagnostic Evaluation

The CSF initially displays inflammatory changes, and MRI reveals signal abnormalities in the medial portions of the temporal lobes. Histological examination reveals neuronal loss, reactive gliosis, and perivascular lymphocytic infiltration predominantly affecting the limbic and insular cortex.

Treatment
There is no known effective treatment. The syndrome sometimes improves with treatment of the primary tumor.

■ Other Paraneoplastic Syndromes

There are paraneoplastic syndromes affecting many different parts of the nervous system, e.g., paraneoplastic *brainstem encephalitis, autonomic neuropathy,* and *myelitis* (206, 574). Further syndromes are listed in Table 2.**87**.

The antibody Anti-Hu is associated with a number of paraneoplastic syndromes; the one originally described under the name "Anti-Hu syndrome" is a sensory polyneuropathy associated with small-cell lung cancer (206, 358). Anti-Ri is histochemically identical with Anti-Hu, but reacts only with central neurons; it causes oculomotor disturbances and, less frequently, cerebellar dysfunction (207).

■ Ischemic and Hemorrhagic Stroke Associated with Neoplasia (74)

Stroke occurs in 15% of cases of cancer (about equally divided between ischemic and hemorrhagic stroke) and is thus the second most frequent cancer-associated disturbance affecting the CNS (after metastases). Some special features of cancer-associated stroke are the following:

- The presentation may be with a diffuse encephalopathic syndrome rather than with an acute focal deficit.
- Stroke may be more likely to be of a particular type (ischemic or hemorrhagic) in the setting of certain primary tumors, patterns of CNS involvement, and modes of antitumor therapy.
- Most strokes in cancer patients have the same etiology and pathogenesis as in persons not suffering from cancer.
- The following causes of stroke are of particular relevance in cancer patients:
  - coagulopathy (disseminated intravascular coagulation, protein C deficiency, thrombocytosis)
  - nonbacterial thrombotic endocarditis
  - vasculitis
  - paraneoplastic syndrome
  - compression or erosion of a blood vessel by tumor
  - leptomeningeal metastasis
  - neoplastic angioendotheliosis
  - tumor embolus (mucin, fragment)
  - infection, sepsis
  - adverse effect of treatment (radiation, chemotherapy, surgery)
  - atherosclerosis
  - thrombotic microangiopathy

Treatment

Stroke in cancer patients is usually treated as in other patients.

Patients with nonbacterial thrombotic endocarditis, and probably also those with disseminated intravascular coagulation, need *second-ary* prophylaxis with heparin, because vitamin K antagonists are ineffective in this situation. Vasculitis can be treated with *corticosteroids* and *cyclophosphamide*, while *plasmapheresis* is beneficial in thrombotic microangiopathy.

Connective Tissue Diseases and Autoimmune Diseases Affecting the Nervous System

Overview:

Connective tissue diseases ("collagenoses") and autoimmune diseases usually affect the skin, joints, and internal organs, but can sometimes primarily involve the nervous system, causing such manifestations as headache, cognitive deficits, seizures, and stroke. Involvement of the peripheral nervous system may cause isolated mononeuropathy, mononeuropathy multiplex, symmetric polyneuropathy, or myositis. Long-term immunosuppressive treatment is usually required.

Connective tissue diseases and autoimmune diseases affect the nervous system in many different ways. Headache and atypical complaints are common in the early phase, before neurologic deficits appear or the disease declares itself through the more usual manifestations affecting the skin, joints, muscles, kidneys, and other organs. Common manifestations in the central nervous system include stroke, seizures, and neuropsychological deficits; in the peripheral nervous system, mononeuropathy multiplex, isolated mononeuropathy, symmetric polyneuropathy, and myositis.

A list of vasculitides affecting the nervous system is found in Table 2.**49**, p. 197. Vasculitis is rarely confined to a single organ. The central or peripheral nervous system may be the site at which the disorder first appears, but even then systemic manifestations are usually evident, such as fever, malaise, or weight loss. The erythrocyte sedimentation rate (ESR) and serum concentration of C-reactive protein (CRP) are usually elevated, and the peripheral blood smear has an inflammatory pattern. Serologic tests and tissue biopsies may aid in establishing the diagnosis. For further discussion of the myositides, see p. 908.

■ Polyarteritis Nodosa (PAN) and Related Diseases (200, 673)

This disease, also called periarteritis nodosa, produces a granulocytic and eosinophilic infiltrate in the arterial wall, with resulting necrosis of the tunica media. Aneurysms that form at the sites of necrosis become thickened by fibrosis. PAN affects multiple organ systems, primarily the kidneys, heart, liver, and gastrointestinal tract.

Cogan's syndrome. This disorder, which primarily affects the cranial nerves, may be a variant of PAN (p. 703) (46, 983).

Churg-Strauss syndrome. Churg-Strauss syndrome is another form of allergic granulomatous angiitis related to PAN. It affects not only the arteries, but also the veins and venules. Its principal manifestations are severe asthma and marked eosinophilia. It more commonly affects the peripheral than the central nervous system; painful mono- or polyneuropathy is typical (919).

Severe atherosclerosis. In severe atherosclerosis, breakdown of an atheromatous plaque may result in embolization of plaque material, containing cholesterol crystals, into all organs of the body, including the brain. The characteristic appearance of ischemia in the toes has given rise to the name "purple (or blue) toe syndrome." Embolization is followed by inflammatory changes in the affected vessels that may be mistaken for a primary vasculitis or PAN (189).

Buerger's disease (thrombangiitis obliterans). This disorder affects young male smokers (723e) and involves inflammatory changes in the small and mid-sized arteries and veins, as well as in the vasa nervorum. Its principal manifestations are intermittent claudication, pain in the legs at rest, ischemic ulcers, thrombophlebitis, Raynaud's syndrome, and sensory deficits (more commonly in the legs than in the arms). Serologic tests are negative.

Clinical Features

PAN begins with nonspecific symptoms and signs such as fever, tachycardia, diaphoresis, weight loss, fatigue, generalized weakness, myalgia, and abdominal complaints. Organ-specific manifestations may, however, be present at the onset of disease. Mono- or polyneuropathy affects half of all patients (p. 606), while central nervous manifestations occur in one-quarter. The latter produce:

- headache,
- seizures,
- vertigo,
- cerebral and (rarely) spinal ischemia and hemorrhage, confusion, and psychosis.

Diagnostic Evaluation

The diagnosis is made by angiography or tissue biopsy.

Treatment

If untreated, PAN generally leads to death through renal failure. In more than 90% of patients, however, long-term remission can be achieved with a combination of *prednisone* (1 mg/kg qd) and *cyclophosphamide* (2 mg/kg p.o. qd with a target white blood count of 3000/µL, or $1 g/m^2$ as a monthly bolus). The treatment must be continued for at least 6 months, and usually longer. *Mesna* should be given concomitantly to prevent nephrotoxicity.

Patients in remission must be followed up regularly. *Azathioprine* (1–2 mg/kg p.o. qd) can be given to prevent recurrences. If recurrence nonetheless occurs, restarting prednisone and cyclophosphamide generally results in remission.

■ Isolated CNS Angiitis
(23, 383, 674)

This disorder, also known as isolated CNS vasculitis and as granulomatous angiitis of the central nervous system (GANS), affects only the CNS – usually only the brain, sometimes also the spinal cord. Some authors classify it among the giant cell arteritides (the other members of this group are cranial arteritis, polymyalgia rheumatica, and Takayasu's arteritis).

Clinical Features
The *major manifestations* are headache and multifocal cerebral ischemia or encephalopathy without focal neurologic signs.

Diagnostic Evaluation
The *CSF* may display inflammatory changes. *Angiography* usually (though not always) reveals vasculitic changes, with stenoses, dilatations, occlusions, and collateral flow. *MRI* reveals multiple foci of ischemia or hemorrhage in the basal ganglia, cortex, and subcortical white matter (359). Leptomeningeal and cortical biopsy are required for definitive diagnosis.

Differential Diagnosis
The major differential diagnoses of isolated CNS angiitis are vasculitides in the setting of herpes zoster, lymphoma, sarcoidosis, and the entire spectrum of chronic meningitis.

▌Treatment
Isolated CNS angiitis has an unfavorable prognosis if untreated. Prednisone and cyclophosphamide are beneficial (for doses, see under PAN, above).

■ Takayasu's Arteritis

This inflammatory disease of the aorta and its branches produces fever, night sweats, and weight loss, as well as neurologic manifestations: headache, orthostatic lightheadedness, transient ischemic attacks, and stroke. Blurred vision on standing up is a characteristic complaint.

▌Treatment
Takayasu's arteritis is treated with *corticosteroids*.

■ Wegener's Granulomatosis
(289, 711, 969)

Clinical Features
Wegener's granulomatosis is a systemic necrotizing inflammatory disorder with vasculitis. It primarily affects the upper and lower respiratory tract and the kidneys. Its *common* neurologic manifestations are:
- headache,
- mono- and polyneuritis,
- cranial neuritis,
- external ophthalmoplegia, and
- hearing loss.

Rarer neurologic manifestations include:
- cerebral ischemia and hemorrhage,
- basilar meningitis,
- cerebritis,
- myelopathy, and
- myopathy.

Diagnostic Evaluation
If the cranial nerves are affected, it must be determined whether this is due to granulomatous disease entering the cranial cavity from the upper respiratory tract (nose), or whether the cranial nerves are primarily affected by vasculitis. MRI is indicated

in this situation. Serologic determination of anti-neutrophilic cytoplasmic antibodies (ANCA), particularly c-ANCA, is a valuable aid to diagnosis. The diagnosis is definitively established by *tissue biopsy* from the respiratory tract and by the demonstration of glomerulonephritis.

Treatment

Wegener's granulomatosis causes death in a few months if untreated. The treatment of choice, a combination of prednisone and cyclophosphamide (for doses, see under PAN, above), usually produces remission. The treatment must be continued for at least 1 year after remission is achieved.

■ Lymphomatoid Granulomatosis

This disorder is another form of granulomatous angiitis predominantly involving the lungs and, less commonly, the skin, kidneys, and central and peripheral nervous system.

Treatment

Most cases of lymphomatoid granulomatosis progress to a lymphoproliferative syndrome and onward to malignant lymphoma. This progression can, however, be prevented by timely treatment with prednisone and cyclophosphamide.

■ Arteritides Associated with Autoimmune Disorders

■ Sjögren's Syndrome (22) (pp. 607 and 909)

Sjögren's syndrome is a slowly progressive autoimmune disease characterized by lymphocytic infiltration of the exocrine glands leading to *sicca syndrome*, with xerostomia and keratoconjunctivitis sicca. Extraglandular manifestations such as arthralgia, Raynaud's phenomenon, and lymphadenopathy appear in one-third of all patients.

Clinical Features

Focal cerebral signs, transverse myelitis, chronic myelopathy, optic nerve involvement, and aseptic meningoencephalitis occasionally appear. Rarer neurologic manifestations are mononeuritis multiplex, symmetric polyneuritis, and myositis.

Diagnostic Evaluation

Anti-Ro (SS-A) autoantibody titers are diagnostically helpful, though nonspecific (22).

Treatment

Sicca syndrome is managed symptomatically – e.g., with artificial tears to prevent corneal ulceration. *Extraglandular manifestations* are treated with *corticosteroids and cyclophosphamide* or *other immune suppressants*.

■ Systemic Lupus Erythematosus (SLE) (228, 33, 483, 670)

Ninety percent of patients suffering from this disorder are women, usually of child-bearing age.

Clinical Features

Nearly all patients have systemic manifestations (e.g., fever, weight loss) as well as involvement of the skin and mucous membranes (butterfly rash, photosensitive dermatitis, oral ulcers, etc.), musculoskeletal system (arthritis, myopathy), heart and lungs (pleuritis, pericarditis, endocarditis) or kidneys (lupus nephritis).

Neurological or psychiatric manifestations appear in 25–75% of patients over the course of the illness, in 3% as the initial manifestation. The most common and often sole neurologic symptom is *migraine-like headache.* Also seen, in decreasing order of frequency, are behavioral abnormalities, cognitive deficits, depression, suicidality, confusion, hallucinations, and psychosis. Possible focal neurologic disturbances include hemiparesis, transverse myelitis, and rarely chorea, athetosis, or ballism. Cranial nerve deficits, mononeuritis, sensorimotor polyneuritis, and polymyositis are relatively common, affecting 15% of patients. *Ischemic stroke* occurs at roughly the same frequency and is usually associated with the lupus anticoagulant, antiphospholipid antibodies (cf. antiphospholipid syndrome, p. 198), or cardiogenic emboli, less commonly with vasculitis. *Seizures* are more frequent in uremic patients.

SLE can be complicated by systemic infection. Neurologic manifestations may be due to opportunistic infections of the CNS (bacterial, fungal, CMV).

Ancillary Tests and Diagnostic Evaluation

The *CSF* is mildly pleocytotic or normal. The *EEG* may be abnormal in patients with psychiatric manifestations, serving to document their organic origin. *CT and MRI* may reveal brain infarcts or multiple, mainly subcortical areas of signal abnormality. The *complete blood count* often reveals anemia, leukopenia, and thrombocytopenia.

Useful *serologic tests* include titers of *antinuclear antibody* (ANA) (a sensitive, but nonspecific screening test) and *anti-dsDNA* and *anti-Sm* antibody (a relatively specific test).

Skin biopsy reveals a specific *lupus band.*

Treatment (and Prevention)

There is no etiologic treatment; non*steroidal anti-inflammatory agents*, *salicylates*, and *antimalarial agents* are frequently used. Neurologic manifestations are treated with *steroids* and sometimes also *cyclophosphamide* (for doses, cf. p. 326). *Azathioprine* is effective, but less so than cyclophosphamide.

Patients with SLE who suffer a stroke have a 50% chance of suffering another one unless specifically treated. Thus, *anticoagulants* are given for prevention of further strokes, as neither steroids nor immune suppressants alter the thrombotic tendency associated with lupus. The course of disease can be monitored by serial determination of the ESR, complement concentration, and anti-dsDNA antibody titer.

Other Disorders of Probable Autoimmune Pathogenesis

This category contains the following disorders:
- rheumatoid arthritis,
- scleroderma,
- ankylosing spondylitis,
- mixed connective tissue disease (Sharp syndrome), and
- ulcerative colitis.

All of these disorders can produce both central and peripheral nervous manifestations.

Differential Diagnosis
Infectious diseases, neoplasia, iatrogenic disorders, and illegal drug use enter into the differential diagnosis of these disorders.

■ Miscellaneous Arteritides
■ Sneddon Syndrome
This syndrome is characterized by strokes, livedo reticularis, and probably antiphospholipid antibodies (577) (p. 198).

■ Malignant Atrophic Papulosis (Köhlmeier-Degos)
This disorder is characterized by cutaneous abnormalities, cerebral, spinal, and peripheral neurologic manifestations, and strokes due to microangiopathy (649).

■ Behçet's Disease
Clinical Features
Behçet's disease is probably of autoimmune pathogenesis and affects multiple organ systems. It produces oral and genital ulceration as well as prominent ocular manifestations (keratoconjunctivitis, iritis, posterior uveitis, optic neuritis) (447, 816c). Arthritis and venous thrombosis may occur. Neurologic and psychiatric manifestations are common, including a multiple-sclerosis-like syndrome, venous sinus thrombosis (p. 193), psychosis, and dementia. Peripheral neuropathy and myositis are also encountered.

Diagnostic Evaluation
MRI reveals a multiple-sclerosis-like picture (18).

▌Treatment▐
The treatment is symptomatic. *Prednisone, azathioprine* or *cyclosporine* are used to treat neurologic manifestations, if present (1037).

■ Retinocochleocerebral Vasculopathy
This is mainly a disease of young women (107); its major manifestations are visual disturbances, hearing loss, and tinnitus, as well as encephalopathy and focal neurologic signs. An inflammatory microangiopathy is presumed to be responsible. The same manifestations are seen in Susac syndrome (an entity of uncertain etiology), Eales disease, and posterior multifocal placoid pigment epitheliopathy (59b, 185c).

■ Sarcoidosis
(175, 480, 858, 909, 1053)
Sarcoidosis is an idiopathic granulomatous disease affecting multiple organ systems. It is most commonly seen in young adults. The organs most often affected are the lungs (90%), followed by the lymph nodes, skin (erythema nodosum), eyes (anterior uveitis more frequently than posterior uveitis), upper respiratory tract, bones, joints, bone marrow, spleen, liver, and nervous system. The disease presents with neurologic manifestations (*neurosarcoidosis*) in only 5% of patients, 97% of whom also have extraneural disease.

Clinical Features
Any part of the nervous system can be affected:
- *Intracranial granulomas* are most commonly found in the meninges of the skull base, in the hypothalamus, and in the pituitary gland.

They are usually small but occasionally reach a large size and exert mass effect. They cause focal deficits, psycho-organic disturbances, and seizures. The basilar meningitis and meningoencephalitis of sarcoidosis may be complicated by hydrocephalus, diabetes insipidus, or other endocrine disturbances, or by cranial nerve involvement.

- *The cranial nerves* are involved in half of all patients, either alone or in combination with other intracranial manifestations. Facial nerve palsy is the most common finding; it may be bilateral (either simultaneous or consecutive) and is sometimes associated with fever and swelling of the parotid gland (Heerfordt's uveoparotid fever, p. 678). Sarcoidosis also commonly affects the trigeminal (sensory deficit, neuralgia), vestibulocochlear (vertigo, hearing loss), and optic nerves (optic neuritis, papillitis).
- *Spinal granulomas* compress or infiltrate the meninges and spinal cord to cause an acute or chronic *myelopathy* (480, 826).
- *Peripheral neuropathy* is seen in up to 18% of cases of neurosarcoidosis. It may take any of several forms, including:
  - mononeuritis multiplex,
  - polyradiculopathy,
  - Guillain-Barré syndrome, and
  - symmetric sensory, motor, or sensorimotor polyneuropathy (1053).

Course

The clinical manifestations of neurosarcoidosis may develop acutely, subacutely, or in slowly progressive fashion. Spontaneous remission is more common than further chronic progression. Patients who have undergone a spontaneous remission can, however, develop new, symptomatic granulomas years later. In such cases, the clinical picture may mimic that of multiple sclerosis.

Ancillary Tests and Diagnostic Evaluation

Sarcoidosis should always be considered in the differential diagnosis of a multifocal process affecting the nervous system. *CSF examination* reveals a chronic inflammatory picture with mild lymphocytic pleocytosis and an elevated protein concentration. Oligoclonal bands may be found, representing both intrathecal production and a disturbance of the blood-brain barrier.

CT is highly sensitive in neurosarcoidosis, *MRI* even more so. Meningeal involvement is best seen on contrast-enhanced T1-weighted images, parenchymal involvement on T2-weighted images. Granulomas may display contrast enhancement. They are usually small, but may occasionally be several centimeters in diameter. Spinal granulomas may encircle the entire spinal cord.

Elevated serum and CSF levels of *angiotensin-converting enzyme* are highly correlated with sarcoidosis, and the serum calcium level is often elevated. *Tuberculin tests* are usually negative, and the *Kveim test* (if available) is positive. Plain radiography reveals typical but nonspecific changes in the lungs and bone.

Neurosarcoidosis is usually accompanied by extraneural manifestations amenable to tissue biopsy for definitive *histologic diagnosis* (e.g., muscle biopsy if myopathy is present). The demonstration of noncaseating granulomas by extraneural biopsy will then obviate the need for a meningeal or brain biopsy. Noncaseating granulomas are, however, not exclusive to sarcoidosis.

Treatment

No controlled studies of the treatment of sarcoidosis are available. Steroids have been found empirically to be of use; in general, they must be given for weeks or months. Treatment usually begins with *prednisone* in a dose of 40 mg/day. If there is no beneficial response, improvement may follow the addition of *cyclophosphamide, azathioprine,* or especially *cyclosporine.*

Renal Failure and the Nervous System (118, 781)

Overview:
Acute renal failure causes uremic encephalopathy. Patients with chronic renal failure and those undergoing dialysis may develop uremic polyneuropathy (p. 604), dialysis dysequilibrium syndrome, or dialysis dementia. Patients who have undergone renal transplantation may develop neurologic disturbances due to long-term immunosuppressive therapy.

■ Uremic Encephalopathy

Uremic encephalopathy is a form of metabolic encephalopathy that produces an impairment of consciousness, cognitive and motor disturbances, asterixis, multifocal myoclonus, and seizures. Severe uremia can cause metabolic coma (p. 334). The severity of uremic encephalopathy is only loosely correlated with the elevation of the blood urea nitrogen and serum creatinine concentrations. Acute renal failure is more likely to cause cerebral manifestations than renal failure that develops more slowly, partly because the brain cannot tolerate rapid changes in electrolyte concentrations (p. 334).

Clinical Features

The initial manifestations of uremic encephalopathy are:
- impaired concentration and attention, and
- somnolence.

Further progression of the encephalopathy may reflect itself in cognitive deficits such as confusion, perceptual disturbances, illusions, or hallucinations, delirium, or impairment of consciousness. Motor disturbances typically appear as well, including dysarthria, unsteady gait, ataxia, intention tremor, asterixis, and multifocal myoclonus.

Asterixis. Asterixis makes it impossible for the patient to retain a given posture. When the patient extends the arms and gently spreads and hyperextends the fingers, irregular, bilaterally asynchronous to-and-fro movements of the fingers appear, along with flexion and extension of the hand and fingers – a rapid phase of flexion, followed by a slower return to the original position. Asterixis can also be observed in the legs and in the face. EMG recordings reveal a momentary loss of tone causing the flexion phase, followed by a return of muscle activity during extension. Asterixis is not specific for uremic encephalopathy, as it is also seen in many other toxic and metabolic disorders.

Multifocal myoclonus. As the level of consciousness progressively declines (usually when the patient becomes stuporous) a multifocal myoclonus appears, in which the muscles twitch suddenly, irregularly, and asymmetrically. The facial and proximal limb muscles are predominantly affected. EMG and EEG reveal that this phenomenon is generated both cortically and subcortically.

Seizures. Seizures usually appear only late in the course of uremic encephalopathy, or as a component of the dialysis dysequilibrium syndrome. The reflexes are usually brisk in uremia, the muscle tone spastically elevated, and the Babinski sign present bilaterally. Papilledema is sometimes found, usually as the result of a concomitant hypertensive encephalopathy (p. 197).

Other neurologic manifestations of uremia. Chronic renal failure can also cause *restless legs syndrome* (p. 895) and *polyneuropathy* (p. 604). The intrinsic muscle reflexes are hypoactive in these disorders, as they are in hyperkalemia. *Autonomic dysfunction*, too, may occur.

Diagnostic Evaluation
EEG reveals slowing of background activity, and there may be triphasic waves reflecting the underlying metabolic disturbance. Spike-wave complexes are also seen at increased frequency, even in the absence of sei-

zures. *CSF examination* may reveal mild pleocytosis and elevation of the protein concentration. There are no *neuropathologic changes* specific to uremic encephalopathy.

Treatment
The neurologic signs of uremic encephalopathy can be reversed by *dialysis*. Seizures are treated with the usual *anticonvulsants*, but in altered doses because uremia alters their pharmacokinetics (*phenobarbital* is the drug least affected by these changes; other drugs must usually be given at different doses). *Diazepam* or *clonazepam* can be used, if necessary, for the symptomatic management of severe myoclonus.

■ **Special Neurologic Sequelae of Chronic Renal Failure**
■ **Dialysis Dysequilibrium Syndrome**
Toward the end of a dialysis session, or a few hours later, the patient may develop diffuse headache, with or without a diffuse encephalopathy manifesting itself as nausea, agitation, delirium, convulsions, or impairment of consciousness, along with exophthalmos and elevated intraocular pressure. The pathogenesis of this syndrome is explained as follows: Dialysis is thought to create an osmotic gradient between brain tissue and the plasma, as the brain tissue already contains nondialyzable "idiogenic osmoles" that have been produced in response to uremia. An abnormality of fluid balance results, in which plasma water is taken up by the brain (p. 334).

▪ Dialysis Dementia (Dialysis Encephalopathy) (565)

Clinical Features

This progressive disorder appears in patients chronically undergoing dialysis. It begins with speech hesitancy, stuttering, mild cognitive dysfunction, myoclonus, and seizures and progresses to severe dementia, usually ending in death.

Diagnostic Evaluation

The EEG reveals bilaterally synchronous slow waves with spikes.

> **Treatment**
>
> *Diazepam* can be used to suppress myoclonus in the early phase of the disorder. Autopsy studies have revealed an elevated concentration of aluminum in the brains of patients with dialysis dementia, and the removal of aluminum has, indeed, been followed by a regression of encephalopathy in a small number of patients so treated to date. This form of therapy involves a change to an *aluminum-free diet*, *removal of aluminum* from the dialysis fluid, and the administration of *desferrioxamine*.

▪ Wernicke's Encephalopathy (p. 310)

> **Treatment**
>
> Dialysis patients occasionally develop Wernicke's encephalopathy, which can usually be reversed by *thiamine* administration (456).

▪ Complications of Renal Transplantation

The immunosuppressive therapy needed to prevent rejection of the renal transplant predisposes both to opportunistic infections (cf. p. 122 and Table 2.**38**) and to primary CNS lymphoma (p. 122).

Electrolyte Disturbances with Neurologic Manifestations; Disturbances of Sodium Concentration

Definition:
Electrolyte disturbances can produce encephalopathy with cognitive deficits and impairment of consciousness as well as neuromuscular manifestations. Hypo- and hypernatremia are accompanied by alterations of the plasma osmolality and impair the functioning of the central nervous system. Hypo- and hyperkalemia cause paralysis and disturbances of intracardiac conduction. Hypocalcemia and hypomagnesemia cause tetany, while hypercalcemia and acid-base disorders cause cerebral dysfunction.

■ Disturbances of Sodium Concentration and Osmolality (35, 639, 891, 951)

The homeostatic regulation of fluid and electrolyte balance, and thus of plasma osmolality, is a prerequisite for the normal functioning of muscle and nerve cells. The blood-brain and blood-CSF barriers protect the central nervous system to some extent against fluctuations in the composition of the extracellular fluid. Such fluctuations in the plasma may or may not be propagated to the CSF and cause neurologic manifestations, depending on the speed at which they develop, the relative permeability of the blood-brain and blood-CSF barriers to the ion(s) in question, and the effectiveness of other compensatory mechanisms in the brain.

The *serum osmolality* is largely determined by the serum sodium concentration and can be roughly calculated with the following formula:

Serum osmolality = 2 [Na] + [glucose] + BUN (all in mmol/L).

The plasma, CSF, and intracerebral extracellular fluid are in osmotic equilibrium with one another. Water diffuses freely across the blood-brain and blood-CSF barriers. Movement of sodium ions requires active transport. Plasma hypo-osmolality thus produces an osmotic gradient with resulting movement of water into the cells, causing tissue edema (cerebral edema); conversely, plasma hyperosmolality causes tissue shrinkage.

Table 2.**88** Important differential diagnoses in the metabolic, toxic, and anoxic encephalopathies, in which neuroimaging studies are usually normal (see also Tables 2.**56** and 2.**91**)

Intoxication (due to medications, illegal drugs, alcohol, or other substances)
Hypoxic-anoxic injury (Fig. 2.**83**)
Metabolic disturbances: <ul><li>Electrolyte disturbances (Na, Ca, Mg, PO$_4$)</li><li>Acid-base disturbances</li><li>Hypo- and hyperglycemia</li><li>Thiamine deficiency</li><li>Renal failure</li><li>Liver failure</li><li>Porphyria</li></ul>
Endocrine disturbances: <ul><li>Hypothyroidism and thyrotoxicosis</li><li>Addison's disease, Cushing's disease</li><li>Hypo- and hyperparathyroidism</li><li>Panhypopituitarism</li></ul>

Both hypo- and hyperosmolar states are clinically manifest as *metabolic encephalopathy* (Table 2.**88**). The critical upper and lower limits of serum osmolality for the development of metabolic encephalopathy are 310 mmol/L and 270 mmol/L for rapid changes, 330 mmol/L and 250 mmol/L for slow changes.

■ **Hyponatremia and Hypo-osmolality** (13b, 35, 639, 951)

> **Definition:**
>
> *Hyponatremia* is an excess of water in relation to sodium, *hypo-osmolality* an excess of water in relation to the totality of dissolved particles.

In hyponatremia and hypo-osmolality, water shifts from the extracellular space into the cells of the brain, causing *cerebral edema*. The intraneuronal potassium concentration falls, the resting membrane potential is decreased, and neuronal excitability increases, while the cerebral blood flow decreases. The most important causes of hyponatremia are inadequate dietary sodium, renal and extrarenal sodium loss, nephrotic syndrome, heart failure, hepatic cirrhosis, cerebral salt-wasting syndrome, and the syndrome of inappropriate ADH secretion (SIADH).

Clinical Features

The clinical manifestations of hyponatremia and hypo-osmolality are headache, nausea, vomiting, hallucinations, impaired attention and concentration, focal and generalized seizures, and rapidly progressive impairment of consciousness, leading, in severe cases, to coma.

Diagnostic Evaluation

Measurement of the serum sodium concentration establishes the diagnosis. CT and MRI reveal cerebral edema, which may, however, be less readily apparent in patients with preexisting brain atrophy.

> ▬▬▬**Treatment**▬▬▬
>
> *NaCl* is given intravenously with the objective of raising the serum sodium concentration by 1–2 mmol/L per hour, or 25 mmol/L over 48 hours. An appropriate target concentration is 125 or 130 mmol/L; excessive or too rapid correction of hyponatremia should be avoided, as this may cause central pontine myelinolysis (p. 336). ("Haste makes waste.") SIADH is treated by concomitant administration of *NaCl and furosemide*.

The diagnosis and treatment of hyponatremia is important, as this electrolyte disturbance can lead, if untreated, to *myelinolysis*, potentially causing severe, irreversible brain damage. A persistent vegetative state may be the result (usually when hyponatremia is combined with hypoxia).

■ **Hypernatremia and Hyperosmolality** (13a, 639, 891, 951)

Definition:
Hypernatremia (as well as the accompanying *hyperosmolality*) reflects a deficit of water in relation to sodium, or, much less commonly, an excess of sodium in relation to water.

The *more common causes* of these disturbances are an inadequate intake of water (e.g., failure to quench one's thirst), renal or extrarenal water loss or combined water and sodium loss, excessive sodium intake (e.g., improper intravenous therapy), decompensated diabetes insipidus, and primary disturbances of osmoregulation (e.g., in old age, or in the setting of certain types of brain tumor). Hypernatremia and hyperosmolality result in movement of water out of the cells of the brain into the CSF and thence into the blood plasma and extracellular fluid, with a resulting *reduction of brain volume*. If the electrolyte disturbance develops slowly, the brain can partly compensate and retain its volume by producing so-called idiogenic osmoles.

Clinical Features
Hypernatremia (like hyponatremia) causes a metabolic encephalopathy that manifests itself in cognitive dysfunction possibly accompanied by focal neurologic signs and a progressive decline of consciousness. It may be further complicated by *subdural hematoma* (a consequence of brain shrinkage), by *thrombosis* in capillaries, cerebral veins, and venous sinuses, and by (typically venous) *intracerebral hemorrhage*.

Diagnostic Evaluation
CT and MRI reveal a reduction in brain volume, which is, however, commonly mistaken for brain atrophy. They also reveal the vascular complications mentioned above, if present.

Treatment
The deficiency of water and (in applicable cases) sodium should be corrected within 48 hours; highly acute water and sodium losses can be corrected more rapidly. Excessively rapid correction and overcorrection must be avoided, as they may lead to seizures, cerebral edema, or even death.

■ **Central Pontine Myelinolysis** (10, 663)

Definition:
This syndrome involves bilaterally symmetric demyelination of the basis pontis, usually also the pontine tectum, and, occasionally, extrapontine structures as well.

Pathogenesis

Fluctuations in electrolyte concentrations, particularly a rapid rise in the plasma sodium concentration, are thought to play the most important role in the pathogenesis of this syndrome.

Clinical Features and Course

This syndrome most commonly affects patients in whom hyponatremia has been rapidly corrected. The patients are usually alcoholics or persons with nutritional disturbances or hepatic disease who enter the hospital because of confusion. They appear to improve at first with intravenous therapy (usually in combination with sedatives) but, over the ensuing days, progressively develop *dysphagia, dysarthria,* and *quadriparesis*, reflecting dysfunction of the corticobulbar and corticospinal pathways. If myelinolysis spreads to involve the pontine tegmentum, oculo- or pupillomotor dis-turbances can result, sometimes producing the locked-in syndrome; the more common abnormalities are *bilateral abducens palsy* or *bilateral gaze palsy*, with small ("pontine") pupils. Consciousness declines, sometimes to coma.

In the typical course of the syndrome, *decerebration* ensues (p. 228), followed by death 2–3 weeks after admission to the hospital.

Nonetheless, there are occasional asymptomatic cases of myelinolysis that can be documented by MRI and CT, as well as other cases in which the paralysis and bulbar signs are only transient.

Diagnostic Evaluation

The definitive diagnosis can only be made at *autopsy* by the histologic demonstration of symmetric, noninflammatory demyelination in the pons, but a presumptive diagnosis can be made in the living patient on

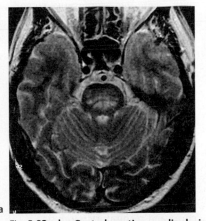
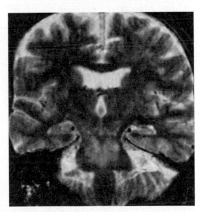

Fig. 2.**82a, b   Central pontine myelinolysis.**
T2-weighted spin-echo images in a 64-year-old man.

a The axial image reveals hyperintense signal in the pons, corresponding to myelinolysis.

b The coronal image shows the hyperintense signal in a butterfly-like pattern, traveling along the pyramidal pathway.

the basis of the typical clinical signs, electrolyte abnormalities, and neuroradiological findings. CT reveals hypodensity of the pons; MRI reveals central pontine T1-hypointensity and T2-hyperintensity (147) (Fig. 2.**82**).

Treatment (and Prevention)

Care should be taken to avoid excessively rapid correction or overcorrection of hyponatremic and hypo-osmolar states, as this can cause central pontine myelinolysis (cf. p. 336).

Extrapontine Myelinolysis

Extrapontine myelinolysis preferentially affecting the corpus callosum is a typical finding in *Marchiafava-Bignami syndrome* (p. 310).

■ Disturbances of Potassium Concentration

The CSF potassium concentration is tightly regulated. Abnormalities of the plasma potassium concentration alter the functioning of muscle and the intracardiac conduction system long before the CSF potassium concentration changes enough to alter the composition of the extracellular fluid in the central nervous system and produce neurologic manifestations. Thus, hypo- and hyperkalemia present mainly with *circulatory signs* and *dyskalemic paralyses* (p. 891).

■ Hypo- and Hypercalcemia

Calcium stabilizes the excitable membranes of muscle and nerve cells. Hypocalcemia thus makes these structures abnormally excitable, and hypercalcemia makes them less than normally excitable. Fluctuations of the calcium concentration in plasma

(like potassium fluctuations) are generally not reflected in the CSF and thus tend to cause peripheral manifestations first (e.g., tetany), long before central nervous manifestations appear. The signs and symptoms of disturbances of calcium balance have already been described (cf. p. 318).

■ Disturbances of Magnesium Balance

Magnesium, a primarily intracellular cation, plays a critical role in the function of a number of enzymes. Its effect on the excitability of nervous tissue is similar to that of calcium.

■ Hypomagnesemia

Hypomagnesemia (defined as [Mg] < 0.8 mmol/L) is caused by inadequate dietary intake or intestinal absorption of magnesium, by renal magnesium wasting, or by endocrine disturbances. Its clinical manifestations include paresthesiae, restlessness, agitation, confusion, convulsions, tremor, myoclonus, and hyperreflexia, which may reach the severity of tetany.

■ Hypermagnesemia

Hypermagnesemia is caused by excessive magnesium intake, usually in combination with renal failure. A serum magnesium concentration above 8 mmol/L is associated with impaired neuromuscular transmission, diminished intrinsic reflexes, and generalized weakness, as well as central nervous depression. Concentrations above 20 mmol/L are associated with coma and respiratory paralysis.

■ Hypophosphatemia (525, 526, 883, 1054)

Phosphate, a mainly intracellular anion, is important for the maintenance of membrane structure and for energy storage. An inadequate dietary intake of phosphate, a shift of extracellular phosphate into the cells, or excessive urinary phosphate loss can lead to *hypophosphatemia* (defined as a serum concentration below 0.3 mmol/L). One of the more common causes is alcoholism; hypophosphatemia in alcoholics often leads to *rhabdomyolysis*.

The neurologic manifestations of hypophosphatemia include *sensorimotor paralyses* resembling Guillain-Barré syndrome and *metabolic encephalopathy* with confusion and impairment of consciousness, possibly leading to coma and death.

■ Acid-Base Disorders

■ Acidosis and Alkalosis

These disturbances may be further classified into:

- metabolic and respiratory acidoses,
- metabolic and respiratory alkaloses, and
- mixed acidoses and alkaloses.

Their causes are manifold and their clinical presentation nonspecific. Deviation of the serum pH outside its normal range (7.35–7.45) causes encephalopathic manifestations including fatigability, impairment of attention, apathy, confusion, and declining consciousness. Severe acidosis or alkalosis causes coma.

Metabolic acidosis may be accompanied by (compensatory) hyperventilation (Kussmaul respiration). The only distinct, clinically recognizable syndrome caused by an abnormality of acid-base homeostasis is the *hyperventilation syndrome*, which reflects the respiratory alkalosis produced by (primary, voluntary) hyperventilation. It begins with perioral and acral numbness and paresthesiae and progresses to tetany, a reflection of elevated neuromuscular excitability. In the brain, hypocapnia causes vasospasm, a decrease in cerebral blood flow, and, finally, loss of consciousness (p. 554).

Hypoxic-Ischemic Encephalopathy (764)

Definition:

Globally diminished cerebral blood flow, a deficiency of oxygen in the blood, or a combination of the two can produce a diffuse hypoxic-ischemic encephalopathy. The disorder is characterized by acute coma and is treated by restoring an adequate flow of oxygenated blood to the brain as rapidly as possible. Timely treatment may bring recovery without lasting damage.

The more common causes of hypoxic-ischemic encephalopathy are primary circulatory failure in myocardial infarction, cardiac arrest, hemorrhagic shock, shock of other etiology, primary respiratory failure followed by circulatory arrest after asphyxiation (drowning, strangulation, aspiration, carbon monoxide poisoning), and respiratory paralysis (neuromuscular disorders, stroke, epilepsy).

Clinical Features and Prognosis

Mild hypoxia causes ataxia and impaired attention and judgment, and severe hypoxia causes loss of consciousness. Cortical function ceases first; brainstem functions (spontaneous breathing, brainstem reflexes) are initially preserved, but these also cease if hypoxia persists (cf. p. 226).

Unless cardiorespiratory function is quickly restored, death ensues (716a) (p. 234).

A brief hypoxic episode with transient loss of consciousness may be followed by a full or nearly full neurologic recovery. Permanent brain damage is likely, however, if the duration of hypoxia exceeds a threshold that lies somewhere between 3 and 5 minutes (p. 151 and Fig. 2.**35**). Patients remaining unconscious for more than 48 hours have an unfavorable prognosis.

Some patients who are successfully resuscitated after a severe hypoxic episode lie motionless thereafter, with preserved brainstem reflexes; their plantar responses are absent, and noxious stimuli evoke decorticate or decerebrate posturing (p.

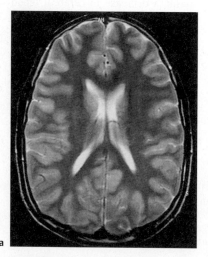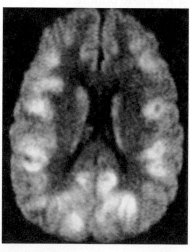

a

b

Fig. 2.**83a, b   Hypoxic brain injury after circulatory arrest.**
The patient is a 20-year-old man in coma.
a The T2-weighted spin-echo image is normal.

b The diffusion-weighted image reveals extensive cortical damage, appearing as hyperintensity.

228). It is difficult to assign a prognosis in such cases. Some of these patients die within 48 hours, while others survive, usually with permanent deficits. Myoclonus and generalized seizures in the first 48 hours after resuscitation are unfavorable prognostic signs, as are nonreactive pupils, absent reflex eye movements, and marked slowing of background activity on the EEG (579, 1026).

Late post-hypoxic manifestations. These encompass the entire spectrum from mild cognitive disturbances to the persistent vegetative state. Conditions of intermediate severity between these two extremes include post-hypoxic dementia (with or without extrapyramidal disturbances such as parkinsonism or choreoathetosis), cerebellar ataxia, visual agnosias, Korsakoff's syndrome, and (rarely) persistent epileptic seizures. Myoclonus as a late post-anoxic manifestation is the defining feature of Lance-Adams syndrome (550). Some patients improve at first, undergo a secondary deterioration, and die 1–2 weeks later; this course of events is known as *delayed post-hypoxic encephalopathy*.

Diagnostic Evaluation

The diagnosis of hypoxic encephalopathy is based on the case history (generally obtained, for obvious reasons, from someone other than the patient), clinical observations of the type described above, and the determination of an arterial P_{O_2} below 40 mmHg, carbon monoxide poisoning, systolic blood pressure below 70 mmHg, or cardiac arrest. Diffusion-weighted MRI in the acute phase reveals abnormal hyperintensity of the cerebral cortex (Fig. 2.**83**).

Treatment

Only a few patients with hypoxic encephalopathy, mostly children, suffer from acute cerebral edema with intracranial hypertension and thus stand to benefit from *measures to lower the intracranial pressure*. The remaining patients can only be given supportive care.

No *medications* have yet been shown to lessen permanent brain damage due to hypoxia. *Hypothermia in the acute phase* may be neuroprotective. Seizures are treated with *anticonvulsants*, myoclonus with *diazepam* or *clonazepam*.

Hepatic and Gastrointestinal Disease and the Nervous System

Overview:

In hepatic disease with portal-systemic venous shunting, the circulating blood is inadequately detoxified in the liver, and an encephalopathy with prominent asterixis results. Acute hepatic failure causes acute encephalopathy with cerebral edema. Pancreatic and intestinal disease can also cause neurologic disturbances.

■ **Hepatic Diseases**

■ **Hepatic Encephalopathy Due to Portocaval Shunting** (3, 593, 777)

In chronic liver disease with portal hypertension, when circulatory shunting from the portal veins to the right atrium has developed spontaneously through collateral channels or has been created surgically through an anastomosis, part of the blood that perfuses the gastrointestinal tract is able to reach the systemic circulation without first being detoxified in the liver. The systemically circulating blood is thus rich in toxins, particularly ammonia. This is the cause of *portocaval encephalomyelopathy*.

Clinical features

Apathy, frequent yawning, somnolence, and mild cognitive impairment are the initial manifestations; the level of consciousness may decline rapidly thereafter to delirium. At this stage, *asterixis* is usually present (p. 271). Hypertonia and hyperreflexia are usually seen, pathological reflexes such as the Babinski sign may appear, and choreoathetosis develops in rare instances. Spastic para- or quadriparesis may also be a prominent finding, either in isolation or together with other signs of encephalopathy, and, if present, is usually irreversible (225). Convulsions are rare. These patients are also at risk of myelinolysis (p. 336).

Diagnostic Evaluation

The *EEG* is usually slowed and reveals bilaterally synchronous triphasic waves. The *serum transaminase concentrations* are usually, though not always, elevated. An elevated *serum ammonia concentration* establishes the diagnosis.

■ **Treatment (and Prevention)** ■

Patients with portocaval encephalomyelopathy are treated with a *low-protein diet, control of gastrointestinal bleeding,* and *lactulose* or *antibiotics,* with the goal of lowering the gastrointestinal production of ammonia and other toxic substances.

■ **Encephalopathy in Acute Hepatic Failure** (594)

Viral infections, hepatotoxins, or Reye's syndrome (p. 296) can cause acute hepatic failure with severe elevation of transaminase concentrations, jaundice, and coagulopathy. The major neurologic manifestation is a progressive decline of consciousness toward coma. Diffuse cerebral edema with intracranial hypertension is a frequently lethal sequela.

■ **Wilson's Disease (Hepatolenticular Degeneration)**

See p. 297.

■ **Pancreatic Diseases**

Diabetes mellitus is the pancreatic disease that most commonly affects the central nervous system, usually through *hyper- and hypoglycemia* (p. 314) or vascular complications (p. 603). In the peripheral nervous system, diabetes can cause mono- and polyneuropathy (p. 598). An islet-cell tumor (insulinoma) can cause chronic, recurrent hypoglycemia, with central nervous effects (p. 113). *Acute pancreatitis* often causes encephalopathic signs because of an electrolyte imbalance, coagulopathy, or other systemic derangement.

- **Intestinal Diseases**
- **Whipple's Disease** (p. 273)
- **Myoneurogastrointestinal Encephalopathy (MNGIE) Syndrome**

MNGIE syndrome consists of mitochondrial encephalopathy together with gastrointestinal disturbances and myopathy (p. 905).

- **Sprue and Other Disorders of Intestinal Resorption**

These disorders can cause polyneuropathy (p. 608). Neurologic manifestations have been described as occurring in 3% of cases of *ulcerative colitis* and *Crohn's disease*: in the former,

mainly peripheral neuropathy, and, in the latter, mainly myelopathy and myopathy, occasionally myasthenia gravis (597). *Sprue* (celiac disease), an inflammatory, atrophic disorder of the small intestine due to gluten hypersensitivity, can cause cerebellar ataxia (p. 280). The latter usually appears in combination with a mild polyneuropathy, but it is occasionally the sole neurologic manifestation or even the sole manifestation of disease, in the absence of gastrointestinal symptoms of gluten hypersensitivity (373c). The diagnosis is supported by demonstration of antigliadin antibodies in the serum.

Hematologic and Vascular Diseases and the Nervous System

Overview:

Hematologic and vascular disorders usually cause cerebrovascular complications such as hemorrhagic and ischemic stroke, less commonly other cerebral manifestations or mono- or polyneuropathies. Leukemia may cause leukemic meningitis, leukoencephalopathy, or paraneoplastic syndromes affecting the nervous system.

- **Leukemia**

Leukemia often causes *cerebrovascular complications* (768) (p. 209) through a wide variety of pathogenetic mechanisms, including coagulopathy, leukostasis, septic embolization, and iatrogenic side effects. These complications include intracerebral hemorrhage, venous sinus thrombosis, thrombotic microinfarction, and territorial infarction. Leukemia also frequently infiltrates peripheral nerves, nerve roots, and the meninges (533).

Leukemic meningitis occurs in nearly one-third of all cases of leukemia, presenting with headache and cranial

nerve deficits, usually affecting the facial, trigeminal, and optic nerves. Other manifestations include meningismus, behavioral abnormalities, signs of intracranial hypertension such as papilledema, paraparesis, and bladder dysfunction. Cytologic examination of the CSF establishes the diagnosis.

Leukemic meningitis must be treated with cytostatic agents given intrathecally (in addition to the systemic therapy given for the primary condition), sometimes in combination with radiotherapy of the neuraxis. This treatment, in turn, may be complicated by a medication- and radiation-induced *leukoencephalopathy*, whose course may resemble that of *progressive multifocal leukoencephalopathy*. A *chloroma* (mass of leukemic cells) may exert local mass effect (e.g., spinal cord compression), and *local leukemic infiltration* may cause many different types of focal neurologic deficit. *Paraneoplastic syndromes* are discussed on p. 320.

The differential diagnosis of neurologic disturbances in patients with leukemia also includes infection, drug and radiation toxicity, electrolyte disturbances, and other metabolic disturbances.

■ Polycythemia Vera
(150, 706, 1039)

Polycythemia is often accompanied by neurologic symptoms such as headache, dizziness, tinnitus, and paresthesiae. Objective findings are present in some 20% patients, most commonly ischemic and hemorrhagic stroke, extrapyramidal signs (parkinsonism, chorea), visual impairment, signs of intracranial hypertension, convulsions, and behavioral abnormalities. A polyneuropathy due to polycythemia vera has also been described. Some of the neurologic manifestations respond favorably to phlebotomy and treatment of the underlying hematologic disorder. Polycythemia may appear as a secondary manifestation of an erythropoietin-secreting hemangioblastoma of the cerebellum.

■ Sickle-Cell Anemia (11a, 12, 391, 907a)

This genetic disease of autosomal recessive inheritance is most common in persons of wholly or partly sub-Saharan African ancestry, but is also found in a variety of other ethnic groups from widely scattered geographic areas. One in 600 black Americans suffers from the disease, and 8% are asymptomatic heterozygotes. Sickle-cell anemia considerably shortens the life expectancy of the sufferer. In persons with the disease, more than half of the hemoglobin in the blood consists of the abnormal hemoglobin S molecule, which, in its deoxygenated state, polymerizes to cause sickling of the erythrocyte, leading in turn to erythrocyte loss (anemia).

Sickle cells also adhere to the vascular endothelium and cause vascular occlusions that account for most of the clinical manifestations of the disease, and, in particular, its neurologic complications. Attacks of acute pain ("sickle-cell crises") occur in the chest, abdomen, back, or extremities; other manifestations include leg ulcers, osteonecrosis, spontaneous abortion, priapism, and splenic infarction. The latter renders sufferers abnormally susceptible to pneumococcal infection, *Salmonella* osteomyelitis, and staphylococcal or *E. coli* sepsis. More than 10% of patients suffer a stroke by the age of 20. Patients at highest risk for stroke can be identified by cerebrovascular Doppler ultrasonography: the risk of infarction rises with increasing flow velocity in the internal carotid and middle cerebral arteries, and the risk of cerebral hemorrhage depends on the degree of injury of the arterial walls. Hemorrhage usually occurs years after infarction.

Treatment

Patients with sickle-cell anemia now live well into their fifth or sixth decade with good medical care. Infants are given *penicillin* as prophylaxis against pneumococcal infection, followed by *antipneumococcal vaccination* at age 2. *Folic acid* is given to prevent megaloblastic erythropoiesis, and *fluids* and *antibiotics* are given whenever the patient develops a fever.

Repeated *blood transfusion* in childhood lessens the risk of a first ischemic stroke and of further strokes, because it lessens the fraction of hemoglobin S in the blood. Vascular complications are significantly less likely when the hemoglobin S fraction is below 30%. Repeated transfusion, however, leads to iron overload, and it remains unknown until what age transfusion is really necessary. *Hydroxyurea* raises the fraction of hemoglobin F and thereby reduces both the frequency of sickle-cell crises and the need for blood transfusion.

A further source of hope is *bone marrow transplantation*, with which there is only limited, but nevertheless highly promising experience to date. This form of treatment appears to prevent chronic problems affecting the lungs and bones, as well as complications in the central nervous system.

■ Pernicious Anemia

See the section on funicular myelosis, p. 441.

Myeloma

Myeloma causes mono- and polyneuropathy (p. 604) and also produces central nervous manifestations through the effects of hypercalcemia (p. 338) and uremia (p. 331).

■ Hereditary Hemorrhagic Telangiectasia (Osler-Weber-Rendu Disease) (370)

This genetic disease of autosomal dominant inheritance is characterized by generalized telangiectases and larger arteriovenous malformations occurring mainly in the nose, skin, lungs, gastrointestinal tract, brain, and spinal cord.

Its *neurologic manifestations* include ischemic stroke, seizures, intracerebral and subarachnoid hemorrhage, and (if the spinal cord is involved) paraplegia.

Patients with pulmonary arteriovenous malformations are at risk for the development of brain abscesses.

Dementing Disorders and Other Neuropsychological Syndromes

Definition:

Because the functions of the brain are localized, a lesion at a particular site in the brain (for example, an infarct, hemorrhage, or tumor) causes a predictable functional deficit – e.g., a specific cognitive impairment or neuropsychological syndrome. If multiple lesions or other disease processes affect the structure and function of brain cells in diffuse, nonlocalized fashion, generalized cognitive impairment usually results. *Dementia* is defined as global impairment or loss of intellectual function. Many different disorders cause dementia; some are treatable. The first part of this section concerns methods of neuropsychological examination for the assessment of cognitive function. In the remainder, the individual syndromes are presented.

Neuropsychological Examination
(87, 198, 374, 403, 665, 765, 850c, 914)

Overview:

The neuropsychological (mental status) examination described in this subsection can be used at the bedside to diagnose and characterize disturbances of language (*aphasia*), the execution of voluntary movement (*apraxia*), memory (*amnesia*), recognition (*agnosia*), spatial construction and orientation, and visuospatial processing. Focal brain lesions typically impair a single neuropsychological function or a small group of related functions, while multifocal or diffuse lesions impair multiple functions simultaneously. Global impairment of cognitive function is termed dementia. The clinical hallmark of dementia is a deficiency of higher, integrative cognitive function.

The *neuropsychological examination* consists of a series of tests of cognitive function and behavior; alternative, synonymous terms for it are "mental status examination" and "neurobehavioral examination." Its purpose is to identify cognitive and behavioral deficits that are due to organic brain dysfunction and to differentiate them from deficits of nonorganic origin. Neuropsychology thus bridges the gap between "classical" neurology and psychiatry. Isolated cognitive deficits can usually be traced back to a particular area of the brain that has become dysfunctional; this is more difficult, however, if a cognitive deficit is relatively diffuse or varies over time. In the latter case, a multifocal or generalized neuropathologic process may be the source of the problem.

Personality changes are often a component of neuropsychological disturbances and are invariably present in dementia. They are often readily apparent to an examiner who is aware of the patient's social environment, level of education, and occupation; the patient may, for example, display unusually slow and circumstantial thought processes, or grossly atypical behavior, in relation to his previous, normal state. Yet the examiner may not be able to detect more subtle changes that are apparent only to persons who interact regularly and intensively with the patient, such as close family members and friends. Thus, thorough history-taking is an essential complement to the mental status examination.

The following types of neuropsychological disturbance interfere with normal attention and well-organized thought processes:

- disturbances of consciousness,
- disturbances of mood (abnormal sadness, impulsiveness, anxiety),
- organic mental illnesses (e.g. schizophrenia, with its delusions, illusions, and hallucinations),
- metabolic and endocrine disturbances, and
- toxic influences (alcohol, illegal drugs, medications).

In any of the above situations, the neuropsychological examination is more difficult to perform, and the patient's attention deficit must be taken into account in the interpretation of its results. Furthermore, the examiner can judge whether a deficit is congenital or acquired only when there is adequate information about the pa-

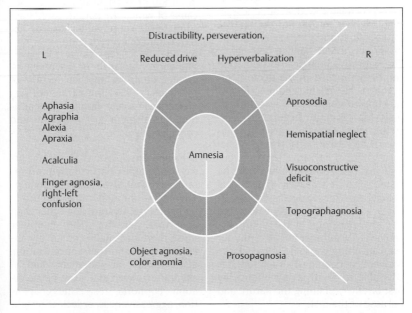

Fig. 2.**84** **Schematic representation of the cognitive deficits that typically result from focal brain lesions** (adapted from Schnider).

tient's previously normal level of function (social environment, level of education, occupation).

Focal brain lesions can cause disturbances of:

- language (*aphasia*),
- the execution of voluntary movement (*apraxia*),
- memory (*amnesia*),
- recognition (*agnosia*),
- spatial construction and orientation, and
- visuospatial processing.

The types of cognitive deficit that result from focal brain lesions are depicted schematically in Fig. 2.**84**. The assignment of deficits to the right and left hemispheres of the brain is valid for all right-handed and most left-handed individuals. The cerebral lateralization of language function is highly correlated with handedness, in that right-hemispheric dominance for speech, though very rare, is found exclusively in left-handed persons.

The neuropsychological examination can be performed in the doctor's office or at the bedside and requires little time to complete. The examiner may, for example, begin with Folstein's mini-mental status examination (p. 363) to obtain a scored, global assessment of cognitive function, but individual functions should always be tested separately as well, or else focal deficits are likely to be missed. Cognitively normal patients generally find the test questions of the neuropsychological examination absurdly or even insultingly simple. Thus, if the patient is not obviously impaired, it is advisable to avoid giving offense by first briefly explaining the nature and purpose of the test.

■ Orientation, Vigilance, Behavior

Orientation. The neuropsychological examination begins with the determination of whether the patient is oriented to person, place, and time. The patient should be able to state his own name, age, and date of birth; the location of the interview (name of hospital or building, floor, department); and the year, possibly also the season, date, day of the week, and time of day. The state of orientation provides a first look into the patient's cognitive condition. Organic brain dysfunction tends to impair orientation to place and time, while leaving orientation to (one's own) person largely intact. A finding of this type reflects an underlying disturbance of attention or short-term memory, because of which the patient cannot assimilate the continually changing external data of everyday life.

Vigilance. Vigilance is discussed in greater detail in another section of this book (p. 566). Impairment of vigilance necessarily implies concomitant impairment of attention and concentration.

Behavior. Focal lesions in certain areas of the brain, particularly prefrontal lesions but also unilateral temporal lobe lesions, may cause practically no neurologic dysfunction other than abnormal behavior. The examiner must, therefore, make note of any abnormality of attention, concentration, distractibility, or judgment, and of any findings such as apathy, perseveration, euphoria, restlessness, agitation, aggressiveness, or lack of insight into the present illness. Illusions and hallucinations should also be noted.

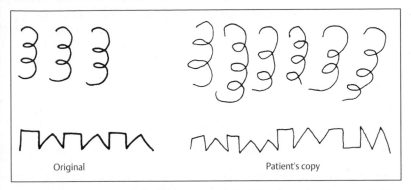

Fig. 2.**85** **Luria loops (above) and alternating square and saw-tooth sequence (below),** as drawn by the examiner (left) and copied by a patient who had sustained a traumatic brain injury with frontal contusions (right).

An *illusion* is a perception of an actual object or sound as being different than it really is; a *hallucination* is a perception of something that is not there. Either may affect any sensory modality – visual, auditory, tactile, olfactory, or gustatory. *Perseveration* indicates a prefrontal functional disturbance and is almost always present when there is a lesion of the frontoorbital cortex. It can often be detected easily by having the patient copy the so-called Luria loops (Fig. 2.**85a**) and alternating sequences (Fig. 2.**85b**). A perseverating patient will draw more than three loops in a single curve, continue drawing curves after the third curve, or do both; on the alternating-sequence test, he will draw one or the other pattern repeatedly, instead of alternating between patterns, as required.

■ Aphasia

Definition:

Aphasia is a disturbance of the reception or expression of language (or both), in which the construction of words and sentences is marred by errors of form, content, and grammar. Aphasia must not be confused with *dysarthrophonia* (p. 384), a disturbance of speech rather than language, in which the sounds and syllables of speech can be distorted, arrhythmic, or even unintelligible, but the language output remains formally correct. The speech of aphasic patients may, of course, be dysarthrophonic as well (as it often is). Aphasia is nearly always due to left-hemispheric dysfunction, except in very rare patients with right-hemispheric dominance for language. It may be present as an isolated deficit, reflecting a focal lesion, or as a component of generalized cognitive impairment, resulting from a multifocal or diffuse lesion. Demented patients practically always suffer from aphasia to some degree.

■ Spontaneous Language Output

The examiner can assess the patient's spontaneous language output unobtrusively throughout the clinical interview, beginning with the taking of the history, or elicit language output directly by asking the patient to describe a pictured scene. The patient's spoken language may be either *fluent* or *nonfluent* (88, 914) (Table 2.**89**):

- *Fluent aphasic speech* retains the normal patterns of intonation and melody (prosody). Its speed exceeds 90 words per minute, sentence length is normal (averaging at least five to eight words), and the patient does not have to make an unusual effort to speak. Its content is abnormal: it consists largely of "filler" words rather than words conveying meaning, and there are frequent literal and semantic paraphasic errors and neologisms. *Paraphasic errors* involve the substitution of one sound, or word, for another. A *literal* (or "phonemic") paraphasic error is the substitution of an individual letter (sound) within a word – "bore" for "door,"

"bed" for "bread," "tagle" for "table," etc. A *semantic* paraphasic error is the replacement of the intended word by a different, semantically related word – "table" for "chair," "dress" for "coat," etc. A *neologism* (in the neurologist's sense) is a nonword used by the patient in place of a real word, such as "luplap" for "syrup."

- *Nonfluent aphasic speech* is produced by the patient with obvious effort. It is slow (fewer than 50 words per minute), and the sentences are short (fewer than five words each). A sentence may consist of only one or two words and lack any grammatical structure. The patient's speech is often dysarthrophonic in addition to being aphasic, and the intonation and melody of speech are abnormal (dysprosodia). The few words that are used tend to be rich in meaning, and "filler" words are rare. Paraphasic errors are rare, and, when they do occur, usually of the literal type.

Table 2.**89** Features of nonfluent and fluent aphasic speech

Feature	Nonfluent aphasic speech	Fluent aphasic speech
Speed	Slow (< 50 words / min)	Normal (> 90 words/min)
Effort	Obviously increased	Normal
Articulation	Dysarthrophonic	Normal
Sentence length	Short (< 5 words)	Normal (> 5 words)
Melody, rhythm	Abnormal, dysprosodic	Normal, prosodic
Content	Many substantives, few "filler" words, agrammatism	Few substantives, many "filler" words
Paraphasic errors	Rare, usually literal	Frequent literal and semantic paraphasic errors and neologisms

Fluent dysphasia is generally due to lesions posterior to the central region of the left (dominant) hemisphere, while nonfluent dysphasia is generally due to lesions anterior to it (Fig. 2.**86**).

■ **Language Comprehension**

The comprehension of language is usually impaired by lesions located posterior to the central region of the left (dominant) hemisphere. The patient's comprehension is tested with tasks that require a minimum of language output, beginning with yes/no questions: "Is it snowing outside?" "Is

it raining?" "Is this a forest?" "Is this a hospital?" The patient can then be asked to perform a motor task, such as pointing to a named object (picture, window, bed, door) or a part of his own body (nose, shoulder, right foot). Next, the ability to understand and carry out *multi-step commands* can be tested: "Stand up, point to the door, turn around once in a circle, and then sit down again." One can also put a number of objects on a table, such as a pen, a pencil, a pair of scissors, and an eraser, and ask the patient to put the eraser between the pen and the pencil, and so forth. For

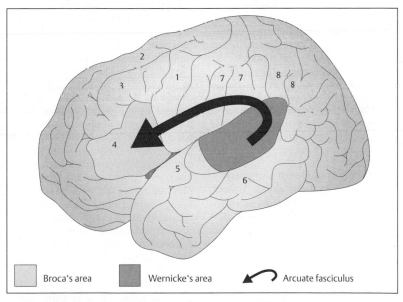

Broca's area   Wernicke's area   Arcuate fasciculus

Fig. 2.**86** **Sites of lesions that cause aphasia.** In the left (language-dominant) hemisphere, lesions of the inferior frontal gyrus cause Broca's aphasia, lesions of the posterior portion of the superior temporal gyrus cause Wernicke's aphasia, and lesions of the arcuate fasciculus cause conduction aphasia.

1 Precentral gyrus
2 Superior frontal gyrus
3 Middle frontal gyrus
4 Inferior frontal gyrus

5 Superior temporal gyrus
6 Middle temporal gyrus
7 Angular gyrus
8 Supramarginal gyrus

obvious reasons, the patient must not be given any visual cues to the tasks proposed (e.g., the examiner must not point to the door himself!).

Progressively complicated multi-step commands offer a convenient means of assessing the severity of impairment of language comprehension.

Among the more sensitive tests of language comprehension are complex sentences and questions such as these: "His hat lay, not on the shelf, but under it. Where was the hat?" or "In the jungle, the hyena was eaten by the wolf. Which animal is dead?"

The interpretation of faulty task performance requires some care, as more than language comprehension is needed to perform these tasks correctly. Patients with disturbed visuospatial processing may be unable to arrange objects in the manner requested, even though they understand the request; apraxic patients may have difficulty pointing and carrying out other tasks; patients who perseverate may get stuck on the first step of a multi-step task and keep on performing it repeatedly.

■ **Repetition of Heard Language**

The patient's ability to repeat a word or sentence spoken by the examiner is impaired to different degrees in different types of aphasia. Repetition can be performed normally only if the receptive and expressive speech areas (Wernicke's and Broca's areas) and the pathway connecting them (the arcuate fasciculus) are intact (cf. Fig. 2.**86**). The patient is given increasingly complex words and sentences to repeat: "Tree." "Locomotive." "He went home." "The locomotive is at the front of the train." "His watch lay not in, but on top of the cabinet." "I thought she would be

coming back home soon." Another useful test is a sequence of "filler" words: "No ifs, ands, or buts." A non-aphasic person should be able to repeat sentences of up to 20 syllables without grammatical or paraphasic errors, omissions, or additions.

Like tests of comprehension, tests of repetition are not purely language tasks, as they require an intact short-term memory. Normal persons can repeat a sequence of five random digits but will, of course, have difficulty if much longer sequences are used.

■ **Naming and Word-Finding**

Naming and *word-finding* are closely related functions that are impaired in nearly all forms of aphasia and thus serve as sensitive tests of language function. An impairment of naming (*anomia*) becomes apparent when the patient is asked to name an object or describe a pictured scene. The things to be named include objects present in the room (clothes, furniture, etc.), parts of objects (the hands, band, or stem of a wristwatch), body parts (chin, shoulder, foot, ankle), common colors (red, blue, green, yellow), less common colors (pink, purple), and faces. If the patient cannot name something, the examiner should point to it and name it. If the patient still cannot name it once this is done, the problem may be *agnosia* rather than, or in addition to, aphasia (p. 357).

(Note, only for the interested: the term *anomia*, an awkward Latin-Greek coinage peculiar to neurology, is not related to the sociologist's *anomie*.)

Word-finding difficulty becomes apparent when the patient is asked to list as many animals as possible, or as many words as possible beginning with the letter A (for example), in one minute. A normal individual will have no trouble naming 10 to 12 animals, or words beginning with A, F, or S (89). Patients with frontal lobe lesions may perform poorly on this task because of perseveration.

■ **Reading**

The ability to read varies greatly among normal individuals, depending largely on the level of education. An acquired impairment of reading ability is called *alexia*. To test reading ability, the patient is asked to read words, sentences, or a short passage out loud. The examiner should note any omissions, additions or substitutions of syllables or words (*paralexic errors*). Comprehension can then be tested with questions about what was read.

Impaired vision and oculomotor disturbances may create the false impression of alexia. Patients with disordered visuospatial perception may not be able to find the right line to read, or the beginning of the line, and be unable to read for this reason.

■ **Writing**

Aphasia impairs reading and writing, as well as speaking. Errors of language content and grammar may be more readily apparent when the patient writes spontaneously, or to dictation, than when he speaks or reads. A suitable test consists of having the patient write sentences of the same type used to test comprehension. Writing one's own name is an overlearned task and thus not particularly useful as a test. *Agraphia* is said to be present when the patient makes basic errors of language, spelling mistakes, or omissions, additions, and substitutions of letters and words (*paragraphic errors*) that would not be expected from his level of education. On the other hand, aphasic patients with or without agraphia usually cannot write complex sentences of the type, "She had been holding her peace far too long anyway." Correct writing of such sentences to dictation practically rules out not only agraphia, but also aphasia.

■ **Disturbances of Spatial Processing**

Definition:
The right hemisphere is dominant for *nonlinguistic spatial processing*. Right-hemispheric lesions often cause neglect of the left side of the body and of space (*hemispatial neglect*).

Useful tests of spatial processing include spontaneous drawing and copying of two- and three-dimensional geometrical figures (Fig. 2.**87**). A patient who can copy or spontaneously produce a drawing of a (three-dimensional) cube or of a house with a gabled roof probably does not have a marked disturbance of spatial processing. Patients who fail to perform these tasks appropriately can be asked to copy and spontaneously draw two-dimensional figures, such as a rhombus, a rectangle, a square, a daisy in a flower pot, or a clock face with numbers and hands indicating a given time. The quality of the resulting performance indicates

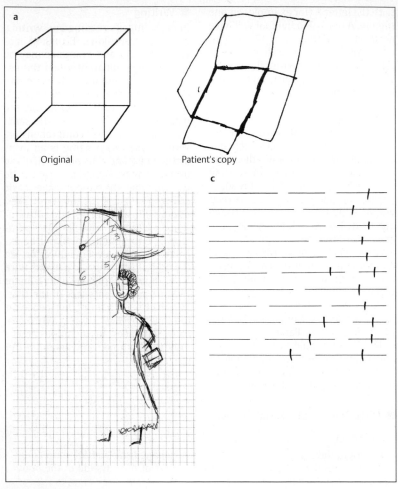

Fig. 2.**87a–c   Spatial processing and neglect.**
a Drawing a cube as a test of spatial processing. The copy was drawn by a patient with a right parietal lesion.
b Drawing of a woman and a clock. The left side of both is missing, indicating severe left hemineglect. The patient had suffered an acute right parietal hemorrhage.
c Line bisection test. A university professor with left hemineglect due to a right-hemispheric astrocytoma.

the severity of the deficit. The following findings are considered to be abnormal:

- rotation of the copy by more than 45° with respect to the original,
- perseveration on a part of the drawing,
- repetition,
- fragmentation,
- distortion or omission of a part of the drawing,
- insertion of the copy into the original, and
- curved lines instead of straight lines and corners.

Many patients with *hemispatial neglect* leave the left side of the paper blank when writing or drawing. Hemispatial neglect may also be apparent when the patient is confronted with the task of *bisecting a given line* or lines: in left hemineglect, the patient bisects only the lines on the right half of the page, and places the bisecting mark, not at the midpoint of each line, but to the right of it. The lines in the left upper quadrant of the page are most consistently neglected. Neglect may affect any sensory or motor modality (for visual neglect, see p. 628; for the extinction phenomenon and sensory neglect, see p. 353) (848). The parietal lobe is the most important anatomic structure for the drawing and copying of figures, but these complex tasks also require adequate functioning of the occipital, temporal, and (in part) frontal lobes, as the figure to be copied must be visually registered, and then conceptually converted into an image and a planned motor activity, before the copy can be successfully executed

■ Apraxia

> **Definition:**
> *Apraxia* is an acquired disturbance of the execution of sequential movements or activities, in the absence of a primary disturbance of motor or sensory function, coordination, comprehension, or attention. Apraxic patients can carry out certain movements or activities spontaneously while being unable to carry out the same movements or activities on command or in imitation of the movements of the examiner.

Ideomotor apraxia is the inability to carry out an individual movement or activity, while *ideational apraxia* is the inability to carry out activities involving multiple steps. *Facial (buccolinguofacial) apraxia* and *limb apraxia* are distinguished from each other by the parts of the body they affect (765).

- Tests of *facial apraxia* include asking the patient to pantomime blowing out a candle, stick his tongue out, lick his lips, drink through a straw, snap his fingers, and make a hissing "sh" sound.
- Tests of *limb apraxia* include asking the patient to salute, thumb his nose or shake his fist at the examiner, or mimic movements such as tooth-brushing, hair-combing, or hammering in a nail. Tests of *ideomotor leg apraxia* include asking the patient to kick a ball, kick away a stick or other piece of debris on the ground, climb over an obstacle, stamp out a cigarette, or push off as

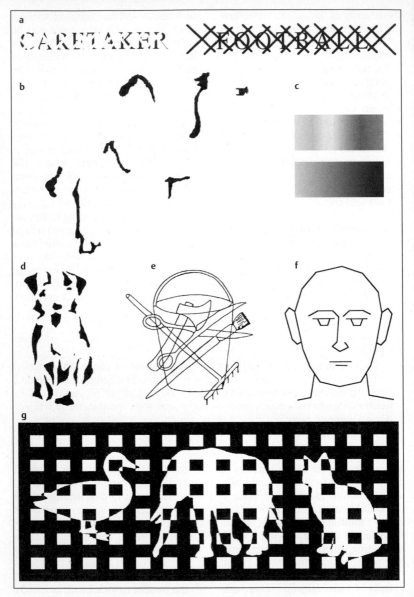

Fig. 2.**88a–g   Tests of visual recognition** (after A. Schnider, 850c).

◀ **a** Masked words.
  b Illusory contours: camel (from K.S. Bowers et al., *Cognitive Psychology* 1990;22:72–110).
  c Color plates for testing of color recognition (e.g., pink, brown, bright green; primary colors are less useful).
  d Fragmentary figure (Street).
  e Overlapping figures (Poppelreuter).
  f Photograph of a well-known individual (e.g. athlete, politician).
  g Masked animal figures.

if with a skateboard. Lesions of the corpus callosum may produce limb apraxia confined to the left side of the body; thus, the left and right sides should be tested separately (p. 384).

• *Ideational apraxia* is the inability to carry out activities involving multiple steps, even though the individ-

ual steps can be performed separately. Two such multistep activities that can be tested are: folding a letter, putting it in an envelope, sealing the envelope, writing an address on it, and affixing a stamp; and opening a tube of toothpaste, removing the toothbrush from its holder, and putting some toothpaste on the toothbrush. These tests are performed with the actual objects at the patient's disposal.

Bilateral ideomotor apraxia is practically always the result of a left-hemispheric lesion (p. 383 and Fig. 2.**92**) and is usually accompanied by aphasia. Ideational apraxia is often accompanied by disturbances of spatial orientation, processing, and planning and is usually encountered as a component of dementia (p. 360)

■ Agnosia (Fig. 2.**88**)

Definition:
Agnosia is a disturbance of recognition, affecting a particular sensory modality, that cannot be explained by a deficit of elementary perception, attention, or cognition.

Visual agnosia. A patient with *visual agnosia* (also termed visual object agnosia) has normal visual acuity, yet cannot recognize an object on sight, and must first feel it in order to name it. The underlying lesion lies in the visual association cortex (areas 18 and 19) of both hemispheres. On the other hand, lesions of the fiber pathway linking the visual association cortex to the speech areas leave the patient still able to recognize an object and demonstrate its use, but unable to name it or the activities for which it is used (*optic aphasia*) (846). *Color a-*

gnosia and *prosopagnosia* are special forms of visual agnosia. Color agnosia, the inability to recognize colors, is produced by lesions of the ventromedial portion of the left occipital lobe, and is to be distinguished from the inability to name colors (color anomia). *Prosopagnosia*, the inability to recognize familiar faces and, usually, complex structures of other kinds as well, is produced by lesions of the inferior portions of the temporal and occipital lobes on the right side, or on both sides (209, 652). *Simultanagnosia* is a disturbance of global recognition, despite a preserved ability to recognize details; it is produced by bilateral parietal or parieto-occipital lesions, and, in milder form, by left occipital lesions.

Patients are tested for visual agnosia by being shown objects or pictures of objects to be named. A patient who cannot name visually presented objects is physically given the objects to manipulate, demonstrate their use, or sort. The task of sorting differently colored strings of yarn is a test for color agnosia; patients with color anomia can perform this task, while those with color agnosia cannot. Prosopagnosia is tested with photographs of the patient's relatives or of famous persons. Patients with prosopagnosia cannot recognize even their closest relatives" faces from photographs. They require other cues, like the sound of the voice, or special visual features such as a characteristic article of clothing, a moustache, etc.

Tactile agnosia Tactile agnosia (or *astereognosia*) is the inability to recognize an object by touch, despite intact primary somatic sensation, and despite the preserved ability to recognize and name the object on sight. It is due to a lesion of the contralateral parietal lobe.

Finger agnosia/Autotopagnosia *Finger agnosia* is a deficit of orientation to one's own body that is confined to the finger's. When the examiner touches one of the patient's fingers (whether or not the patient is looking), the patient cannot state which finger was touched. This finding is usually due to a lesion at the junction of the left parietal and occipital lobes. *Autotopagnosia* is the more general inability to name a part of one's own body after the examiner touches it, or to point to it after the examiner names it.

Anosognosia Anosognosia is the failure to recognize one's own neurologic deficit. Affected patients behave as if they were not blind, deaf, hemiparetic, or otherwise impaired, as the case may be. They will also minimize the deficit or even actively deny it.

■ **Memory and Amnesia**
■ **Memory**

Definition:
Memory is the cognitive faculty by which information is stored and retrieved. Memory makes learning possible. It is subdivided into *short-term* and *long-term memory;* the latter, in turn, is subdivided into *recent* and *old memory.* These distinctions are somewhat arbitrary.

Short-term memory, or *working memory,* as it is sometimes called, is closely related to attention. Its content is soon lost unless it is refreshed by repetition and transferred to long-term memory. A person given the task of repeating a word or a series of numbers, for example, need only retain these data for a short time. More difficult tasks, e.g. complex calculations, require data storage for at least a few seconds.

The neurological examiner usually gains an impression of the patient's attention span and short- and long-term memory while taking the case history, even before proceeding to the mental status examination *per se*, in which these functions are directly tested. To test *verbal short-term memory*, for example, one can give the patient 10 words to remember that belong to three different semantic groups, such as

- dog, lion, tiger,
- sky, boat, blue, sea,
- field, forest, green.

After the examiner says the entire sequence slowly two or three times, the patient with intact memory should be able to repeat nine or all 10 of the given words. He should still be able to do so 15 or 20 minutes later (delayed recall).

Old memory can be tested with biographical information from the patient's childhood or adolescence, supplied by a third party (usually a relative), or with facts about the patient's family (e.g., age and names of spouse and children). One can also ask about dates in history, political events (e.g., wars), or famous people such as presidents, prime ministers, sportsmen, musicians, singers, and movie stars. The results must be interpreted in the light of the patient's premorbid intelligence.

■ Amnesia

Definition:

Amnesia is a deficit of memory, i.e., the storage or retrieval of consciously processed information. *Anterograde amnesia* is the inability to learn new information from the moment a brain injury occurred; *retrograde amnesia* is the inability to remember information stored before the injury occurred.

Impaired acquisition of new memories (anterograde amnesia) accompanies lesions of diencephalic or limbic structures. Anterograde amnesia is more severe and longer-lasting if the underlying lesion is bilateral (p. 377).

■ Higher Cognitive Function

Overview:

The higher cognitive functions, such as the use of acquired verbal and nonverbal knowledge, abstract thinking, problem-solving, calculations, and social behavior, are preserved only when the underlying neuropsychological mechanisms are intact and interact normally. These functions are what enables the individual to cope successfully with life in his or her particular social and occupational setting.

Higher cognitive function is only partly testable by neuropsychological examination. The patient's fund of knowledge and intellectual ability can be assessed with direct questioning, arithmetical tasks, proverb interpretation, and the like, and social behavior is best assessed by questioning the patient's family. The patient's fund of knowledge and intellectual ability can also be assessed with so-called intelligence tests, such as the Wechsler Adult Intelligence Scale (WAIS) (1001).

The patient is asked questions of increasing difficulty regarding plants, animals, geography, culture, and history; persons of normal intelligence answer such questions variably well, depending on their level of education. Arithmetical tasks of increasing difficulty include, for example, oral addition, subtraction, multiplication, and division of one- and then two-digit numbers, and written calculations with still larger numbers. Proverb interpretation requires good general knowledge and an ability to think in the abstract. Asked to interpret the proverb, "People who live in glass houses shouldn't throw stones," a normal individual might say, "Don't criticize other people, because you're not perfect either," or the like. An excessively concrete response – "It might break the glass" – reveals a deficit of abstract thinking.

Higher cognitive functions depend on the integrity of the cerebral cortex and of subcortical structures such as the limbic system. Often, disturbances of higher functions are not localizable to any specific brain area and reflect underlying diffuse pathologic abnormalities, as in Alzheimer's disease.

If the neurologic and neuropsychological examination is normal, the patient is unlikely to have a brain lesion. If an isolated abnormality is found, there is probably a focal lesion. If behavioral abnormalities, memory impairment, and other deficits as well are found, the patient is probably suffering either from congenital mental retardation or from an (acquired) dementing disorder. The patient's deficits may need to be assessed in standardized fashion by a neuropsychologist for medicolegal or insurance-related purposes, but the interpretation of the findings remains the task of the physician, who is responsible for diagnosing the illness that has brought them about.

Dementia and Dementing Disorders (198, 199, 688, 849, 1018)

Definition:

Dementia is a progressive impairment of cognitive function that eventually becomes severe enough to interfere with social behavior and with the patient's work. Memory, language expression and learning, spatial-constructive abilities, visual recognition, affect, behavior, and higher cognitive and abstract thinking are all impaired, to varying degrees. Most cases of dementia are due to Alzheimer's disease.

Epidemiology

Some 1% of persons aged 60 to 64, but 30% to 40% of those over 85, suffer from dementia. The age-specific prevalence of dementia roughly doubles every 5 years after age 60. Persons with a large fund of knowledge and varied interests are less likely to become demented in old age (910).

Diagnostic Criteria and Psychopathological Signs of Dementia

The diagnosis of dementia implies that all of the following are present:

- *Memory impairment,* affecting recent memory more severely than old memory, which may remain intact much longer.
- *Personality change,* manifesting itself as inappropriate, coarse, or rude behavior, a decline of interests, lack of patience in carrying out everyday tasks, deficient social interaction, lack of critical ability, (sometimes) an exaggerated opinion of oneself and a loss of distance, lability of affect, irritability, anxiety, and occasionally hypochondriacal, depressive, or paranoid features.
- *Impairment of abstract thinking and judgment, language (aphasia), execution of motor tasks (apraxia), recognition (agnosia), and perception.* The presence of such deficits is often revealed by the case history: for example, the patient may no longer be able to manage his own finances, cope with the intellectual demands of his job, learn new material, orient himself in unfamiliar surroundings, or maintain a proper sense of time. Neuropsychological examination (p. 372) reveals disturbances of higher cognitive function as well as evidence of aphasia, alexia, agraphia, apraxia, agnosia, and impaired spatial processing. In the early phase of dementia, some aspects of cognitive function may be only mildly impaired, or not at all: aphasia, for example, may be limited to anomia with rare paraphasic errors. In such cases, the abnormality must be demonstrated by asking the patient to produce a word list (e.g., animals) or to take down a relatively long passage to dictation.

Neurologic Signs of Dementia

Neurologic signs are found frequently, but not invariably. A number of *primitive reflexes* are usually abnormally elicitable in advanced dementia. Most of these reflect diffuse frontal lobe dysfunction, e.g., the glabellar tap reflex, snout, sucking, and chewing reflexes, the nuchocephalic (head retraction) reflex, and the palmomental and grasp reflexes (374).

Impairment of motor function may be manifest as a stooped, parkinsonian posture, slowing of movement, rigidity, ataxia, tremor, chorea, and uni- or bilateral spasticity or central paresis. The patient's speech may be hypophonic and dysarthric.

Cortical Versus Subcortical Dementia

Dementia may be classified as cortical, subcortical, or mixed (198, 439). Subcortical dementia is marked by prominent motor disturbances, which, in cortical dementia, are either absent or only a late manifestation. Patients with subcortical dementia think and move slowly and appear apathetic or depressed. Patients with cortical dementia, on the other hand, often seem carefree or even disinhibited, and cortical disturbances such as aphasia, apraxia, agnosia, and impaired spatial processing and perception are prominent. The disturbance of memory seems mainly to involve recall in subcortical dementia, attention and storage in cortical dementia.

Alzheimer's disease is the classic example of cortical dementia, while the dementia of progressive supranuclear palsy is an example of subcortical dementia.

Mental Retardation Versus Dementia

Mental retardation is a condition in which the intellectual faculties never develop normally. The retarded individual has an undifferentiated personality and a sphere of interests limited to the immediate concerns of everyday life. As for language, the patient's sentences are simply constructed, and his written language is marred by frequent spelling errors. In contrast, a demented patient's previous personality may still be partly discernible, depending on the stage of disease, through his choice of words, manner of writing, and fragments of preserved knowledge.

Delirium

Delirium is an acute confusional state (590) to which elderly, demented patients are predisposed, consisting mainly of a disturbance of attention. It is further characterized by abrupt onset after a brief prodrome, impairment of memory, incoherent conversation, abnormal flight of ideas, hallucinations, illusions, disturbances of the sleep-wake cycle, and, often, decreased wakefulness. Delirium is usually a manifestation of systemic illness.

The Diagnosis of Dementia

The diagnosis of dementia is based on a thorough case history, including interview of persons close to the patient, as well as neurologic and neuropsychological examination. The *Mini-Mental Status Test* (Table 2.**90** can be used for initial screening and

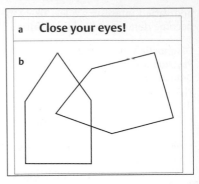

Fig. 2.**89a, b   Two illustrative tasks from the Mini-Mental Status Test** (Schnider). **a** Question 28. The patient is asked to read and carry out this command. **b** Pentagons to be copied.

for semi-quantitative follow-up assessment. In this test, a normal person scores the maximum value of 30 points; persons with benign senile forgetfulness score at least 24 points. A score of 23 points or less suggests dementia. This test, however, may fail to reveal specific types or subtle degrees of cognitive impairment and thus cannot be used as a substitute for a thorough neuropsychological examination.

Etiologies of Dementia and Their Relative Frequency

The more common etiologies of dementia are listed in Table 2.**91**.

Table 2.**90**   Mini-Mental Status Test (after 309)

Name of patient: ....

Date of birth: ....

Date of examination: ....

      1 point for each correct answer

Orientation in time

1.   "What day of the week is it?" ....

2.   "What is today's date?" ....

3.   "What is the current month?" ....

4.   "What is the current season?" ....

5.   "What year is it?" ....

Orientation to place

6.   "Where are we (hospital, old age home, etc.)?" ....

7.   "On what floor?" ....

8.   "In what city?" ....

9.   "In what state (province, canton, etc.)?" ....

10.   "In what country?" ....

Retentiveness

"Please repeat the following words."
(To be spoken at 1 word per second; to be performed only once)

11.   "Lemon, ...

12.   key, ...

13.   ball." ....

Attention and calculations

14.   "Please count from 100 backward by 7's" (serial-7 test) ....

15.   1 point for each correct subtraction ....

16.   Maximum 5 points ....

17.   – – – ....

18.   – – – ....

(Cont.) →

Table 2.**90**   *(Cont.)*

Recent memory

19.   "Which 3 words ....

20.   did you repeat earlier?" ....

21   1 point for each word correctly recalled ....

Language, naming

22.   "What is this?" (show a pencil) ....

23.   "What is this?" (show a watch) ....

24.   "Please say after me: 'No ifs, ands, or buts.'" ....

Language comprehension, motor execution

25.   "Take this piece of paper in your hand, ...

26.   fold it down the middle, ...

27.   and put it on the ground." ....
        (each command to be given only once)

Reading

28.   "Please do what it says on this card." ....
        (Cf. Fig. 2.89a)

Writing

29.   "Write any sentence." ....
        (the patient is given a piece of paper
        and something to write with)

Drawing

30.   "Please copy this drawing." (Cf. Fig. 2.89b) ....
        (all 10 edges of the two pentagons must
        be drawn, and the pentagons must overlap,
        for the patient to receive 1 point for this task)

Level of wakefulness: ....

Total points achieved: ....

Table 2.**91**   Causes of dementia (cf. references 199, 688, 1018)

Degenerative diseases of the nervous system:
- Alzheimer's disease[1]
- Pick's disease
- Frontal lobe degeneration
- Parkinson's disease[1]
- Progressive supranuclear palsy[1]
- Pantothene kinase-associated neurodegeneration (formerly Hallervorden-Spatz disease)
- Hereditary ataxias
- Progressive myoclonus epilepsy[1]
- Lewy body disease
- Corticobasal degeneration

Cerebrovascular diseases:
- Multi-infarct syndrome[1]
- "Strategic" infarcts[1]
- Binswanger's disease[1]

Infectious diseases:
- HIV, AIDS-dementia complex[1]
- Other viral encephalitides and post-viral encephalopathies[1]
- Prion diseases:
  - Kuru
  - Creutzfeldt-Jakob disease
  - Gerstmann-Sträussler-Scheinker syndrome
  - Familial fatal insomnia
  - familial progressive subcortical gliosis
- Syphilis (progressive paralysis)[2]
- Brain abscesses[2]
- Whipple's disease[2]

Metabolic disorders affecting the brain:
- Wilson's disease[2]
- Disorders of lipid, protein, urea, and carbohydrate metabolism[1]
- Leukodystrophies

Neoplasia:
- Primary brain tumors, metastases[1]
- Paraneoplastic encephalopathies[1]

Epilepsy:
- Progressive myoclonus epilepsy[1]
- Frequent seizures
- Status epilepticus[2]

Systemic diseases, endocrine disorders, and deficiency states:
- Hypothyroidism, encephalopathy of Hashimoto's thyroiditis[2]
- Hypopituitarism[2]
- Hepatic encephalopathy[1]
- Uremic encephalopathy[2]
- Hypoxic brain injury
- Hypoglycemia[1]
- Electrolyte disorders[1]
- Hypercalcemia, hyperparathyroidism[2]
- Vasculitis, connective tissue disease[2]
- Vitamin B_{12} deficiency[2]
- Pellagra[2]
- Wernicke's encephalopathy[1]
- Jejunoileal bypass[2]

Toxic conditions:
- Alcoholism[2]
- Heavy metal poisoning[2]
- Carbon monoxide poisoning
- Organic solvent poisoning[1]
- Medication toxicity[2]

Mental illnesses:
- Depression[2]
- Schizophrenia[2]
- Hysteria[2]

Hydrocephalus:
- Obstructive hydrocephalus[2]
- Malresorptive hydrocephalus[2]

Trauma:
- Open trauma with destruction of brain tissue
- Closed trauma with brain contusions[1] and/or subcortical shear injuries[1]
- Dementia pugilistica[1]
- Diseases that simultaneously cause epilepsy and dementia[1]

Demyelinating diseases:
- Multiple sclerosis[1]

1) Preventable or (occasionally) curable, or manifestations may improve with medical treatment.
2) Generally curable or, at least, treatable.

Table 2.**92** Etiologies of dementia and their relative frequencies, after Cummings and Benson (198)

Etiology	n	%
Alzheimer's disease	612	44.9
Alcoholism	68	5.0
Multi-infarct	181	13.3
Infectious	11	0.8
Metabolic	39	2.9
Neoplasia	31	2.3
Hydrocephalus	34	2.5
Toxic	8	0.6
Trauma	15	1.1
Hypoxia	2	0.1
Subdural hematoma	3	0.2
Huntington's disease	16	1.2
Parkinson's disease	6	0.4
Miscellaneous	127	9.3
Mental illnesses	130	9.5
Not demented (misdiagnosis)	80	5.9
Total	1363	100

Table 2.**93** Ancillary tests in dementia

Initial evaluation:
- MRI of brain, possibly also CT
- ESR, CRP
- complete blood count and smear
- Na, K, Ca
- BUN
- glucose
- Serum electrophoresis
- Hepatic enzymes
- HIV, syphilis serology
- TSH
- Vitamin B_{12}, folic acid

Further tests as indicated:
- EEG
- Cerebrovascular ultrasound
- ECG, Holter monitoring
- Lumbar puncture (cell count, protein, IEP, other specific tests)
- SPECT or PET
- Antibodies: ANA, anti-dsDNA, anti-Ro (= SSA), cANCA, rheumatoid factor, anti-Hu, anti-Yo, anti-Ri
- Heavy metals, specific toxicological tests
- Intestinal biopsy
- Ammonia
- Cortisol
- Thyroid function tests
- Copper, ceruloplasmin
- Lyme, herpes simplex, and other serologies
- Lactate, pyruvate
- Urine screening for amino acids and disorders of carbohydrate metabolism
- Genetic analysis

■ **Alzheimer's Disease** (198, 530)

Definition:

This disease, described by Alois Alzheimer in 1907 and sometimes also called senile dementia of Alzheimer type (SDAT), is characterized by cortical dementia progressing rapidly over a few years. Neurologic signs other than dementia do not appear until the disease is at an advanced stage.

Epidemiology and Genetics

Alzheimer's disease affects persons over age 65, women more commonly than men. It affects persons under 65 much less commonly, and those under 45 hardly ever, unless they have trisomy 21 (Down syndrome): persons with trisomy 21 who reach the age of 30 or older regularly display both clinical and neuropathological features of Alzheimer's disease. In this subgroup of patients, the pathogenesis of dementia is likely to be related to excessive production of amyloid precursor protein, which is encoded on the triplicated chromosome 21.

Some 5–10% of cases of Alzheimer's disease are familial. Mutations in a number of different genes have been found in pedigrees with familial Alzheimer's disease, including the amyloid precursor protein gene on chromosome 21, the presenilin-1 gene on chromosome 14q, the presenilin-2 gene on chromosome 1, and the apolipoprotein E gene on chromosome 19q (798). Mutations of the presenilin genes cause autosomal dominant Alzheimer's disease, usually appearing before age 60. Mutations of the apolipoprotein E gene usually do not produce clinically evident dementia till old age, in persons with either familial or sporadic Alzheimer's disease (579a).

Pathoanatomy and Pathophysiology

The brain is diffusely atrophic, particularly in the temporal and parietal lobes. Brain atrophy may not yet be grossly evident in early Alzheimer's disease. Histologic examination reveals Alzheimer tangles, senile plaques, loss of cells (mainly neurons) and, often, amyloid angiopathy (p. 194). The latter finding and the fact that familial Alzheimer's disease is sometimes due to a mutation of the amyloid precursor gene suggest that amyloid protein plays a central role in the pathogenesis of the disease. Presenilin mutations are associated with elevated serum concentrations of Aβ-amyloid and are thus probably related in some way to amyloid precursor protein; apolipoprotein E probably also plays a role, as mutations of this substance can also cause familial Alzheimer's disease (800).

The nucleus basalis of Meynert is regularly found to be degenerated in Alzheimer's disease. This structure has a widely distributed cholinergic projection to the cerebral cortex, particularly the frontal lobes. The cerebral acetylcholine content is diminished, probably as an effect, rather than a cause, of neuron loss. Attempts to treat Alzheimer's disease with acetylcholine substitution, employing acetylcholine precursors or cholinomimetics, have met with varying success.

Clinical Features

Nonspecific complaints such as headache, dizziness, restlessness, insomnia, anxiety or agitation, generally impaired performance, or a depressive mood dominate the clinical picture in the initial stage of the disease before the impairment of memory and other specific cognitive deficits become apparent. Over several months or years, forgetfulness, aphasia, apraxia, disturbances of spatial processing and orientation, impairment of abstract thinking, confusion, disorientation, and other cognitive deficits appear and gradually worsen until the patient is no longer able to cope with his previous everyday activities.

The patient's external appearance and personality remain intact for a relatively long time. If the patient is well cared for and dressed by family members, his actual physical helplessness may not be externally evident. It is only in the later stages of the disease that the neuropsychological deficits begin to be accompanied by *neurologic deficits*, such as pyramidal and extrapyramidal motor disturbances and abnormalities of muscle tone and posture, that make the patient's illness immediately visible. In advanced disease, there may be stereotypic repetition of words or phrases, stereotyped movements such as picking at the bedclothes, wiping movements, or rocking, multifocal myoclonus, or generalized seizures. Finally, language may be entirely lost, and the patient may become entirely dependent on nursing care.

Diagnostic Evaluation and Differential Diagnosis

The diagnosis is based on the clinical manifestations of slowly progressive dementia and the exclusion of other, specific brain diseases causing dementia by means of a thorough history, clinical examination, and ancillary testing.

SPECT and PET studies most often reveal hypometabolism and a decrease in regional cerebral blood flow in the temporal and parietal lobes of patients with Alzheimer's disease, but predominantly frontal abnormalities in most other types of dementia. SPECT and PET cannot, however, be used as specific tests for Alzheimer's disease.

CT and MRI reveal progressive brain atrophy. CSF and blood tests are normal. Stepwise progression of deficits or sharply focal neurologic disturbances should arouse suspicion that the cause of dementia is something other than Alzheimer's disease, even though marked spasticity, ataxia, and other focal deficits can be present in rare cases (17).

| Treatment |

There is no etiologic treatment for Alzheimer's disease. *Tacrine* was the first cholinomimetic drug that was found to improve cognitive functioning in some patients, but it can be hepatotoxic (220, 524). *Donepezil* and *rivastigmine* (99b, 99c) are better tolerated; they improve cognition, behavior, and global function in Alzheimer's disease of mild to intermediate severity. *Metrifonate* is another effective agent (677a), and *co-dergocrine* has been found to elevate patients' mood and improve their capacity for attention.

The most important component of treatment, however, is symptomatic management. Patients feel most at ease in familiar surroundings. Nocturnal confusion may be improved to some extent by a *night light*; *antidepressants* can be given to counteract depressive mood, but care should be taken to use only those that have no anticholinergic effect, such as *fluvoxamine*. Insomnia can be treated with short-acting *benzodiazepines* or *chloral hydrate*. *Neuroleptics* such as *haloperidol* may improve agitation and stereotypic behavior, but may also further compromise cognitive function.

■ **Pick's Disease** (693)

Definition:

Pick's disease is much less common than Alzheimer's disease. It usually appears in men aged 40 to 60; most cases are sporadic, though there are a few families with an autosomal dominant hereditary form (420). Pick's disease is a type of system atrophy and has been classified by some authors among the frontal lobe degenerations.

Pathoanatomy

Macroscopically, there is an often asymmetrical atrophy of the cortex and subcortical white matter of the frontal or temporal lobes, or both. The areas most commonly affected are the fronto-orbital cortex, the temporal pole, and the temporobasal region. Microscopically, these changes correspond to widespread neuronal loss and gliosis. Argyrophilic intraneuronal inclusions (Pick bodies) are sometimes, but not always, found.

Clinical Features

Behavioral abnormalities, particularly a loss of social etiquette, are prominent in the beginning. Intelligence and orientation tend to be preserved in the early stages, which are often characterized by impulsiveness, disinhibition, and inappropriate jocularity (*Witzelsucht*), or else by loss of drive and initiative (apathy, abulia) or even hyperphagia. Neuropsychological deficits reflecting frontal and temporal lobe dysfunction appear later, particularly memory impairment, amnestic aphasia, and pali- and echolalia, which may progress to a total loss of language function.

Sensory abnormalities or disturbances of spatial perception are not a component of Pick's disease, though focal neurologic manifestations, such as pyramidal tract signs, are common. Pathological reflexes (grasp, suck, snout) are generally present. Bilateral

atrophy of the mediobasal temporal structures, if present, can lead to compulsive placement of objects in the mouth, as in Klüver-Bucy syndrome (p. 387).
In its late stage, Pick's disease consists of severe dementia with extrapyramidal akinesia.

Diagnostic Evaluation and Differential Diagnosis

Pick's disease is a diagnosis of exclusion, as there are no tests that can demonstrate it definitively other than brain biopsy and necropsy. *Neuroimaging studies* (CT or MRI) reveal the focal brain atrophy that is characteristic of this disease and serve to rule out other entities that present similarly, such as fronto-orbital tumor, butterfly glioma, and frontal lobe stroke.

Treatment

Symptomatic management and, if necessary, psychotropic drugs for sedation.

■ Focal Cortical Atrophies

The diseases, other than Alzheimer's disease and Pick's disease, that produce focal cortical atrophy are usually associated with gliotic or spongiform changes. Their clinical features depend mainly on the particular area of the brain that is affected. Some of these diseases are hereditary.

Frontal lobe degeneration. Frontal lobe degeneration (a class of disorders, one of which is Pick's disease) begins with personality changes, abnormal social behavior, aphasia, and dysarthria, which may progress to total mutism (146). Primitive reflexes and extrapyramidal signs such as rigidity and akinesia are seen in later stages.

Primary progressive aphasia. This disorder begins with aphasia, which progresses until, finally, dementia sets in (666).

Posterior cortical atrophies. Patients with these disorders may present clinically with Balint (p. 379) or Gerstmann syndrome (p. 376) (86).

■ Lewy Body Disease

Lewy bodies are PAS-positive intraneuronal inclusion bodies seen in the brains of persons with Parkinson's disease, typically in the substantia nigra. Patients who are also demented, and have Lewy bodies in the cerebral cortex, are said to be suffering from *Lewy body disease.*
The clinical picture may be dominated either by parkinsonism (tremor, rigidity) or by dementia. Lewy body disease is more a neuropathological than a clinical entity. The density of Lewy bodies is correlated with the severity of dementia (387a). Lewy bodies sometimes appear in combination with Alzheimer plaques and tangles *(the Lewy body type of Alzheimer's disease).*

■ Cerebrovascular Dementia

Cerebrovascular disturbances are the next most common cause of dementia after Alzheimer's disease. Dementia is typically produced by multiple subcortical infarcts secondary to microangiopathy or embolic disease (p. 191), though even a single stroke raises the risk of dementia several times over (931). Brain infarction causes dementia because of the loss of brain tissue. Not only the volume of lost tissue, but also its precise location are critical. Thus, dementia may appear after a single infarction in the thalamus or angular gyrus ("strategic infarct"), but only after multiple infarction in other areas.

MRI-signal abnormalities of white matter due to cerebrovascular disease are associated with a decline of cognitive function (330a, 968d), though the quantitative correlation is rather loose.

Cerebrovascular dementia, in contrast to dementia of other types, tends to be of acute onset and to progress in stepwise fashion. It can also transiently improve. The following are typical manifestations: transient aphasia, pseudobulbar palsy (p. 384), gait impairment (characteristically with a small-stepped, wide-based gait — "marche à petits pas"), extrapyramidal motor signs, and other focal neurologic deficits.

These patients tend to have exaggerated emotional reactions, bursting into tears unexpectedly or laughing inappropriately. Neuropsychological examination often reveals mainly frontal dysfunction, e.g. prominent aphasia, but the findings are otherwise comparable to those of dementia of other causes. The patient's ability to learn new material is usually more severely impaired than old memory. Many patients with cerebrovascular dementia have vascular risk factors, such as arterial hypertension and smoking, and concomitant vascular disease elsewhere in the body (coronary artery disease, occlusive peripheral vascular disease).

Specific Syndromes of Individual Lobes of the Brain

Overview:
Lesions of individual lobes of the brain produce specific symptoms and signs.

Different areas of the cerebral cortex subserve different (localized) functions and are of different cytoarchitectural makeup; it follows that focal lesions cause specific symptoms and signs that are characteristic of their location. Not only the site of the lesion itself is important, but also its interactions with other, functionally linked cortical and subcortical structures. Even a lesion confined to the white matter tract connecting two cortical regions can produce classic neurologic findings (the so-called *disconnection syndromes*).

In functional terms, the cerebral cortex is divided into somatotopically organized primary motor and sensory areas and modality-specific and polymodal association areas (Fig. 2.**90**).

Another group of structures anatomically comprising the so-called *limbic lobe* form a functional unit called the *limbic system* (318, 319, 486,665).

Lesions of the primary cortical areas produce elementary deficits such as paresis, hypesthesia, or visual field cut (scotoma), while lesions of the association areas cause more complex, modality-specific disturbances. A lesion of the motor association area, for example, impairs not only the raw strength of a specific group of muscles, but also their spatially and temporally coordinated joint activity that is needed to generate a purposeful and effective movement. Another example, this time on the sensory side, is prosopagnosia (discussed on p. 357), in which the patient cannot recognize faces despite perfectly adequate vision; the problem is that complex forms cannot be grasped in their entirety and cannot be integrated into a unitary concept. Finally, the polymodal association areas subserve the integration of sensory information from all of the different modalities and are the substrate of the so-called higher cortical functions.

The anatomical subdivision of the brain into frontal, parietal, temporal, and occipital lobes does not reflect any sharp functional or cytoarchtitectural segregation along the same boundaries. It nevertheless remains in universal descriptive use as a vestige of the pioneer days of classical neurology (19th century).

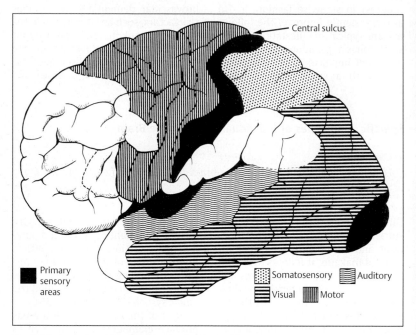

Fig. 2.90 Functional localization in the brain. The primary sensory areas are colored black. Adjacent to them are the modality-specific somatosensory, auditory, and visual association areas. The white zone posterior to the central sulcus comprises the angular and supramarginal gyri and is probably a polymodal sensory association area. The primary motor cortex occupies most of the precentral gyrus; anterior to it lie the premotor cortex and the supplementary motor area. The inferior frontal gyrus of the left (dominant) hemisphere contains the motor speech area. The white area anterior to the motor areas is the prefrontal cortex. (From H.J. Freund, "Funktionelle Organisation," in K. Kunze, *Lehrbuch der Neurologie,* Stuttgart: Thieme, 1992.)

■ Frontal Lobe Syndromes

The frontal lobe comprises:

- the primary motor, premotor, and supplementary motor cortex;
- the frontal eye field,
- the motor language area (Broca's area),
- the frontopolar and prefrontal cortex,
- the fronto-orbital cortex, and
- the cingulate cortex (frontal part).

The insula (of Reil) separates the frontal lobe from the temporal lobe, while the central sulcus separates it from the parietal lobe. The important landmarks for the identification of the central sulcus in CT or MR images are depicted in Fig. 2.**91** (261). The frontal lobe projects via the pyramidal tract to the motor neurons of the cranial nerve nuclei and spinal cord, as well as to the cerebellum, basal ganglia, limbic system, temporal lobe, and contralateral frontal lobe. Afferent fibers reach the frontal lobe from practically all parts of the brain, as every motor activity requires the integration of sensory feedback data for its smooth execution.

Neurologic Signs

Lesions of the *primary motor cortex* produce *contralateral spastic paresis* with exaggerated intrinsic reflexes, diminished extrinsic reflexes, and a Babinski sign (Table 2.**94**). The more superficial the lesion, the more circumscribed the paresis. Thus, a small lesion in the precentral gyrus may produce a monoplegia of the contralateral leg or opposite side of the face. Indeed, such pareses may be so limited in spatial extent that they may simulate a peripheral nerve lesion such as a radial nerve palsy (hand drop) or a peroneal nerve palsy (foot

drop, great toe drop), especially because a pure, isolated lesion of the precentral gyrus actually causes, not spasticity, but a diminution of muscle tone (flaccid paresis).

The innervation of the distal muscles of the arm and leg by the primary motor cortex, by way of the pyramidal tract, is purely contralateral, while the axial and proximal limb muscles are both ipsi- and contralat-

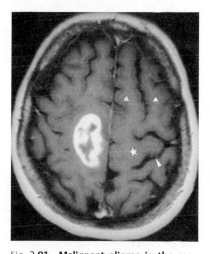

Fig. 2.**91 Malignant glioma in the central area** (axial T1-weighted MRI). The patient had a monoparesis of the left arm. The marked cortical areas are the superior frontal gyrus (open triangle), middle frontal gyrus (solid triangle), precentral gyrus (star), and central sulcus (arrowhead) of the uninvolved (left) hemisphere. The superior frontal gyrus is easily recognized by its course parallel to the midline. The first gyrus that turns away from the midline, making an acute angle, is the precentral gyrus. Its posterior border is formed by the central sulcus, which usually, as here, does not reach all the way to the midline. The tumor of the right hemisphere is thus located in the parasagittal portion of the precentral gyrus (primary motor cortex).

Table 2.**94** Major features of frontal lobe syndromes

I Unilateral frontal lobe lesion, left or right:
• Contralateral spastic hemiparesis
• Loss of drive and initiative, tact, and propriety; mildly elevated mood
• Disinhibition of primitive reflexes
• Anosmia (in fronto-orbital lesions)
II Left frontal lesion:
• Right spastic hemiparesis
• Motor aphasia, agraphia
• Bilateral limb apraxia and bucco-linguofacial apraxia
III Right frontal lesion:
• Left spastic hemiparesis
• Left limb apraxia
IV Bifrontal lesions:
• Spastic para- or quadriparesis
• Spastic (pseudobulbar) palsy
• Urinary dysfunction
• Abulia, akinetic mutism, impersistence, perseveration, imitative behavior

erally innervated by the *premotor cortex.* Therefore, unilateral *lesions of the premotor cortex* often cause no more than transient, contralateral, mainly proximal weakness, with good distal function and limb apraxia. The synergistic innervation of muscle groups, in tightly regulated temporal sequence and with appropriately graded strength of each participating muscle, is impaired, so that the speed, rhythm, and fluidity of movement are impaired. The interaction of the proximal muscles of the two sides may also be abnormal: the patient may have trouble making windmill movements with his arms or bicycling movements with his feet.

Lesions of the supplementary motor cortex produce contralateral hypokinesia and apraxia, as well as difficulty initiating movement, but no rigidity or tremor. *Lesions of the frontal eye fields* produce a transient contralateral gaze palsy, and *lesions of Broca's area* produce motor aphasia and agraphia. The snout, suck, grasp, and palmomental reflexes are present. The lips and jaws are reflexively closed when touched. These reflexes are, in fact, subserved by the parietal lobe but are normally suppressed by the frontal cortex, only to appear again when the frontal lobe is dysfunctional ("disinhibition"). An object laid in the patient's hand is compulsively palpated or tightly held, and, if the examiner tries to take it away, the hand follows it like a magnet. *Interruption of the frontopontocerebellar projection* produces a contralateral ataxia that mainly affects the leg.

Neuropsychological Signs

For aphasia and agraphia, see pages 379 and 384; for apraxia, see p. 355. The *prefrontal cortex* plays a major role in the planning and execution of motor activities, the suppression of external stimuli, and the organization of short-term memory. The *fronto-orbital cortex* projects extensively to the limbic system. The *olfactory cortex* is directly connected to the hippocampus and amygdala of the temporal lobe. *Lesions of the prefrontal and fronto-orbital cortex* produce disturbances of personality and neuropsychological changes, particularly in the area of affective behavior. Loss of drive, spontaneity, and activity leads to indifferent-passive, inattentive and uninterested behavior. The patient lacks initiative, stops thinking for himself, and fails to be interested in or even respond to those around him. The most striking behavioral abnormalities are inattention, impersistence, and perseveration. Impersistence is defined as the inability to maintain any given position for more than a moment, e.g., the inability to keep the arms outstretched. The loss of drive is often misinterpreted as depression.

Involvement of the *frontobasal* structures markedly impairs affective behavior. Differentiated affective responses of the type that facilitate social interaction are lost. The patient's affect becomes progressively blunted as primitive, impulsive behaviors are released; the patient becomes inappropriately jocular, can no longer conform to basic social etiquette, and finally develops an affective dementia. Motor testing reveals perseveration or impersistence. Perseverating patients retain any given posture for an abnormally long time, and, if a limb is passively moved a few times by the examiner, will keep on repeating the movement actively thereafter. Patients with impersistence cannot keep their arms outstretched; as soon as the posture is established, the arms are pulled back again. Patients may mimic the examiner's gestures (echopraxia, imitative behavior) or repeat heard words and phrases (echolalia). They may resist passive movement of the extremities *(Gegenhalten)* in a manner similar to that seen in catatonic schizophrenia.

Urinary dysfunction is another sign of frontal lobe dysfunction that is produced especially by lesions of the posterior portion of the superior frontal gyrus. It may be manifest merely as frequent urination (pollakisuria) or as episodic, sudden, unexpected, and embarrassing incontinence of urine or stool. *Olfactory dysfunction* indicates a fronto-orbital process. Slowly progressive, unilateral frontal lobe lesions often escape clinical attention until they are quite advanced.

Signs of Frontal Lobe Excitation

These signs are described in the section on partial seizures (p. 527)(271).

■ Parietal Lobe Syndromes

The parietal lobe is bounded by the central sulcus anteriorly and the parieto-occipital sulcus posteriorly. Its most anterior part, the postcentral gyrus, contains the primary somatosensory cortex, which is somatotopically organized and subserves the perception and discrimination of stimuli such as touch, pressure, position, noxious stimulation, temperature, and vibration.

Further posteriorly, the sensory association area is responsible for the analysis, integration, and interpretation of the data it receives from the primary somatosensory cortex, the localization of stimuli, and the differentiation of different shapes, weights, etc. The polymodal association area (angular and supramarginal gyri) subserve the integration of somatosensory information with that derived from other sensory modalities.

Neurologic Signs (Table 2.95)

Parietal lobe lesions produce contralateral *hypesthesia* in the elementary sensory modalities, i.e., touch, pain, temperature, and vibration. Hypesthesia is usually more marked in the extremities than on the trunk. Involvement of the more posterior areas of the parietal lobe (sensory association cortex) produces a deficit of

Table 2.**95**   Major features of parietal lobe syndromes

I	Unilateral parietal lobe lesion, left or right:
	• Contralateral hemihypesthesia
	• Mild hemiparesis
	• Parietal ataxia
	• Homonymous hemianopsia or
	• Inferior quadrantanopsia
	• Unilateral impairment of optokinetic nystagmus

II	Left parietal lesion:
	• As in I
	• Sensory aphasia
	• Gerstmann syndrome
	• Bilateral apraxia
	• Tactile agnosia
	• (occasionally) as in III, but on the opposite side

III	Right parietal lesion:
	• As in I
	• Extinction phenomenon (left)
	• Left visual neglect
	• Neglect of the left side of the body and extracorporeal space
	• Anosognosia
	• Impaired spatial processing
	• Dressing apraxia

IV	Biparietal lesions:
	• As in I–III
	• Markedly impaired orientation and spatial processing
	• Ataxia

the more complex sensory modalities, i.e., two-point discrimination, graphesthesia, position sense, stereognosis, and autotopognosia (see p. 358).

These sensory disturbances are generally accompanied by a mild hemiparesis. The "parietal-hand" phenomenon, however, is due not to weakness, but rather to the lack of sensory feedback guiding its movement, resulting in *parietal ataxia*, which may make it practically unusable. Involvement of the subcortical white matter, if present, affects the optic radiation to produce a contralateral, inferior homonymous *quadrantanopsia* or *hemianopsia*. The normally present optokinetic nystagmus is diminished for stimuli in the affected half of the visual field (contralateral to the lesion).

Neuropsychological Signs

The neuropsychological signs produced by a parietal lobe lesion depend on the hemispheric dominance of the individual patient. *Lesions of the language-dominant parietal lobe* produce aphasia or alexia. Lesions of the angular gyrus produce *Gerstmann syndrome*, defined as the combination of agraphia, acalculia, bilateral finger agnosia, and right-left confusion. Further signs may include bilateral *tactile agnosia* (i.e., astereognosis) and bilateral ideomotor and ideational *apraxia*.

Lesions of the nondominant parietal lobe impair the perception of extrapersonal space and (in some cases) topographical memory. Much more commonly than lesions on the dominant side, such lesions produce sensory extinction or neglect, impaired spatial processing, and dressing apraxia. Neglect may be the only clinical finding indicating a parietal lobe lesion. Larger lesions often produce anosognosia (p. 358).

Signs of Parietal Lobe Excitation

These are seen in epilepsy (p. 529) and migraine (p. 811).

■ **Temporal Lobe Syndromes**

The temporal lobe is separated from the frontal lobe and the anterior portion of the parietal lobe by the insula; there is no clear boundary separating it from the posterior portion of the parietal lobe and the occipital lobe. It comprises, laterally, the superior, middle, and inferior temporal gyri; basally, the occipitotemporal gyri; superiorly, the transverse temporal gyri (of Heschl); and, medially, the hippocampal formation. A major internal structure of the temporal lobe is the optic radiation, which passes over the lateral aspect of the temporal horn, and is shaped like a fan (p. 629).

Table 2.**96** Major features of temporal lobe syndromes

I	Unilateral temporal lobe lesion, left or right:
	• Homonymous superior quadrantanopsia or sector anopsia
	• Emotional disturbances, behavioral abnormalities
	• Olfactory, gustatory, auditory, or visual hallucinations
II	**Left temporal lesion:**
	• As in I
	• Word agnosia, word deafness
	• Wernicke's aphasia, anomic aphasia
	• Amusia
	• impaired ability to learn verbally presented material
III	**Right temporal lesion:**
	• As in I
	• Amusia
	• Impaired spatial perception
	• Agnosia for visual, nonverbal material
	• Impaired ability to learn visually presented material
IV	**Bitemporal lesion:**
	• As in I-III
	• Deafness
	• Apathy, affective indifference
	• Impaired learning and memory
	• Amnesia, Korsakoff's syndrome, Klüver-Bucy syndrome

Neurologic Signs (Table 2.96)

Temporal lobe lesions produce a non-congruent contralateral superior quadrantanopsia or sector anopsia.

Neuropsychological Signs

Hippocampal lesions produce *disturbances of memory and learning* that are disproportionately severe in relation to other types of cognitive disturbance. The explicit memory is affected (p. 358). Bilateral lesions produce a more severe deficit than unilateral lesions. Bilateral lesions of the primary auditory cortex (transverse temporal gyri of Heschl) or of its afferent input from the medial geniculate body produce *cortical deafness.* Lesions of the auditory association area impair the recognition of complex auditory sequences, such as words or music. Either a right- or a left-sided lesion can produce *amusia.* Left-sided lesions produce *word agnosia and sensory aphasia* (p. 379), while right-sided lesions produce *agnosia for visually presented nonverbal material.*

Patients with sensory aphasia may occasionally suffer from uncontrollable outbursts of emotion. The primary vestibular cortex is posterolateral to the primary auditory cortex; lesions in it impair optokinetic nystagmus. Lesions of the inferolateral temporal cortex do not produce a clearly defined deficit. Left-sided lesions produce word-finding difficulty or impair the learning of verbally presented material, while right-sided lesions impair the learning of visually presented material. Bilateral lesions of the primary auditory cortex cause deafness (396c).

Signs of Temporal Lobe Excitation

Temporal lobe epilepsy is described in the section on epilepsy (p. 524). Auditory hallucinations, as in schizophrenic patients, involve activation of the primary auditory cortex (234b).

■ Occipital Lobe Syndromes

The occipital lobe is bounded medially by the parieto-occipital sulcus; its lateral and basal boundaries, separating it from the parietal and temporal lobes, are not precisely defined. The primary visual cortex (striate cortex, Brodmann area 17) is located at the occipital pole and in the banks of the calcarine fissure; it projects to the unimodal visual association cortex (parastriate cortex, areas 18 and 19). From here, efferent fibers project to the angular gyrus, the temporal lobe, the frontal motor cortex and the limbic system, and across the corpus callosum to the opposite hemisphere.

Neurologic and Neuropsychological Signs (Table 2.97)

Unilateral lesions of the occipital lobe produce *contralateral, homonymous visual field defects* (p. 626). Visual acuity is impaired only if there are bilateral lesions. Bilateral lesions also cause *cortical blindness* or an *impairment of color perception*. Patients with cortical blindness have preserved pupillary reflexes; they may fail to be aware of the deficit and even deny it when asked about it (*Anton's syndrome*). Some cortically blind patients remain able to see flashing lights or moving objects. *Altitudinal hemianopsia* is a rare consequence of bilateral occipital lobe lesions. An upper altitudinal hemianopsia is produced by lesions of the lower bank of the calcarine sulcus, a lower altitudinal hemianopsia by lesions of its upper bank.

Table 2.**97** Major features of occipital lobe syndromes

I	**Unilateral occipital lobe lesion, left or right:** • Contralateral homonymous hemianopsia or quadrantanopsia • Visual agnosia • Visual illusions • Elementary visual hallucinations
II	**Left occipital lesion:** • As in I • Alexia without agraphia • Color agnosia
III	**Right occipital lesions:** • As in I • Impaired visual orientation and topographical memory
IV	**Bioccipital lesions:** • As in I-III • Cortical blindness • Altitudinal hemianopsia • Impaired color perception • Anton syndrome • Prosopagnosia, simultanagnosia

Visual agnosia (= visual object agnosia). In the various types of visual agnosia, the patient is unable to recognize and name a visually presented object, despite intact visual acuity, visual fields, and language (p. 357). The object can, however, be immediately recognized and named as soon as it is smelled, heard, or palpated. Individual types of visual agnosia may be restricted to particular classes of objects. They are commonly accompanied by alexia and homonymous hemianopsia.

Prosopagnosia and *color agnosia* may be thought of as special types of visual object agnosia (209, 652). Prosopagnosia is due to right-sided or bilateral lesions of the inferior temporo-occipital cortex, while color agnosia is due to left-sided lesions of the ventromedial portion of the occipital lobe. The loss of topographical memory and of the sense of being in a familiar place may be a type of visual agnosia (552). *Simultanagnosia* is a characteristic feature of Balint syndrome, which is due to a lesion in the visual association cortex. Such patients can recognize parts of objects but not the entire visual field at once. They are also unable to perceive the motion of objects in the visual field.

Signs of Occipital Lobe Excitation

These signs consist of visual illusions (metamorphopsias) and visual hallucinations (see the section on epilepsy, p. 529) and arise, for example, in epilepsy, migraine, and delirium of various causes. Visual illusions may involve the shape, size, color, or motion of an object, which may appear to be too large (macropsia), too small (micropsia), present in two or more "copies" (polyopsia), bent or distorted, too near, too far, obliquely or incorrectly placed, or spatially reversed; objects may also appear to move though they are stationary, or they may seem to reappear (palinopsia). Such phenomena can also be produced by lesions in the occipitotemporal and occipito-parietal border zones.

There are two types of visual hallucinations. *Elementary hallucinations* consist of single or multiple flashes, colors, colored dots, stars, circles, or other geometric shapes, which may be stationary or mobile. *Complex hallucinations* consist of objects, persons, or animals. The causative cortical disturbance lies near the occipital pole for elementary hallucinations, farther forward toward the temporal lobe for complex hallucinations.

Neuropsychological Syndromes

■ Types of Aphasia (87, 210, 765)

Definition:

Aphasia is a neurological impairment of language. Expressive aphasia affects the ability to organize and express one's thoughts in the symbols and grammatical forms of normal language, while receptive aphasia affects the ability to understand words and sentences, whether they are spoken or written. Aphasia is almost always due to a left-hemispheric lesion (339); "crossed aphasia" from a right-hemispheric lesion is very rare.

The examination of the aphasic patient is discussed on p. 349. In this section, the different types of aphasia will be presented, as summarized in Table 2.**98**.

■ Broca's Aphasia

The major manifestation of Broca's aphasia is nonfluent, agrammatical spontaneous language, with many literal (phonematic) paraphasic errors and dysarthrophonia. The patient's language output consists mainly of nouns and is poor in verbs and adjectives, creating a telegraphic effect. The patient's utterances, though terse, often convey a good deal of information. Repetition of spoken words and reading aloud are just as impaired as spontaneous language, but language comprehension is not impaired, or, at any rate, much less so. Most Broca's aphasics also suffer from right hemiparesis. Written language, in those patients who are still able to write despite the hemiparesis, is affected in the same way as spoken language.

The responsible lesion involves the posterior portion of the left inferior frontal gyrus (area 44) and the adjacent cortical areas (areas 47, 46, and 9). Lesions restricted to area 44 produce only a transient disturbance of speech, in which comprehension and the production of written language remain intact. This condition is known as *aphemia* (841).

■ Wernicke's Aphasia

Wernicke's aphasia is the linguistic "opposite number" of Broca's aphasia. Its major manifestations are a marked impairment of language comprehension and fluent, but paraphasic spontaneous language. The melody and rhythm of speech (prosody) and its speed are normal or barely abnormal. The patient's spontaneous language is marred by frequent literal and semantic paraphasic errors and neologisms, and content-bearing nouns are rare. Broken-off sentences, interjections, and faulty word placement are frequent (paragrammatism). Deficits of comparable severity are found in repetition of spoken words and sentences, naming, reading, and writing. Most Wernicke's aphasics concomitantly suffer from emotional disturbances. They are usually agitated and anxious.

The responsible lesion involves the posterior portion of the superior temporal gyrus (auditory association cortex, area 22), the supramarginal gyrus (area 40), the angular gyrus (area 39), the posterior portion of the middle temporal gyrus (area 37), or a combination of these areas. Thus, Wernicke's aphasics are usually not hemiparetic, but there may be a concomitant hemianopsia if the lesion penetrates into the subcortical white matter as far as the optic radiation.

Wernicke's aphasics are not uncommonly misdiagnosed as psychotic if they become agitated or frustrated through their inability to communicate, or when they develop paranoid ideas.

■ Conduction Aphasia

The major manifestation of conduction aphasia is impaired repetition. Language comprehension is preserved and language output is fluent, though there are frequent phonematic paraphasic errors. Naming is also impaired. There is usually a concomitant contralateral facial or faciobrachial paresis, or contralateral faciobrachial sensory deficit. The responsible lesion involves the supramarginal gyrus, from which the arcuate fasciculus originates, and possibly also the primary auditory cortex (areas 41 and 42), the insular cortex, and the underlying subcortical white matter. Conduction aphasia is a type of disconnection syndrome (p. 383).

■ Global Aphasia

Global aphasia combines the characteristics of Broca's and Wernicke's aphasia. Globally aphasic patients are capable neither of formulating language, nor of understanding it. Their utterances are confined to a few auto-

Table 2.**98**   Differential diagnosis of aphasia

Spontaneous speech	Comprehension	Repetition	Diagnosis	Associated findings	Localization
Nonfluent	Intact	Deficient	Broca's aphasia	Right hemiparesis	Inferior frontal gyrus
		Intact	Transcortical motor aphasia	–	Anterior and superior to Broca's area, possibly overlapping with Broca's area
	Deficient	Deficient	Global aphasia	Right hemiparesis	Territory of middle cerebral artery
		Intact	Anomic aphasia	–	Poorly localizable
Fluent	Intact	Deficient	Conduction aphasia	(Sometimes) hemiparesis or hemisensory deficit, mainly affecting face and arm	Arcuate fasciculus
		Intact	Transcortical sensory aphasia	–	Posterior or inferior to Wernicke's area
	Deficient	Deficient	Wernicke's aphasia	No paresis; emotional disturbances, anxiety, agitation, paranoia	Auditory association cortex, often also angular and supramarginal gyri

matically repeated words or syllables (automatic speech). Cursing or the automatic recitation of learned series (numbers, days of the week) is sometimes preserved. Most patients with global aphasia concomitantly suffer from right hemiparesis or hemiplegia.

The classic cause of global aphasia is an infarct involving the entire territory of the middle cerebral artery, including Broca's and Wernicke's areas and the perirolandic (central) region. It is less commonly caused by embolic infarction of Broca's and Wernicke's areas with sparing of the perirolandic region, in which case there is no hemiparesis.

■ **The Transcortical Aphasias**

The transcortical aphasias are characterized by intact oral repetition. Language production is deficient in *transcortical motor aphasia*, while language comprehension is deficient in *transcortical sensory aphasia*. Watershed-zone infarcts are the most common cause of the transcortical aphasias. Lesions responsible for the motor type are near Broca's area, while lesions responsible for the sensory type are near Wernicke's area.

■ **Anomic Aphasia**

In anomic aphasia, language dysfunction is almost entirely restricted to word-finding and naming difficulty. The patient's spontaneous speech may contain paraphasic errors. Anomic aphasia is poorly localizable. It can be produced by posteroinferior frontal lobe lesions, by lesions of the middle and inferior temporal gyri, or by lesions of the parietotemporal transition zone. Lesions in the last-named location also cause agraphia and alexia.

Aphasia can also be caused by lesions of the thalamus or of the head of the caudate nucleus and the anterior portion of the internal capsule. These *subcortical aphasias* typically impair language comprehension and are accompanied by dysarthria.

▨ **Treatment** ▨

The course of aphasia largely depends on its etiology and the site and extent of the underlying lesion. PET studies have shown that recovery from aphasia involves a functional reorganization of the brain, in which noninjured areas, including homotopic areas of the contralateral hemisphere, are activated and assume some of the function of the lesioned area (1008). Speech therapy can improve aphasia to some extent. The treatment plan should be developed individually for each patient by a team composed of speech therapists, neuropsychologists, and neurologists (850, 870).

■ Disconnection Syndromes (340)

Definition:
The concept of the disconnection syndromes was introduced by Hugo Liepmann, a former student of Carl Wernicke (585, 586). It was his idea that a lesion of the pathway connecting two neural structures can have the same effect as a lesion of the structures themselves. The involved pathways may be association fibers, i.e., fibers connecting different cortical areas in one hemisphere, or commissural fibers, i.e., fibers connecting homotopic areas in the two hemispheres.

■ Ideomotor Apraxia

For a definition of ideomotor apraxia, see p. 355. Auditory or visual information travels by way of the arcuate fasciculus to the left motor association cortex (Fig. 2.**92**), in which a program for the movement to be executed is generated and then sent onward to the motor cortex. The last-mentioned connection is through ipsilateral association fibers for movements of the right side of the body, and across the corpus callosum to the contralateral (right) motor association cortex and then to the (right) motor cortex for movements of the left side of the body. Thus, lesions of the arcuate fasciculus or the left mo

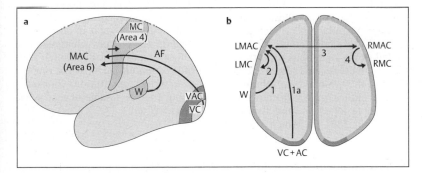

Fig. 2.**92a, b Neural pathways involved in disconnection syndromes** (after Poeck).
a Lateral view.
b Axial view (schematic).

AF   Arcuate fasciculus
L   Left
MAC Motor association cortex
MC   Motor cortex
R   Right
VAC Visual association cortex
VC   Visual cortex
W   Wernicke's area

1   Verbal–motor association fibers in arcuate fasciculus
1a   Visual–motor association fibers in arcuate fasciculus
2   Association fibers between LMAC and LMC
3   Commissural fibers between LMAC and RMAC
4   Association fibers between RMAC and MRC

tor association cortex produce bilateral limb apraxia, but lesions of the corpus callosum or of the right motor association cortex produce only unilateral (left) limb apraxia. Buccolinguofacial apraxia is produced by lesions of the association fibers or motor association cortex representing the facial musculature. Right-sided lesions generally do not cause facial apraxia, because most facial muscles receive bilateral cortical innervation.

■ Anterior Corpus Callosum Syndrome

The anterior corpus callosum syndrome consists of *agraphia and apraxia* as well as *tactile agnosia of the left hand*. It can be produced by (for example) a glioma or infarct involving the commissural fibers of the corpus callosum (334, 845), or by surgical transection of the anterior portion of the corpus callosum (callosotomy). A similar clinical picture can arise if the same fibers are interrupted in the more lateral portion of their course – i.e., in a subcortical position in the cerebral hemisphere. A lesion of the corpus callosum is also responsible for *alien hand syndrome* (239, 292, 338), in which the left

hand (of a right-handed patient) behaves in a strange and uncontrollable way, so that it is perceived as not belonging to the patient, and bimanual coordination is not possible.

■ Alexia without Agraphia

Infarction in the territory of the posterior cerebral artery on the left side is the classic cause of this syndrome. The lesion deprives the left inferior parietal lobe of visual afferent input from both sides of the brain: from the left side, because the left visual cortex is destroyed; and from the right side, because information from the right visual cortex must reach the left parietal lobe by way of the splenium and the subcortical white matter on the left side, which are also involved by the lesion. The result is that visual language input (i.e., reading) is impossible. Most patients, however, can still name objects and recognize individual letters. They can also write meaningful sentences spontaneously or on command, but they cannot read words or sentences. A patient may be able to write "constitution," for example, but then be unable to read what he has written.

■ Dysarthrophonia, Pseudobulbar Palsy, and Nonneurological Language Impairment

Definition:
In these disorders, the patient uses normal linguistic symbols (words) and grammar, but his speech is nevertheless unintelligible, or nearly so, because of deficient articulation, voicing, or action of the respiratory muscles.

Language impairment of nonneurologic origin can be mistaken for aphasia. Also distinct from aphasia is *dysarthrophonia*, a disturbance of speech articulation, voicing, and speech-related breathing. Dysarthrophonia does not affect the linguistic form and content of speech.

The following diseases and syndromes should be kept in mind in the differential diagnosis of aphasia:

- *Nonneurological language impairment* is seen in schizophrenia; in catatonia, in the form of mutism; as slow, monotonous speech in depression; and as aphonia (whispering) in hysteria. Pseudo-aphasic hysterical patients, unlike true aphasics, usually communicate normally by reading and writing – a clinical picture seen in only one true neurologic disorder, namely aphemia (see p. 379).

- *Dysphasia* is a disturbance of language development, rather than an acquired language impairment; stuttering is one form of dysphasia.

- *Dysfunction of the speech-forming structures* alters the sound and clarity of speech, but not the choice of words and the cogency of the patient's language. Some examples include hoarseness in diseases of the larynx, closed nasal speech due to tonsillar hypertrophy or tumors of the epipharynx, or open nasal speech due to cleft palate. Further examples are open nasal speech, worsening with fatigue, in disorders of neuromuscular transmission such as myasthenia gravis, and neurogenic paralysis of the muscles of speech due to lower cranial nerve dysfunction. Bilateral palatal weakness, vocal cord paralysis, or hypoglossal nerve palsy causes severe dysphonia (e.g., in cranial polyradiculitis), but unilateral weakness is usually well compensated.

- *Lesions of the medullary cranial nerve nuclei* cause "bulbar speech," which is nasal, slurred, and poorly articulated and may sound as if the patient had a marble in his mouth. A poor distinction between *r* and *l* is typical. This disturbance is the most obvious clinical manifestation of bulbar paralysis, and also of brainstem involvement by amyotrophic lateral sclerosis (p. 434) – in the latter case, however, there may be an additional spastic component of dysarthria. Unilateral brainstem lesions usually produce only transient hoarseness (e.g. Wallenberg syndrome, p. 178).

- *Supranuclear palsy of the speech muscles bilaterally*, as in pseudobulbar palsy (p. 178), produces a type of dysarthrophonia that is acoustically nearly indistinguishable from that of bulbar palsy. Pseudobulbar palsy is usually due to cerebrovascular disease and, unlike bulbar palsy, tends to appear suddenly.

- *Bilateral lesions of the frontal operculum*, i.e., of the frontal areas that bilaterally innervate the lower cranial nerve nuclei (p. 715), cause central diplegia of the oral and pharyngeal musculature, known as Foix-Chavany-Marie syndrome (613, 847). Unilateral left-sided lesions produce aphemia (p. 379).

- *Cerebellar disease* may affect the coordinating and regulating role of the cerebellum in motor function, including speech, with the result that syllables and words are produced at irregularly varying volume and speed. An explosive speech pattern, called scanning dysarthria, is the result. This is typically encountered in multiple sclerosis.

- *Parkinson's disease and other disorders of the basal ganglia:* Parkinsonian hypokinesia manifests itself in soft, monotonous, often slowed and poorly modulated speech (bradylalia, or, in extreme cases, mutism). Logoclonus (paroxysmal repetition of final syllables) and iteration (repetition of entire words) are rare manifestations of extrapyramidal disease; they more commonly accompany diffuse cerebrovascular disease and dementia of other causes.

- *Spasmodic or spastic dystonia* is a type of focal dystonia that can be treated with medication or botulinum toxin injections (1022).
- *Lesions of the periventricular/periaqueductal gray matter, the intrala-minar thalamic nuclei, the fronto-orbital cortex, or the limbic system* can produce a generalized loss of drive, including the motivation to speak – in the extreme case, akinetic mutism – without necessarily impairing consciousness. Possible etiologies include viral encephalitis and paraneoplastic limbic encephalitis (p. 322), bilateral midbrain and diencephalic strokes, or vasospasm after subarachnoid hemorrhage.

■ Amnesia and Other Disturbances of Explicit Memory

Overview:

The acquisition of new verbal and nonverbal information (explicit memory) depends on an intact limbic-diencephalic system. Dysfunction of this system causes anterograde and retrograde amnesia but does not impair implicit memory, i.e., the faculty of learning and consolidating motor skills. Thus, amnesia is not associated with an impairment of motor function.

The memory tests described on p. 359 all concern *explicit (or declarative) memory,* whose anatomical substrate is the limbic-diencephalic system. Explicit memory is the faculty of acquiring and integrating new information, which is ultimately stored in the cerebral cortex. Explicit memory may also be defined as memory for conscious content, while *implicit (or procedural) memory* is that which enables the unconscious learning and consolidation of motor skills. Implicit learning usually occurs through visual stimuli and with the participation of the association cortex. A further system, based on a frontostriatal network, serves as "working storage" for the acquisition of motor abilities and skills (324). The *limbic-diencephalic system* comprises the vmediobasal temporal lobe (hippo-campus, amygdala), medial thalamic nuclei, hypothalamus, septal and preoptic areas, and orbitofrontal cortex, and the pathways interconnecting them, including the fornix and the mammillothalamic tract. Unilateral lesions of these structures usually produce only mild and transient disturbances of explicit memory, while bilateral lesions can produce severe and lasting disturbances, including both retro- and anterograde amnesia. Extensive neocortical lesions disturb the consolidated content of long-term memory, producing dementia (p. 360).

Confabulation. Spontaneous confabulation ("making up" of memories, i.e., the involuntary generation of "memories" that do not, in fact, correspond to past events) reflects a selective disturbance of the temporal organization of the content of memory (850b, 850d). The basic problem is an inability to suppress the intrusion of irrelevant information into the content of memory. Spontaneous confabulation can be observed with lesions of the orbitofrontal cortex, the basal forebrain, the amygdala, and the perirhinal cortex. Evoked confabulations, i.e., those that are produced by asking the patient to recall an event from memory, seem to represent a "normal" compensatory strategy in the setting of memory impairment, and are of no localizing value. Disorientation, as may occur in amnesia or delirium, is similarly due to an inability to follow temporal sequences (850a). Thus, disoriented patients jumble together the traces of different events in memory and cannot tell which of them is actually happening at present. Yet disoriented patients are not necessarily incapable of forming new memories, as a specific temporal context may not be required for this process.

Transient global amnesia (TGA, amnestic episode). This syndrome reflects transient, bilateral dysfunction of the hippocampus, thalamus, cingulate gyrus, or fronto-orbital cortex. It is a disturbance of explicit rather than implicit memory, in contrast to Alzheimer's disease, which impairs both (p. 367). It usually affects middle-aged persons (688).

The sufferer is unable to lay down new memories (anterograde amnesia) or to remember anything that happened in the preceding days, weeks, or even months or years (retrograde amnesia); he has a vague understanding of what the trouble is and seems mildly disturbed, anxious, and perplexed. He constantly tries to reorient himself and repeatedly asks the same questions. Nonetheless, he can still carry out most everyday activities, including complex ones. The general physical examination is normal. Anterograde amnesia clears first, and then retrograde amnesia, slowly, over the course of a few hours or days. After recovery, amnesia remains only for the amnestic episode itself. Recurrences are relatively rare (ca. 3% per year).

The etiology of transient global amnesia is unknown, and probably heterogeneous. The vascular risk profile of affected patients differs from that of patients with TIAs, and epilepsy is slightly more frequent in the further course of TGA patients than in that of TIA patients (424). Migraine, traumatic brain injury, oxyquinoline preparations, Ketalar (ketamine) and diazepam and its derivatives may provoke an episode of TGA. PET and SPECT reveal hypo- or hyperperfusion in the left temporal lobe of some, but not all, patients with TGA. A diffusion-weighted MRI study revealed hippocampal hyperintensity in seven of 10 TGA patients, on the left side in four and bilateral in three (914a), which normalized once the TGA resolved. This finding suggests that cellular edema is present during TGA and that amnesia in this disorder may be due to a spreading depression of hippocampal neural activity.

Klüver-Bucy syndrome. This unusual behavioral syndrome consists of a tendency to put any object whatsoever in the mouth and explore it orally or eat it. Patients with Klüver-Bucy syndrome have an indifferent affect, usually with reduced drive, and are easily distracted by any external stimulus. They are "psychically blind," i.e., incapable of recognizing objects by sight. Sexual disinhibition manifests itself as frequent and inappropriate masturbation and promiscuity. The syndrome is produced by bilateral lesions of the medial temporal lobes, which also render the patients permanently unable to lay down new memories.

Korsakoff syndrome. This syndrome, too, a consequence of alcoholism and other nutritional disorders, is a disturbance of explicit memory reflecting dysfunction of the limbic-diencephalic system (p. 386).

Further differential diagnoses of amnesia are listed in Table 2.**99**.

Treatment

The treatment of amnesia is based on its etiology.

Table 2.**99** Causes of transient and permanent amnesia (after ref. 11)

Amnesia of acute onset with incomplete recovery:
- Bilateral hippocampal infarction
- Bilateral thalamic infarction
- Bilateral infarction of the territory of the anterior cerebral artery
- Vasospasm after rupture of an aneurysm of the anterior communicating artery
- Carbon monoxide poisoning
- Diencephalic, orbitofrontal, or mediobasal contusions

Amnesia of acute onset and brief duration:
- Transient global amnesia
- Temporal lobe epilepsy
- Concussion

Amnesia of subacute onset, usually with incomplete recovery:
- Wernicke-Korsakoff syndrome
- Herpes simplex encephalitis
- Tuberculosis and other basal meningitides
- Paraneoplastic limbic encephalitis

Slowly progressive amnesia:
- Tumors involving the wall of the third ventricle and the limbic cortex
- Early Alzheimer's disease and other neurodegenerative diseases involving the temporal lobes

3 Diseases Mainly Affecting the Spinal Cord

Characteristics of Diseases of the Spinal Cord

Overview:

The typical *history* of diseases of the spinal cord consists of slowly progressive impairment of gait, often of a poorly defined nature; bladder dysfunction; sensory abnormalities affecting the lower limbs only, or the lower half of the body below a particular level on the trunk; band-like pain or a feeling of constriction on the trunk; and back pain at the level of the lesion. Patients frequently complain of an electric shock-like sensation traveling from the neck or back downward, possibly into the extremities, on flexion of the neck or certain other movements of the trunk (Lhermitte sign, p. 470), and rarely of restless legs.

Physical examination typically reveals spastic para- or quadriparesis, with hypertonia, hyperreflexia, and pyramidal tract signs (though any of these findings may be absent in individual cases); a sensory deficit below a particular level on the trunk; in some cases, spinal muscular atrophy (perhaps with fasciculations); normal function of the cranial nerves; and normal function of the upper limbs as well, for lesions at thoracic or lower levels.

Ancillary tests, particularly neuroimaging studies, are essential aids to the diagnosis of spinal cord diseases.

Ancillary Tests in Diseases of the Spinal Cord

Neuroimaging of the Spine and Spinal Cord

Plain films provide a projectional view of the bony structures of the spine. *Tomographic studies* (CT, MRI) enable cross-sectional and three-dimensional views of both the musculoskeletal and the neural structures. *Dynamic studies,* such as plain films in flexion and extension, can provide evidence of spinal instability (254).

MRI and CT

MRI and CT are the most useful imaging studies of the spinal cord itself. MRI is generally more informative than CT for study of the cervical or thoracic region, though CT with fine cuts can be as good as MRI, or better, in the lumbar region, particularly when clinical evidence points to a monoradicular lesion, as it depicts bone more clearly. *Acute paraparesis or paraplegia* requires prompt evaluation by MRI, or, if MRI is unavailable, by myelography with post-myelographic CT. *Acute processes of the conus medullaris and cauda equina* are best studied by MRI, though CT and myelography can also be used to rule out a mass lesion.

Myelography

Myelography involves injection of water-soluble, radiopaque contrast medium into the spinal subarachnoid space, followed by plain spinal radiography. This relatively invasive technique is used far less often today than in previous decades, having been replaced by MRI for most applications. Like MRI, it is useful for the diagnosis or exclusion of the following:

- disk herniation and other degenerative changes of the spine that may compress the spinal cord or spinal nerve roots,
- tumors (extradural, intradural-extramedullary, and intramedullary),
- nonneoplastic masses (e.g., hamartoma), arachnoid fibrosis, or syringomyelia,
- abnormal blood vessels in arteriovenous malformations and highly vascularized tumors,
- dilated nerve root sleeves and cysts.

A *lumbar puncture* is performed on the sitting or lying patient and 10–15 mL of nonionic, water-soluble contrast medium is injected into the subarachnoid space. Anteroposterior and lateral views of the spine are obtained. Spinal stenosis and nerve root compression are sometimes detectable only by comparing myelographic images taken with the patient lying and standing *(dynamic myelography)*.

Tarlov cysts fill with contrast medium only after a certain latency—i.e., they are visible only on later images in a sequence taken in the standing position.

Whenever the plain myelogram is abnormal, a *post-myelographic CT* is likely to yield additional useful information.

Side effects of lumbar puncture and contrast medium injection are uncommon. If they occur, they most often consist of headache, nausea, and vomiting; confusion, seizures, and ana-

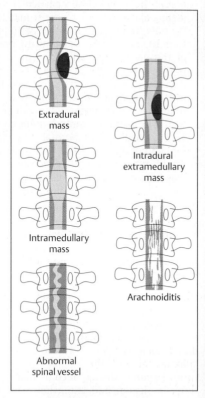

Fig. 3.**1 Myelographic findings** (schematic representation).

phylactic reactions are rare (515). Symptomatic intracranial hypotension is a potential complication of lumbar puncture.

Myelography can only detect pathological processes that alter the configuration of the spinal subarachnoid space. The more common types of myelographic abnormalities are depicted schematically in Fig. 3.**1**.

Spinal Angiography

Spinal angiography is indicated for the evaluation of spinal vascular malformations and highly vascularized spinal tumors. It is an invasive and relatively labor-intensive technique, as it requires separate, individual catheterization and contrast injection of all of the arteries supplying the spinal cord (vertebral arteries, costocervical trunk, thyrocervical trunk, intercostal arteries, internal iliac arteries). It is usually performed only when MRI and myelography have revealed abnormal vessels and a neurosurgical or interventional neuroradiological procedure is being considered (238, 928).

Evoked Potentials (p. 473)

Somatosensory evoked potentials (SEP, p. 476) and *motor evoked potentials* (MEP, p. 478) are performed with the aid of electrical and magnetic stimulation.

▌Classification of Spinal Cord Syndromes

Spinal Cord Transection Syndrome (Para-/Quadriplegia, Para-/Quadriparesis)

- Sensory level below which all sensory modalities are more or less deficient (cf. Fig. 3.**3**);
- paraspasticity or paraparesis;
- urinary dysfunction (neurogenic bladder, automatic bladder, cf. p. 396);
- possible segmental neurological deficit at the level of the lesion, such as:
  - segmental reflex deficit (cf. Tables 10.**4** and 10.**5**),
  - segmental muscle weakness (cf. Tables 10.**4** and 10.**5**),
  - accompanying muscular atrophy,
  - occasionally, reversal of reflexes indicating the level of the lesion: when the lesion is between L2 and L4, elicitation of the Achilles reflex may induce simultaneous flexion of the knee; lesions at C5–C6 may cause reversal of the supinator reflex.

Spinal Cord Hemisection Syndrome (Brown-Séquard Syndrome)

See Table 3.**1**.

Central Cord Syndrome (Segmentally Limited)

- Ipsilateral spasticity below the level of the lesion,
- bilateral, segmental dissociated deficit of temperature sensation (due to interruption of fibers decussating in the anterior commissure) (Fig. 3.**2**),

Table **3.1**   Brown-Séquard syndrome

Affected structure	Ipsilateral deficit	Contralateral deficit
Pyramidal tract	Paresis	
Vasomotor fibers of the lateral columns	Warmth and erythema of the skin, possibly absent sweating	
"Overload" of the contralateral spinothalamic pathway by tactile stimuli?	Transient superficial hyperesthesia	
Posterior columns	Loss of deep pressure and vibration sense	
Anterior horn cells, anterior root	Segmental atrophy and flaccid paresis	
Posterior root	Segmental anesthesia and analgesia	
Lateral spinothalamic tract		Severe impairment or loss of pain and temperature sensation (dissociated sensory deficit)
Anterior spinothalamic tract		Mild hypesthesia to light touch

- possible dissociated sensory deficit in the entire body below the level of the lesion (if the spinothalamic pathways are affected bilaterally),
- possible segmental muscle weakness and atrophy and loss of reflexes if the anterior horn cells are affected,
- largely intact sensation to light touch and deep pressure (because the posterior columns are spared),
- urinary dysfunction.

Syndrome of Lesions of the Anterolateral Portion of the Spinal Cord (e.g., ischemia in the territory of the anterior spinal artery)

- Paraspasticity or paraparesis,
- dissociated sensory deficit below the level of the lesion,
- (rarely) exclusively segmental dissociated sensory deficit,
- intact sensation to light touch and deep pressure,
- urinary dysfunction.

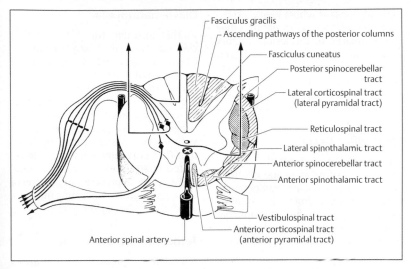

Fig. 3.**2 Cross-section of the spinal cord with important pathways.** "X" marks the site of the lesion responsible for a dissociated sensory deficit

Long Tract Signs

- E.g., isolated spastic paraparesis (as in spastic spinal paralysis, cf. p. 432),
- sensory deficit for deep pressure (as in tabes dorsalis, p. 112, or funicular myelosis, p. 441),
- combinations of the above.

Other Spinal Cord Syndromes

- For example, spinal muscular atrophy due to a lesion of the anterior horn,
- combined spinal muscular atrophy and pyramidal tract involvement in amyotrophic lateral sclerosis (p. 434).

Congenital and Perinatally Acquired Lesions of the Spinal Cord

Overview

Incomplete closure of the neural tube may lead to spina bifida occulta (usually in the form of incomplete formation of the laminae of L5 and S1, often with a tuft of hair over the area), meningocele, myelomeningocele, or meningomyelocystocele. The latter two types of malformation are often accompanied by hydrocephalus and Arnold-Chiari malformation (p. 43), and occasionally also by syringomyelia.

Meningocele

Operative repair of meningocele in the first few hours of life enables survival of the vast majority of treated patients, most of whom would otherwise die of CNS infection or other causes related to the lesion. Factors unfavorably affecting survival and long-term neurologic function include paralysis of the lower extremities at a high level, marked kyphosis, and associated hydrocephalus.

Spina Bifida Occulta

This condition is generally asymptomatic and often an incidental finding on lumbar spine radiography. Rarely, pressure from the spinous process of L5 on an incompletely formed S1 lamina causes back pain and sciatica (de Anquin's syndrome).

Complex Spinal Dysraphism

Complex cases of spinal dysraphism may involve a dermal sinus, a lipoma, intraspinal adhesions, or a tethered spinal cord (see below), with or without incompletely formed vertebral arches. Such cases are almost always accompanied by abnormal pigmentation of the skin over the lesion, which is sometimes hairy as well. Affected children often suffer from incontinence, pedal deformities, abnormal reflexes, and distal weakness. The spinal plain radiograph is almost always abnormal in some way—e.g. spina bifida, sacral deformity, or enlarged spinal canal. MRI establishes the diagnosis.

Diastematomyelia

In this disorder, the spinal cord is cleft into two halves by a bony or cartilaginous spur protruding into the spinal canal from its ventral aspect backward. There are usually other skeletal or spinal cord deformities as well. The disorder is associated with congenital deformities of the feet and with weakness and urinary dysfunction that gradually worsen as the affected child grows. Surgical removal of the spur can prevent progression of the neurologic deficits, but cannot reverse those already present.

Tethered Cord Syndrome

A similar symptomatic picture arises when the spinal cord is too tightly anchored to the caudal end of the sacral canal by an excessively short filum terminale. The diagnosis is made by MRI and, in some cases, myelographic CT. Treatment by surgical division of the filum terminale to undo the tethering can sometimes, but not always, bring improvement.

Birth Trauma

Trauma to the spinal cord in the birth process occurs mostly, but not exclusively, with breech delivery. The amount of force on the cervical spine is the critical factor. The spinal cord may actually be torn, or there may be traumatic contusions or hematomata within it.

Spinal Cord Trauma

Fundamentals of (Complete) Spinal Cord Transection Syndrome

Acute Total Spinal Cord Transection

At first, there is flaccid paraplegia with diminished or absent reflexes and without pyramidal tract signs (this is the stage of spinal shock, or, diaschisis, in von Monakow's term). The bladder and bowel are paralyzed. The findings in this acute stage are explained by the loss of the tonic effect of corticospinal excitation on the motor neurons of the anterior horn, whose resting potential therefore changes by 2–6 mV in the direction of increased stability. The acute stage usually lasts no more than 3 weeks; in exceptional cases, it may last as long as 6 weeks.

Later Stages of Spinal Cord Transection, and Slowly Progressing Lesions Causing Paraparesis

Some of the phenomena described here are due to an oversensitivity of spinal neurons below the level of the lesion. These neurons are deprived of their (partly inhibitory) nerve supply from supraspinal centers and thus discharge more readily in response to afferent impulses coming from below.

Paraparesis or paraplegia. Weakness or paralysis with elevated muscle tone, enhanced reflexes, and pyramidal tract signs.

Sensory disturbances. Sensory spinal cord transection syndrome with anesthesia below a particular segmental level (sensory level).

Spinal cord automatisms. These include the *retraction reflex*, which may be elicited by the Marie-Foix grasp, i.e., intense passive flexion and supination of the foot; *positive support reactions* (magnet reactions), such as extension of the leg in response to pressure on the sole of the foot or alternating flexion of one leg and extension of the other; and *mass reflex* with defecation, urination, sweating, and a rise in blood pressure.

Trophic disturbances. Trophic changes are especially evident in the skin. These changes, when combined with pressure ischemia secondary to immobility, can progress within hours to decubitus ulcers.

Hypotension. Patients in the acute stage of spinal cord transection syndrome with a lesion above T6 (spinal shock) become hypotensive when the upper body is elevated. The cause is the interruption of the central component of the sympathetic vasomotor pathway. Vasomotor fibers exit the spinal cord by way of the motor roots above the mid-thoracic level.

Paroxysmal hypertension. Episodes of hypertension may be produced by (unnoticed) overdistension of the bladder. This phenomenon develops 8–12 months after the initial injury and may pose a risk of complications, such as cerebral or other hemorrhage. Hypertensive episodes are accompanied by headache, sweating, and confusion.

Bladder Function

Anatomy

The neural substrate of bladder function comprises the following:
- cortical representation of the bladder and lateral control center in the anterior pons,
- spinal center at levels S2–S4,
- parasympathetic efferent fibers traveling through the S2–S4 roots and the pelvic nerve to the detrusor and the internal vesical sphincter,
- sympathetic efferent fibers traveling through the lower thoracic and upper lumbar roots and the sympathetic chain to the internal vesical sphincter,
- somatic motor efferent fibers traveling through the S2–S4 roots and the pudendal nerve to the external vesical sphincter (which consists of striated muscle), and
- sensory afferents by way of the hypogastric, pelvic, and pudendal nerves.

Physiology

Micturition is a spinal reflex that can be released or inhibited by higher (cerebral) centers, which exert their action through autonomic pathways in the lateral columns of the spinal cord. It is thus normally subject to voluntary control.

Bladder Dysfunction

Spinal cord transection and other neurologic disorders can cause the following types of bladder dysfunction:

Uninhibited neurogenic bladder. This condition is caused by congenital or acquired lesions of the cerebral cortex and pyramidal tract. The impulse to urinate, when it comes, cannot be resisted, though urination can usually be voluntarily initiated. Incontinence occurs only occasionally, and there is no residual urine in the bladder. Like automatic bladder (see below), uninhibited neurogenic bladder can be a complication of multiple sclerosis and pernicious anemia.

Reflex neurogenic (automatic) bladder. The sacral urinary centers and their afferent and efferent connections are intact, but there is a complete anatomical or functional interruption of the suprasegmental reflex pathway. This situation is found in lesions of the spinal cord above the conus medullaris, in multiple sclerosis, and in pernicious anemia, as well as in the normal infant, in whom the suprasegmental pathway is not yet active. Once a certain filling volume is reached, the bladder automatically empties, retaining relatively little residual urine. Patients with this condition should optimally void every 3–6 hours. Though voiding cannot be initiated or stopped by volition, it can be initiated by various physical maneuvers (manual pressure above the symphysis, stroking the medial aspect of the thigh, etc.). Provocative testing by intravesical instillation of ice water induces strong contractions that can be measured by cystomanometry, while in autonomic bladder (see below), the pressure curve is flat.

Deafferentated bladder. This condition is due to interruption of the afferent pathway arising in the bladder and traveling through the pelvic nerves; tabes dorsalis, which affects the posterior roots, is a classic cause. The deafferentated bladder cannot contract in response to distention and is therefore overfilled, hypotonic, and thin-walled. The small amount of contraction that is still present reflects an intrinsic response of the vesical smooth muscle to stretch. "Sensory paralytic bladder" would thus be a valid alternative name. The functional result is overflow incontinence. Causes other than tabes dorsalis include pernicious anemia, diabetes mellitus, multiple sclerosis, and syringomyelia.

Deefferentated bladder. This condition reflects isolated dysfunction of the motor arm of the vesical reflex arc and might alternatively be called "motor paralytic bladder." It is seen in poliomyelitis, in some cases of polyradiculitis, and in other disorders. Bladder function usually renormalizes spontaneously in such patients; if not, overflow incontinence develops.

Denervated (autonomic) bladder. Both arms of the vesical reflex arc are dysfunctional, either because of peripheral lesions or because of a lesion of the spinal bladder center in the conus medullaris. The bladder is flaccid and distended, and the patient suffers from overflow incontinence. Over time, minor contractions of the denervated vesical smooth muscle appear, sometimes followed by a shrinking of the bladder and hypertrophy of the vesical wall. Thus, unlike the deafferentated bladder, the denervated bladder manifests a certain amount of hyperactivity, due to a denervation-induced hypersensitivity of the vesical smooth muscle. Denervated bladder can be a conse-

quence of trauma, infection, arachnoiditis, myelomalacia, spina bifida, and tumors of the cauda equina. The bulbocavernosus reflex (cf. Table 10.**4**) is useful for the diagnosis of lesions in the S2 and S3 segments and the corresponding afferent and efferent pathways, and aids in the differentiation of neurogenic and strictly urological disturbances of micturition.

Clinical Features of Spinal Cord Trauma

Trauma affecting the vertebral column (even that due to exclusively axial mechanical stress) can produce a lesion in the spinal cord with or without accompanying damage to the vertebrae, intervertebral disks, or spinal ligaments. The following types of spinal cord injury can occur:

■ Spinal Cord Concussion

This term refers to signs of focal spinal cord injury arising at the moment of a spinal trauma, often a fall on the back during athletic activity. The manifestations may be purely sensory, but are more often mixed motor and sensory, and there may initially be a complete spinal cord transection syndrome identical to that of the acute shock phase seen in other patients with irreversible, complete spinal cord transection syndrome. The difference is that spinal cord concussion resolves spontaneously and completely, usually within hours and, at most, within 3 days (1056).

■ Spinal Cord Contusion

This term refers to the traumatic destruction of spinal cord tissue by direct mechanical compression or hemorrhage, which may be the result of:

- a dislocated vertebral fracture,
- a free bony fragment,
- a herniated intervertebral disk, or
- a (repositioned) subluxation of one vertebra on another.

There may be no evident traumatic pathology in spinal tissues other than the spinal cord; MRI reveals the area of contusion. The initial clinical presentation is usually that of complete spinal cord transection. There is often improvement thereafter, its extent depending on the severity of the initial injury and the persistence (if present) of the causative mechanism, e.g. bony compression, after the moment of injury. In a group of patients with spinal cord contusion who were very carefully followed by an experienced medical team, spontaneous improvement was found in 57% and 25% of those who had presented with incomplete and complete spinal cord transection syndrome, respectively. Early recovery of nociceptive sensation seems to be a favorable prognostic sign for motor recovery.

The level of the injury to the vertebral column often does not correspond exactly to the neural level of spinal cord damage. The clinically determined spinal level of dysfunction is frequently at C5, T4, T10, or L1 even if the bony lesion is two or more segments away. Indirect spinal cord injury through post-traumatic ischemia is presumably the reason. As the syndrome improves, the clinical spinal level often drops one or more segments.

■ Myelomalacia

This term refers to ischemic injury to the spinal cord occurring secondarily hours or days after trauma. Some 4–5% of patients with traumatic spinal cord transection develop *syringomyelia* extending cranially from the level of injury, months or years after the initial trauma. The mechanism by which syringomyelia develops is unknown. An increasing neurologic deficit is an indication for neurosurgical treatment.

■ Spinal Cord Compression

The spinal cord can be mechanically compressed by a herniated intervertebral disk, a bone fragment, or a *spinal epidural abscess or hematoma* (638). An epidural hematoma may arise spontaneously, as a complication of anticoagulation or medical procedures (lumbar puncture), or after apparently insignificant trauma or not particularly strenuous exercise. Intense local back pain is felt at first, followed within hours or days by neurologic signs of spinal cord involvement. Spontaneous hematomata often develop at the site of a congenital anomaly of the spine, e.g., a Klippel-Feil deformity.

■ Hematomyelia

Hematomyelia is a confluent hematoma in the central region of the spinal cord, usually extending over several segments. It typically produces a partial spinal cord transection syndrome, often with a dissociated sensory deficit in the dermatomes of the affected segments and spasticity below the level of the lesion, or else a Brown-Séquard syndrome (p. 392). Trauma is the most common cause, including trauma with a predominantly axial mechanical stress (fall onto the buttocks, nosedive into shallow water). The neurologic deficit commonly worsens over the ensuing hours and days, while its clinically determined level rises. Local pain is common. The lower cervical cord is a preferred site. The CSF is often, but not always, bloody or xanthochromic. *Spontaneous hematomyelia* is much rarer, and is often due to a vascular malformation (p. 423). MRI is the preferred initial diagnostic study.

■ Conus Medullaris Syndrome

The conus medullaris lies at the level of the first lumbar vertebra. A pure *conus medullaris syndrome* is characterized by disturbances of urination (denervated autonomic bladder, cf. p. 307), defecation, and sexual function, with sphincter weakness. A dissociated sensory deficit in the lower three or four sacral segments and the coccygeal area, or hypesthesia to all sensory modalities in this region (saddle hypesthesia), is occasionally seen. Motor function is often intact, though the glutei may be weak, and pyramidal tract signs need not be present. The bulbocavernosus reflex is absent (cf Table 10.4).

Conus medullaris syndrome can be caused by trauma, neoplasm, or ischemia (due to, e.g., an abdominal aortic aneurysm).

Cauda Equina Syndrome

Cauda equina syndrome can be caused by spinal fractures but is most often due to lumbar disk herniation at the level of the cauda equina (i.e., at L2–L3 or below). Unlike conus medullaris syndrome, cauda equina syndrome is often painful. There is flaccid weakness of the lower extremities with hypesthesia in all sensory modalities (usually in a saddle pattern), areflexia, and sphincter weakness, but no pyramidal tract signs. The clinical manifestations in the individual case depend on which roots are af-

fected; those that have already exited from the spinal canal above the level of the lesion are, of course, spared (cf. Table 10.3).

Figure 3.3 is a schematic depiction of the clinical findings in lesions of the spinal cord and cauda equina at various levels.

Practical Approach to Acute Traumatic Spinal Cord Transection

Diagnostic Evaluation

- *Neurological examination* to determine the level of the lesion. *Note:* the patient should only be moved with extreme caution.
- *Plain radiography of the spine* at the suspected level of injury (and any other levels that might be injured, according to the history of the trauma). The lateral image is likely to be the most informative.
- *MRI and (possibly) CT* for assessment of the spinal canal and spinal cord.
- *Note:* A lumbar puncture and (cautious) Queckenstedt test were a component of the immediate management in the pre-CT era, but are rarely, if ever, necessary today. The presence or absence of blood in the spinal fluid has no additional diagnostic or prognostic value.

Surgery

Immediate neurosurgical exploration via laminectomy is indicated as an emergency measure if the MRI or CT documents ongoing compression of the spinal cord in a patient with a complete or incomplete spinal cord transection syndrome immediately after the injury, or an incomplete

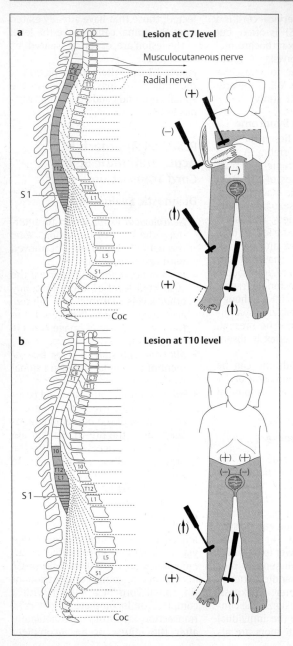

Fig. 3.**3a–d Clinical findings in lesions of the spinal cord and cauda equina at various levels** (after Mumenthaler, 692a).

a

Lesion at C7 level

Musculocutaneous nerve

Radial nerve

b

Lesion at T10 level

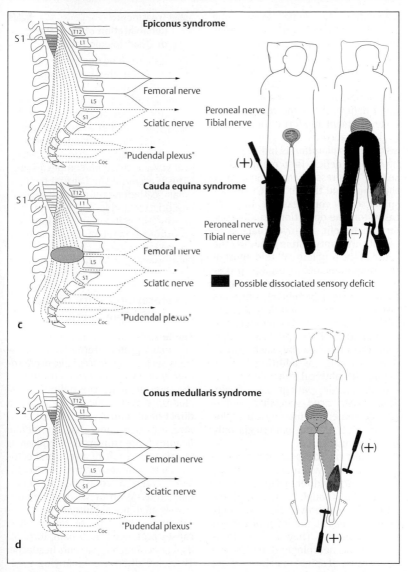

Epiconus syndrome

Femoral nerve

Peroneal nerve
Tibial nerve

Sciatic nerve

"Pudendal plexus"

(+)

Cauda equina syndrome

Peroneal nerve
Tibial nerve

Femoral nerve

Sciatic nerve

(−)

Possible dissociated sensory deficit

"Pudendal plexus"

c

Conus medullaris syndrome

Femoral nerve

(+)

Sciatic nerve

"Pudendal plexus"

(+)

d

Fig. 3.**3c** a. **d**

transection syndrome some time later. Unfortunately, such operations usually bring no immediate change in the neurologic deficit, which is nearly always due to spinal cord contusion. In rare cases, however, improvement can follow evacuation of a spinal epidural hematoma or the removal of a bone fragment hindering blood flow to the spinal cord.

Secondary exploration is indicated if a neurologic deficit first manifests itself, or progresses, some time after the injury, and the MRI or CT reveals spinal cord compression. In such cases, too, the operation usually confers no benefit, as myelomalacia or spinal cord contusion is generally the cause of the problem. All told, most of the numerous neurosurgical procedures performed in spinal cord trauma are not beneficial, some are possibly beneficial, and very few are definitely beneficial. The biomechanical properties of the spine can be further compromised by such procedures, causing an additional delay before the physical rehabilitation of the paraplegic patient can begin. Thus, experienced specialists generally recommend neurosurgical exploration for traumatic paraplegia only in exceptional cases.

Orthopedic surgical procedures are always indicated when bone fragments or subluxations directly compress the spinal cord (though such procedures hardly ever improve the neurologic deficit, except at the level of the conus medullaris). They are also indicated if the neurologic deficit worsens because of spinal instability, if the spine is unstable without (yet) any new or worsening deficit, and to treat post-traumatic spinal pain, so that the patient's mobilization and rehabilitation may proceed more rapidly.

**Treatment:
Rehabilitation of the Para- or Quadriplegic Patient**

Rehabilitation begins at the time of injury. From the very beginning, the patient must be correctly positioned, and repositioned every 2 hours, to prevent decubitus sores. It is also essential to prevent overdistension of the bladder, cystitis, and chronic cystitis leading to vesical stones and renal complications. This is accomplished at first by regular catheterization with strict aseptic technique and later by intermittent self-catheterization; recently, suprapubic drainage has come into wide use. Motor rehabilitation will not be discussed here.

Acceleration Injury of the Spine (Whiplash Injury)

The term "whiplash" is controversial, and many prefer alternative designations such as *cervicocephalic acceleration trauma* or *distortion trauma of the cervical spine*. The definition excludes cases in which there is also a direct head injury, which is not at all rare at present, now that automobile headrests are universal. Whiplash is usually the result of a rear-end collision, less commonly a front-end collision; rear-end collisions are more dangerous. With or without demonstrable anatomical injury to the cervical spine, this type of injury often causes prolonged neck pain, torticollis, cervicobrachialgia, and headache. There are often accompanying vegetative manifestations such as dizziness and blurred vision (345b), sexual dysfunction, persistent neuropsychological deficits, and neurasthenic phenomena.

Many of these manifestations can be explained as the result of chronic, painful tension on the capsular and ligamentous apparatus of the cervical spine. The chronic pain, in turn, may account for all of the neuropsychologic deficits, obviating the need to postulate a structural lesion of the brain. Pathological afferent input from the sensory receptors of the damaged cervical spine may modify the functioning of the brainstem center responsible for the correlation and integration of vestibular, visual, and sensory impulses (345b). The radiological findings may be entirely normal or consist of no more than an extended posture of the cervical spine with restricted mobility and degenerative changes unrelated to the accident. In occasional cases, acceleration trauma causes an acute cervical central cord syndrome that resembles hematomyelia in its acute presentation, but is more likely to resolve. There may also be a very brief loss of consciousness followed by long-lasting, complex psychopathological changes, even in the absence of direct head trauma. Such phenomena were long unjustly dismissed as "accident neurosis"; recent studies have revealed a typical clinical syndrome whose pathogenesis remains unexplained, but which is real rather than "psychogenic" (778). Nonetheless, this does not automatically imply major or permanent disability, even if the symptoms persist for a long time. Finally, it should be clear that the subjective intensity of whiplash symptoms can be affected by many factors other than the accident itself, e.g., the solicitous attitude of the patient's family, excessive diagnostic testing and therapeutic intervention, claims to monetary compensation, and lawsuits.

The diagnostic evaluation of acceleration injuries of the cervical spine is notoriously difficult, particularly as a medicolegal matter. The more important elements of such an evaluation are listed in Table 3.2.

Table 3.**2** Important aspects of the history and physical examination in acceleration injuries of the cervical spine

Category	To be determined
History:	
• The accident as such	Type(s) of automobile, relative speed, additional front-end impact if any, crumple zones, damage to automobile(s)
• Mechanism of injury	Seat belt, head rest (how positioned), seat back
• Posture at moment of injury	Upright, diagonal, head turn
• Expectation of accident	Collision anticipated, support grip, muscle tension

(Cont.) →

Table **3.2**   *(Cont.)*

Category	To be determined
• Immediate effects	Loss of consciousness, external injury (seat-belt injury, scalp abrasions)
• Behavior immediately after accident	Exited vehicle independently, who informed whom of accident, vehicle towed or driven home?

• Signs and symptoms thereafter:
  – Neck pain
  – Headache
  – Cervical mobility
  – Shoulder pain
  – Arm pain
  – Dizziness
  – Mental symptoms
  – Cervical root manifestations
  – Long tract manifestations
	When did they begin?

• What happened to other passengers?	Their position at time of accident, etc.
• Present life situation—personal, occupational	
• Insurance and other economic issues	
Physical examination	
• Head	Position at rest, spontaneous movement, mobility on direct testing
• Cervical spine	Mobility (rotation, flexion/extension, lateral flexion, turning of head in maximal flexion and extension)
• Mobility of individual segments of cervical spine, tested manually	Blocking, zones of irritation
• Ocular motility	Nystagmus
• Musculature	Paravertebral muscle tenderness, shoulder girdle tenderness
• Sensation	Occipital scalp, angle and neck of the mandible, dermatomes of the upper limbs, possible dissociated deficit on trunk or limbs
• Motor function	Segmental weakness in the upper limbs, paraparesis

(Cont.) →

Table 3.**2** *(Cont.)*

Category	To be determined
• Reflexes	Diminution of individual reflexes in the upper limbs
• Long tract signs	Paraparesis, hyperreflexia, pyramidal tract signs, urinary dysfunction
• Neuropsychological deficits	Memory, concentration, fatigability, irritability, impaired performance of complex tasks, neurasthenic reactions, depression

▌Tumors and Other Masses Compressing the Spinal Cord

General Aspects

Slowly progressive mechanical compression of the spinal cord causes a gradually worsening spinal cord transection syndrome. The warning signs of spinal cord compression are listed in Table 3.**3**.

Table 3.**3** Clinical features possibly indicating spinal cord compression

Progressive feeling of stiffness or fatigue in the legs
More or less rapidly progressive impairment of gait
Urinary dysfunction
Sensory disturbances in one or both legs
Band-like abnormal sensation around the thorax or abdomen
Back pain

The following are characteristic clinical features of spinal cord compression:

- *Motor function* is most prominently affected. Thus, a slowly growing mass may cause an isolated paraparesis with pyramidal tract signs and no sensory abnormality.
- Careful examination, however, usually reveals a predominantly distal *sensory deficit,* particularly involving epicritic touch and vibration sense. A precisely definable sensory level is not always present at the onset of symptoms.
- *Urinary dysfunction* is a relatively late sign.
- Radicular, *band-like sensations* sometimes point to the level of the lesion.
- The lack of individual *cutaneous abdominal reflexes or intrinsic muscle reflexes* may also provide a clue to the level of the lesion.

- *Pain in the lower limbs*, resembling sciatica, may be produced by spinal cord tumors at any level, including cervical and thoracic.
- The *cranial nerve examination* is normal in diseases affecting only the spinal cord. Occasionally, a spinal cord tumor causes an elevation of the CSF protein concentration, leading, in turn, to papilledema.
- *Spinal deformities* such as gibbus may accompany spinal cord tumor, or the spinous processes in the region of the tumor may be tender to percussion.
- *Plain radiography of the spine* may reveal bone destruction, widening of the spinal canal, destruction of the laminae or spinous processes, or a vertebral hemangioma.
- *MRI* is of crucial diagnostic value; in some cases, myelographic CT is a useful adjunctive study. Obviously, these tests are useful only if images are obtained from the level of the lesion; thoracic lesions will be missed on cervical spine MRI, etc.
- *SSEP* with stimulation above and below the level of the lesion can reveal the level.

The symptoms and signs may fluctuate to some degree, but masses compressing the spinal cord do not spontaneously regress and practically always require neurosurgical resection. Temporary improvement may result from the administration of corticosteroids, which relieve pressure on the cord through their anti-edematous effect.

Types of Mass Compressing the Spinal Cord

Intraspinal Extramedullary Tumors (851a)

Clinical Features and Diagnostic Evaluation

The diagnosis of a spinal cord tumor may be strongly suggested by history and physical examination (see above) but can be made definitively only by MRI or, in exceptional cases, myelography and post-myelographic CT. Some MR images of spinal lesions are shown in Fig. 3.**4**. The three most common types of intraspinal extramedullary tumor are neurofibroma, meningioma, and metastasis.

Neurofibroma. These lesions account for about one-third of all intraspinal extramedullary tumors. They are most commonly found in the lower thoracic and lumbar regions, but may occur anywhere. Because they grow from a nerve root, they commonly cause radicular pain and radicular deficits. Those that arise in the intervertebral foramen widen the bony margins of the foramen (as seen in MRI or in semi-oblique plain views) and grow both intra- and extraspinally (hourglass or dumbbell neurofibroma); such lesions are well seen by CT (Fig. 3.**5**). Spinal neurofibroma may be an isolated occurrence or a manifestation of neurofibromatosis (von Recklinghausen's disease, p. 36).

Meningioma. These benign, durally based tumors account for a further third of intraspinal extramedullary tumors. They often grow very slowly and may not be noticed by the patient until they finally produce high-grade spinal cord compression. They are

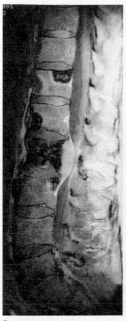

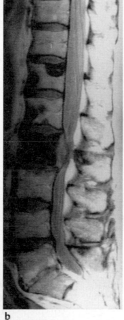

a   b

Fig. 3.**4a–f**   **MR images of masses involving the spinal cord and cauda equina.**

a, b *Metastatic carcinoma of the prostate.* There are osseous metastases and an epidural soft-tissue mass at the L4 level compressing the dural sac.

a   T1-weighted gradient-echo image.

b   T2-weighted spin-echo image.

c, d *Cervical disk herniation.* A herniated C5–C6 intervertebral disk compresses the dural sac and lightly indents the spinal cord.

c   T1-weighted spin-echo image.

d   T2-weighted spin-echo image.

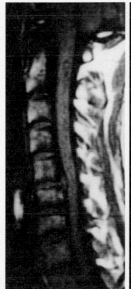

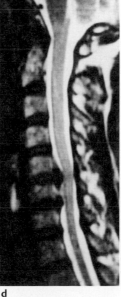

c   d

Fig. 3.**4e–f** →

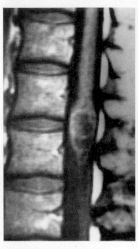
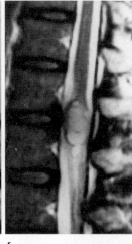

Fig. 3.**4e–f**
e, f *Intramedullary tumor (ependymoma) in the conus medullaris.* Note the expansion of the spinal cord.
e   T1-weighted spin-echo image.
f   T2-weighted spin-echo image.

e   f

most commonly found at thoracic levels. Their appearance on imaging studies is highly characteristic—a round, contrast-enhancing tumor growing out of the dura mater (Fig. 3.**6**).

Metastasis. Metastases are usually located in the vertebral bodies and compress the spinal cord secondarily (cf. Fig. 3.**4**). The primary tumor is in the lung in one-third of cases, the breast in almost a further third, else-

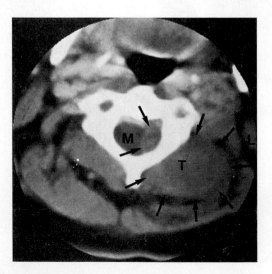

Fig. 3.**5** **Neurofibroma.** CT image of a neurofibroma at the C4 level, left (arrow). The intraspinal portion of the tumor displaces the cervical spinal cord (M) to the right. (Reprinted with the kind permission of Dr. H. Spiess, Institute of Neurological Computed Tomography, Zurich, Switzerland.)

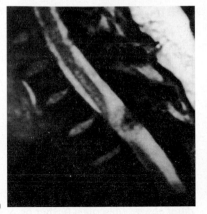 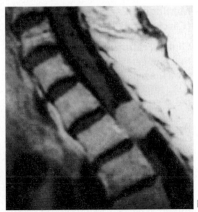

Fig. 3.**6**   **Meningioma in the thoracic spinal canal.** Sagittal MR images. Note the intradural extramedullary location of the tumor.
a T2-weighted image.

b T1-weighted image after contrast administration.

where in one-quarter, and occult in ca. 10%. Vertebral metastases are the presenting manifestation of cancer in almost half of the cases in which they are found. Two-thirds of patients have back pain or radicular pain as their first symptom; the description of a band (or half-band) of pain radiating from dorsal to ventral is particularly characteristic. Yet it is usually weakness in the legs that brings patients to medical attention. Sphincter disturbances appear relatively late. Plain radiographs of the spine are abnormal in 80–90% of cases, particularly those due to breast cancer. Vertebral metastases are typically hypointense on T1-weighted MRI.

Treatment

Benign tumors such as neurofibroma and meningioma can be cured by radical neurosurgical excision. Spinal metastases are treated with a combination of surgery and radiotherapy, or with radiotherapy alone. The latter method is usually preferred when there are multiple lesions. The prognosis depends on the type of primary tumor. When it is lung cancer, only one-third of cases respond to treatment, and only a small percentage of patients are still alive 1 year later. In breast cancer, half of cases respond to treatment, and one-third of patients are still alive 1 year later.

Meningeal Carcinomatosis (Carcinomatous Meningitis)

Clinical Features

In meningeal carcinomatosis, the leptomeninges are diffusely studded with tumor tissue over multiple spinal segments (51b). The clinical presentation is with neurologic signs reflecting spinal cord involvement, severe pain, and signs of polyradiculopathy, particularly affecting the cauda equina. The CSF protein concentration and cell count are elevated, the CSF glucose concentration is low, and tumor cells are found in the sediment. The condition is most commonly due to cancer of the stomach, lung, or breast. Sarcomatous meningitis may be a variant form of medulloblastoma.

Prognosis

Patients with meningeal carcinomatosis have a very poor prognosis. The median survival time after diagnosis is approximately one month.

Intramedullary Tumors

Histology and Clinical Features

Intramedullary tumors are much rarer than extramedullary tumors. *Astrocytoma*, the most common histologic type, may affect so a long segment of the spinal cord (or even its entirety). *Ependymoma* is rarer and is usually found toward the caudal end of the cord. Intramedullary tumors rarely metastasize.

The signs and symptoms depend on the site and extent of the tumor within the spinal cord.

■ **Treatment** ■
Intramedullary tumors, even very extensive ones, can often be resected neurosurgically under the operating microscope with a surprising degree of radicality.

Nonneoplastic Spinal Cord Compression

■ Intraspinal Mass

Two types of intraspinal mass that have already been mentioned are *epidural hematoma* (see p. 398) and *epidural abscess* (described further on p. 414).

■ Spinal Cord Compression from Lesions of the Spine

Vertebral body hemangioma. Vertebral body hemangioma can produce local pain with percussion tenderness of the spinous processes, radicular pain, or spinal cord compression. It most commonly occurs in the midthoracic spine and is often found on MRI as an incidental finding of no clinical importance. It is hyperintense in both T1- and T2-weighted images.

Other, rarer causes of spinal cord compression. Slowly progressive spinal cord compression can be caused by kyphoscoliosis and, more rarely, by chondrodystrophy, vertebral deformities in pseudohypoparathyroidism, and osteopenia with kyphosis. Kyphoscoliosis can often be remedied by orthopedic surgery. Adolescent kyphosis (Scheuermann's disease) is another rare cause of spinal cord compression.

Herniation of the spinal cord. Herniation of the spinal cord through a dural defect is rare (236b, 999e). It is usually a spontaneous event, though it may be post-traumatic in rare cases. The result is a progressive spinal cord transection syndrome, less commonly a Brown-Séquard syndrome. The diagnosis is made by MRI (999e).

Cervical spondylosis. Cervical spondylosis can cause myelopathy, particularly when the spinal canal is congenitally narrow or in patients with rheumatoid arthritis who have chronic atlantoaxial subluxation. Posterior osteophytes compress the spinal cord directly and also harm it indirectly by compromising its blood supply through the spinal and radicular arteries. The clinical picture is characterized by radicular motor deficits, which are sometimes present in multiple segments because the motor roots run diagonally (even in the cervical spine), and thus a lesion at a single level may affect more than one root at the same time. There are often poorly characterizable sensory deficits in the upper limbs; these may be distributed sporadically or like a glove (because of involvement of spinal cord tracts) and are not always dermatomal (988). There may be a misleading thoracic sensory level on the trunk (8a). The sensory deficit in the hands may create the impression of astereognosis. There are also marked deficits of pain and temperature sensation, ataxia due to involvement of the spinocerebellar tracts, spasticity of the lower limbs with pyramidal tract signs, spasticity of the upper limbs (sometimes even when the lesion lies lower in the cervical spine, because of compromise of the anterior spinal artery). Rarely, involvement of the anterior horn cells causes fasciculations of the upper limb muscles only, raising the differential diagnostic question of spondylotic myelopathy versus amyotrophic lateral sclerosis. Occasionally, the Lhermitte sign can be evoked (an electric sensation running down the back on flexion of the neck) (84c). In spondylotic myelopathy, the antero-posterior diameter of the spinal canal usually measures 13 mm or less. MRI is the best means of establishing or excluding the diagnosis (903) (Fig. 3.**7**).

Lumbar puncture is no longer a routine part of the diagnostic work-up. A Queckenstedt test performed with maximal flexion and extension of the neck usually does not indicate an impediment to CSF flow, and the CSF protein concentration is normal or only mildly elevated.

The syndrome of *intermittent claudication of the cervical spinal cord* is a special form of cervical spondylotic myelopathy with variable clinical manifestations, seen in patients with a congenitally and/or spondylotically narrowed cervical spinal canal (see above). The degree of tension of the spinal cord in the cervical spinal canal plays a role in the generation of symptoms; thus, they may tend to arise preferentially when the neck is flexed or extended during intense physical activity. The mechanical effect is transmitted to the spinal cord by the dentate ligaments (575i). The clinician must beware of automatically diagnosing cervical spondylotic myelopathy in any elderly patient with chronically progressive spastic paraparesis, even though this is the most common cause. Other etiologies, such as multiple sclerosis, are not at all rare.

Treatment

Cases in which the diagnosis of cervical spondylotic myelopathy can be made unequivocally can be treated with a generous neurosurgical decompression of the spinal cord by multilevel laminectomy, or with vertebral body fusion from an anterior approach (84c). If the clinical presentation is relatively acute, improvement can be achieved in some two-thirds of cases, otherwise in only about one-third. The surgical outcome is disappointing in cases with spastic quadriparesis.

Clinical manifestations of cervical spondylosis other than spinal cord compression. See p. 729.

Myelopathy due to stenosis of the thoracic spinal canal. This rare but well-defined clinical syndrome can appear even in the absence of the spinal diseases listed on p. 730. Progressive spastic gait impairment, sensory deficits, and (sometimes) urinary dysfunction appear over the course of several months or years. Intermittent claudication forces the patient to stop walking or change his posture from time to time. MRI is the best means of making the diagnosis (CT is the second choice). A generous posterior decompression via laminectomy is the treatment of choice.

Thoracic disk herniation with spinal cord compression from an anterior direction should be treated by diskectomy, through one of several approaches that have been described. Laminectomy in such cases tends to worsen the myelopathy and should not be performed.

A number of conditions entering into the **differential diagnosis** of spinal cord compression are listed in Table 3.**4**.

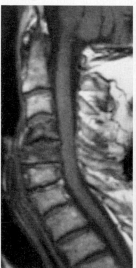 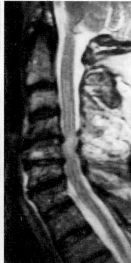

Fig. 3.7a, b   Cervical spondylosis with myelopathy.
Sagittal MR images. The spinal canal is narrowed at the level of the spondylotic degenerative changes, and the subarachnoid space anterior and posterior to the cord is obliterated. Note the mild signal abnormality within the cord at this level.
a T1-weighted image.
b T2-weighted image.

Table 3.4 Differential diagnosis of spinal cord compression

Disease	Characteristics of differential diagnostic importance	Ancillary tests possibly required
Multiple sclerosis	Early relapse or stepwise progression, cranial nerve involvement (look for internuclear ophthalmoplegia), absent or imprecise sensory level, possible urinary dysfunction (urgency)	MRI of brain and spinal cord, CSF examination for oligoclonal bands, visual evoked potentials
Familial spastic spinal paralysis	Family history, purely motor, affects upper as well as lower limbs, possibly enhanced jaw jerk reflex, no urinary dysfunction	CSF studies, MRI of spinal cord
Dural arteriovenous fistula	Rapidly progressive paraparesis, more or less purely motor	MRI, possibly spinal angiography
Arteriovenous malformation of the spinal cord	Possible stepwise progression, sudden exacerbation of deficits (cf. Table 3.5)	CSF possibly xanthochromic, MRI of spinal cord, spinal angiography
Adrenoleukodystrophy	Affects males, very slowly progressive spastic paraparesis, hyperpigmentation or other signs of Addison's disease, family history may be positive	Serum cortisol level, elevated concentration of long-chain fatty acids
Transverse myelitis	Acute	Lumbar puncture (inflammatory CSF picture), MRI of spinal cord
Lathyrism	Increasing spastic paraparesis with simultaneous involvement of anterior horn cells	Evaluate nutritional status
Hyperthyroidism	Systemic signs of hyperthyroidism (rare)	Thyroid function tests
Syringomyelia	Dissociated sensory deficit, trophic disturbances of muscles and/or joints	MRI
Amyotrophic lateral sclerosis	Rarely purely spastic paraparesis at onset, enhanced jaw jerk reflex, no sensory deficit, no urinary dysfunction	EMG
Funicular myelosis	Posterior column signs always present, no clear spinal level	Vitamin B_{12} level, possibly also vitamin B_{12} resorption test

Infectious, Allergic, and Toxic Diseases of the Spinal Cord and Its Coverings

Infectious Diseases of the Spinal Cord

Bacterial Infections

Intramedullary abscess. Abscesses within the substance of the spinal cord are very rare.

Spinal subdural abscess. Spinal subdural abscesses are clinically characterized by back pain, radicular signs and symptoms, long tract signs, and, finally, the sudden onset of paraplegia. The syndrome commonly follows an antecedent infectious process, often osteomyelitis of a vertebral body. The erythrocyte sedimentation rate is usually elevated. Early diagnosis and operative treatment are decisive for a good outcome.

Spinal epidural abscess. One in 250–350 patients hospitalized with a neurologic disease suffers from a spinal epidural abscess. The condition can arise at any age. A primary source of infection can be identified in about half of all cases—e.g., furuncle, pulmonary infection, abortion, osteomyelitis, endocarditis, otitis, etc. The responsible organism is usually *S. aureus*. The spinal manifestations usually arise two to four weeks after the primary infection, typically beginning with severe back pain accompanied by fever and an elevated sedimentation rate. There follow radicular signs and, in nearly all cases, a spinal cord or cauda equina compression syndrome. The CSF is always abnormal (inflammatory changes). Plain films, CT and MRI may demonstrate discitis if present, but MRI is the crucial diagnostic study, as only MRI can reveal the abscess itself and the resulting spinal cord compression. Spinal cord compression by an epidural abscess is generally regarded as an indication for immediate neurosurgical treatment; antibiotic treatment is begun concomitantly. Antibiotic treatment alone is appropriate in some cases, but neurosurgical consultation is imperative.

Poliomyelitis

Epidemiology

This endemic and epidemic viral disease is spread by oral ingestion of virus particles derived from the stool or respiratory secretions of an infected person. The virus produces neurologic manifestations in only 1–2% of infected persons. The incidence of poliomyelitis is now practically zero in countries in which active vaccination is practiced.

Histopathology

The disease affects the central gray matter, particularly the anterior horn ganglion cells of the spinal cord, which are acutely lost and replaced with gliotic scar tissue.

Clinical Features

An *incubation period* of 3–20 days is generally (though not always) followed by a nonspecific febrile *prodromal phase*, and then, several days later, by the *main phase* of the disease, characterized by fever, a general feeling of illness, headache, and meningeal signs. *Weakness* develops after

1–4 days and progresses over a few hours or days to marked paresis or paralysis. Paresthesiae or other purely sensory abnormalities are not part of the clinical picture of poliomyelitis, though there may be pain and tenderness in the involved muscles. Spinal poliomyelitis is the most common form, but there are also occasional cases with predominant or even exclusive involvement of the brainstem, producing (for example) dysphagia, facial palsy, and ophthalmoplegia. The encephalitic form of the disease is extremely rare.

CSF Findings

The second (main) phase of the disease is marked by CSF pleocytosis, with 100 or more cells per cubic millimeter—predominantly polymorphonuclear neutrophils at first, with a rapid transition to lymphocytic predominance. The cell count falls over the ensuing 1–2 weeks, while the CSF protein concentration rises, sometimes creating the picture of so-called "albumino-cytologic dissociation" ordinarily considered characteristic of Guillain-Barré syndrome.

Differential Diagnosis

The differentiation of poliomyelitis from Guillain-Barré syndrome is discussed below on p. 575. The anterior horn cells can also be affected by viral illnesses other than poliomyelitis, including certain types of *echovirus* and *coxsackievirus* infection. The pathogen can be determined only by virologic testing.

Prognosis

Cases with brainstem involvement and respiratory paralysis have a poor prognosis, with a mortality of up to 50%. In other than cases, the neuro-logic manifestations may begin to regress as soon as the paralytic phase has reached its peak, and there may be substantial or complete regression within a few weeks. The presence of any degree of residual motor function at the peak of the paralytic phase is a good prognostic sign. Once a few months have passed, the likelihood of further improvement is low. Paralysis usually resolves incompletely, leaving a variable degree of residual weakness, muscular atrophy, and areflexia, as well as stunted growth of the affected limb(s) if the illness strikes in early childhood.

Vaccination

Poliomyelitis vaccination is currently performed with the live oral vaccine of Sabin. Its use has led to the near complete disappearance of paralytic cases in many countries of the world. Paralysis as a complication of vaccination is exceedingly rare.

Special Clinical Phenomena

Post-polio syndrome (PPS). The various symptom complexes that have been described under this name are phenotypically and pathogenetically diverse (377a, 478e). The rare cases of *progressive paresis* arising years after acute poliomyelitis are associated with *spinal muscular atrophy,* which can be documented by electromyography and by muscle biopsy. Fortunately, the progression is usually limited and rarely life-threatening. *Amyotrophic lateral sclerosis* develops extremely rarely in the aftermath of poliomyelitis, probably as a coincidental second illness rather than a true late complication. It is conceivably due to secondary loss of previously damaged anterior horn cells, or else it may be the expression of an accompanying myopathy (204, 669). In rare cases of poliomyelitis, persistence of the poliovirus can be demonstrated (478e). MRI reveals hyperintensity of the anterior horns (779a).

The term "post-polio syndrome" is also used to refer to conditions that do not involve worsening paresis, including:

- excessive *fatigability* of post-polio patients or
- a more *complex constellation of findings* including pain, respiratory abnormalities, and dysfunctional temperature regulation.

Poliovirus antibody titers are usually negative in such cases (659). Such patients do not, as a rule, have an abnormal personality structure. No effective treatment is known (203a). Pyridostigmine (949b) and other medications have been tested, with a negative result.

Bronchial asthma (Hopkins syndrome). This syndrome, originally described by Hopkins, affects children under 10 who have been vaccinated against poliomyelitis. An acute asthma attack is followed within a few days by the sudden appearance of muscle weakness and atrophy in an extremity (the precise location is variable) (670a, 863c). There is no sensory deficit. Pain and meningeal signs are occasionally present. The CSF is pleocytotic with an elevated protein concentration. The leading hypothesis as to the pathogenesis of this syndrome is that the anterior horn cells are selectively damaged by hypoxia arising during the asthma attack; supportive evidence has been obtained both from histological study (670a) and from MRI (35a).

The paresis resolves incompletely, if at all.

Myelitis
General Aspects

Myelitis is a general term for inflammatory processes affecting the spinal cord, either in isolation or in the context of a systemic infectious illness, an allergic reaction, or an (allergic) demyelinating disease. Most myelitides involve multiple spinal cord tracts simultaneously, with or without concomitant encephalomyelitis, and can produce more or less complete spinal cord transection syndromes, sometimes in more than one level at the same time. In extreme cases, they can cause para- or quadriplegia (see below).

Myelitis is a rare sequela of leptospirosis, rickettsial diseases, measles, mumps, herpes simplex infection, and other viral diseases (604a). Though HIV-I more often causes encephalopathy, it occasionally causes myelopathy even in the absence of brain involvement (268b). Cutaneous herpes zoster in an immunocompromised patient may be followed 1–2 weeks later by a viral myelitis of variable spatial distribution and extent (229); we have seen this also in elderly patients without known immune compromise. Locally endemic spastic paraparesis in certain (tropical) countries is strongly associated with the presence of antibodies to HTLV-I, which indicates that this retrovirus is highly neurotropic (p. 123). Myelitis is also occasionally a postvaccinial (smallpox, rabies) or paraneoplastic phenomenon (p. 320). Finally, there remain many cases in which the etiology cannot be determined.

Transverse Myelitis

Epidemiology

The incidence of transverse myelitis is ca. 4.6 cases per 1 million individuals per year (461). The disease can strike at any age; two peaks in its age-related incidence are found between the ages of 10 and 20 and after age 40 (496a). Men and women are affected with equal frequency. There is no seasonal dependence.

Clinical Features

The illness usually begins with fever, myalgia, back pain, and a band-like paresthesia around the trunk, and progresses within 24 hours in about half of all cases to a more or less complete spinal cord transection syndrome. The temporal course of progression varies, however, from 5 minutes to several weeks, and progression may also occur in stepwise fashion (496a, 571b). Recovery occurs, if at all, within a few weeks or at most 3 months. An episode of pure transverse myelitis is only rarely followed by further neurologic manifestations; in particular, long-term study of such patients has shown that transverse myelitis only very rarely represents the first episode of multiple sclerosis, unless oligoclonal bands are present in the CSF.

Transverse myelitis together with optic neuritis constitutes *neuromyelitis optica (Devic's syndrome)* (p. 484). In our opinion, the creation of a separate diagnostic category for *progressive necrotizing myelopathy* (496a, 858a) carrying a very poor prognosis, as distinct from transverse myelitis in demyelinating disease, is not justified.

Toxic Myelopathies

Myelopathy in Heroin Addicts

Heroin addicts are subject to a number of neurologic complications:
- brachial plexus neuropathy,
- polyradiculitis,
- polyneuropathy,
- injection trauma of a peripheral nerve,
- rhabdomyolysis,
- brain abscess,
- mycotic aneurysm,
- intracerebral hemorrhage,
- tetanus,
- seizures.

Myelopathy, which concerns us here, usually arises immediately after self-injection of heroin, sometimes when the patient awakens from a period of unconsciousness. The clinical picture is generally of an acute thoracic spinal cord transection syndrome, which is most often complete, though sometimes only partial. The prognosis for recovery is poor. The pathogenetic mechanism is unclear; possible mechanisms include hypertension, hyperextension of the head in drug-induced coma, toxic or allergic factors, emboli, and vasculitis. The consumption of other illegal street drugs can produce the same syndrome.

Myeloneuropathy Due to Nitrous Oxide Abuse

Persons who abuse nitrous oxide regularly over a period of months or years, and rarely also persons who are repeatedly accidentally exposed to it (including dentists!), may develop the following neurologic manifestations:
- polyneuropathic sensory disturbances in the limbs,

- ataxia,
- sexual dysfunction,
- hyperreflexia,
- pyramidal tract signs,
- sphincter disturbances,
- cognitive disturbances.

The prognosis for recovery is poor.

Other Toxic Myelopathies

The epidemic form of *tropical spastic paraparesis* is largely due to the toxic effects of staples of the local diet (978)—e.g., the grass pea *Lathyrus sativa* (lathyrism) and cyanide-laden cassava.

Ergotism may also lead, by a neuro-vascular mechanism, to spastic paraparesis with only minor sensory involvement, as well as to cerebral manifestations (901a).

For *myelopathy in alcoholism,* see p. 308.

Circulatory Disorders of the Spinal Cord

Blood Supply of the Spinal Cord

The blood supply of the spinal cord is shown schematically in Figs. 3.**8** and 3.**9**.

Radicular arteries are present in the fetus at every segmental level, but most of them regress over the course of development so that, by adulthood, the spinal cord is supplied by only six to eight anterior and posterior segmental arteries. The largest of these is the great radicular artery, also called the artery of Adamkiewicz (Fig. 3.**8a**), which enters the spinal canal between T10 and L2, usually on the left side. All of the segmental arteries enter the spinal canal through the intervertebral (neural) foramina and follow the course of the nerve roots into the subarachnoid space. They communicate with each other on the surface of the spinal cord through the single anterior spinal artery and the paired posterior spinal arteries. These three arteries that run longitudinally

down the cord anastomotically connect the supplying radicular arteries and are connected with each other through the transversely oriented, circular vasocorona (Fig. 3.**9**).

An essential feature of the blood supply of the spinal cord is that the flow of blood in the longitudinal arteries may be in either direction, depending on the local vascular geometry and momentarily prevailing pressure relationships. The vascular border zones are at a particularly high risk of ischemia.

Spinal Cord Ischemia Due to Deficient Arterial Blood Flow

Pathogenetic Mechanism

Ischemic necrosis of the spinal cord (*myelomalacia*) is analogous to ischemic necrosis of the brain (cerebral infarction, stroke). Other vascular disturbances of the spinal cord include intramedullary hemorrhage and subacute or chronically progressive man-

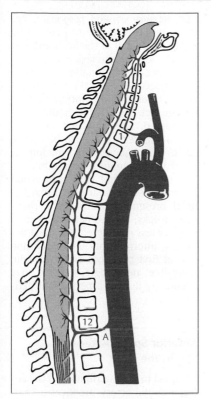

Fig. 3.**8** **Blood supply of the spinal cord (longitudinal section)** (after Lazorthes).
A = great radicular artery (artery of Adamkiewicz).

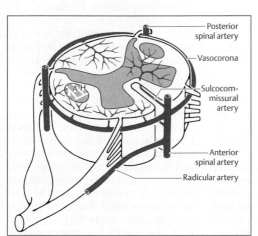

Fig. 3.**9** **Blood supply of the spinal cord (cross-section)**.
L   Leg
A   Arm
H   Hand

ifestations of highly variable type (paraparesis, chronic anterior horn involvement). The common vascular disturbances of the spinal cord and their clinical features are listed in Table 3.**5**.

Histopathology

Arteriosclerosis can affect the large supplying arteries, but not the vessels of the spinal cord themselves. The latter display no more than adventitial fibrosis, which does not cause vascular occlusion. Circulatory events causing anoxia and ischemia of the spinal cord produce symmetrical infarcts of the spinal gray matter that are most pronounced at lumbosacral levels. Spinal cord infarction due to venous thrombosis is rare (517) (p. 423).

Clinical Features

The clinical expression of spinal cord ischemia depends on its extent and duration. Intermittent hypoperfusion can cause transient, fully reversible deficits, while lasting hypoperfusion can produce an infarct, whose clinical manifestations are determined by its location.

Intermittent Hypoperfusion of the Spinal Cord

Intermittent hypoperfusion causes repeated, transient episodes of paraparesis, pyramidal tract signs, paresthesiae in the lower limbs, and sensory abnormalities. If such disturbances appear only while the (typically elderly) patient is walking, they are designated *intermittent claudication of the spinal cord*. Intermittent hypoperfusion of the spinal cord may be due to incompletely compensated heart failure or to atherosclerosis. So-matosensory evoked responses, i.e., the cerebral response to stimulation in the lower half of the body, may reveal the level of the lesion even if the neurological examination between episodes is normal. MRI can also reveal corresponding intramedullary changes (cf. Fig. 13.**1**). It should be remembered, however, that intermittent paraparesis may also be due to an arteriovenous malformation or dural arteriovenous fistula (606).

A complete spinal cord transection syndrome of vascular origin that has been present for days, or perhaps even weeks, can sometimes regress more or less completely. On the other hand, intermittent hypoperfusion that at first produces only transient, reversible neurologic deficits may eventually lead to a permanent deficit.

Anterior Spinal Artery Syndrome

Ischemia in the distribution of the anterior spinal artery produces a characteristic syndrome. Prodromal pain and band-like paresthesia around the trunk may be present for hours or days before weakness sets in. Flaccid paraplegia develops over the course of several minutes to one hour (rather than with apoplectic suddenness) and is accompanied by a dissociated sensory deficit, in which pain and temperature sensation are disturbed, but touch, position sense, and vibration sense are preserved. This sensory deficit usually affects the entire body below the level of the lesion, but may be limited, in rare cases, to the level of the lesion itself. There is also dysfunction of the sphincters. The examiner who fails to test pain, tempera-

Table 3.5 Common causes and clinical features of circulatory disorders of the spinal cord

Type	Features	Causes	Remarks
Infarction	More or less complete spinal cord transection syndrome	E.g., radicular artery occlusion, rarely embolization (e.g. of cartilage), atherosclerosis, aortic dissection	Usually of sudden onset, sometimes with stepwise progression over hours or days; improvement is rare
Anterior spinal artery syndrome	Usually total motor deficit below lesion, with sensory level for pain and temperature sensation	As above; also anterior spinal artery occlusion, possibly because of direct arterial compression	
Intermittent ischemia	Partly or completely reversible spinal cord transection syndrome, possibly recurrent	Stenosis of supplying arteries, heart failure, arteriovenous malformation; may be exercise-dependent	Usually seen in older patients, sometimes presents as intermittent claudication of the spinal cord (p. 420), must be differentiated from multiple sclerosis
Progressive ischemia	Spinal cord transection syndrome developing over days, weeks, or months	E.g., dural arteriovenous fistula	MRI, possibly spinal angiography to demonstrate the lesion

ture sensation, and rectal tone may falsely conclude that the paralysis is psychogenic, as pyramidal tract signs are initially absent.

The neurologic manifestations may be explained as arising from the territories of the anterior spinal artery and the sulco-commissural arteries. If the syndrome affects the cervical spinal cord, it may present with bilateral paresis of the upper limbs (783c) or, rarely, with cluster-like headache and facial pain (223a). MRI is useful for the demonstration of spinal cord infarcts and vascular anomalies, if present. Any of the vascular disorders mentioned above may be the ultimate cause of anterior spinal artery syndrome, which may also be due to direct compression of the artery by a mass—e.g., a herniated intervertebral disk. Spontaneous regression of deficits is unusual, and very rarely complete.

Posterior Spinal Artery Syndrome

Ischemia in the distribution of the posterior spinal artery is quite rare. Its clinical expression is clearly distinct from anterior spinal artery syndrome. Severe paraparesis is accompanied by a deficit of posterior column sensation.

Sulco-commissural Artery Syndrome

An infarct in the territory of the sulco-commissural artery involves one half of the spinal cord at a given level up to the midline and is thus clinically manifest as Brown-Séquard syndrome.

Total Myelomalacia

Total myelomalacia is an infarct that involves the entire cross-section of the spinal cord at a given level. Infarction is often rapid (though not necessarily apoplectic) and accompanied by pain. The neurologic deficit may progress to become complete over the course of several days and usually remains more or less complete, though certain exceptions have already been mentioned above. Many cases that are diagnosed as necrotizing myelitis or acute transverse myelitis actually belong in this category. Sometimes the lesion is at the level of the conus medullaris (p. 401).

Central Cord Infarction

On occasion, transverse infarction of the spinal cord at a given level (with a corresponding spinal cord transection syndrome, possibly including a dissociated sensory deficit) is combined with infarction of the central portion of the cord in the caudally adjacent segments. Central cord involvement inactivates the lower motor neurons of the caudal segments and produces the paradoxical picture of flaccid paraparesis with areflexia and absent pyramidal tract signs, which is unexpected in the setting of a transverse cord lesion. The flaccid weakness indicates permanent loss of spinal motor neurons and thus precludes the possibility of motor recovery.

Chronically Progressive Vascular Myelopathy

Chronically progressive vascular myelopathy may be the result of chronic hypoperfusion of the spinal cord due to atherosclerosis, a venous disturbance, or an arteriovenous malformation (see below). It can present with paraparesis. If the anterior horn cells are among the structures affected by hypoperfusion, the clinical presentation may closely resemble that of amyotrophic lateral sclerosis, and electromyographic studies may also seem to support this (erroneous) diagnosis (528). Electrophysiologic signs of an anterior horn cell lesion can be found in chronic hypoxia—e.g., that accompanying chronic respiratory insufficiency (966). For posthypoxic pathoanatomical changes, see the relevant discussion above.

Spinal Cord Ischemia Due to Venous Disturbances

Venous Infarction of the Spinal Cord

Hemorrhagic or nonhemorrhagic *venous thrombosis* is a rare cause of spinal cord ischemia (517). A spinal cord transection syndrome develops either progressively or in stepwise fashion. An inflammatory disorder of the spinal veins (i.e., *spinal phlebitis*) can also cause spinal cord transection syndrome.

Arteriovenous Malformations and Fistulae of the Spinal Cord (586c)

Definition:
These congenital anomalies consist of simple arteriovenous shunts (fistulae) or more complex arteriovenous malformations. One-third are located in the dura mater and two-thirds are intradural, including in the spinal cord itself (801). (*Angioma racemosum venosum* was an earlier term for such lesions.) Arteriovenous fistulae are found mainly at lower lumbar levels. This type of lesion is probably the cause of the syndrome that was previously designated as *angiodysgenetic myelomalacia* (spinal varicosis, necrotizing myelitis of Foix and Alajouanine).

Clinical Features

The signs and symptoms usually appear in the second, third, or fourth decade of life, most commonly at the thoracolumbar junction. Their onset is typically sudden or subacute but may be progressive, with highly variable speed of progression (526a). Rapidly progressive paraparesis leading to a rapid decline in the distance the patient is able to walk is a characteristic presentation of dural arteriovenous fistulae (36, 1035). The initial symptom is often local and radicular pain, which is then followed more or less rapidly by a spinal cord transection syndrome. Men are much more commonly affected than women. Urinary dysfunction is often present early in the course of the disorder (a point of differential diagnostic significance, as it is generally only a late finding in spinal cord compression by tumor or other mass lesions). The transection syndrome may be complete or incomplete, e.g. Brown-Séquard syndrome.

The clinical manifestations may make their appearance in the context of trauma, physical stress, or menstruation. An intermittent neurologic deficit with more or less complete recovery between episodes is a not uncommon alternative mode of presentation. The deficit always returns at the same level as before (in distinction to the deficits of multiple sclerosis).

A vascular malformation of the spinal cord (or, in rare cases, a spinal cord tumor) may cause an *acute subarachnoid hemorrhage* (p. 215). Back pain and neurologic deficits referable to the spinal cord point to a spinal, rather than intracranial, source of bleeding.

Ancillary Tests

The CSF is pleocytotic and its protein concentration is elevated in 75% of cases; xanthochromia is rarer. MRI reveals the vascular malformation, and possibly also a spinal cord infarct (if present), though acute hemorrhages are more easily seen on CT. Contrast myelography reveals tortuous veins on the surface of the spinal cord in ca. 80% of cases (subdural contrast injection may lead to erroneous interpretation). Spinal angiography practically always demonstrates the pathological vessels.

Differential Diagnosis

If the spinal cord transection syndrome develops rapidly, the alternative diagnosis of *myelitis* may have to be considered; if it arises slowly, *spinal cord compression by an enlarging mass;* if it is intermittent, *multiple sclerosis.* The correct diagnosis is usually indicated by the fact that the deficit always remains in the same place, and by the accompanying pain. *He-*

matomyelia has been described above (p. 398).

Prognosis

Cases in which the malformation has caused acute infarction of the spinal cord or intramedullary hemorrhage have a poor prognosis, though in some cases (mainly of dural fistulae) early treatment may yield clinical improvement. If the deficit is progressive or intermittent, or if there is spastic paraparesis that has not yet progressed to paraplegia, surgical or endovascular treatment should be provided promptly before a worse and most likely permanent deficit develops.

Treatment

Microneurosurgical excision of vascular malformations of the spinal cord is rapidly giving way to *interventional neuroradiological treatment* ("embolization") via the supplying vessels (see also under cerebral arteriovenous malformations, p. 213). Successful treatment is possible in some 80% of cases of dural arteriovenous fistula and in some 50% of intramedullary processes (801).

Degenerative and Heredodegenerative Diseases Mainly Affecting the Spinal Cord

Diseases Affecting the Anterior Horn Cells

General Features

The features of the spinal muscular atrophies are summarized in Table 3.**6**.

Pathophysiology and Special Features

■ The Motor Unit

The ganglion cell of the anterior (motor) horn, together with its axon and axonal branches, is the *peripheral motor neuron* (lower motor neuron) of the corticospinal pathway. A *motor unit* is the set of muscle fibers innervated by a single ganglion cell (cf. Fig. 14.**2**). The fibers in a motor unit contract synchronously. The number of fibers per motor unit varies from muscle to muscle; motor units in the extraocular muscles comprise only 10–12 fibers, those in the gastrocnemius as many as 1600. Each motor unit occupies a portion of the cross-sectional area of the muscle in question; in the human biceps brachii muscle, for example, the cross-sectional area occupied by a motor unit is about 20 mm^2. The individual fibers of the motor unit are arranged within this area in apparently random fashion. All of the fibers of a single motor unit are of the same histochemical type.

■ Denervation and Reinnervation

If a motor ganglion cell should be lost (e.g., because of spinal muscular atrophy), the corresponding axon degenerates and all of the fibers of the motor unit are *denervated*. New processes sprout from the axons of neighboring, still intact ganglion cells and partially *reinnervate* the denervated fibers. Two results are that the intact motor units are enlarged and the new motor units that result consist of multiple *subunits*. If ganglion cells continue to be lost, a single muscle fiber can undergo denervation and reinnervation multiple times. These processes form the basis of the changes that can be detected by muscle biopsy and electromyography (cf. Fig. 14.**2**).

■ Electromyography

The electromyogram of a normal muscle reveals the normal bi- and triphasic course of the action potentials of single motor units. Maximal voluntary muscle contraction results in the summation of the action potentials of many units at once, causing a full *interference pattern*. In patients with *chronic neurogenic muscular atrophy*, the enlarged motor units (see above) are reflected by abnormally high, sometimes polyphasic potentials, and maximal voluntary contraction produces only a sparse interference pattern. Myopathies affect muscle fibers belonging to multiple motor units and thus reduce the size of each motor unit, without (at first) reducing the number of units; thus, the electromyogram in myopathies reveals low-amplitude, fragmented individual potentials and, with maximal voluntary contraction, a full (but low-amplitude) interference pattern (cf. Fig. 14.**2**).

Table 3.6 General features of the spinal muscular atrophies

Phenomenon	Course	Ancillary studies	Remarks
Weakness: • Increasing • Often symmetrical • Sometimes focal	Slowly progressive, often over years, initially focal but increasingly symmetrical over time	EMG characteristic ENG: normal velocity, motor potential decreased Serum muscle enzymes usually normal or mildly elevated in chronic cases when so-called accompanying myopathic changes are present	Hereditary and sporadic forms
Muscle atrophy			
Fasciculations			
Muscle tone: • Flaccid		Muscle biopsy reveals typical grouping of atrophic fibers (and sometimes accompanying myopathic changes)	
Reflexes: • Diminished/absent • Enhanced in ALS		CSF normal (protein rarely elevated)	
Pyramidal tract signs • Absent • Present in ALS			
Sensation • Always normal			

■ Muscle Biopsy

The first and most basic diagnostic distinction made possible by muscle biopsy is that between neurogenic muscular atrophy and primary myopathy. If a *neurogenically altered* motor unit (i.e., one that already consists of multiple subunits because of the cycle of denervation and reinnervation) is denervated a further time, the groups of fibers that make up its subunits all become atrophic to a similar degree, as muscle biopsy will reveal. The atrophic subunits generally take an elongated polygonal shape, and they remain structurally intact. Their nuclei are peripheral and appear normal. There is no increase in the amount of connective tissue. In *primary myopathy*, on the other hand, the affected fibers are randomly distributed throughout the muscle and atrophic to a variable extent; most retain their original round shape and manifest various structural changes, without being atrophic (waxy degeneration, loss of longitudinal and transverse striations, clump-like or granular degeneration, macrophage infiltration, etc.). The nuclei are often increased in number and centrally located, and may be arranged in rows. There may be an increase in the amount of connective and fatty tissue, and inflammatory infiltrates are found (even in myopathies other than polymyositis). The individual types of primary myopathy have specific histopathologic features that often enable a precise etiologic diagnosis from the muscle biopsy alone; these will be mentioned in the relevant clinical sections below (cf. Fig. 14.**3**). Abnormalities resembling those found in primary myopathy—changes of fiber structure, an increase in the amount of connective tissue, and cellular infiltrates – are sometimes seen in cases of spinal (and other neurogenic) muscular atrophy, particularly when the disorder has taken a slowly progressive course. These are referred to as "accompanying myopathic changes." In such cases, the serum creatine kinase level is often elevated as well.

■ Fasciculations

Chronic loss of anterior horn ganglion cells is associated with involuntary, synchronous contractions of motor units, called fasciculations. These are visible with the naked eye, but are generally seen only if the examiner looks for them. They can be provoked or enhanced by vigorous tapping on the affected muscle or, even better, by the intravenous injection of 10 mg of edrophonium chloride. Fasciculations are typical but not pathognomonic of chronic loss of anterior horn cells, as they can also be due to radicular or peripheral nerve lesions. Benign fasciculations may accompany systemic infectious illness and indeed sometimes appear spontaneously, without any known cause; sometimes fasciculations due to a lower motor neuron lesion can only be told apart from benign fasciculations through other, accompanying neurologic signs, or after observation of their further course. The electromyographic correlate of fasciculations consists mainly of arrhythmic and polyphasic potentials of variable configuration, with signs of denervation and reinnervation. Long-term observation has shown that patients with fasciculations as an isolated sign are not at risk of developing spinal muscular atrophy or any other progressive illness, even if the fasciculations are very widespread, e.g., in the calves (101, 103). For the combination of myalgia and fasciculations, see p. 845.

■ Contraction Fasciculations

The enlargement of the (still preserved) motor units in the process of denervation and reinnervation has the consequence that motor recruitment may bring far too many muscle fibers into synchronous contraction than are needed for a given movement. The patient's movements may therefore make excessively large excursions; for example, an outstretched finger may twitch irregularly ("signe de l'index," "contraction fasciculations").

Clinical Syndromes

The "degenerative" conditions discussed here, some of which are familial, are often difficult to distinguish on initial clinical examination from the rarer symptomatic forms of spinal muscular atrophy due to cancer, dysproteinemias, certain types of intoxications, and disorders of carbohydrate metabolism. Spinal muscular atrophy can also be an element of the clinical picture of many other neurologic diseases that are discussed in other parts of this book, among them amyotrophic lateral sclerosis, Parkinson's disease–dementia complex, Creutzfeldt-Jakob disease, Friedreich's ataxia, intraspinal masses, orthostatic hypotension, and others. Hexosaminidase deficiency usually produces a complex syndrome with encephalopathy, ataxia, and complex neurologic manifestations, but can also produce pure spinal muscular atrophy.

Classification

It is reasonable to classify the spinal muscular atrophies (SMA) by specific features of their age-dependent clinical course, but, however they are classified, there will be cases of a transitional type that seem not to fit into any particular category. A classification of SMA according to their severity has been proposed, in which the disorder is of type I, II, IIIa, IIIb, or IV depending on the age of onset and the maximal motor skills attained by the patient (Table 3.7). Although there is, in reality, a continuous spectrum of disease states, many cases will fall into one of five traditionally identified diagnostic categories, which are listed with their salient features in Table 3.8 and described individually in the following sections.

Table 3.7   Classification of spinal muscular atrophies by severity, after Zerres (1047)

Type	Definition	Mean age of onset (range)
I	Never sat unaided	2.3 months (0–10)
II	Sits unaided, never walked	4.4 months (0–18)
IIIa	Walks with assistance	7.8 months (3–30)
IIIb	Walks unaided	5.6 years (3–24)
IV	Walks unaided	7 years (3–54)

Table 3.**8**   Diseases causing chronic loss of anterior horn ganglion cells (spinal muscular atrophies)

Name	Structures involved	Clinical features	Special features	Etiology
Infantile spinal muscular atrophy (Werdnig-Hoffmann)	Anterior horn ganglion cells	Muscle atrophy and weakness, hypotonia, fasciculations of the tongue	Infants and toddlers, rapidly fatal	Autosomal-recessive (?); gene on chromosome 5
Pseudomyopathic spinal muscular atrophy (Kugelberg-Welander)	Anterior horn ganglion cells	Muscle atrophy and fasciculations, progressive gait impairment, no bulbar signs	Children and adolescents, proximal, usually begins in the lower limbs, slow progression	Irregularly dominant; gene on chromosome 5
Adult spinal muscular atrophy (Aran-Duchenne)	Anterior horn ganglion cells	Muscle atrophy, weakness, and fasciculations	Young adults, begins distally (hands)	Usually sporadic rather than hereditary, of undetermined etiology; occasionally associated with syphilis
Proximal spinal muscular atrophy of the shoulder girdle (Vulpian-Bernhardt)	Anterior horn ganglion cells	Muscle atrophy, weakness, and fasciculations affecting the muscles of the shoulder girdle	Adults, slow progression	Unknown; occasionally associated with syphilis
Amyotrophic lateral sclerosis (with or without true bulbar palsy)	Anterior horn ganglion cells, possibly also motor neurons of the cranial nerve nuclei and cerebral cortex	Muscle atrophy, weakness, fasciculations, bulbar palsy with dysphagia and dysarthria, spasticity, pyramidal tract signs	Adults, rapidly progressive and lethal; juvenile (familial) cases are rare and relatively benign	Usually sporadic, occasionally familial

■ Infantile Spinal Muscular Atrophy (Werdnig-Hoffmann)

Genetics

The inheritance pattern of this genetic disorder is probably autosomal recessive; it may affect multiple siblings even if the parents and other ascendants are unaffected. As in other forms of spinal muscular atrophy, the genetic defect lies on the long arm of chromosome 5, between the sites D5 S629 and D5 S557 (229a, 329a, 997). The most important of the various genes on chromosome 5 associated with spinal muscular atrophy is probably the one designated SMN (for "survival of motor neurons"), which is partly or wholly absent in patients with spinal muscular atrophy (809).

Clinical Features

In rare cases, the disorder is already apparent prenatally because of a paucity of fetal movement in the womb, or because of an associated arthrogryposis multiplex congenita. It otherwise becomes manifest at birth or in infancy, most commonly between the ages of 6 and 12 months. The child is flaccid and weak, lies with flexed arms ("jug-handle posture") and floppy, extended legs, shows some distal residual movement, and cries abnormally softly. Paradoxical breathing and, later, dysphagia indicate involvement of the cranial nerve nuclei. Fasciculations are mainly seen in the tongue; fasciculations and muscle atrophy are difficult to detect in the extremities because of the normal infantile fat pad.

Prognosis

The prognosis is poor, as most of these children die before the age of 4 years, and many die earlier. Yet there are cases with much slower progression, and survival past the age of 20 years is occasionally seen.

Differential Diagnosis

Other diseases to be considered in the differential diagnosis include congenital muscular dystrophy, Foerster's astatic-atonic syndrome, cerebral palsy, and rare myopathies (some of which are benign). Hypotonia and paucity of movement at birth or in the first few months of life used to be referred to as amyotonia congenita (of Oppenheim), but this term is no longer recommended, as it masks a wide diversity of underlying etiologies.

Treatment

Werdnig-Hoffmann disease, like other forms of spinal muscular atrophy, has no known effective treatment. Many experimental treatments have been found to be ineffective, among them intravenous immunoglobulin (271b).

■ Pseudomyopathic Spinal Muscular Atrophy (Kugelberg-Welander)

Genetics

This disorder is a relatively common form of spinal muscular atrophy that is usually inherited in an autosomal recessive pattern, less often in an autosomal dominant pattern. The responsible gene is on chromosome 5.

Clinical Features

Unlike children with Werdnig-Hoffmann disease, children with this disorder can usually walk normally at first, as the disease usually becomes evident between the 2nd and 10th year of life with proximal muscular atrophy and weakness, mainly in the legs in most cases. Disappearance of the knee-jerk reflex is an early sign. Pseudohypertrophy of the calf may be seen, and fasciculations are practically always present. Pyramidal tract signs and bulbar signs are usually absent, though there are exceptions (e.g., ophthalmoplegia in rare cases). Cardiac abnormalities, including abnormal intracardiac conduction and congestive heart failure, have been described.

Ancillary Tests

In this slowly progressive disorder, electromyography and muscle biopsy enable the definitive demonstration of a neurogenic muscle atrophy. As in chronic denervating diseases of other types, biopsy often additionally reveals accompanying myopathic changes; in such cases, the serum creatine kinase concentration may be elevated.

■ Adult Spinal Muscular Atrophy (Aran-Duchenne)

Clinical Features

Spinal muscular atrophy of adulthood of Aran-Duchenne type is usually nonfamilial, though there are very rare familial cases. The onset of disease is in the third decade of life or later. The disorder is characterized by a symmetrical, distal muscular atrophy that usually begins in the hands and is accompanied by fasciculations. Marked reduction of muscle mass may be associated with a deficiency of gluconeogenesis, leading to hypoglycemia (145).

Course

The disorder progresses slowly, first in a distal-to-proximal direction along the upper limbs and then in the trunk and lower limbs. It may continue to progress for decades; such chronic cases have also been called *poliomyelitis chronica* (an unfortunately misleading term, not to be confused with post-polio syndrome, p. 415).

Differential Diagnosis

The most important entities in the differential diagnosis of Aran-Duchenne spinal muscular atrophy are *HSMN types I and II* (p. 595) and *chronic polyneuropathy*. The latter is distinguished by the presence of sensory abnormalities.

Treatment

No treatment is known to be effective against spinal muscular atrophy per se. Polyneuropathy with multiple conduction block (p. 581) and the rare cases of an autoimmune disorder with anti-G_{M1} antibodies (754) may respond to plasmapheresis and immune suppression. The very rare cases of progressive amyotrophy due to parathyroid adenoma are also amenable to treatment (249).

■ Adult Proximal Spinal Muscular Atrophy (Vulpian-Bernhardt)

This disorder is considered to be a separate hereditary disease entity whose inheritance pattern is probably autosomal recessive. Its onset occurs, on average, in the fourth decade of life. It is characterized by symmetrical weakness and atrophy that remain confined to the trunk and proximal muscle girdles of the extremities over many years. It progresses very slowly, leading eventually to gait impairment but not to a reduction of life expectancy.

■ Rarer Types of Spinal Muscular Atrophy

A symmetrical type of spinal muscular atrophy affecting mainly the upper limbs has been described (496b). *Kennedy disease* (507a) is a type of spinal muscular atrophy accompanied by bulbar signs, fasciculations mainly in the face, muscle cramps, areflexia, and diminished conduction of sensory impulses in peripheral nerve. Pyramidal tract signs, overt sensory dysfunction, and cerebellar signs are absent. The disease progresses very slowly and has little or no effect on life expectancy. It affects men in young adulthood and is caused by a genetic defect on the long arm of the X chromosome in the vicinity of the androgen receptor gene.

Monomelic amyotrophy is a rare type of muscular atrophy affecting only one limb. Its etiology and pathogenesis are unknown; it is perhaps a type of spinal muscular atrophy. It begins in mid-adulthood, progresses slowly, and does not spread to the other limbs.

Spastic Spinal Paralysis (1044, 1017c)

Definition

The term *spastic spinal paralysis* excludes symptomatic spastic paralysis due to other disease processes affecting the spinal cord (see below) and refers to a collection of primary disorders, most of them genetic, characterized by spastic weakness and hyperreflexia, without any sensory abnormality. These disorders were previously called *primary lateral sclerosis* (771b).

Genetics

The mode of inheritance is autosomal dominant in two-thirds of cases but may rarely be autosomal recessive (386, 387, 521). Men and women are equally frequently affected. The defect is most often on chromosome 2p, on which the spastin gene is located. Several other loci, on 4 different chromosomes, have been identified to date in individual families (699c, 709a, 1017c).

Frequency

Among 672 patients referred to a university neurology department because of spastic paraparesis, only 16 were given the final diagnosis of familial spastic spinal paralysis; a further 44 were given the diagnosis of spastic spinal paralysis of indeterminate etiology. This fact alone makes clear that the differential diagnosis of this syndrome is much more important than its diagnosis *per se.*

Clinical Features

Spasticity of the lower limbs begins in childhood and progresses very slowly till the patient reaches old age. The initial symptom is an effortful, dragging gait. Often, the patient can still pursue gainful work despite marked spasticity. Twenty percent of patients have additional findings, such as muscle atrophy, fasciculations, ataxia, extrapyramidal signs, optic atrophy, and dementia. There are occasional cases with distal sensory neuropathy and trophic changes.

Histopathology

Pathologic examination usually reveals only a degeneration of the pyramidal tracts in the lateral columns of the spinal cord (Strümpell's "primary sclerosis of the lateral columns"), beginning just below the pyramidal decussation. Occasionally, the anterior corticospinal tract and the posterior columns are involved as well.

Treatment

Spastic paraparesis without identifiable, treatable etiology is managed with *physical therapy, antispasmodic agents,* and, where indicated, *local injections of botulinum A toxin* into the spastic muscles (252).

Differential Diagnosis of Progressive Spasticity

One of the rare symptomatic forms of progressive spastic paraparesis is *ectodermal dysplasia* (Bloch-Sulzberger), also known as *incontinentia pigmenti.* This disease tends to affect multiple members of the same family; most patients are female. Affected infants have linear pigmented areas on the trunk and running vertically along the posterior thigh; these later turning into atrophic scars. Dental anomalies, corneal opacification, cataracts, alopecia, and nail changes are common. The IQ is usually low. Progressive para- or quadriparesis begins in adolescence.

A familial metabolic disturbance causing *hyperglycinemia* produces spastic paraparesis accompanied by atrophy of individual calf muscles, pes cavus, and loss of the Achilles reflexes (a clinical picture similar to that of Friedreich's ataxia or neurogenic muscle atrophy).

Spastic paraparesis rapidly progressing to paraplegia is also seen in *aminoaciduria.*

Lathyrism (caused by a toxin in the grass pea, a dietary staple in some poor areas of the world) is characterized by leg cramps, paresthesiae, tremor of the limbs, pollakisuria, memory impairment, fasciculations, and rapidly progressive paraparesis, without any sensory abnormality.

The X-linked disorder *adrenoleukodystrophy* (p. 295) may present as a pure (familial) spastic spinal paralysis (616, 679). The progressive spastic paraparesis of *HIV myelopathy* has already been mentioned (pp. 119, 122). *Spinal arteriovenous malformations* and even *intracranial dural arteriovenous fistulas* draining into the spinal venous plexus can produce myelopathy, occasionally in the form of a pure, progressive spastic para- or quadriparesis. These lesions are amenable to treatment by embolization or neurosurgical resection.

The acute myelopathy of *heroin addicts* has already been mentioned (p. 417). The autosomal recessive *Sjögren-Larsson syndrome* is characterized by severe, congenital ichthyosis in combination with spastic quadriparesis, dementia, and (sometimes) peripheral neuropathy and dysalbuminemia. In *Rud syndrome,* on the other hand, congenital ichthyosiform erythrodermia is accompanied by oligophrenia and epileptic seizures, but there is no spasticity.

Spastic paraparesis is a feature of *alcoholic myelopathy* (p. 418), *leukodystrophy* (p. 288), *adrenal insufficiency* (including adrenoleukodystrophy, p. 295), and *multiple sclerosis* (p. 465). *Primary lateral sclerosis* is due to atrophy of the precentral cortex, but is clinically manifest as progressive spastic quadriparesis.

Amyotrophic Lateral Sclerosis (ALS)

Definition:
As its name implies, this disease is characterized by a combination of muscle atrophy (due to loss of spinal anterior horn ganglion cells) and spasticity with pyramidal tract signs (due to involvement of the lateral columns of the spinal cord). Other names for it include "Charcot's disease" (after an early describer), "motor neuron disease," and "Lou Gehrig's disease" (after a famous patient).

Epidemiology

This disorder usually begins between the ages of 40 and 65. It affects men roughly three times as often as women. It rarely strikes children or adolescents. Its incidence is two to four cases per 100,000 individuals per year.

Etiology and Pathogenesis

Most cases are sporadic, though a small minority (5–10%) are familial, of genetic etiology (144a). Roughly one-fifth of these familial cases are due to one of the 70 or so different mutations that have been identified to date in the *SOD1* gene, which encodes the enzyme superoxide dysmutase (791e). Pedigrees with autosomal dominant inheritance have been described (679a).

Some families are afflicted with a *familial, juvenile, relatively benign form of amyotrophic lateral sclerosis* that begins in childhood and may progress slowly over several decades. Another inherited form is found among the Gomoro people on the Pacific island of Guam; in this population, ALS is 100 times more common than in Europe.

The combination of amyotrophic lateral sclerosis with parkinsonism and dementia has already been mentioned (p. 245); it has been suggested that this may be due to an intoxication. Most cases in the temperate zones are sporadic.

Many hypotheses as to the pathogenesis of ALS have been proposed (37a, 192, 281, 981b), but none has yet been convincingly substantiated.

Clinical Features

Symptoms. The patients themselves usually first complain of *weakness*, which, despite a notion common among neurologists, is not necessarily only distal, and may begin proximally. The problem may remain unilateral for many months. Later, weakness is noted in other muscle groups as well. Sometimes patients will note *muscle atrophy*, often in the intrinsic muscles of the hand. Often, they will not mention certain other symptoms until asked about them directly, such as *painful muscle cramps* (frequently in the thighs, usually at night but sometimes only with active muscle contraction), dating back to the very onset of weakness or even before it, or *fasciculations* in individual muscles.

Signs. Neurological examination reveals *paresis* that may be asymmetrical and can be more pronounced either proximally or distally. Systematic testing generally reveals weakness in

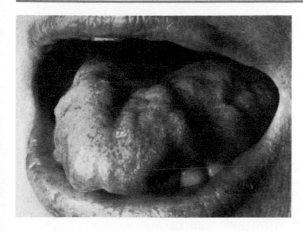

Fig. 3.**10** **Bilateral glossal atrophy and paresis in true bulbar palsy due to amyotrophic lateral sclerosis (ALS)** in a 65-year-old woman. (From M. Mumenthaler, *Atlas der klinischen Neurologie*, 2nd ed., Berlin: Springer, 1986.)

multiple muscle groups. The paresis may resemble that of myasthenia and, indeed, respond to cholinesterase inhibitors. *Fasciculations* must be deliberately sought and patiently watched for. They can be provoked or enhanced, if necessary, by vigorous tapping on the muscle, or by the intravenous injection of a cholinesterase inhibitor (edrophonium chloride 10 mg, see p. 924). Paresis may be present for a long time before *muscle atrophy* becomes grossly evident.

In addition to the above findings, *spasticity, hyperreflexia, and pyramidal tract signs* must be present to satisfy the diagnostic criteria for amyotrophic lateral sclerosis (as opposed to spinal muscle atrophy). The presence of relatively brisk reflexes in clearly paretic muscles suffices to arouse the suspicion of ALS. Spasticity is often relatively mild and evident only in an advanced stage of the disease; it is often partially canceled out by the concomitant spinal muscular atrophy with lower-motor-neuron paresis ("pseudoneuritic form of ALS"). Thus, spasticity may be surprisingly minor or even totally absent, despite marked pyramidal

tract signs. In other cases, however, spasticity may appear before the anterior horn ganglion cells are affected, so that the disease initially has the appearance of a spastic spinal paralysis (or pseudobulbar palsy). Sphincter function is unaffected, and sensation is entirely intact. As the disease progresses, the muscles of respiration are increasingly affected, with a corresponding decline of pulmonary function.

Bulbar signs—slurred speech, dysphagia, and flaccid facial paresis—usually do not appear till later in the course of the disease, though they are prominent from the beginning in roughly one-quarter of cases. The tongue moves less than normal, is atrophic (Fig. 3.**10**), and displays fasciculations; rapid or large-amplitude movements of the lips are difficult to execute (bulbar palsy). Eye movements are not affected.

Involvement of the corticobulbar tract leads to enhancement of the *intrinsic muscle reflexes of the face* (snout reflex, nasopalpebral reflex, jaw jerk). *Involuntary laughing and crying* are also a feature of bulbar palsy. These phenomena should not be confused with affect incontinence, as they do not reflect an underlying emotion of happiness or sadness on the patient's part.

ALS sometimes occurs in combination with *focal brain atrophy of Pick type*, with additional clinical manifestations including aphasia and frontal lobe signs.

Ancillary Tests

The *CSF* is normal. The most important diagnostic test is *electromyography*, which reveals fasciculations and fibrillation potentials, a reduced number of motor units, higher than normal (sometimes extremely high) motor unit potentials, and practically normal conduction velocity in peripheral nerve. Motor evoked potentials, if abnormal, indicate degeneration of the central motor neurons. Neurophysiologic tests can also be used in longitudinal follow-up (937a) to monitor the progression of the disease.

Muscle biopsy reveals the typical picture of neurogenic muscle atrophy and, not uncommonly, accompanying myopathic changes (in such cases, the serum creatine kinase level is elevated).

MRI occasionally reveals global atrophy of the spinal cord, as well as signal changes at various points along the intracranial course of the corticospinal pathway (818).

Prognosis

Inexorable progression leads to death within 5 years in about half of all patients, and 60% of those with bulbar palsy die within a year. There are cases with a more protracted course, however; 6% of patients are still alive at 10 years from diagnosis, and remissions are sometimes seen.

Treatment

There is still no etiologic treatment for ALS. *Riluzol* has been shown to increase life expectancy slightly compared to placebo, and to affect mortality favorably (over the period of the study) in the subgroup of patients with bulbar signs (85, 549b, 650, 791d). A dose of 100 mg qd is recommended (549b). The early placement of a *PEG* (percutaneous endoscopic gastrostomy) in patients with dysphagia does not alter the course of the disease, but does prolong survival by about 6 months on average.

Differential Diagnosis

Purely motor paresis with muscle atrophy may be seen in various types of myopathy. *Fasciculations* may reflect a radicular lesion or no lesion at all (benign fasciculations, p. 428). *Spasticity* is a feature of very many neurologic diseases, e.g. spastic spinal paralysis (p. 432).

A difficult problem in differential diagnosis arises only *when spasticity is present in combination with muscle atrophy and/or fasciculations*. This combination may appear as a paraneoplastic phenomenon, in which case its course is more protracted than that of ALS; it can also be a consequence of diabetes mellitus, hyperparathyroidism, mercury or lead poisoning, trauma, electric trauma, (rarely) polyglucosan body disease (p. 295), and gastrectomy.

Chronic progressive vascular myelopathy was mentioned above on p. 422. Muscle atrophy and spasticity are also present in combination in a small minority of cases of Creutzfeldt-Jakob disease. Syphilis (20) can produce a syndrome similar to ALS, as can macroglobulinemia with para-proteinemic involvement of the nerve roots. A neuroimmunological mechanism is also at work in *multifocal acquired demyelinating neuropathy*; this disorder affects only motor function (at least at first), causing fasciculations and muscle cramps, and can easily be mistaken for ALS (742). It is also known as multifocal motor neuropathy (MMN). Electroneurography reveals multiple conduction blocks. For further details, see p. 581.

Hyperthyroidism can cause muscle atrophy with paresis, fasciculations, and enhanced reflexes, creating the impression of ALS. Lyme disease, too, can produce the clinical picture of motor neuron disease (405a). A tumor or malformation at the craniocervical junction may produce bulbar signs, bulbar atrophy, involuntary laughing, and pyramidal tract signs; these phenomena may continue to progress slowly for years, particularly in the case of a meningioma.

Spinocerebellar Ataxias

Definition:
Most of the spinocerebellar ataxias are hereditary disorders—i.e., spinocerebellar heredoataxias. These diseases are first manifest in childhood or adolescence and progress slowly thereafter. The underlying lesion is in certain pathways of the spinal cord and certain areas of the cerebellum, occasionally also in the optic nerve and other central nervous structures. They present with varying clinical syndromes; their more common manifestations include ataxia, gait impairment, dysarthria, and reflex abnormalities.

Classification

Harding's classification of the spinocerebellar ataxias by pattern of inheritance and age of onset (386) is reproduced in Table 3.**9**. Thanks to continuing advances in molecular biology and genetics, the pathogenesis of more and more of these diseases is rapidly becoming known (446a, 851b). For example, a mutation of the α-tocopherol transfer protein gene on

chromosome 8q produces a particular adult-onset form of spinocerebellar degeneration (354c), while type II spinocerebellar ataxia is due to a mutation of chromosome 12 (699a).

Major Types

A number of the hereditary ataxias have already been discussed above in the section on cerebellar diseases (p. 318); several more are introduced here.

■ Friedreich's Ataxia

Definition:
Friedreich's ataxia is a familial, progressive degeneration of the spinocerebellar and corticospinal tracts and the posterior columns, of autosomal recessive inheritance.

Table 3.**9**   Classification of hereditary disorders causing ataxia and spastic paraparesis (from Harding, ref. 386)

Designation		Inheritance pattern	Decade of life
1	**Diseases of known cause**		
1.1	*Metabolic diseases*		
1.1.1	*Progressive ataxias*		
	Abetalipoproteinemia (Bassen-Kornzweig disease)	Autosomal recessive	1st, 2nd
	Hypobetalipoproteinemia	Autosomal recessive	2nd, 4th
	Hexosaminidase deficiency	Autosomal recessive	1st
	Glutamate dehydrogenase deficiency	Autosomal recessive	2nd to 6th
	Cholestanolosis	Autosomal recessive	Ataxia 3rd to 6th
1.1.2	*Intermittent ataxias*		
	Pyruvate dehydrogenase deficiency	Autosomal recessive	1st
	Hartnup disease	Autosomal recessive	1st
	Intermittent branched-chain ketoaciduria	Autosomal recessive	1st
	Urea cycle enzyme deficiencies (ornithine transcarbamylase deficiency, citrullinemia, argininemia, argininosuccinyl aciduria)	Autosomal recessive/ X-linked dominant	1st
1.2	*Diseases with faulty DNA repair*		
	Ataxia telangiectasia (Louis-Bar syndrome)	Autosomal recessive	1st
	Xeroderma pigmentosum (de Sanctis-Cacchione syndrome)	Autosomal recessive	2nd
	Cockayne syndrome	Autosomal recessive	1st
2	**Diseases of unknown cause**		
2.1	*Cerebellar ataxias of early onset (before age 20)*		
	Friedreich's ataxia	Autosomal recessive	1st, 2nd
	Early-onset cerebellar ataxia with preserved reflexes	Autosomal recessive	1st, 2nd
	With hypogonadism, possibly deafness and/or dementia	Autosomal recessive	1st–3rd
	With congenital deafness	Autosomal recessive	2nd, 3rd
	With deafness in childhood and mental retardation	Autosomal recessive	1st
	With retinal pigment degeneration, possibly retardation/dementia/deafness	Autosomal recessive	1st
	With optic atrophy and retardation, possibly deafness and spasticity (Behr syndrome)	Autosomal recessive	1st

(Cont.) →

Table 3.**9** *(Cont.)*

Designation		Inheritance pattern	Decade of life
	Marinesco-Sjögren syndrome (with cataract and retardation)	Autosomal recessive	1st
	With myoclonus (Ramsay Hunt syndrome)	Autosomal recessive/ autosomal dominant	1st, 2nd
	X-linked recessive spinocerebellar ataxia	X-linked	1st, 2nd
	Cerebellar ataxia with essential tremor	Autosomal dominant	1st–3rd
2.2	*Cerebellar ataxias of late onset (after age 20)*		
	Cerebellar ataxia with optic atrophy/ ophthalmoplegia/dementia/ amyotrophy/extrapyramidal signs (probably including Azorean ataxias)	Autosomal dominant	3rd–5th
	Cerebellar ataxia with retinal pigment degeneration and possibly ophthalmoplegia and/or extrapyramidal signs	Autosomal dominant	2nd–4th
	Pure cerebellar ataxia of late onset	Autosomal dominant	6th, 7th
	Cerebellar ataxia with myoclonus and deafness	Autosomal dominant	Ataxia in 2nd to 5th

Genetics

The inheritance pattern is autosomal recessive. The underlying defect is an intron triplet repeat in a gene located on the short arm of chromosome 9 (97a, 282a). Patients with Friedreich's ataxia have 200 to 900 GAA repeats, as compared to 7–22 repeats in normal individuals; the result is a disturbance in the synthesis of the protein frataxin (161a, 739a). This leads, in turn, to neuron loss, by a yet undetermined mechanism. Detection of the triplet mutation by molecular genetic techniques enables presymptomatic diagnosis as well as the identification of asymptomatic, heterozygous carriers.

Clinical Features

Friedreich's ataxia is more common in men than in women. The disease usually becomes apparent at about the same age in affected siblings, but sometimes at markedly different ages from generation to generation, even within the same family. The onset is usually in the first or second decade of life; the patient may have had difficulty learning to walk, or may have developed a progressive gait impairment only later. An unsteady, broad-based, slapping gait with frequent falls is always the first sign of the disease. Clumsiness of the hands and slurred speech develop over the ensuing years. The findings in advanced cases include:

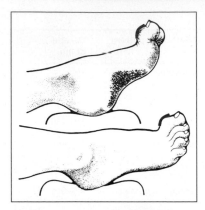

Fig. 3.**11** **Characteristic configuration of the feet in Friedreich's ataxia.**

- ataxia,
- broad-based, unsteady gait,
- explosive speech with an irregular rhythm,
- impairment or loss of position and kinesthetic sense and vibration sense, with little or no impairment of sensation to light touch or pinprick,
- the typical "Friedreich foot": pes cavus with hammer-toe (Fig. 3.**11**),
- scoliosis,
- (sometimes) nystagmus, hypotonia, areflexia,
- and, in later stages, Babinski signs, muscular atrophy, dysphagia, and bulbar signs.

Optic atrophy has also been described in rare cases, and careful examination often reveals oculomotor and vestibular dysfunction. Dementia is rare. The electrocardiogram may indicate myocardial damage; pathological study often reveals extensive interstitial fibrosis of the myocardium with focal degeneration of muscle fibers. The disease progresses inexorably, usually leading to total disability after a number of years, though there are cases in which the progression is much slower.

Treatment

Only *physostigmine* seems to be of therapeutic value in Friedreich's ataxia and other types of spinocerebellar atrophy.

■ Roussy-Levy Syndrome

These authors described a progressive *"dystasie aréflexique héréditaire"* with a probably autosomal dominant inheritance pattern, characterized by bilateral pes cavus, gait impairment, and areflexia in the absence of sensory disturbances, amyotrophy, dysarthria, or cerebellar signs. Posterior column signs and tremor are present in some cases, while pyramidal tract signs, sphincteric disturbances, and skeletal anomalies are exceptional findings.

■ Familial Clubfoot with Areflexia

Sir Charles Symon described the inherited disorder consisting of these, and only these, abnormalities. It causes practically no disability.

■ Rarer Types of Spinocerebellar Ataxia

A *hereditary ataxia of purely posterior-column type* has been described. *Alipoproteinemia* (p. 296) is characterized by ataxia, areflexia, and occasionally pyramidal tract signs. *Transitional states* sharing the characteristics of Friedreich's ataxia and other syndromes (e.g. Charcot-Marie-Tooth disease, p. 588) are also found. For *sensory radicular neuropathy with distal limb analgesia,* see p. 456. The hereditary ataxias are listed in Table 3.**9**.

Metabolic Disorders Mainly Affecting the Spinal Cord

Vitamin B$_{12}$ Deficiency and Funicular Myelosis

Pathophysiology

Vitamin B$_{12}$ is obtained in the diet from meat (particularly liver) and, to a lesser extent, from eggs and dairy products. It plays a role in many metabolic processes, including nucleic acid synthesis. Vitamin B$_{12}$ (also called "extrinsic factor") binds to a secretory product of the mucosal glands of the gastric fundus ("intrinsic factor") to form a hematopoietic factor. Only in this form can it be taken up through the small intestinal mucosa to participate in metabolic processes throughout the body. Inadequate resorption of vitamin B$_{12}$ leads to a deficiency state characterized by megaloblastic anemia and neurologic abnormalities.

Causes

Vitamin B$_{12}$ deficiency is usually due to *inadequate resorption,* either because of a deficiency of intrinsic factor (gastric mucosal atrophy, carcinoma, total gastrectomy) or because of a condition affecting the small intestine (sprue, steatorrhea, terminal ileitis, extensive bowel resection). *Abnormal consumption* of the vitamin in the small intestine occurs in infection with the fish tapeworm *Diphyllobothrium latum* and in abnormal bacterial colonization of the intestine. Inadequate intake of vitamin B$_{12}$ is exceedingly rare, e.g. in persons who follow an unbalanced and strictly vegetarian diet. Even when little or no vitamin B$_{12}$ is consumed in the diet, the body's stores can last for ca. $2^{1}/_{2}$ years before a deficiency develops.

Clinical Features

General and hematologic manifestations include:

- abdominal symptoms,
- fatigue,
- burning of the tongue,
- glossitis,
- (sometimes) hepatosplenomegaly,
- hyperchromic megaloblastic anemia with macrocytosis, leukopenia, relative lymphocytosis, and thrombocytopenia,
- yellow serum, and
- straw-yellow coloration of the skin.

True pernicious anemia with neurologic manifestations is always accompanied by histamine-refractory achylia (i.e., gastric hyposecretion), except in a minority of childhood cases.

The severity of the neurologic abnormalities need not parallel that of the hematologic changes; there may be marked neurologic deficits even in the absence of anemia. The most characteristic finding is a marked proprioceptive deficit, which may develop very rapidly or very slowly; there are often changes in other sensory modalities as well. In some cases, the patient may become unable to walk in a matter of weeks. In more slowly progressive cases, *abnormal sensations in the lower limbs* may be present for months before the patient's mobility is impaired; an initially symmetric paresthesia and dysesthesia is typical. Later, *gait ataxia* develops. Neurological examination generally reveals a marked deficit of position and vibration sense, as well as tactile hypesthesia and hypalgesia, which can rapidly progress to total anesthesia. The intrinsic muscle reflexes are diminished, and pyramidal tract signs are usually present; cases without pyramidal tract signs are sometimes referred to as the "tabetic" or "polyneuritic" form of the disorder. Careful examination reveals evidence of *polyneuropathy* in two-thirds of cases; this may be due, at least in part, to a concomitant vitamin B_1 deficiency. *Lhermitte's sign* (p. 470) is rarely seen. A *decline of visual acuity* with central scotoma occurs rarely, usually in men. Vitamin B_{12} deficiency is a major pathogenetic factor in so-called tobacco-alcohol amblyopia (p. 625).

Mental abnormalities appear in about 4% of patients, always accompanied by objective neurologic signs. They may include:

- neurasthenic symptoms,
- depression,
- confusional states,
- paranoid psychosis,
- amnestic syndromes,
- dementia.

The *CSF protein concentration* may be elevated. Nonspecific electroencephalographic *changes* are found in most cases, but their extent does not parallel the severity of the clinical findings.

Diagnostic Evaluation

Hematologic work-up and evaluation for *achylia* are important for the diagnosis, but the decisive step is the direct demonstration of vitamin B_{12} deficiency by measurement of the *serum vitamin B_{12} concentration* (normal value, 100–900 ng/L). If the value is in the borderline low range, measurement of the serum methylmalonic acid and hemocysteine levels may enable a secure diagnosis. The vitamin B_{12} concentration may be

normal in partially treated cases; the diagnosis can then be made by the *vitamin B_{12} resorption test* (Schilling test). If the orally administered, labeled vitamin B_{12} passes through the bowel without being resorbed, less than 10% of it will appear in the urine—generally even less than 5%, in true pernicious anemia.

Histopathology

An initially reversible demyelination is followed by irreversible axonal degeneration and secondary glial proliferation. In the spinal cord, these changes occur first in the posterior columns, predominantly at midthoracic levels, and then later in the pyramidal and other long tracts. In the brain, there are multiple, small perivascular foci of demyelination.

Treatment

Treatment must be initiated immediately whenever funicular myelosis is suspected. It begins with daily injections of 1 mg of vitamin B_{12} for 2 weeks to replenish the body's stores. Thereafter, injections can be given once a month.

Prognosis

The prognosis is good if treatment is initiated while the disease is still at an early stage, in which the major symptom is a subjective abnormality of sensation and the ataxia and paraparesis are only mild. In later stages, the neurologic deficits are irreversible.

Differential Diagnosis

Subacute ataxia is produced by intoxications of various kinds, e.g., phenytoin overdose, and by acute polyneuropathies, such as porphyria. The *combined involvement of multiple long tracts of the spinal cord* may be a paraneoplastic manifestation (p. 320). Hypokalemia (e.g., of renal origin) occasionally causes a proprioceptive deficit, spasticity, and pyramidal tract signs; so, too, can a portocaval shunt, in rare cases (p. 342). For adrenoleukodystrophy, see p. 295.

Syringomyelia and Syringobulbia

Pathological Anatomy
The defining feature of *syringomyelia* is a tubular or slit-like intraparenchymal cavity (syrinx) extending over several segments of the spinal cord. *Syringobulbia*, a similar finding in the medulla (possibly reaching into the pons), is much rarer. The cavity is filled with yellowish fluid. In a cross-sectional view of the spinal cord, the cavity usually extends from one posterior horn to the other, and comes near the anterior gray commissure. Thoracic syringes sometimes involve the posterior horn on only one side. In syringobulbia, there is often a slit-like cavity extending ventrolaterally from the floor of the fourth ventricle. The syrinx wall is often irregular. The neurons and glia around the syrinx show degenerative changes, and the myelin in its vicinity is poorly stained. Fibrous gliosis is a late finding. The syrinx is partly lined with ependyma only if it is continuous with the central canal. In contrast, *hydromyelia* is simply a dilatation of the central canal of the spinal cord. The hydromyelic cavity is fully lined with ependyma.

Pressure from the syrinx on the surrounding axons leads to secondary degeneration of the ascending and descending long tracts. Sometimes, instead of a cavity, only a column of gliosis is found. Syringomyelia is a rare component of von Hippel-Lindau disease (p. 34). For syringomyelia after spinal cord trauma, see p. 398.

Early Manifestations
The onset of symptoms and signs is usually in the 2nd or 3rd decade of life. *Infantile syringobulbia,* on the other hand, may present soon after birth with stridor and dysphagia. It is often accompanied by other anomalies such as spina bifida or a malformed craniocervical junction. Torticollis may also be present at an early age (see below).

Common and Typical Manifestations
The following symptoms and signs are all consequences of the location of the syrinx in the spinal cord.
- Pressure from the syrinx on the ascending and descending long tracts causes *sensory disturbances* from the level of the lesion downward, and *spastic paraparesis* with pyramidal tract signs, respectively.
- Pressure from the syrinx on the anterior horn ganglion cells causes *muscular atrophy* and weakness, usually over several segments, possibly with fasciculations.
- Destruction of the decussating pain and temperature fibers in the anterior spinal commissure causes a *segmental dissociated sensory deficit* (see Fig. 3.**2**).
- If the syrinx replaces or impinges on all of the entering sensory fibers

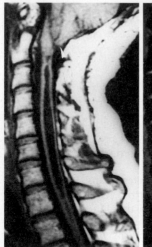
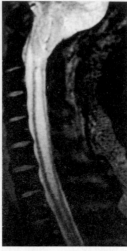

a   b

Fig. 3.**12** **Syringomy-elia accompanying Arnold-Chiari malformation.** MR images. Note the low-lying cerebellar tonsils (arrowhead in **a**).
a T1-weighted spin-echo image. The cavity in the cervical spinal cord is hypointense.
b T2-weighted spin-echo image. The cavity is hyperintense.

of the posterior roots at the level of the lesion, there will be *segmental hypalgesia in all sensory modalities* in the corresponding segments.

- *Pain* is a common symptom, and frequently the initial symptom.
- Destruction of the intermediolateral cell column at upper thoracic levels produces marked *autonomic dysfunction,* with a disturbance of sweating, edema of the hands, etc. The latter, in combination with frequent (painless) injuries and infections, may produce a succulent hand with *mutilation of the fingers* (Morvan type).
- *Arthropathies* are seen in ca. 20% of patients and are likewise due to autonomic and trophic dysfunction.
- *Kyphoscoliosis* is usually a secondary complication.
- *Common accompanying findings* include spina bifida, basilar impression, dolichocephaly, peaked palate, etc. Fixed torticollis in a child may be an early sign of the disorder.

The most common symptoms and signs are listed in Table 3.**10**.

Ancillary Studies
MRI reveals the intramedullary cavity (Fig. 3.**12**), enabling assessment of its size and location. The cavity may also be seen in the later images of a myelogram with postmyelographic CT; this study requires prior knowledge of the level of the lesion so that the CT sections can be obtained at the correct level.

Pathogenesis
The putative causes of syringomyelia are summarized in Table 3.**11**.

Course
The disorder is either slowly progressive, or stable for a prolonged period. Transient improvement of long tract signs does rarely occur, apparently because of a transient drop of pressure within the syrinx. Progression is due both to enlargement of the syrinx and to a steady rise in the pressure

Table 3.**10** Common manifestations of syringomyelia

Symptom or sign	Localizing significance	Remarks
Spastic para- or quadri-paresis	Pressure from cavity on pyramidal tracts	May be unilateral or more prominent on one side
Muscular atrophy	Destruction of anterior horn ganglion cells	Segmental, usually unilateral
Sensory level	Pressure from cavity on all ascending sensory fiber tracts	Differential diagnosis: external compression of spinal cord
Uni- or bilateral dissociated sensory deficit below a particular level	Lesion of the ascending spinothalamic tract on one or both sides	Particularly characteristic
Segmental loss of all sensory modalities	Cavity near a dorsal root entry zone	Usually unilateral
Pain	Lesion of sensory fibers entering the spinal cord, or of ascending spinal cord pathways	
Segmental dissociated sensory deficit	Cavity near the anterior spinal commissure, impinging on the decussating spinothalamic fibers	Bilateral or, less commonly, segmental on one side
Autonomic dysfunction	Lesion of the intermediolateral cell column of the upper thoracic cord, or of the lateral horns	Dysfunctional sweating, succulent edema, lysis of epiphyses, arthropathies
Trophic disturbances	As above	Marked spondylosis, mutilation of fingers
Kyphoscoliosis	Due to weakness of back muscles	Usually late in course, rarely congenital
Associated anomalies	Part of a disorder of embryonal development	Basilar impression, Arnold-Chiari malformation, spina bifida, hydrocephalus

within it. One-third of patients have a benign course (614).

Treatment

Marked progression is an indication for neurosurgical intervention. *Ventriculoperitoneal shunting* may be performed, on the assumption that the enlargement of the syrinx is due to pulse-synchronous CSF pressure waves that are transmitted from the cerebral ventricular system to the syrinx by an open communication between the fourth ventricle and the cervical spinal cord. If syringomyelia is seen in combination with fourth ventricular outflow obstruction, as in Arnold-Chiari malformation, then the treatment usually consists of *decompression of the posterior fossa and craniocervical junction,* possibly with mechanical opening of the closed foramina of Magendie and Luschka. In some cases, a direct opening of the syrinx cavity is indicated (Puusepp's operation), perhaps with insertion of a catheter to form a *syringosubarachnoid shunt.* Another possibility, in case the cavity extends all the way down to the filum terminale (perhaps in association with tethered cord), is to sec-

tion the filum to create a *"terminal ventriculotomy."* Radiation therapy was used decades ago to combat the pain of syringomyelia but is no longer considered a valid form of treatment for this nonneoplastic disease.

Of all of the treatments mentioned, posterior fossa decompression appears to yield the best results, but truly satisfactory long-term follow-up is lacking (614).

Differential Diagnosis

Syringomyelia must be distinguished from other intramedullary processes, such as *tumor, hematomyelia,* and *radiation-induced myelopathy. Noonan's syndrome* consists of an intramedullary cyst in the upper cervical spinal cord in combination with Arnold-Chiari malformation, mental retardation, short stature, a short neck, and other deformities (421). A dissociated sensory deficit can be produced not only by syringomyelia, but also by a thalamic process, a dorsolateral medullary lesion (e.g. Wallenberg syndrome), Brown-Séquard syndrome, or any of the disturbances of nociception discussed below on p. 456.

Table 3.**11** Putative pathogenetic mechanisms of syringomyelia

Mechanism	Supporting evidence
Disorder of embryonal development	Distribution of cavities between alar plate and basilar plate, associated anomalies of midline fusion
Birth injury	Observed association between syringomyelia and difficult delivery
Impaired outflow of CSF from the fourth ventricle	Occurrence in combination with other disorders, e.g. Arnold-Chiari malformation, hydrocephalus; development of syringomyelia after basilar meningitis
Trauma	Development of progressive syringomyelia, after a latency period, cranial to a traumatic spinal cord contusion (4.5% of cases)

Other Diseases of the Spinal Cord

Radiation-Induced Myelopathy

Of the two forms of radiation-induced myelopathy, the one that develops after a short latency has the better prognosis; it can develop rapidly, but generally regresses in a few months. Lhermitte's sign is a typical finding. The late form, arising months or years after radiation therapy, is irreversible (505a).

Decompression Myelopathy

Myelopathy is sometimes the sole manifestation of decompression sickness (Caisson's disease); dysesthesiae and paraparesis or Brown-Séquard syndrome may appear in the absence of tinnitus or vertigo. The symptoms may begin up to 6 hours after decompression and should be treated by immediate recompression (17a).

Other Diseases of the Spinal Cord

Radiation-Induced Myelopathy

Decompression Myelopathy

4 Autonomic and Trophic Disorders

Definition:

The autonomic nervous system regulates the vitally important functions of the internal organs of the body, in a manner largely independent of voluntary movement and conscious sensory perception (Table 4.1). It consists of two component systems, sympathetic and parasympathetic. Dysfunction of the autonomic nervous system manifests itself in abnormalities of cardiac activity, blood pressure regulation, respiration, gastrointestinal function, urination, sexual function, and sweating (32, 571c). Autonomic function is impaired in many diseases affecting the central and peripheral nervous systems. There are also a number of diseases that predominantly or exclusively affect the autonomic nervous system itself.

Table 4.1 Typical manifestations of autonomic dysfunction

Function	Pathological phenomena
Blood pressure	Orthostatic hypotension, syncope
Heart rate	Hypotension not accompanied by reflex tachycardia
Pupillary light response and accommodation	Pupils fixed in midposition
Sweating	Absent sweating
Salivation and lacrimation	Diminished or absent salivation and lacrimation leading to dryness of oral mucosa and conjunctiva
Micturition	Incontinence, overflow
Gastrointestinal activity	Constipation, diarrhea
Male sexual function	Impotence, retrograde ejaculation

Table 4.2 Diagnostic tests for autonomic dysfunction (after Fuji et al. and Weidmann)

Function	Test	Technique	Normal findings
Blood pressure regulation (entire reflex arc)	Orthostatic hypotension on standing, or lying on tilt table	Measurement of blood pressure in the horizontal position at 8, 9, and 10 minutes, then change of position, then remeasurement every 2 minutes for 10 minutes	Systolic BP unchanged or lower, diastolic BP higher; heart rate increased by 10 to 20/min
Blood pressure regulation (sympathetic efferent arm)	Cold pressure test	Immersion of hand and forearm in ice water (4°C) for 1 minute; measurement of BP (and, optionally, ECG) before and after till maximal response is noted	BP rises, heart rate falls
	Hand grip test	The patient squeezes a hand manometer with 30% of maximal force of contraction for at least 3 minutes; measurement of BP before and during contraction	BP rises (diastolic by at least 10 mmHg)
Pupillary reactivity (norepinephrine storage in sympathetic nerve terminals)	Pupillometry	Instillation of 0.2 mL of 2.5% tyramine solution into the conjunctival sac	Mydriasis
Pupillary reactivity	Pupillometry	2.5% methacholine in conjunctival sac	No miosis
Heart rate (vagal efferent arm)	Atropine test	0.04 mg/kg atropine i.v., measure heart rate	Heart rate rises
	Beat-to-beat variation	Measurement of successive RR intervals in the ECG during 30 seconds of deep breathing	Respiratory variation of instantaneous heart rate of at least 10 beats/min

Table 4.**2** Diagnostic tests for autonomic dysfunction (after Fuji et al. and Weidmann)

Function	Test	Technique	Normal findings
Heart rate (vagal afferent arm)	Carotid sinus test	Unilateral carotid sinus massage with simultaneous ECG recording	Heart rate falls
Sweating	Heat test / Pilocarpine iontophoresis	Heating arc / 20 mg pilocarpine	Generalized sweating / Localized sweating
Lacrimation	Schirmer test	Local anesthesia of the conjunctiva with 2 drops of 0.4% oxybuprocaine and insertion of a piece of filter paper (5 mm × 50 mm) into the conjunctival sac	At least 30 mm wet at 5 min; less than 15 mm or a difference of more than 30% between the two sides is considered abnormal
Salivation	Secretion test	Catheterization of parotid duct	0.4–0.8 mL/min

Anatomy

The basic anatomy of the autonomic nervous system is shown schematically in Fig. 4.**1**.

General Symptomatology

The typical manifestations of autonomic dysfunction (32, 58, 571c, 842) are listed in Table 4.**1**. Diagnostic tests for autonomic dysfunction are listed in Table 4.**2**.

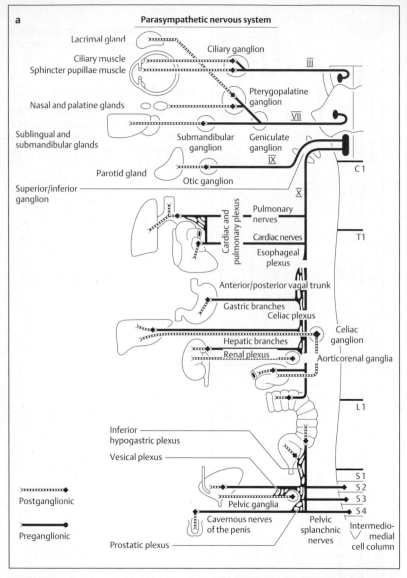

Fig. 4.**1a, b   Diagram of the sympathetic and parasympathetic nervous system.**

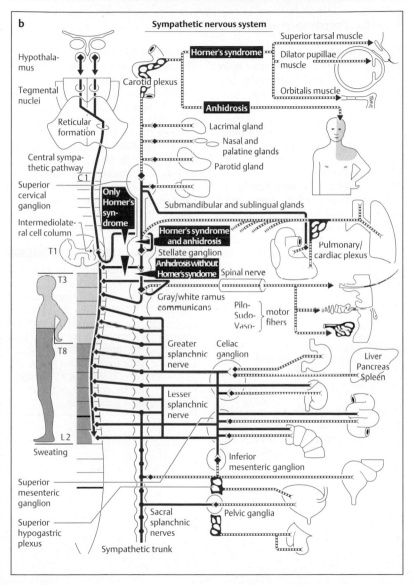

Fig. 4.**1 b**

Acute Pandysautonomia

Pathogenesis

This rare acquired disorder is an acute form of peripheral neuropathy that affects pre- or postganglionic autonomic fibers with a varying degree of selectivity. A small number of cases have been found to be due to infection with Epstein-Barr virus.

Clinical Features

The disorder is characterized by orthostatic hypotension, unchanging heart rate, absent sweating and lacrimation, dry mucous membranes, unreactive pupils fixed in midposition, impotence, constipation, and a hypotonic bladder. Weakness and reflex abnormalities are absent. Dysesthesia and pain may be present, as may hypoventilation and sleep apnea syndrome.

Course

Subacute onset over several weeks, then spontaneous and usually complete remission over many months.

Diagnostic Evaluation

The CSF protein is occasionally elevated. Sural nerve biopsy reveals a diminished number of myelinated fibers.

Differential Diagnosis

The most important item in the differential diagnosis is botulism; the disorder may also be mimicked by polyneuropathies of other origin with predominant involvement of the autonomic fibers–e.g., diabetic polyneuropathy (p. 598). Autonomic dysfunction is seen in HIV infection (607c) and as a component of Adie's syndrome (517a); it can also be a transient secondary manifestation of a tumor of the fourth ventricle (706a) or of Guillain-Barré syndrome (751c).

Treatment

As this disorder tends to regress spontaneously, treatment is often unnecessary. Until improvement occurs, patients should adapt their behavior to avoid provoking orthostatic hypotension. In the rare cases that fail to improve, *intravenous immune globulin* has been found to be effective (399a, 660a). Dysesthesiae can be treated with *carbamazepine or gabapentin*.

Familial Dysautonomia (Riley-Day Syndrome)

Pathogenesis

This rare autosomal recessive disorder is probably due to an impairment of noradrenaline synthesis. Nearly all patients are of Eastern European Jewish descent.

Pathology

The CNS is structurally normal, but pathological changes are found in the peripheral autonomic ganglia and plexuses. There are a diminished number of unmyelinated and small myelinated fibers in peripheral sensory nerves.

Clinical Features

The illness manifests itself in infancy, e.g., with dysphagia and resulting failure to thrive. Dysautonomia is the defining feature of the disease, but it has other manifestations as well. Absent lacrimation while crying, orthostatic hypotension, excessive sweating, dysphagia, ataxia, dysarthria, diminished or absent pain sensation, and emotional lability are practically constant findings, often accompanied by abnormal temperature regulation, absent deep tendon reflexes, vomiting, frequent bouts of pneumonia, and stunted growth.

Prognosis

The prognosis is poor. Fewer than half of all patients survive into adulthood.

Botulism

Pathogenesis

This disease is due to toxins of the anaerobic organism *Clostridium botulinum,* which grows in canned food. It may also result from growth of the organism in soft tissue wounds.

Clinical Features

The typical signs of botulism include impaired accommodation, oculomotor disturbances, dry mouth, bulbar signs, and phenomena resembling polyneuropathy.

Intoxications with botulinum B toxin, in particular, may take a relatively benign course, with exclusive involvement of the cholinergic autonomic pathways (impaired accommodation, dry mouth, and diminished lacrimation) that slowly resolves over the course of several months.

Insensitivity to Pain

Congenital Insensitivity to Pain

This entity includes a number of different clinical variants that have been designated by various terms, e.g., "pain asymbolia."

Congenital Sensory Neuropathy with Anhidrosis

Pathology
In this disease, there is cell loss in the spinal ganglia, while only mild abnormalities are found in the CNS.

Clinical Features
This familial form of insensitivity to pain is usually accompanied by anhidrosis. Self-mutilation and fever are invariably found in early childhood.

Diagnostic Evaluation
A particular familial variety of this disease is characterized by a loss of myelinated fibers with a mosaic-like distribution of Schwann cells, as revealed by sural nerve biopsy. Evoked potential studies document dysfunction of the first sensory neuron.

Sensory Radicular Neuropathy

(acropathie ulcéro-mutilante Thévenard, acrodystrophic neuropathy)

Pathology
Changes are found mainly in the spinal ganglia but also in the peripheral nerves, posterior roots, and posterior columns of the spinal cord.

Clinical Features
This hereditary disorder of autosomal dominant inheritance may appear in childhood but usually appears between the ages of 10 and 40. Its major feature is a dissociated sensory deficit of the feet, associated with ulceration. There are also disturbances of the other sensory modalities, as well as lancinating pains, absent deep tendon reflexes, deafness, muscle atrophy, and involvement of the upper limbs. An elevated serum IgA concentration has been repeatedly described, apparently due to increased production in the jejunal mucosa.

Pain Asymbolia

The acquired disorder known as pain asymbolia is characterized by a loss of defense reactions to painful stimuli anywhere on the body, and by an inappropriate emotional response to these stimuli. It is due to a lesion that interrupts the connection between the sensory cortex and the limbic system (94).

Sympathetic Syndromes

Anatomy and Pathophysiology

The *central sympathetic pathway* probably originates in the hypothalamus; this is where fibers conveying impulses reflecting the individual's emotional state, which descend from the contralateral cerebral cortex, presumably converge with thermoregulatory fibers. From the hypothalamus, fibers of the central sympathetic pathway descend uncrossed into the spinal cord, where they descend further in the lateral column and finally terminate to form a synapse onto the second sympathetic neuron in the intermediolateral cell column between T3 and L2/L3. The axon of the second neuron exits the spinal cord through the anterior root of the corresponding thoracic or upper lumbar segment: the T2–T4 roots supply the sudomotor innervation of the head and neck, T5–T7 that of the thorax, axillae, and upper limbs, and T8–L2 that of the remainder of the trunk and the lower limbs. Each fiber then leaves the anterior root through the corresponding white ramus communicans and enters the sympathetic chain, forming a synapse onto the third neuron in one of the sympathetic chain ganglia. The axon of the third neuron travels over a gray ramus communicans into a spinal nerve root and continues with the sensory portion of a peripheral nerve into the skin (mainly into the sweat glands).

Sweating, piloerection, and vasomotor function are thus controlled by nerve fibers that travel through the sympathetic chain and enter their peripheral end organ by way of sensory nerve branches (Fig. 4.**1**).

Typical Manifestations

Disturbances of Sweating

A lesion of sensory or mixed peripheral nerve(s) causes, not only a sensory deficit, but also a simultaneous *local impairment of sweating* in the area of distribution of the affected nerve(s). The abnormality can be demonstrated with a sweating test (cf. p. 746). Anhidrosis of half of the face without Horner's syndrome is known as harlequin syndrome (188a, 248); it may be accompanied by local flushing, and may be provoked by exercise. *Excessive local sweating,* too, may appear paroxysmally, usually reflecting compensatory hyperhidrosis after partial sympathectomy or localized sympathetic dysfunction elsewhere in the body. It can be produced by hypothalamic disease; by various diseases of the spinal cord, including syringomyelia, tabes dorsalis, tumors, and trauma; and also by peripheral nerve lesions (e.g. due to a cervical rib), as well as by vertebral osteoma, bronchial carcinoma, pleural endothelioma, teratoma of the testes, and so-called sudoriparous nevus.

> **Treatment**
>
> Intradermal injections of botulinum A toxin are effective against excessive local sweating (541a). A rare idiopathic form of this disorder seems to respond to treatment with *clonidine.*

Horner's Syndrome

Horner's syndrome is the clinical manifestation of sympathetic denervation of the eye – in some cases also the remainder of one side of the face, and a variable portion of the ipsilateral upper limb.

Horner's syndrome confined to the eye is characterized by the clinical triad of ptosis, miosis, and enophthalmos. The lack of anhidrosis indicates that the sympathetic chain is intact and that the lesion affects the C8 through T2 roots, as the sudomotor pathway follows the roots below T2 and then ascends in the sympathetic chain. If, however, Horner's syndrome is accompanied by anhidrosis of the face, neck, and arm on the same side, then the lesion is at the level of the stellate ganglion or the carotid plexus. The sudomotor fibers to the face then follow the course of the external carotid artery, while the sympathetic fibers to the eye travel along the internal carotid artery. Thus, carotid dissection (for example) can cause Horner's syndrome without affecting sweating in the face. If sweating is impaired on one side of the body above the waist, but Horner's syndrome is absent, the lesion is in the sympathetic chain just below the stellate ganglion.

Pharmacologic testing can also help to determine the site of the lesion and

Table **4.3**   Differential diagnosis of ptosis according to site of lesion (after Sturzenegger [921])

Type of ptosis	Cause	Special features	Particular etiologies, other remarks
Connective tissue	Old age	Age > 50, familial, bilateral, slow progression	Wide tarsus, normal ocular motility and pupillary reactivity
Myogenic	Dystrophy of extraocular muscles	Very slow progression, sometimes accompanied by oculomotor dysfunction or diplopia	Graefe's chronic progressive ocular myopathy, Kearns-Sayre syndrome with cardiac involvement (oculopharyngeal progressive external ophthalmoplegia)
	Myotonic dystrophy (Steinert)	Flaccid facial musculature, distal limb atrophy	
	Myositis	With proptosis and impaired ocular motility, sometimes generalized muscle involvement	
	Myotonia and paramyotonia	Variable, symmetric, e.g. in response to cold	

(Cont.) →

Table 4.**3** *(Cont.)*

Type of ptosis	Cause	Special features	Particular etiologies, other remarks
Synapto-genic	Myasthenia gravis	Often unilateral, variably severe	Positive Simpson test (see p. 663)
	Botulism	Impaired accommodation, dysphagia	
Neuro-genic	Cortical	Ptosis always mild	Contralateral to a frontal lobe lesion
	Supranuclear (midbrain)	Usually bilateral, sometimes combined with Parinaud's syndrome	Multiple sclerosis, encephalitis, hemorrhage, Wernicke's encephalopathy
	Paradoxical innervation	Congenital, unilateral	Duane syndrome (lateral rectus palsy with narrow palpebral fissure on adduction) Marcus-Gunn syndrome (ptosis at rest, disappears with mouth opening or sideways movement of the jaw)
	Sympathetic	As a component of Horner's syndrome	E.g. in Wallenberg syndrome
	Nuclear	Congenital	E.g. in Möbius syndrome with ophthalmoparesis
	Peripheral	Usually accompanied by third nerve palsy	E.g. in faulty regeneration after third nerve palsy
Pseudo-ptosis	Local orbital changes	Usually due to abnormalities of the globe	E.g. phthisis bulbi (after uveitis), microphthalmia
	Faulty reinnervation after facial nerve palsy	Mass innervation of the facial muscles	
	Blepharospasm	Symmetric, intermittent	
	Cataplexy	Unilateral, transient	Accompanied by other components of the cataplexy-narcolepsy syndrome
	Psychogenic		

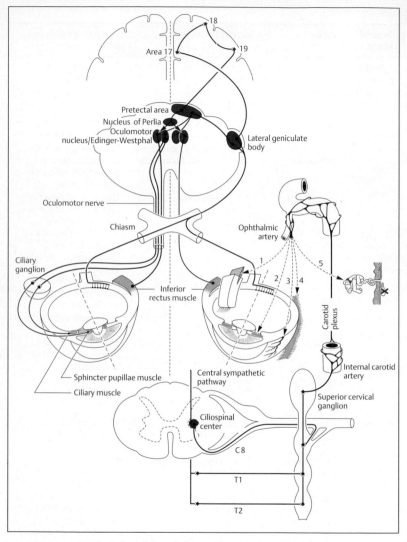

Fig. 4.**2**   **Innervation of the pupil and the anatomical basis of ptosis and Horner's syndrome** (after Mumenthaler [692a]).
1   Superior tarsal muscle
2   Dilator pupillae muscle
3   Conjunctival vessels
4   Orbitalis muscle
5   Sweat gland (anhidrosis)

to establish the diagnosis of true Horner's syndrome as opposed to physiological anisocoria, which is found in 15–30% of normal individuals and even more commonly in the elderly. Bilateral Horner's syndrome is also occasionally encountered (890a). Figure 4.2 provides an overview of the innervation of the pupil.

Ptosis

Ptosis deserves mention here because it is an important finding in differential diagnosis, though its causes are by no means limited to sympathetic denervation of the eye. Numerous diseases of muscle and, above all, of the central nervous system can cause ptosis, as listed in Table 4.3. For further information, see p. 662.

Raeder's Paratrigeminal Syndrome

In this syndrome, a process lying in between the sella turcica and the Gasserian ganglion causes a loss of function in both the sympathetic and the trigeminal pathway, and possibly diplopia as well. The typical findings are unilateral miosis, mild ptosis, facial pain, weakness of the masticatory muscles, and (possibly) oculomotor nerve palsy.

Lesions of the Sympathetic Chain

An infiltrating paravertebral tumor is the most common type of lesion affecting the sympathetic chain and may cause anhidrosis of the thorax or the lower limbs in the absence of a sensory deficit. Conversely, if a sensory deficit is found in the sacral or caudal lumbar segments, a lack of sweating in the same area rules out a proximal root lesion (e.g., compression from a herniated disc) as the cause. The lesion must lie further distally, e.g., in the lumbar plexus, because the sudomotor fibers for the lower limb all exit the spinal cord above L2–L3 and pass through the sympathetic chain to reach the peripheral nerves (cf. Fig. 4.1). For sympathetic chain lesions in Horner's syndrome, see above.

Trophic Disorders

Definition:
Trophic disorders are those that affect the physical condition of bodily tissues, particularly with respect to their volume, consistency, superficial structure, degree of moisture, and so forth. The trophic state of a part of the body depends on numerous factors including mechanical stress and mechanical activity, nerve supply (both somatic and autonomic), perfusion, general nutritional state, and metabolic processes.

In this section, we will briefly discuss trophic disturbances of various organ systems that may be a sign of neurologic disease.

Skin. The skin is affected by various trophic disorders, including progressive facial hemiatrophy (of Romberg). Certain endocrine disorders affect the texture of the skin all over the body (hypopituitarism, hypothyroidism). Scleroderma causes localized hardening and retraction of certain areas of the skin, occasionally taking the classic "coup de sabre" form on the face and scalp.

Subcutaneous fat. Generalized depletion of subcutaneous fat is seen in various disorders, e.g., anorexia nervosa, hypothalamic tumors in children (Russell syndrome), or progeria. *Isolated atrophy* of the facial fat pad of Bichat, which is occasionally a familial condition, gives the face a death's-head-like appearance. *Progressive lipodystrophy* (Morgagni-Barraquer-Simons syndrome) involves loss of fatty tissue from the upper half of the body (104a). Localized loss of subcutaneous fat from the thigh may be seen in diabetics as a consequence of repeated local insulin injection. *Localized augmentation of subcutaneous fat* is seen in lipomas, in benign symmetric lipomatosis around the neck and shoulders (Madelung's disease), and, together with pain, in adiposis dolorosa (Dercum's disease). The subcutaneous fat can also become calcified in scleroderma or in calcinosis universalis, which affects young girls.

Nails and hair. Irritative disturbances of peripheral nerves may cause the nails to grow abnormally rapidly or slowly. In the latter case, the striations are usually exaggerated. Shelf-like thickening and advancement of the nail bed is seen accompanying peripheral nerve injuries and is known as Alföldi's sign. Polyneuropathy due to arsenic or thallium poisoning may produce characteristic, transversely running white stripes in the nails (Mees lines). Prematurely white hair is seen in progeria.

Ulcers. Cutaneous ulcers can be due to ischemia but are also seen in various types of polyneuropathy, particularly diabetic polyneuropathy. Ulcers on the face are seen in various disorders, including trigeminal neuropathy. Disorders that impair pain sensation are often complicated by cutaneous ulceration: among these are syringomyelia, leprosy, congenital insensitivity to pain, Thévenard's syndrome, and Lesch-Nyhan syndrome.

Joints and bones. Destruction of large joints occurs in tabes dorsalis, syringomyelia, and other disorders causing reduced sensitivity to pain. The small, distal joints, particularly the interphalangeal joints of the toes, are vulnerable to destruction in polyneuropathy (particularly diabetic). Osteopenia is seen in Sudeck's dystrophy (now included in the comprehensive term, complex regional pain syndrome).

Muscle. *Muscular atrophy* may be a misdiagnosis in extremely thin individuals; genuine muscular atrophy may be a sign of anterior horn disease or primary myopathy. Isolated atrophy of individual muscles should raise suspicion of a peripheral nerve lesion. Congenital aplasia of a single muscle can also occur, particularly the pectoralis major or the thenar muscles. *Generalized muscular hypertrophy* may be the result of congenital myotonia (Thomson type), bodybuilding, the consumption of anabolic steroids, or congenital hypothyroidism.

Hypertrophy of individual muscles, e.g., of the calf muscles bilaterally, is seen in Duchenne muscular dystrophy as well as in certain subtypes of chronic spinal muscular atrophy of Kugelberg-Welander type. Hypertrophy of a single muscle can also result form chronic unilateral (radicular) denervation, in which case it is accompanied by fasciculations (632). *Calcification and ossification* of muscle occur in traumatic para- and quadriplegia, in myositis ossificans, and as the result of repetitive mechanical trauma (e.g., "saddle calcifications" in horseback riders).

Individual parts of the body. Entire body parts may display trophic abnormalities. Macrocephaly (megalencephaly) without hydrocephalus is usually genetically determined, while microcephaly is only rarely familial and generally reflects a developmental disorder. Macromelia of a single limb may be due to lymphangioma or to the so-called hemi-three syndrome (hypertrophy, areflexia, abnormal temperature sensation, and scoliosis without syringomyelia, often in the setting of familial neural tube closure disorders) (715). Macromelia is also seen in Klippel-Trénaunay syndrome, including that due to arteriovenous malformations of the spinal cord. Micromelia is usually congenital but is sometimes due to a contralateral acquired parietal lobe lesion, or to poliomyelitis.

5   Demyelinating Diseases

Definition

Myelin is an electrically isolating sheath around nerve cell processes that is composed of many tightly wound layers of cell membrane. It plays an important role in the conduction of nerve impulses. This section deals with diseases characterized by alteration and degeneration of the myelin sheath, particularly in the CNS. Some myelin diseases are due to inborn errors of enzymatic metabolism that affect the generation and breakdown of myelin. The leukodystrophies, discussed above on p. 290, are of this type. Most, however, arise only later in life from causes that are not well understood, though immune processes are often a major factor. These diseases impair axonal conduction, producing motor and sensory deficits whose severity and potential reversibility depend on the etiology and extent of demyelination. In some demyelinating diseases, the deficits tend to be progressive and irreversible.

Multiple Sclerosis (76c, 185a, 185b, 714b, 778a)

Definition

Multiple sclerosis (MS) is a demyelinating disease of the CNS (i.e., the brain and/or spinal cord). Myelin degeneration in MS is due to autoimmune processes. Certain hereditary factors and environmental influences, possibly including viral infection, also seem to play a role. A relapsing and remitting course is typical: the neurologic deficits of MS tend to be present for a limited time and then improve partially or completely, only to be followed by new deficits later on. Each relapse may be associated with a different type of deficit than in previous relapses, and may leave a variably severe residual deficit after remission. In the later course of the disease, the deficits—particularly weakness and spasticity—tend to progress slowly, uninterrupted by remission. In a minority of cases, spasticity and weakness are slowly progressive from the beginning.

Typical Clinical Features (185b, 512)

The typical clinical features of multiple sclerosis are summarized in Table 5.**1**.

Table 5.**1**   Clinical features of multiple sclerosis

Symptoms and signs	Remarks
Repeated attacks	• Separated in time • After each attack, either complete recovery or residual deficit
Diverse sites in CNS affected	• Multiple, distinct sites may be involved in a single attack • different sites involved in each attack • Rarely, the clinical manifestations of successive attacks are similar (particularly when the lesions are in the spinal cord)
Progressive neurological impairment	• Cumulative progression with worse residual deficits after each attack • Steady progression independent of attacks (particularly in late-onset disease)
Common symptoms and signs:	
• Lhermitte's sign	An early sign
• Urge incontinence	Patients usually report this only when directly asked about it
• Retrobulbar neuritis	Severe, usually unilateral loss of visual acuity developing over a few hours or days and lasting 1–2 weeks
• Diplopia	Usually due to abducens palsy, practically always reversible
• Nystagmus	Oscillopsia
• Internuclear ophthalmoplegia (INO)	Often subjectively asymptomatic; sometimes produces oscillopsia, hardly ever diplopia
• Spastic paraparesis	Usually a late sign; slow progression
• Spastic-ataxic gait	Highly characteristic sign of advanced MS

Epidemiology

Multiple sclerosis is one of the more common neurological diseases in the temperate zones of the world. Its prevalence (i.e., the fraction of the population suffering from MS at a given moment in time) is highest in northern and central Europe, in Russia, Canada, and the northern states of the USA, in New Zealand, and in southwestern Australia. In these areas, the prevalence of MS reaches 30–110 cases per 100,000 inhabitants; in other areas of the world, it is lower than five per 100,000. The incidence of MS (i.e., the number of new cases per year) is four to six per 100,000 inhabitants per year. In populations of mixed ethnic origin, the highest incidence and prevalence are in persons of European ancestry. Persons migrating from a high-incidence to a low-incidence area as children (below the age of 15) take on the low risk associated with their new country, while those migrating as adults bring the high risk of their home country with them.

MS is found in more than 1% of all autopsies in Switzerland and Germany; the prevalence seems to have increased in recent decades. In the Faeroe Islands, not a single case of MS was registered before 1939, but 24 cases were registered between 1943 and 1960, after the islands had been occupied by British troops during the Second World War.

The extent of familial clustering has been variably estimated at 3% to 12%. In any case, it is known that a person's risk of contracting MS is 15 times greater if a parent or sibling is already affected.

Clinical Features

General Clinical Features

The disease makes its first appearance in young adulthood in two-thirds of all cases, less commonly at older ages or in childhood (805a). In about 60% of cases, individual *bouts of illness* (attacks, relapses) lasting a few weeks at a time occur at irregular intervals over the course of many years. The attacks affect different areas of the CNS each time and thus cause variable clinical manifestations. In the initial phase of the disease, the deficits associated with each attack tend to resolve more or less completely (*relapsing-remitting course*). Later on, there tend to be increasingly severe residual deficits after each attack (*progressive relapsing course*) (540b), and, finally, the patient's condition, especially spasticity, tends to worsen without intervals of improvement in between (*secondary progressive course*). Certain findings of the CSF examination allow a statistically significant distinction between relapsing-remitting and secondary progressive MS (478a). This is the commonest pattern of the disease, but others are also found: *frequent attacks* occurring one after the other and leading, over a few months or years, to cumulative, severe disability (540b); *benign forms* causing only mild disability for decades (398); and, finally, *primary progressive MS* (189a) without relapses or remissions, most often seen in patients who become ill after age 50 or in whom mainly the spinal cord is affected (714a). The sooner such patients reach a value of 8 on Kurtzke's Expanded Disability Status Scale (EDSS; see Appendix), and the more neurological systems are involved, the worse the prognosis (189a). Multiple sclerosis tends to involve specific areas of the CNS, giving rise to *typical clinical manifestations*, including retrobulbar neuritis, internuclear ophthalmoplegia, nystagmus, cerebellar ataxia, intention tremor, spastic paraparesis and spastic-ataxic gait impairment (these will be discussed in more detail below.) The EDSS provides a means of assessing the patient's disability quantitatively.

Specific Clinical Features

■ Ocular Signs

Retrobulbar neuritis is characterized by a severe decline of visual acuity appearing over a few days, usually in one eye at first. The patient can often not even count fingers with the affected eye. The eye may be painful, and eye movement may be accompanied by light sensations. The fundus and optic disc are normal at first ("neither the patient nor the doctor sees anything"). If the inflammatory process affects the distal portion of the optic nerve, the clinical picture of papillitis may develop, followed in 3–4 weeks by optic atrophy, particularly temporal pallor of the disc (a sign that is often too readily diagnosed by the non-specialist). Visual acuity usually begins to improve in 1–2 weeks and may return to normal. One-third of patients who have suffered an attack of retrobulbar neuritis develop other signs of multiple sclerosis within 5 years, and 45% of patients within 15 years; the percentage is higher if retrobulbar neuritis appears very early or recurs soon after the initial attack, or if the CSF findings are abnormal. Patients who go on to develop multiple sclerosis are more often HLA-RT-1a-positive than other

patients. In one study, isolated retrobulbar neuritis was the initial symptom in 19% of a group of patients with MS (894b). Among women with MS, those who had retrobulbar neuritis as their initial symptom have a better prognosis for long-term survival (894b). Two large studies of patients with clinically isolated retrobulbar neuritis revealed that about one-half of them had at least one clinically silent MR signal change in the CNS of the type seen in multiple sclerosis. Such signal changes indicate a higher risk of developing MS in the years to come, though by no means all such patients went on to develop MS over the duration of follow-up (4 years and 6 years), and some patients without such signal changes did develop MS (455, 455a). Thus, the MRI findings in a case of isolated retrobulbar neuritis, whatever they may be, do not make it any easier for the physician to decide what to tell the patient about the risk of MS. On the other hand, the presence of oligoclonal bands in the CSF clearly confers a higher risk of developing MS (340a, 455a). For treatment, see p. 480.

Bilateral, simultaneous retrobulbar neuritis has an entirely different clinical significance. In a study with 30 years of follow-up, no children with this condition went on to develop MS, and only very few adults did. For *visual evoked potentials*, see below. For the *Marcus Gunn pupillary phenomenon* and the swinging flashlight test in retrobulbar neuritis, see p. 662. *Uveitis* in MS is less common than retrobulbar neuritis but nonetheless 10 times more frequent than in the general population.

Disturbances of ocular motility are common in MS. Transient *diplopia* often occurs in the early phase of illness, commonly because of an abducens palsy. In later stages, clinical and oculographic diagnostic techniques reveal abnormal saccades and pursuit movements in some 80% of MS patients; internuclear ophthalmoplegia is found in one-third (p. 649), while "one-and-a-half" syndrome is rarer (p. 649). These oculomotor disturbances are often accompanied by *nystagmus*, which, once it has arisen, generally does not regress. Dissociated nystagmus–i.e., nystagmus that is different in the two eyes—is a particularly characteristic sign. Nystagmus due to MS, unlike that due to other causes, worsens when the body temperature is raised, as may be documented by electronystagmography; indeed, in some cases, nystagmus is only present at higher temperature. Ocular ataxia may occur as a paroxysmal phenomenon (see below).

■ Brainstem Signs

Trigeminal neuralgia arises in 1.5% of MS patients and is thus 300 times more common in this group than in the general population. It is twice as likely to be bilateral in MS patients than in others. Often, background pain is present in between paroxysmal attacks, and there may also be pain outside the distribution of the trigeminal nerve, facial nerve palsy, or other accompanying signs pointing to a pontine lesion. MS-related trigeminal neuralgia responds to treatment with a prostaglandin E analogue (782). Sudden deafness (247) or an acute attack of vertigo resembling an acute vestibular crisis can also rarely be the initial sign of MS.

■ Cerebellar Signs

Cerebellar signs are found in one-quarter of cases. *Ataxia* is often prom-inent; the gait is often not only spastic, but also ataxic. A particularly impressive and characteristic finding is *intention tremor* accompanying goal-directed movement, as revealed by, e.g., the finger-nose-finger test (see Fig. 2.**78**, p. 276). This form of tremor is due to a lesion of the dentate nucleus or its efferent projection. *Dysdiadochokinesia and dysmetria* are usually seen in addition to spasticity and exaggerated deep tendon reflexes. *Scanning dysarthria* with explosive speech is also characteristic (p. 384).

■ Pyramidal Tract Signs

More than 80% of MS patients suffer from spastic paraparesis with bilateral *pyramidal tract signs and hyperreflexia*. If spastic paraparesis remains absent in long-term follow-up, the diagnosis of MS should be questioned. Progressive paraparesis may be the only manifestation of (monosymptomatic) MS, particularly in late-onset disease, and tends to progress rapidly in such cases (430). *Absence of the abdominal cutaneous reflexes* may be an expression of spastic paraparesis. This is of no informative value as an isolated finding, as these reflexes are absent in some 20% of normal adults, but is significant if seen in combination with exaggerated intrinsic reflexes of the abdominal wall muscles. *Spastic gait* is typical of advanced MS, as mentioned above, and often has an ataxic component as well.

■ Sensory Disturbances

These are present in an early stage of disease in about half of all patients. Impaired vibration sense in the lower limbs is especially common. Abnormal spontaneous sensations (*paresthesiae*) and abnormal, spontaneous or evoked unpleasant sensations (*dysesthesiae*) may appear; a limb or limbs may be abnormally sensitive to touch. Severe *astereognosis* may be found in the hands. A dissociated sensory deficit is a rare finding. About one-quarter of MS patients suffer from *pain* (181, 679b, 973) either on the trunk or in the extremities; pain is an early symptom of MS in about 20%. Acute radicular pain is the initial manifestation of MS in a small percentage of patients (779). About 20% of patients with MS complain of back pain (679b).

■ Seizures and Similar Phenomena

An increased frequency of *epileptic seizures* in MS patients has been reported, and contested, by many authors. In our own patients with MS, we have found epilepsy to be about 4 times more common than in the general population. *Tonic brainstem seizures* (see p. 557) should arouse the suspicion of MS, particularly in younger patients, as they may be an early sign of the disease. The same can be said of *paroxysmal loss of muscle tone* with falling (drop attacks) and also of *paroxysmal dystonia.* Rare patients experience repeated attacks of *paroxysmal dysarthria with sudden ataxia* that last for 15–45 seconds each. *Ocular ataxia* may be present intermittently. The potential diagnosis of MS should be thought of in every case of *trigeminal neuralgia,* particularly in younger patients, and particularly when the pain is not always on the same side (see above).

■ Bladder and Bowel Dysfunction

These problems arise in about 20% of patients before their first hospitaliza-tion. Disturbances of micturition are the initial symptom of MS in 2% of patients, and the sole symptom for some length of time in about 10%; they are present at some point in the course of disease in 75% of patients, and permanent in 50% (314). These disturbances range from a hyperreflexic bladder with involuntary emptying to incomplete emptying with accompanying risk of infection. *Urge incontinence* is characteristic, i.e., a sudden, practically uncontrollable urge to void; other types of incontinence are less common.

■ Mental Disturbances

MS patients often display inappropriate euphoria and lack of insight into their illness. As the disease progresses, frank psycho-organic changes often become evident. These progress to dementia in one-quarter of cases, particularly those with a chronic, protracted course (310). Mental disturbances can also be the initial manifestation of MS, usually in combination with brainstem signs (295, 981); we have also seen psychosis as an early sign of MS. Yet investigation of patients in the early phase of MS reveals mental abnormalities in only about 3%.

■ Special Manifestations and Special Forms of MS

Lhermitte's sign is typical, though not pathognomonic, of MS; it is seen in about one-third of patients and is present in half of these on presentation of the disease. It consists of a feeling resembling an electric shock running down the spine, and perhaps into the arms and legs, that can be provoked by forceful flexion of the neck. In our experience, MS patients generally notice this phenomenon themselves and should thus be asked about it directly during history-taking, before the examiner attempts to elicit it with a provocative maneuver. Any other pathological process affecting the cervical spinal cord may also produce Lhermitte's sign, including tumor, arachnoiditis, atlantoaxial subluxation (e.g., in rheumatoid arthritis), radiation-induced myelopathy, chemotherapy, and funicular myelosis (1003). For Lhermitte's sign after traumatic brain injury, see p. 54.

Forceful flexion of the neck rarely induces a transient worsening of spastic paraparesis and gait disturbance; this is known as *McArdle's sign.*

In very rare cases, MS is accompanied by a *peripheral neuropathy* with muscle atrophy (particularly in the hands), areflexia, and even fasciculations. In a few such cases, MRI has revealed correspondingly located plaques in the cervical spinal cord (964). The frequency of peripheral neuropathy in MS as defined by both clinical and neurophysiological criteria has been estimated at 10% (1045). Younger patients with the *hemiplegic type* of MS can become acutely hemiplegic over the course of a few hours, without pain or impairment of consciousness. Complete recovery usually follows in a few days or weeks.

Abnormal fatigability of muscle, similar to that of myasthenia gravis, is seen in rare cases of MS. Cholinesterase inhibitors bring both clinical and electrophysiological improvement. *Abnormal generalized fatigability* is also sometimes reported, even when other signs of neurologic disease are only modest, or even totally absent. Some cases of this type may respond to amantadine and modafinil (see below). The symptoms of MS commonly worsen in a warm environment or with a *rise in body temperature* (Uhthoff's phenomenon). This may be explained as the clinical correlate of a reversible block of conduction in partially demyelinated fibers. Such patients may be able to climb into, but not out of, a hot bath, or may be admitted to the hospital during an acute febrile illness because of a supposed relapse. This phenomenon can be exploited for diagnostic purposes: for example, the ability to discriminate two barely separated light flashes in time may be found to depend on body temperature.

The characteristic findings in MS are depicted schematically in Fig. 5.**1**.

Ancillary Tests

Imaging Studies

MRI is the most important ancillary test for establishing the diagnosis of MS (511). It can reveal plaques as small as 2 mm in diameter (Fig. 5.**2**). Not every signal abnormality on MRI is necessarily due to MS. The MR image is said to be positive for MS when a single contrast-enhancing lesion is found, or nine T2-hyperintense lesions, one or more infratentorial lesions, one or more subcortical lesions, or three or more periventricular lesions. Spinal cord lesions count the same as brain lesions.

Areas of signal abnormality that enhance with Gd-DTPA contrast represent fresh foci of inflammation with disruption of the blood-brain barrier. Such foci do not enhance any more once the acute MS attack is over, but they may remain visible as scars on T2-weighted images or, if brain tissue is lost, as "black holes" on T1-weighted images. The volume of the lesions seen on T2, the number of "black holes," and the extent of brain atrophy are correlated with the degree of neurological impairment (352c). MRI is an expensive test and thus should be used–outside of research–only for the initial diagnosis of MS. The physician must beware of interpreting every signal anomaly on MRI as evidence of MS if there is no clinical correlate to support this diagnosis. CT is less useful than MRI but can occasionally reveal contrast-enhancing plaques. MRI is also useful for monitoring the course of MS and its response to treatment in research studies. MRI does not yet play an established role in the follow-up of response to treatment in the individual patient.

CSF Examination

A lumbar puncture should be performed whenever needed to establish the diagnosis. There is no evidence of any adverse effect of lumbar puncture on the course of the disease. The *total CSF protein concentration* is elevated in about one-third of patients but rarely exceeds 75 mg/dL. *Immunoelectrophoresis* reveals significant increases in the concentrations of IgG, IgA, and IgM, which are less marked under steroid treatment or in the remission phase. Intrathecal production of antibodies is demonstrated in some 70% of cases by an elevated IgG concentration and, in some 90% of cases, by *oligoclonal bands,* which can be visualized by iso-

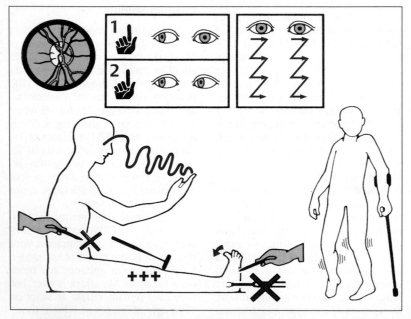

Fig. 5.1 **Schematic representation of the major neurologic findings in multiple sclerosis** (after Mumenthaler [692a]).

electric focusing. Oligoclonal bands are absent in some 5% of cases of clinically definite MS but will appear in the subsequent course of some of these cases. The absence of oligoclonal bands seems to be associated with a relatively benign course (1046b). The *total cell count* is mildly elevated in just under half of all MS patients, hardly ever exceeding 40 cells/mm^3, while plasma cells–absent in normal CSF – are seen in nearly two-thirds of cases. There is no regular correlation among these individual abnormal CSF findings.

Evoked Potentials

Evoked potentials (375, 911) can demonstrate the presence of a lesion in motor and/or sensory nerve path-

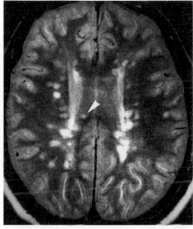

a Axial T2-weighted spin-echo image.

Fig. 5.**2a–c Foci of multiple sclerosis.** Brain MRI in a 24-year-old man. The T2-weighted images reveal multiple, mostly periventricular areas of signal abnormality (plaques) in the white matter. The corpus callosum and brainstem are characteristic plaque sites (arrowheads in a and b). Scattered "active" plaques display contrast enhancement (c).

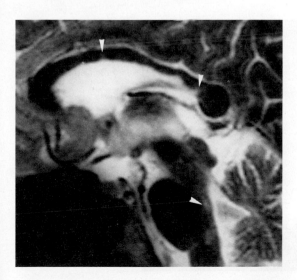

b Sagittal T2-weighted spin-echo image.

ways, but are uninformative regarding the type of lesion. *Visual evoked potential* studies (VEP, p. 475) usually reveal a prolonged latency of the cortical potentials evoked by visual stimuli (Fig. 5.**3**); this is the case in nearly all patients who have had clinically overt retrobulbar neuritis, and in perhaps 70 % of those who have not. Additional recording of *auditory evoked potentials* (AEP) yields abnormal findings in a further group of MS patients with brainstem lesions. Abnormal *somatosensory evoked potentials* (SEP) imply a lesion of sensory pathways (Fig. 5.**4**). Finally, *magnetically evoked potentials* (MEP; 470, 607a, 607b, 801a) can be used to demonstrate a slowing of central motor conduction, particularly with the aid of the triple stimulation technique (TST, Fig. 5.**5**).

■ **Other Ancillary Tests**

Other tests can usually be dispensed with. In about one-third of cases, *EEG* reveals non-specific abnormalities

that are not correlated with any particular mental disturbance. *Serum testing* may reveal an increased concentration of gamma-globulin, and other changes detectable by immunoelectrophoresis, but only during an acute MS attack. Serologic tests are currently not useful in clinical diagnosis.

Prognosis

Longitudinal studies of MS patients and control populations of comparable age structure have shown that a first attack of MS reduces the patient's chance of surviving 10 years by 20%. Most MS ppatients, however, have a normal or only slightly shortened life span. Patients with paraparesis and bilateral Babinski signs are more likely to have an unfavorable course of disease. Other poor prognostic factors are late onset of disease (but only in patients with primary or secondary progressive MS), cerebellar

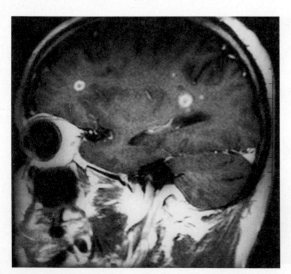

c Parasagittal T1-weighted spin-echo image after intravenous contrast administration.

and brainstem signs, rapid initial progression, and a short interval between the first and second attack (263a).

When MS begins at an advanced age, its progression tends to slow significantly within a few years of onset (812). The claim that men have a worse prognosis than women is inadequately supported (556). The relapse rate of MS has been estimated at 0.5 relapses per year in the first 5 years from onset. The patient's condition 5 years after onset—particularly with regard to cerebellar and pyramidal tract signs—is closely correlated with his or her condition at 10 and 15 years. In a group of male patients with a secure diagnosis of MS, 8% had

died of the disease or its consequences within 10 years of onset, and 20% within 20 years. A hyperacute course of MS, with death occurring within weeks, is encountered in rare cases, particularly in neuromyelitis optica (see below) and when there is rapid progression of brainstem signs. Nonetheless, about one-third of patients are without major disability 10 years after the onset of the disease, and a few remain so at 25 years and beyond. There are thus *benign forms* of MS, which are characterized by complete or near-complete remission after each relapse (however frequent they may be), without significant progression in between (120).

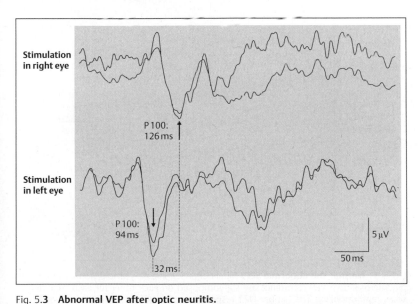

Fig. 5.**3** **Abnormal VEP after optic neuritis.**
A 34-year-old woman with multiple sclerosis and low visual acuity in the right eye. Abnormal VEP on the right. Two VEP recordings are shown superimposed on each other for each side. The latency of the P100 response is normal (94 ms) after left-sided stimulation, but markedly prolonged (126 ms) after right-sided stimulation. These findings are consistent with a demyelinating lesion of the right optic nerve due to retrobulbar neuritis.

The physician may be asked by a life insurance company to predict the course of MS in an individual patient, but this is very difficult (752a). The life expectancy of severely disabled patients is largely a function of the nursing care they receive.

Pathologic Anatomy

MS is characterized by foci of demyelination (plaques) and, later, destruc- tion of axons and neuronal cell bodies. These changes can appear anywhere in the central nervous system but have a predilection for the periaqueductal area, the floor of the fourth ventricle, and subpial areas of the spinal cord. Foci of total demyelination are often sharply demarcated, while subtotally demyelinated areas may merely appear pale. The neurons in the gray matter are often intact and the astrocytes slightly in-

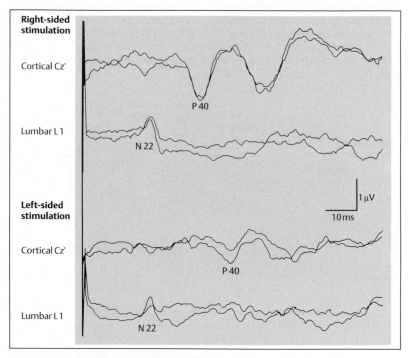

Fig. 5.**4   Normal and abnormal SEP.** Tibial nerve SEP in a 41-year-old woman with multiple sclerosis. Two VEP recordings are superimposed on each other for each condition to show reproducibility. The lumbar N22 response to tibial nerve stimulation is normal on both sides. The cortical P40 response is normal after right-sided stimulation, delayed and diminished in amplitude after left-sided stimulation. Thus, the central sensory transmission time (difference between the latencies of P40 and N22) is normal on the right, abnormal on the left. These findings are consistent with a demyelinating lesion of the spinothalamic (or lemniscal) pathway.

creased in number. Old plaques in the white matter are gray and hardened, with marked glial proliferation, fibrillary gliosis, and an increased density of reticulin fibers. These multiple and sclerotic foci give the disease its name.

Etiology and Pathogenesis

Causes of Multiple Sclerosis

The causes of MS remain inadequately understood despite intensive research (405b, 778a). Many hypotheses have been formulated. The possible role of genetic factors is unclear (288a, 815a), though these may partly explain the few familial cases (see above). Most MS patients in Europe bear the histocompatibility antigens HLA-A3, B7, DW2, and DR2. During an MS attack, the number of suppressor T-cells in peripheral blood is diminished

The two hypotheses with the strongest experimental support at present are that of a *slow viral infection* and that of an *autoimmune mechanism*. Evidence for the former hypothesis is derived from an Icelandic study in which brain tissue from MS patients was injected into sheep; scrapie (an ovine prion disease) appeared in the sheep 18 months later. There is also much evidence suggesting a pathogenetic role for herpes simplex virus (type I) infection in childhood, leading either to clinically silent persistence of the virus or to an abnormal, initially latent immune status. A later viral infection, perhaps with herpes simplex virus (type II), might then provoke the autoimmune reaction that causes MS. The most important evidence for an autoimmune mechanism is derived from an animal model of the disease called *experimental al-*

lergic encephalomyelitis (EAE), which closely resembles human MS, and has a similar relapsing and remitting course. EAE is due to a delayed sensitization reaction to "encephalitogenic" CNS proteins. Sensitized lymphocytes play an important role in this cell-mediated immune process.

Current knowledge is consistent with the following *hypotheses* guiding further research:

- An infection of the neuroglia in childhood is followed by persistence and periodic reactivation of the infective agent. Its primary effect is on oligodendrocytes, causing demyelination; gray matter changes and antibody production are secondary effects. On the other hand, lymphocytic changes may reflect an independent effect of the infective agent on lymphocytes.
- An infection provokes a cell-mediated autoimmune reaction against normal or virally infected components of the central nervous system.
- Multiple sclerosis has more than one cause (which may explain the heterogeneity of its clinical manifestations and course).

Provocative Factors

The cause of MS being unknown, it is not surprising that a variety of toxic substances and other external influences have been said to provoke the initial or subsequent attacks of the disease. Large-scale studies have failed to support such a role for *traumatic brain injury* or *lumbar discectomy* (885). In the rare case of an MS attack closely preceded by a traumatic lesion at a corresponding site in the CNS, a causal connection can be hypothesized, but not proved. A

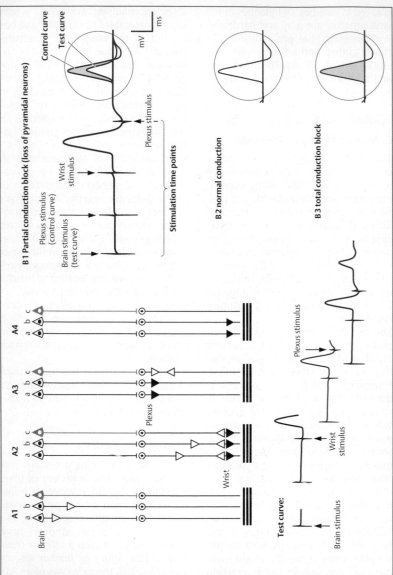

Fig. 5.5 **Technical basis of the triple stimulation technique** (TST). (Modified from Magistris et al., *Brain* 1999; 122: 265–79.

Left side (A): The pyramidal tract is schematically represented by three corticospinal neurons (a, b, c) with monosynaptic connections to three α-motor neurons (a major simplification of the complex segmental wiring pattern). The muscle fibers of the three motor units are represented by horizontal lines. One of the three corticospinal neurons is abnormal and fails to conduct. The white triangles represent action potentials that are not seen in the final recording, while the black triangles represent those that do contribute to the recorded response.

A1 After a magnetic stimulus to the brain, action potentials descend in axons (a) and (b).

A2 The two action potentials due to the magnetic stimulus are not synchronous. A short time after the stimulus to the brain, the peripheral nerve at the wrist is maximally stimulated, so that a summated muscle potential is generated, and antidromic action potentials travel centripetally. Antidromic action potentials traveling up axons (a) and (b) meet the descending action potentials in these axons and cancel them out, while the antidromic action potential in (c) continues along its way.

A3 Finally, a short time later, a third external stimulus is given, this time at the brachial plexus. The resulting synchronized action potentials can travel unhindered down axons (a) and (b) to the muscle, but are blocked in axon (c) when they collide with the antidromic action potential.

A4 Thus, in axons (a) and (b), which had originally been asynchronously activated by the brain stimulus, two synchronized action potentials travel toward the muscle, but no action potential reaches the muscle from axon (c). Recording of the test curve is supplemented by recording of a control curve in which the sequence of stimulation is plexus-wrist-plexus (i.e., the brain is not stimulated), with appropriately adjusted interstimulus intervals.

Right side (B): Possible results of the TST. In each of the three figures (B1, B2, B3), three curves are superimposed: the test curve, the control curve, and the response to stimulation at the wrist alone. The area shaded in red represents the central motor conduction deficit.

plaque may appear at a site of previous brain trauma. It seems that *pregnancy and delivery* may shorten the interval to the next attack, without increasing the overall frequency of attacks; attacks are rarer during pregnancy but more frequent in a brief period thereafter (99, 185d, 805). MS is thus not, in general, a medical indication for termination of pregnancy.

Treatment

We will discuss separately the treatment of individual MS attacks, the long-term treatment of relapsing-remitting and chronic progressive disease, and, lastly, the treatment of individual manifestations of MS, such as spasticity.

■ Treatment of an Acute MS Attack

Treatment

High-dose corticosteroid administration is an established form of treatment for an acute MS attack. It shortens the duration of the attack but has no effect on the further course of the disease. A possible treatment protocol consists of *methylprednisolone*, 500 mg i.v. qd for 5 days (877a). The rapid therapeutic effect probably results from a reduction of CNS edema and reconstitution of the blood-brain barrier; both of these effects can be seen by MRI (510).

In highly active disease, the combination of *mitoxantrone and methylprednisolone* has been found more effective than methylprednisolone alone (263a). *ACTH* was used earlier with good effect but has largely been abandoned because of its frequent side effects.

Oral prednisone alone is not invariably effective (77b). Acute retrobulbar neuritis is less likely to be followed by an MS attack within 2 years if it is treated with methylprednisolone, 250 mg i.v. q6h for 3 days, followed by prednisone, 1 mg/kg p.o. qd for the following 2 weeks (77c). This treatment protocol does not, however, alter the long-term prognosis (77d).

■ Treatment of Frequent MS Attacks

Treatment

Both clinical (449, 450) and radiological studies have amply documented the effectiveness of the immune modulator β-interferon in patients with frequent attacks or with residual neurologic impairment after each attack. Interferons reduce the annual frequency of attacks by about 30% and slow the progression of the disease. The recommended dose of β-interferon-1b is 0.25 mg s.c. every other day. The recommended dose of β-interferon-1a is 22 μg or (if tolerated) 44 μg s.c. three times weekly, or 30 μg i.m. once a week. Treatment with either of these medications should be begun as early as possible (771c).

The side effects of these injections include local pain at the injection site, which can be treated with *analgesics*, as well as flu-like symptoms and fatigue (995b), which can be treated with a *phosphodiesterase inhibitor* (786a). The question whether one interferon preparation is better than the others or

▶

leads less frequently to the generation of neutralizing antibodies has not yet been clearly answered. About one-third of patients develop neutralizing antibodies within 18 months. Among such patients, the treatment is more likely to fail if antibodies are present in two successive assays 3 months apart (450a). Termination of interferon therapy should be considered if clinical progression of the disease has been continuous for 6 months or more, or if three or more attacks requiring corticosteroids or hospitalization have occurred within 1 year (744a).

A number of studies suggest a limited therapeutic role for *azathioprine* (354, 736c). The synthetic polypeptide *copolymer-1*, at a daily dose of 20 mg s.c., appears to be somewhat less effective than β-interferon, but it causes less inflammation at the injection site and rarer flu-like side effects (211a, 471, 1006).

In patients with worsening relapsing-remitting or secondary progressive MS, *mitoxantrone* can be given as an alternative to interferon and copolymer (392c). In a randomized, controlled multicenter trial, mitoxantrone at a dose of 12 mg/m^2 daily was generally well tolerated and slowed the progression of disability and clinical exacerbations. As mitoxantrone is cardiotoxic, however, patients can only take it for a limited time. Another promising drug is natalizumab (667b). In a placebo-controlled trial, patients with relapsing multiple sclerosis had fewer inflammatory brain lesions and fewer relapses over a six-month period if they were treated with natalizumab.

A combination of multiple, individually effective medications should also be considered (488b). Monthly *intravenous administration of immunoglobulins* has been shown to be effective (290a). Vaccination with *autologous irradiated T-cells* reactive to myelin basic protein yielded encouraging results in a small group of patients with either relapsing-remitting or progressive disease (654). The immune modulator *linomide* also seems to be effective (482a).

■ Treatment of Chronic Progressive MS

Treatment

The treatment of the chronic, progressive form of MS is even more difficult. In one study, β-*interferon-1b* at a dose of 0.25 mg s.c. every other day was found to delay the progression of the disease (287a). *Cyclophosphamide* is also said to be effective against this form of MS, but this is less well documented than for β-interferon; in one large-scale study, both cyclophosphamide and *plasmapheresis* were found to be completely ineffective. Chronic administration of *methotrexate* in a low dose of 7.5 mg p.o. once per week, or of *azathioprine* 100–150 mg p.o. qd, appears to slow the progression of the disease (353, 354, 1006).

Innumerable unconventional treatments have been claimed to be effective in the treatment of MS (as is the case with all inexorably progressive diseases). Clear scientific evidence is lacking for the *Evers*

▶

low-fat diet and all other treatments of this kind. Some have actually been proven ineffective, including *hyperbaric oxygen therapy* (582).

Thus, despite a few encouraging successes, it must be admitted that MS remains a progressive disease for which the optimal treatment remains to be found (354a).

■ Treatment of Individual Manifestations of MS

Treatment

• *Spasticity:*
Spasticity is commonly the major manifestation of MS that requires specific treatment. Medications that can be used include diazepam, the GABA derivative baclofen (10–100 mg po qd, usually in the evening), tizanidine (12–20 mg p.o. daily), and gabapentin (300–400 mg daily) (251a). Severe spasticity rarely responds adequately to these oral medications. In such cases, continuous intrathecal application of baclofen through a permanently implanted catheter and pump is the method of choice, though this, too, has its problems (182, 696a, 747b). Spasticity of individual muscles or even of entire limbs can be treated locally by intramuscular injection of botulinum A toxin (252, 336). Contractures can be treated, if necessary, by adductor tenotomy.

• *Urinary dysfunction:*
Urinary dysfunction is common in MS (see p. 470). The treatment depends on the type of urinary dysfunction. The patient with a hyperreflexic bladder can be made to void regularly with the aid of provocative maneuvers. The patient whose bladder empties incompletely, with frequent episodes of incontinence, can be treated with emepronium bromide, 200 mg p.o. tid or qid.

• *Fatigue:*
Fatigue in MS patients responds to amantadine 100 mg p.o. bid (544a), and occasionally to modafinil or tolterodine 2 mg p.o. bid.

• *Other manifestations:*
Paroxysmal phenomena, including trigeminal neuralgia, tonic brainstem seizures, episodic pains and dysarthria, and ocular ataxia can be treated with carbamazepine, oxcarbazepine, or gabapentin (437b, 894a). Intention tremor may be so severe as to be disabling; it may respond to isoniazid (814a) and can otherwise be treated with stereotactic neurosurgical procedures—either thalamotomy or chronic thalamic stimulation through an implanted electrode, though the improvement in overall function is transient (431a). Specialized neurologic rehabilitation and regular physiotherapy and exercise also play an important role, as does appropriate psychological counseling. Treating physicians, nurses, and therapists should maintain a good rapport with their patients by being honest, reassuring, and dependable.

Differential Diagnosis

The major alternative diagnoses to be considered depend on the particular neurologic manifestations in the individual case:

- *Cranial nerve deficits* may be due to various types of focal lesion, such as a dermoid tumor of the skull base, a tumor of the cerebellopontine angle (perhaps with accompanying ataxia and nystagmus), a tumor at the foramen magnum, an optic glioma or sphenoid wing meningioma with optic atrophy, a brainstem astrocytoma, brainstem encephalitis, etc.
- *Hemiplegia* may be due to a brain tumor or stroke.
- *Spastic paraparesis* may be due to a spinal cord tumor or cervical spondylotic myelopathy.
- *Recurrent paraparesis* may be due to a vascular malformation of the spinal cord.
- *Simultaneous cerebellar and pyramidal tract signs,* and possibly also brainstem signs, may be due to a mass or malformation of the brainstem or craniocervical junction. Such processes are often misdiagnosed as MS. Vascular malformations of the brainstem, too, may cause fluctuating neurologic signs with onset in middle age or later.
- *Involvement of multiple areas of the central nervous system* may be due to systemic diseases such as systemic lupus erythematosus (944), sarcoidosis, vascular diseases, toxic encephalomyelopathy, hypothyroidism, or funicular myelosis.
- *Involvement of the eye and of the central nervous system* may be due to vasculitis or an intoxication. Uveitis is found together with neurologic abnormalities in *uveoencephalomyelitis* (Vogt-Koyanagi-Harada syndrome), a rare, presumably viral syndrome that presents with uveitis, impairment of gait, leukodermia, patches of white hair, encephalitis, and fluctuating meningeal signs.
- *Behçet's disease* causes aphthous ulcers, ocular manifestations, and central nervous manifestations, particularly brainstem encephalitis. There is evidence that the CNS disturbances are due, at least in part, to multiple foci of ischemia, secondary to vasculitis. Myopathy is an occasional component of Behçet's disease.
- An eye disease known as *Eales disease,* characterized by recurrent retinal and vitreous hemorrhages, periphlebitis, and vascular occlusion, is occasionally followed by a severe, subacute myelopathy, or, more rarely, by encephalopathy (1000).

Other Demyelinating Diseases

Concentric Sclerosis (Baló's Disease)

Pathologic Anatomy

Concentric bands of demyelination are found, with myelinated zones in between. There are also small foci of demyelination resembling those of MS.

Clinical Features

This disease, also known as *encephalitis periaxialis*, affects persons of both sexes and all age groups (171). It progresses slowly. It often begins with focal deficits, then progresses to increasingly severe weakness and dementia. Sometimes there are signs of intracranial hypertension.

Diffuse Sclerosis (Schilder's Disease)

Children with this disease suffer a rapid mental and neurological decline because of extensive, symmetrical demyelination mainly affecting the centrum semiovale. The disease is considered a type of leukodystrophy.

Acute Disseminated Encephalomyelitis (ADEM)

This disease is presumed to be an acutely progressive variant of multiple sclerosis. As in MS, there are foci of demyelination in the brain and spinal cord with axonal destruction and perivascular lymphocytic infiltration. The illness begins acutely, often with fever, leukocytosis, and CSF pleocytosis with up to 300 cells per cubic millimeter, and may simultaneously in-volve the peripheral nervous system as well. A developmentally immature form of myelin basic protein appears to play a role in the pathogenesis of ADEM (1033c). This disease often progresses rapidly, leading to death within a few weeks, but there can also be a full recovery.

Neuromyelitis Optica (Devic's Disease)

Pathologic Anatomy

Both optic nerves are commonly involved, with either retrobulbar neuritis or papillitis. Myelitis is present as high as the cervical spinal cord, or, not infrequently, the brainstem.

Clinical Features

This disease is characterized by transverse myelitis and optic nerve involvement occurring within a short time of each other. Like ADEM, it, too, can be considered a special, acute presentation of multiple sclerosis; MRI in Devic's disease reveals multiple cerebral foci of demyelination (581). It can, however, remain restricted to the spinal cord and optic nerves, with either a monophasic or a relapsing course (1029b). The latter has the worse prognosis. The disease usually arises very acutely in children or adolescents, with the spinal and ocular manifestations appearing simultaneously or in rapid succession (either may come first).

Prognosis

The prognosis for vision is poor. Spinal cord involvement responds only partially to corticosteroids, and there is usually a residual paraparesis (581).

Subacute Myelo-optic Neuropathy (SMON)

Pathologic Anatomy

This disease is regularly associated with pathologic changes in the anterior and posterior spinal nerve roots, and in the posterior root ganglia. There is also a symmetric demyelination of the corticobulbar tracts and posterior columns of the spinal cord, with axon degeneration, particularly at cervical levels, as well as occasional demyelination of the optic nerve.

Pathogenesis

Ingestion of oxyquinoline preparations is thought to play a role in the pathogenesis of this disease, though only 75% patients were found to have taken these in one study; viral infection is another possible cause. Oxyquinoline-related cases of SMON are very rare outside of Japan; perhaps Japanese are particularly susceptible to the disease because of a genetic enzymatic particularity or because of other, as yet undetermined environmental factors. Ingestion of large amounts of oxyquinoline has also been followed, in some reported cases, by amnestic episodes. *Thallium poisoning* causes a similar clinical syndrome.

SMON is said to belong to a group of demyelinating diseases known as the "central distal axonopathy syndromes."

For amnestic episodes after oxyquinoline ingestion, see p. 387.

Clinical Features

Japanese authors have described a form of subacute myelo-optic neuropathy that is not uncommon in Japan. The neurologic manifestations appear a few days or weeks after nonspecific gastrointestinal symptoms or, in rare cases, after abdominal surgery. Ascending paresthesiae are accompanied by weakness of the lower limbs and, in about one-third of cases, optic neuritis. A fatal outcome is rare, but so is complete recovery; most patients remain significantly disabled, and recurrences have been described.

Hereditary Demyelinating Diseases

See p. 290.

6   Injury to the Nervous System by Specific Physical Agents

Overview

The nervous system may be injured by a number of physical agents other than direct mechanical trauma. The tissues of the central and peripheral nervous system conduct electricity and are thus susceptible to *electrical injury*. Divers who ascend too rapidly from the depths are vulnerable to *decompression injury*, i.e., diffuse or focal CNS ischemia due to the embolization of gas bubbles formed in the bloodstream. *Radiotherapy* of various bodily tissues often affects the nervous system as well; the resulting neurological injuries, which may not appear till many months after radiotherapy, may involve either the central or peripheral nervous system, with a predilection for the brachial plexus. *Hypothermia* can cause peripheral nerve injury.

▌Electrical Injury

Physical Factors

The effects of lightning and man-made electricity on the nervous system (137) depend on the following factors:
- the intensity of the current,
  - which is given by the ratio between electromotive force and resistance; the resistance is, in turn, determined by
  - the size, shape, and type of tissue through which the current passes;
- the duration of the current; and
- the sites at which the current enters and exits the body.

Mechanism

Electricity can injure the nervous system by:

- the direct, immediate effect of the local burn,
- later changes at the burn site, with secondary involvement of nervous tissue by scarring;
- current flow through well-conducting portions of the nervous system, causing (for example):
  - acute loss of consciousness and epileptic seizures,
  - paresis and paralysis,
  - delayed epileptic seizures.

Clinical Features

Heat at the site of current entry produces a *burn* that may directly involve the underlying nervous tissue. This generally occurs when a person is struck by lightning or comes in contact with high-tension wires

(>5000 V). Burns can, however, be produced by household alternating current as well (100–220 V), if the electrical resistance at the site of entry is low (e.g., when the skin is wet) and if the current is applied for a long enough time.

The nervous system is a relatively good conductor of electricity and is thus susceptible not only to direct electrical burns and coagulation necrosis, but also to injury from current that meets nervous tissue along its path through the body.

Current flow through the brain. Current passing through the brain can cause loss of consciousness and generalized seizures. If the current also heats the tissues appreciably, permanent injury may result, e.g. hemi- or quadriplegia, cerebellar injury, parkinsonism, or secondary epilepsy.

Current flow through the spinal cord. Current passing through the spinal cord (e.g., the cervical spinal cord, as it flows from one arm to the other) can cause a more or less complete *spinal cord transection syndrome.* An amyotrophic-spastic syndrome has also been described as a sequela of electrical injury. It has been hypothesized that electrotrauma may, in some cases, contribute to the pathogenesis of classic amyotrophic lateral sclerosis.

Peripheral nerve injury. Electrical injuries of peripheral nerves are rare: paresthesiae, sensory disturbances, or lower-motor-neuron weakness were found in only 3.6% of 10,000 cases of electrical injury (137). Peripheral nerve injury may be of two types, either a burn or a reversible nerve-trunk palsy. The neurologic signs often regress, but are permanent in some cases.

Evidence for causality. The physician may be asked for a medicolegal determination whether a particular neurologic abnormality is the result of an electrical injury. The inference of a causal relationship is secure only if:
- the neurologic lesion is at a site that was demonstrably the point of entry of current or lay in the current path;
- and (preferably) the symptoms arose immediately after the event.

A causal relationship cannot be inferred if the neurologic abnormality arose only later; if, once it was present, it progressed in severity; or if it can be ascribed to another neurologic disease. Non-specific neurologic manifestations such as headache, autonomic lability, and neurasthenic complaints are at most an indirect effect of electrical injury, due to a fright reaction.

Gas Embolism

Gas emboli arise when gas bubbles are formed or introduced in the venous or arterial system (495a). Most cases are iatrogenic.

Venous Gas Embolism
Pathogenesis

Air enters the venous system when a vein is open to the air and the intravenous pressure is lower than the atmospheric pressure. Venous air emboli travel via the heart to the pulmonary arteries and block blood flow to the lungs. They can be produced during surgical procedures on the head with the patient in the sitting position, and especially during heart surgery.

Clinical Features

The classic "mill-wheel" heart murmur is produced by turbulent flow of blood mixed with air in the heart and great vessels. The air bubbles can be seen with ultrasonography. Paradoxical air embolism into the systemic arteries can occur if the foramen ovale is open, or if the volume of air in the veins is very large; for the manifestations of arterial emboli, see below.

Arterial Gas Embolism

Pathogenesis

Arterial gas emboli may arise during cardiac surgery with extracorporeal circulatory bypass, or in the setting of decompression barotrauma (Caisson's disease). In a diver who ascends too rapidly from the depths, the gases–mainly nitrogen – that are dissolved in the blood may become supersaturated upon rapid decompression and come out of solution to form bubbles, which then embolize. Divers with a patent foramen ovale or other type of right-left shunt are at elevated risk for this syndrome; in such cases, the foramen ovale can be prophylactically closed with a surgical or endovascular procedure (1028d). Incidentally, such procedures have also been found to reduce the frequency of migraine.

Clinical Features

The most common manifestations are transient headache, nausea, and vomiting after the ascent. Rarely, there may be an acute spinal cord transection syndrome of variable severity. The *diffuse brain ischemia* produced by arterial gas embolism may manifest itself later with epileptic seizures, neuropsychological abnormalities, or neurasthenic and psychosomatic symptoms.

Treatment

Decompression syndrome should be treated with *immediate recompression*, even if the signs and symptoms are already several hours old. Additional treatment with *hyperbaric oxygen* some time later, even after a delay of 48 hours to 8 days, can promote the improvement of spinal cord manifestations (if present). Further recommended measures in the acute phase are *intravenous fluid therapy* for hemodilution and *heparinization* (495a).

Injury Due to Ionizing Radiation

General Aspects

Radiation therapy can injure the brain, the spinal cord, and the peripheral nerves. The extent of injury depends on:

- the radiation dose per session and the total dose,
- the treatment field,
- and the timing of the treatment sessions.

An empirical measure of the injurious potential of radiation therapy is given by the NSD (normalized standard dose), which is calculated according to the following formula:

$$NSD_{RET} = TD \times N^{-0.24} \times T^{0.11}$$

Here the NSD is expressed in RET (rad equivalent therapy), TD stands for the total dose in rads, N the number of individual doses, and T the duration of treatment. The latency of radiation injury may be months or years, depending on the NSD.

Radiation Injury to the Brain

Mechanism

Radiation necrosis of the brain may occur with a dose of 2800 rad (28 Gy) or more. As already mentioned, the extent and latency of radiation injury are strongly dose-dependent.

Pathological Anatomy

Fibrinoid necrosis of blood vessels, with extravasation of plasma and erythrocytes, is accompanied by lymphocytic infiltration and massive necrosis of nervous tissue, particularly in the white matter.

Differential Diagnosis

Because radiation therapy is usually given to treat a tumor, radiation necrosis of the brain generally requires differentiation from recurrent tumor. Cerebral ischemia is sometimes the indirect result of radiation therapy, when it is due to radiation-induced occlusion of large vessels such as the middle cerebral artery or the internal carotid artery in the neck.

Radiation Injury to the Spinal Cord

The spinal cord, too, like the brain, can be injured by either conventional photon-beam or high-energy electron-beam radiotherapy. Signs of spinal cord dysfunction generally appear only if the dose used is 3500 rads or higher, given over a period of 28 days or less. Radiation myelopathy has been described after radiotherapy for tumors of the pharynx and neck, lymphoma, mediastinal tumors, and lung tumors. It most commonly arises about 1 year after treatment, though the latency may vary from 2 months to 5 years, and rarely longer. The pathoanatomic changes, which mainly affect the white matter of the spinal cord, consist of spongiform demyelination with astroglial reaction in the early phase, and focal or diffuse demyelination with necrosis in later phases. Vessel walls are regularly affected by changes ranging from fibrinoid necrosis with extravasation to telangiectasis. The neurons are often relatively well preserved.

Clinical Features

The clinical presentation of radiation myelopathy is highly varied. *Cervical myelopathy,* the most common syndrome, usually presents with *paresthesiae in the legs,* which may remain the only symptom or may later be accompanied by *Lhermitte's sign* (which usually resolves spontaneously). Other patients suffer from *progressive para- or quadriparesis.* More than half of all patients develop a more or less pure *Brown-Séquard syndrome.* Proprioception is disturbed more often than superficial sensation.

There is some evidence that radiation therapy may induce a form of myelitis accompanied by myoclonus in the lower limbs. This process, when it occurs, may remain stable at a relatively mild degree of severity, but unfortu-nately tends to progress to a more or less complete spinal cord transection syndrome over a period of weeks to months. About half of the affected patients die months or years later from the complications of the myelopathy, while in others the myelopathy can remain stable or even regress.

> **Treatment**
>
> In the absence of an etiologic treatment, only symptomatic treatments are available, e.g., *carbamazepine* to relieve dysesthesia.

Radiation Injury to the Peripheral Nervous System

See p. 764.

Hypothermic Injury

General Aspects

Generalized hypothermia is rarely the result of cold exposure alone; usually other factors are at work that have rendered the patient unable to protect himself adequately against the cold (e.g., alcohol or drug abuse or mental illness).

Clinical Features

Central nervous system. The depth of hypothermia determines the extent to which the patient's consciousness is impaired and his pulse, blood pressure, and respiratory rate are depressed. Severe hypothermia can cause cardiac arrest. The pupillary reflexes and the intrinsic muscle reflexes are diminished, while muscle tone may be increased, and pyramidal tract signs may appear. Meningismus may develop even though the CSF is normal. If the patient survives, there are generally no permanent neurologic sequelae other than those associated with the underlying illness, if any.

Peripheral nervous system. Animal experiments have shown that hypothermia alters the fine structure of peripheral nerves and causes a slowing or blockade of impulse conduction. Weakness and sensory disturbances due to hypothermic peripheral nerve injuries were described in soldiers who fought in the trenches during the two World Wars, and in shipwreck survivors. The thick, myelinated fibers are most susceptible to this type of injury. Myocardial cooling during open heart surgery causes hypothermic injury to the phrenic nerve in 7% of cases; such injuries are not always fully reversible.

Treatment

Resuscitation and *warming* are the essential components of treatment for hypothermia. Severely hypothermic patients may be rewarmed by *extracorporeal cardiopulmonary bypass*, if necessary (993a). Therapeutic success is possible even in cases of extremely deep hypothermia (343b).

7   Epilepsy, Other Episodic Disorders of Neurologic Function, and Sleep Disorders

Epilepsy

Definition:

Epilepsy is characterized by attacks of impaired neurologic function, nearly always combined with loss of consciousness and/or other paroxysmal motor, sensory, or autonomic phenomena. Each seizure is produced by an abnormal electrical excitation of brain tissue that can usually be detected during the seizure as an abnormal pattern on the electroencephalogram (EEG). There are different types of epilepsy that are caused by different structural and functional (metabolic) anomalies of the brain.

History

Epilepsy was well known in the ancient world, both in medical practice and in everyday life. The Greek term *epilepsia* is derived from the verb *epilambanein,* "to lay hold of, seize, attack" (cf. English *seizure*). It is easy to see how the sufferer's obvious lack of self-control during the fit or seizure gave rise, in many different cultures, to the notion of possession by a supernatural being – either an evil spirit or, sometimes, a beneficent one. The Latin term *morbus sacer* ("the holy disease") reflects this primitive conception. Yet Hippocrates, the founder of rational medicine (5th–4th cent. BC), already understood epilepsy correctly as the product of a sick brain. The notion of epilepsy as divine punishment prevailed once again throughout the Christian Middle Ages and was not definitively discarded until the Enlightenment.

The Swiss physician *Samuel Auguste Tissot* described practically all forms of epilepsy in his *Traité de l'épilepsie* of 1770 (491a). The British neurologist *John Hughlings Jackson* proposed in 1873 that epilepsy was due to excessively strong electrical discharges of the gray matter of the brain. Two years later, in Liverpool, *Richard Caton* was able to confirm this hypothesis by direct measurement of cerebral electrical activity in rabbits and monkeys. In this era, too, the antiepileptic activity of bromide was discovered (1857).

Further antiepileptic drugs were developed in the first half of the 20th century – phenobarbital in 1912 and diphenylhydantoin (phenytoin) in 1938. The first human EEG was recorded by *Hans Berger* of Jena, Germany, in 1924 (who gave due credit to Caton). By mid-century, the Montreal neurosurgeon *Wilder Penfield,* in collaboration with the neurologists *Her-*

bert Jasper and *William Lennox,* had succeeded in using direct intraoperative observation and electroencephalography to correlate the normal function of various brain regions with the clinical phenomenology of epilepsy.

Etiology and Pathogenesis

Etiology

In principle, any brain – even a healthy one – can generate an epileptic seizure under certain conditions that render the gray matter unusually excitable. A single febrile seizure in early childhood, for instance, does not qualify as "epilepsy." The term, in its proper sense, refers to a lasting tendency to generate seizures. The cause may be a structural abnormality of the brain, such as a developmental anomaly, a scar due to trauma during the birth process or at any later time, ischemia, focal infection, or tumor. In other cases, epilepsy is due to a metabolic disturbance, such as hypoglycemia, or to a toxic condition, such as alcoholism. The cause of epilepsy often remains unidentified.

Pathogenesis

Epilepsy reflects the abnormal functioning of cerebral neurons. In general, a neuron receives both excitatory and inhibitory influences from other neurons, and fires an action potential only when the overall effect of the excitatory postsynaptic potentials (EPSPs) outweighs that of the inhibitory postsynaptic potentials (IPSPs). Intraneuronal recordings from epileptic foci have revealed a membrane depolarization of abnormally high amplitude that provokes the firing of a series of action potentials at high frequency, followed by hyperpolarization. This type of electrical event, which can be considered a giant EPSP, is called a *paroxysmal depolarization shift* (PDS).

A PDS occurring in the midst of a population of neurons is reflected on the EEG by spikes followed by a slow wave (spike-wave complex). Such complexes may be the initial EEG correlate of a clinically observable seizure. It is not yet known with certainty where these complexes arise; thalamocortical and intracortical

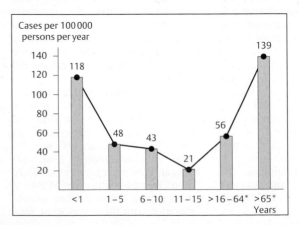

Fig. 7.**1 Incidence of epilepsy by age** (after Schmidt and Elger; data from Camfield et al. and Forsgren et al.). The incidence of epilepsy is highest in the first year of life and after age 65, and lowest in early adulthood.

generation have both been hypothesized. The following processes play an important role in neuronal depolarization and repolarization:

- calcium and sodium influx and potassium efflux,
- excitatory amino acids such as glutamate,
- and inhibitory neurotransmitters such as GABA.

These processes are the basis of various kinds of anticonvulsant therapy. Some medications lessen the sodium influx, others potentiate GABA-ergic inhibition, and others selectively block calcium channels.

Epidemiology

Epilepsy is one of the more common types of neurologic disease. It affects 0.5% to 1% of persons. The onset of epilepsy is more common in the first year of life and after age 65 (Fig. 7.1). Persons with affected family members are more likely to develop epilepsy. If one parent suffers from idiopathic epilepsy, the child's risk is 1 : 25; if one parent suffers from symptomatic epilepsy, the child's risk is 1 : 67. The risk is higher than 1 : 25 if both parents are affected.

Ancillary Diagnostic Tests in Epileptology

We will first discuss the more important diagnostic tests before proceeding to the classification and clinical features of epilepsy.

Electroencephalography
(320, 491,708)

EEG, the most important diagnostic study in epileptology, provides information about the *function*, rather

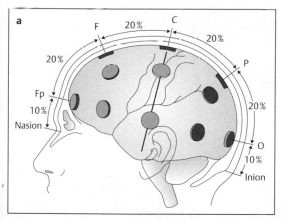

a Lateral aspect.
The electrodes are mounted at the specified intervals between the nasion and the inion.

Fig. 7.**2a–d** **Electrode placement in the 10-20 system** (a–c from K.F. Masuhr and M. Neumann, *Neurologie* (Stuttgart: Hippokrates, 1992); **d** from H. Kunkel, Das EEG in der neurologischen Diagnostik, in H. Schliack, H.C. Hopf, *Diagnostik in der Neurologie* (Stuttgart: Thieme, 1988). The EEG recording from any given electrode reflects the electrical activity of the underlying brain area. Fig. 7.**2b–d** ▶

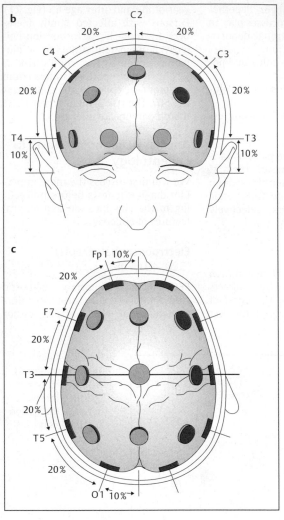

b Frontal aspect. The preauricular points are the reference sites for the placement of the central transverse row of electrodes. C2 is the intersection of the central transverse and longitudinal rows.

c Superior aspect.

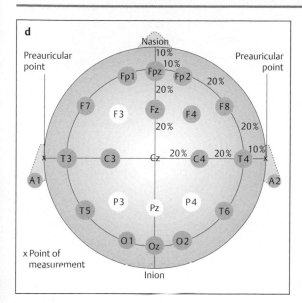

d The names of the electrodes in the 10–20 system.

than the structure, of the brain. It registers changes in electrical potential that represent the net effect of the EPSPs and IPSPs in the cerebral cortex. It also indirectly reflects the function of the thalamus and the midbrain reticular formation, which are responsible for the maintenance of the sleep-wake cycle.

The standard EEG is recorded through electrodes mounted on the scalp according to the *10–20 system* (Fig. 7.**2**). It is a general property of electrical potential that it is not well-defined as an absolute quantity, but can only be measured as a difference between two points. Thus, the EEG is obtained either as a *bipolar recording* (in which potential differences are measured between the scalp electrodes) or as a so-called *monopolar recording* (in which the difference is measured between each scalp electrode and a reference electrode). The ECG is recorded simultaneously with the EEG on the same sheet of paper.

Potential differences at the scalp are on the order of 10–100 µV, while potential differences at the surface of the brain (without the attenuation produced by the skull and scalp) are about ten times higher. EEG activity in different frequency ranges is conventionally designated by Greek letters, as follows:

- sub-δ waves, < 1 Hz;
- δ waves, from 1 Hz up to (but not including) 4 Hz;
- θ waves, from 4 Hz to 8 Hz;
- α waves, from 8 Hz to 13 Hz;
- β waves, > 13 Hz.

The normal EEG in the awake adult with eyes closed consists of sinusoidal oscillations in the range of 8–13 Hz (i.e., α rhythm), maximally intense over the occipital lobes. Faster (β) activity is seen over the

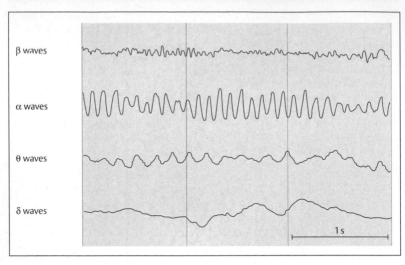

Fig. 7.**3**   **EEG rhythms in various frequency ranges.**

Table 7.**1**   Pathological EEG rhythms and their clinical significance

EEG finding	Clinical significance
Focal slow activity	Localized cerebral lesion – e.g., infarct, hemorrhage, tumor, abscess, encephalitis
Intermittent, rhythmic slow waves	Thalamocortical dysfunction; metabolic or toxic disturbance, obstructive hydrocephalus, deep-seated process near the midline, posterior fossa lesion; a nonspecific finding in patients with generalized epilepsy
Generalized arrhythmic and polymorphic slow activity	Diffuse encephalopathy of metabolic, toxic, infectious, or degenerative origin
Epileptiform discharges – e.g., focal or generalized spikes, sharp waves, or spike-slow-wave complexes	Focal or generalized epilepsy (or clinically silent predisposition to seizures)
Low-voltage activity	Hypoxic-ischemic brain injury, degenerative brain disease, extra-axial lesion such as subdural hematoma (focal low voltage)
Flat-line EEG	Consistent with, but not diagnostic of, death ("brain death")

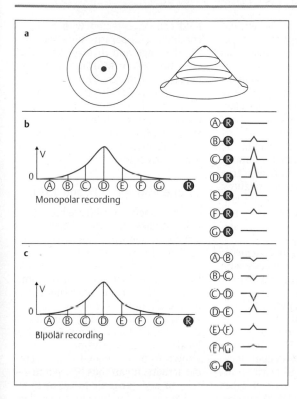

Fig. 7.**4a–c**
Schematic illustration of a sharp wave.

a A sharp wave is produced by the rapid rise and decline of a "hill" of negative potential at the brain surface.

b In a *monopolar recording,* the electrode directly over the peak has the highest potential.

c In a *bipolar recording,* phase reversal is seen over the peak.

frontal lobes, when the eyes are open, during mental activity, or after the ingestion of barbiturates or diazepam. Slower (sub-δ, δ, and θ) activity is seen during sleep or in the presence of diffuse or generalized pathologic processes. Some degree of temporal θ activity is normal in older persons.

Typical EEG rhythms in various frequency ranges are shown in Fig. 7.**3**. Figure 7.**4** shows how the site of origin of a sharp wave can be localized in mono- and bipolar EEG recordings. The sharp wave is best understood as a hill of (negative) potential centered on a particular point on the surface of the brain. The spatial localization of a slow-wave focus is performed in analogous fashion.

Hyperventilation, photostimulation, and *sleep deprivation* are all *provocative methods* by which focal disturbances of brain function can be accentuated to increase the diagnostic yield of EEG (518a). Sleep deprivation puts most patients into a superficial stage of sleep, in which the likelihood of a paroxysmal electrical disturbance is greatest.

A number of pathological EEG rhythms and waves and their clinical significance are summarized in Table 7.**1**.

A valuable technique in the evaluation of patients with epilepsy, particularly those for whom neurosurgical treatment is under consideration, is *simultaneous EEG and video monitoring*. By playing back each seizure at reduced speed and noting the electroencephalographic events corresponding to each phase of the seizure, the clinician can make a number of valuable determinations, among them the distinction between true epileptic and psychogenic seizures. The former generally have an unchanging, stereotyped pattern, while the latter vary from seizure to seizure.

Subacute EEG recording and telemetry, performed over days or weeks with or without accompanying video monitoring, maximizes the chance of capturing a seizure for analysis (263).

Invasive neurosurgical treatment of epilepsy is often preceded, as a final diagnostic step, by EEG recording through electrodes at deeper locations, placed by a semi-invasive surgical procedure: the various types used include sphenoidal electrodes, foramen ovale electrodes, and stereotactically implanted epidural or intracerebral ("depth") electrodes. *Electrocorticography* (ECoG) is the recording of the EEG from the brain surface itself, either through a previously implanted strip or grid electrode, or directly during an open neurosurgical procedure. ECoG enables the localization of abnormal electrical activity with maximal accuracy.

Magnetoencephalography

The electrical activity of neurons generates a magnetic field oriented perpendicularly to the direction of current flow. Variations in the magnetic field can be detected with a superconducting apparatus enclosed in a Faraday cage and displayed together with the EEG or MRI in a single, superimposed image. This enables the highly precise localization of epileptic foci, which is useful in the presurgical evaluation of candidates for epilepsy surgery. Magnetoencephalography is available in only a small number of academic centers.

CT and MRI (pp. 132 and 133)

CT and, especially, MRI are indispensable studies for the detection of structural abnormalities of the brain and meninges. They may reveal potential causes of epilepsy – including, for example, low-grade astrocytoma, cortical dysgenesis, cavernoma, or mesial temporal sclerosis.

Functional MRI (fMRI) enables a three-dimensional representation of local cerebral perfusion, which is known to be correlated with electrical activity. It can thus be used to detect an epileptogenic focus, or to localize important functions (e.g., language) in the brain before resective surgery for epilepsy.

Radioisotope Studies

Isotope diagnosis. SPECT and PET both involve measurement of the γ-radiation (i.e., photons) emitted by intravenously administered radioactive isotope tracers.

Single photon emission computed tomography (SPECT). SPECT enables measurement of regional cerebral perfusion, oxygen and glucose consumption, and blood volume and can thus be used as a test of brain function. It makes use of radioactive technetium or iodine compounds as tracers – e.g., ^{99m}Tc-HMPAO or ^{133}I-iodo-amphetamine (IMP). Central benzodiazepine receptor ligands such as ^{11}C-flumazenil can be used to detect areas of neuronal damage (425). SPECT generally reveals increased regional blood flow at the epileptogenic focus during a seizure, and decreased regional blood flow in the interictal period.

Positron emission tomography (PET). This technique requires a cyclotron close by for the production of the short-lived radionuclides that emit positrons, such as ^{11}C, ^{14}O, and ^{18}F. It is used to generate tomographic images of local cerebral blood flow (CBF), cerebral blood volume (CBV), oxygen consumption (CMRO$_2$), glucose consumption (CMRGlu), and intracellular pH (pH$_i$). It enables the performance of biochemical studies in vivo. Coupling of these radioactive tracers with specific biologically active chemicals, such as DOPA, enables the investigation of specific metabolic processes in the brain (890).

PET and SPECT have vastly increased our understanding of the pathophysiology of numerous diseases of the brain (65). Their primary use in epileptology at present is as part of the preoperative evaluation of candidates for epilepsy surgery.

Classification of Epilepsy (491, 628a, 844a, 904b)

Epilepsy may be classified in various ways:
- by etiology:
  - idiopathic, genetic, genuine
  - symptomatic, due to an acquired lesion of the brain
  - cryptogenic

- by clinical pattern (Table 7.**2**):
  - generalized
  - partial (focal, localized)
  - unclassifiable
  - series of seizures, status epilepticus
- by site of epileptogenic focus:
  - frontal lobe seizures
  - temporal lobe seizures
  - parietal lobe seizures
  - occipital lobe seizures
- by EEG pattern
- by age of onset (e.g., late-onset epilepsy, beginning after age 30).

Epileptic seizures are episodic disturbances of brain function. When epileptic seizures occur repeatedly and without provocation, the patient is said to be suffering from *epilepsy* in the proper sense of the term, while seizures that occur only occasionally and under special circumstances, such as sleep deprivation or alcohol withdrawal, are called *provoked seizures*. A single seizure does not constitute epilepsy. The *suspicion* of epilepsy may, nonetheless, be raised by a single seizure if an EEG obtained thereafter reveals the typical interictal pattern of a particular variety of epilepsy.

In *focal* (partial) epilepsy, the abnormal electrical discharges are confined to a portion of the cerebral cortex. Partial seizures are further subdivided into *simple* and *complex* types: consciousness is preserved in the former, altered (usually impaired) in the latter. Partial seizures with secondary generalization may be impossible to distinguish from primarily generalized seizures from their clinical appearance alone.

Epilepsy due to some other pathologic process, such as a tumor, is called *symptomatic epilepsy*. Epileptic

Table 7.**2**   Classification of epileptic seizures as proposed by the International League Against Epilepsy

1	**Partial (focal, localized) seizures**
1.1	*Simple partial seizures (without alteration of consciousness)*
1.1.1	With motor signs Focal motor without Jacksonian march Focal motor with Jacksonian march Versive Postural Phonatory (vocalization without interruption of speech)
1.1.2	With somatosensory or specific sensory symptoms (elementary hallucinations) Somatosensory Visual Auditory Olfactory Gustatory Vertiginous
1.1.3	With autonomic symptoms or signs Epigastric sensations Pallor Sweating Blushing Gooseflesh Pupillary dilatation
1.1.4	With mental symptoms and/or disturbances of higher cerebral function (almost always involving alteration of consciousness – i.e., generally seen in complex partial epilepsy) Dysphasia Dysmnesia (e.g., déjà vu) Cognitive (twilight states, altered sense of time) Affective (anxiety, excitement) Illusions (e.g., dysmorphopsia) Structured hallucinations
1.2	*Complex partial seizures (with disturbance of consciousness, sometimes beginning with simple manifestations only)*
1.2.1	simple partial onset, followed by disturbance of consciousness with simple partial features, followed by disturbance of consciousness with automatisms
1.2.2	Disturbance of consciousness at onset Isolated disturbance of consciousness Automatisms

(Cont.) →

Table 7.**2** Classification of epileptic seizures as proposed by the International League Against Epilepsy (continued)

1.3	*Partial seizures with secondary development of generalized tonic-clonic (GTC) seizures (= GTC seizures with partial or focal onset; partial seizures with secondary generalization)*
1.3.1	Simple partial seizures with secondary generalization
1.3.2	Complex partial seizures with secondary generalization
1.3.3	Simple partial seizures that develop into complex partial seizures and then become generalized
2	**Generalized seizures**
2.1	*Absence seizures* Only disturbance of consciousness With automatisms With mild clonic component With atonic component With tonic component With autonomic component
2.2	*Atypical absences* Altered muscle tone may be more prominent On- and offset often gradual
2.3	*Myoclonic seizures* Single Multiple
2.4	*Clonic seizures*
2.5	*Tonic seizures*
2.6	*Tonic-clonic seizures*
2.7	*Atonic seizures*
3	**Unclassifiable seizures**

patients who are neurologically normal in between seizures and have no structural abnormality on MRI are said to have *idiopathic epilepsy* (sometimes confusingly called *genuine epilepsy*), which has a genetic basis in some, though by no means all, cases. Epilepsy is said to be *cryptogenic* ("of hidden cause") when it is thought to be symptomatic, but the underlying disorder cannot be determined with current diagnostic methods.

The following sections provide an overview of epileptology based on a clinical classification of seizure type. The revised classification of the International League Against Epilepsy is reproduced in Table 7.**2**. The designations that have been chosen for many types of seizure phenomena are quite complicated and of debatable usefulness. Each of the individual clinical types of epilepsy is associated with specific EEG characteristics and a specific etiology (or etiologies).

Individual Seizure Types

■ Generalized Seizures

Somewhat less than half of all seizures are generalized (the rest are focal). Tonic-clonic seizures are the most common kind of generalized seizure.

■ Generalized Tonic-Clonic Seizures

These seizures, also known as *grand mal seizures* and *primarily generalized tonic-clonic seizures*, are characterized by sudden loss of consciousness, tonic extension of the entire body, and then generalized clonic jerking (p. 508). Some patients with grand mal seizures have at least 90% of their seizures within 2 hours of waking up, while others have them exclusively during sleep. Generalized tonic-clonic seizures may begin at any age.

Absence (Petit Mal) Seizures

Absence seizures, another type of generalized seizure, are characterized by a brief disturbance of consciousness that ends as suddenly as it begins. Ninety percent of absence seizures last less than 30 seconds. Most are accompanied by motor phenomena such as eyelid flutter or mild facial myoclonus, and automatisms may be seen in longer-lasting absence seizures. Motor phenomena are by no means obligatory, however, and falls are uncommon. Absence seizures ac-

companied by abnormalities of muscle tone or autonomic disturbances, and those in which consciousness is gradually rather than suddenly impaired, are called *atypical absence seizures*. Absence seizures are most common in children of a particular age group. The EEG shows characteristic changes. Absence seizures require specific medical treatment.

Myoclonic Seizures

These are characterized by brief, rapid muscle twitches on one or both sides of the body, which, when they occur bilaterally, may be either synchronous or asynchronous. The clinical spectrum ranges from fine twitching of the face, arm, or leg to massive, bilateral spasms of the entire body. Two age-dependent types of myoclonic seizure are *impulsive petit mal seizures* and *myoclonic-astatic seizures*.

Clonic, Tonic, and Atonic Seizures

Myoclonic and tonic seizures sometimes occur as fragments of tonic-clonic seizures; tonic seizures also occur as fragments of tonic-axial seizures. Atonic seizures, also called drop attacks, involve a sudden loss of muscle tone, causing the patient (usually a child) to fall to the ground. A less severe atonic seizure may merely cause a momentary bobbing of the head. Tonic and atonic seizures are the main types of seizure that cause falls.

■ Partial (= Focal) Seizures

The terms "partial" and "focal" seizure are synonymous. Seizures of this type are caused by a focal abnormality in the brain and are not associated with a loss of consciousness or with a generalized tonic-clonic convulsion (unless they become secondarily generalized). *Simple partial seizures* involve either motor or sensory phenomena (or both), while *complex partial seizures,* by definition, involve an altered state of consciousness, perhaps with automatisms and autonomic manifestations as well. A partial seizure of either type may become secondarily generalized.

■ **Simple Partial Seizures**

Simple partial seizures are the expression of an ictal electrical discharge that remains confined in or near the cortical area in which it arises (the epileptogenic focus). Nearly any neurologic manifestation can be the mode of presentation of a simple partial seizure. Purely sensory simple partial seizures are evident only to the patient and not to those around him; such seizures are called *auras.* Motor simple partial seizures are, of course, evident to other persons as well.

The manifestations of simple partial seizures range from simple, elementary movements (Jacksonian seizure, adversive seizure), to unilateral sensory disturbances, to emotional disturbances, hallucinations, and misperceptions. Any type of simple partial seizure may develop secondarily into a complex partial or generalized seizure. In such cases, the initial simple partial seizure is termed the aura of the seizure that follows it.

■ **Complex Partial Seizures**

Complex partial (focal) seizures are characterized by a disturbance of consciousness and a bilateral spread of seizure activity, at least in the limbic system or frontobasal cortex. Patients usually also manifest automatisms, such as the stereotyped repetition of a particular movement, rubbing or wiping movements, chewing, lip-licking, lip-smacking, or abnormal breathing. There may be turning of the eyes, head, or torso to one side or complex stereotyped performances. There may also be involuntary phonation or vocalization, dysarthria, or *speech arrest* – i.e., inability to speak while the ability to understand spoken language is preserved.

Complex partial seizures usually last 1–2 minutes. The patients do not remember these seizures afterward, but most do describe an aura at the beginning of the seizure, most commonly a vague feeling of warmth arising in the epigastrium and ascending retrosternally into the neck. Rarer types of aura include gustatory, olfactory, auditory, or visual hallucinations or a "dreamy state" – i.e., a change in the perceived familiarity of one's surroundings: déjà vu, jamais vu, déjà entendu, jamais entendu. These terms, by the way, should be used in their original, scientific meaning, rather than as they are popularly misconstrued. Thus, déjà vu is the patient's (inaccurate) feeling that a currently experienced, but unfamiliar thing has been seen somewhere before. It is not the reliving of an earlier experience.

■ **Unclassifiable Seizures**

The clinical history often provides an insufficient basis for classification of the seizure type. In such cases, the seizures may be termed (at least provisionally) unclassifiable.

Clinical Patterns of Epilepsy and Epileptic Syndromes

The initial diagnostic question in any patient presenting with "seizures" is whether the seizures are, in fact, epileptic. A thorough clinical history will help answer this question and provide clues as to the specific type of seizure present. The questions to be asked of the patient himself, *and of witnesses,* if any, in the aftermath of a seizure are listed in Table 7.**3**, while the physical examination of the patient in the aftermath of a seizure should include at least the elements listed in Table 7.**4**. Important questions for clinical history-taking in patients with known epilepsy are listed in Table 7.**5**; a model algorithm for the classification of seizure type is shown in Fig. 7.**5**.

Table 7.**3** Questions for history-taking in the aftermath of a seizure

1 About the current seizure:
- Premonitory signs?
- Amnesia?
- Loss of consciousness?
- Manner of waking up?
- Postictal fatigue?
- Injury?
- Tongue-biting?
- Urinary or fecal incontinence?
- Provocative factor?

2 Past history:
- Family history of epilepsy?
- Past events possibly causing brain damage?
  - Perinatal injury (left-handedness, strabismus, psychomotor delay)?
  - Meningitis, encephalitis?
  - Head trauma?
- History of impaired consciousness?
  - Febrile seizure(s) in childhood?
  - Unconsciousness?
  - Bedwetting (possibly due to nocturnal grand mal seizures)?
  - Twilight states? (ask specifically about partial complex seizures and déjà vu)
- If there have been seizures in the past:
  - When was the first one?
  - When was the most recent previous one?
  - How frequent?
  - What kind of seizure?
  - EEG obtained? If so, with what result?
  - Antiepileptic medications taken, if any:
    Which medications?
    Dosage?
    Taken regularly as directed?
    How effective?
    Side effects?

Table 7.**4** Important points for physical examination in the aftermath of a seizure

1 Evidence that a seizure has occurred
- Clinical:
  - Tongue bite
  - Urinary or fecal incontinence
  - Conjunctival hemorrhage
  - External injury
  - Fractured bone
  - Shoulder dislocation
- Laboratory:
  - Elevated CK
  - Elevated prolactin (a few minutes after the event)

2 Clues to the cause of the seizure:
- Clinical:
  - Focal neurologic signs (indicate brain lesion)
  - Signs of intracranial hypertension, esp. papilledema
  - Mental changes
  - General medical illness, heart disease
- Laboratory:
  - CT
  - EEG no sooner than 24 hours after the event (acute postictal changes are nonspecific)

Any particular type of seizure may have a number of possible causes and may be found in multiple epilepsy syndromes. Thus, the diagnosis of the particular epilepsy syndrome that is present requires not only a phenome-

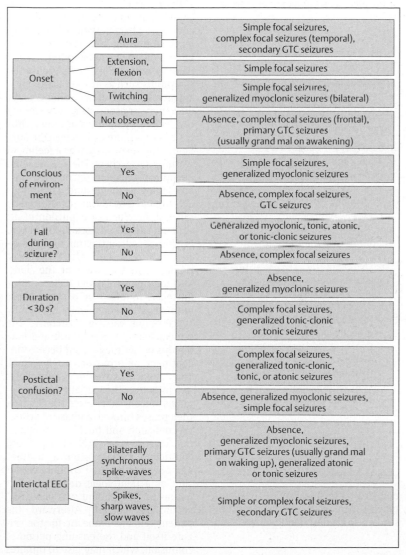

Fig. 7.**5** **Algorithm for the classification of individual seizures** (after Schmidt and Elger)

Table 7.**5**   Questions for history-taking in a patient with known epilepsy

1 Family history

2 Possible causes of an acquired brain lesion

- Birth trauma or hypoxia?
- Meningitis, encephalitis?
- Head trauma?

3 Previous ictal events

- Febrile seizure(s) in childhood?
- Bedwetting (possibly due to nocturnal grand mal seizures)?

4 Details of previous seizures

- When was the first one?
- When was the most recent one?
- Frequency?
- Precipitating factors?
  - Sleep deprivation?
  - Alcohol?
  - Visual stimuli (television)?
- Type of seizure:
  - Aura?
  - Impairment of consciousness?
  - Motor phenomena?
  - Onset in a specific part of the body?
  - Tongue-biting?
  - Other injuries?
  - Urinary or fecal incontinence?
  - Amnesia?
  - Postictal fatigue or confusion?
  - Postictal weakness?
- Antiepileptic medications
  - Which medications?
  - Dosage?
  - Taken regularly as directed?
  - How effective?
  - Side effects?

nological classification of seizure type(s), but also various ancillary studies, to be described below.

■ **Grand Mal Epilepsy**
(Generalized Tonic-Clonic Seizures)

Clinical Features

Grand mal epilepsy is the "classic" and most characteristic form of epilepsy and thus also the form best known to the general public. Many patients report nonspecific prodromal symptoms such as anxiety, irritability, a general feeling of not being well, or difficulty concentrating, preceding the seizure by minutes or hours. Others report a more or less specific aura before the seizure, such as a feeling of warmth in the chest. The seizure itself begins with sudden unconsciousness and falling to the ground, sometimes accompanied by a shout (produced by forceful, involuntary expulsion of air through the closed vocal folds). There is generalized contraction of the muscles, with respiratory arrest, cyanosis, rigidity, and extension of the body. This *tonic phase,* lasting 10 seconds or longer, is followed by a *clonic phase* with generalized, usually bilaterally synchronous muscle twitching. The patient foams at the mouth and may bite his or her tongue and become incontinent of urine or (rarely) stool. The clonic phase generally lasts 2–5 minutes. The patient briefly remains unconscious after the seizure, then passes through a phase of postictal confusion and finally regains normal consciousness. (Note: the word "postictal" means "after a seizure" and does not by itself connote confusion or a neurologic deficit. Inexact use, as in "The patient was postictal," should be avoided.) Afterward, the patient remains amnestic for the seizure itself and the ensuing period of confusion, which may last 10 minutes or longer. The physician examining the patient immediately after a seizure should look for a bite on the lateral edge of the tongue, as this is usually the only abnormality present. Focal neurologic signs in the postictal period, such as an arm or leg paresis that gradually resolves over a few hours (*Todd's postictal paresis*), are evidence of a partial seizure with secondary generalization, and are thus usually due to symptomatic, rather than idiopathic, epilepsy.

Patients with frequent seizures gradually undergo a change of personality, characteristically becoming cognitively slowed, complicated, overprecise, and "sticky," though abnormal agitation and irritability may also be found. Such changes usually do not arise in patients who respond well to appropriate antiepileptic medication.

EEG and Other Ancillary Studies

EEG. The interictal EEG is normal in almost one-quarter of patients with generalized epilepsy and shows characteristic features of epilepsy in only about 50%. These consist of episodic, synchronous, high-amplitude slow waves in all leads, with a few sharp waves and spikes (Fig. 7.**6**). During a grand mal seizure, however, the EEG is abnormal throughout. The ictal EEG occasionally shows a focal, rather than generalized, epileptic discharge at first, even if the clinical seizure phenomena are generalized from the start (see below). If the EEG is normal, the next diagnostic step is *EEG after sleep deprivation* or *subacute EEG recording and video monitoring,* with special electrodes if necessary (see p. 508).

CSF examination. In patients with frequent generalized seizures, CSF pleocytosis is occasionally found, typically with only a few cells but rarely with as many as 100 per microliter.

Serum tests. The serum creatine kinase concentration is elevated after a grand mal seizure, reaching its peak 24–48 hours later. The serum prolactin concentration is elevated 20–60 minutes after a generalized seizure (but never after a psychogenic seizure).

Etiology and Precipitating Factors

Grand mal seizures are often due to an abnormality in the brain that is not detectable by currently available methods of structural imaging ("genuine" epilepsy, primary generalized epilepsy). Hereditary influences often play a role in such cases. Grand mal seizures may also be symptomatic of another process, which may be of any of the types listed below as possible causes of focal seizures; in such cases, the ictal EEG reveals a focal seizure with secondary generalization. *External influences* are of varying importance in individual cases. Possible *precipitating factors* include sleep deprivation and repetitive photic stimulation (strobe light in a discothèque, driving through an artificially lit tunnel, television, etc.). Seizures tend to occur more frequently just after the patient has woken up.

The onset of epileptic seizures during *pregnancy* is more common than that of eclamptic seizures and usually occurs between the 26th and 36th weeks of gestation. Epileptic seizures in the puerperal period may be a manifestation of cerebral venous or venous sinus thrombosis (p. 545). Pregnant women should be treated prophylactically with folate and B vitamins, as both antiepileptic medication (especially phenytoin) and pregnancy itself can cause folate deficiency and osteopenia (for antiepileptic drugs and fetal malformations, see p. 545).

Alcohol can precipitate seizures in epileptic patients and can itself be the cause of epilepsy. Thirty percent of patients with delirium tremens have epileptic seizures, usually before the delirium sets in, and usually 12 or

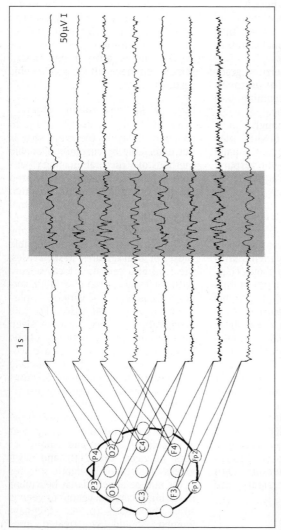

Fig. 7.6 **Interictal EEG in a patient with grand mal epilepsy.** Paroxysmal, generalized, partially atypical spikes and waves are seen simultaneously in all leads.

more hours after the last consumption of alcohol ("rum fits"). Alcoholism can also lead to the development of true epilepsy, with repeated seizures.

Other causes of generalized epileptic seizures are discussed elsewhere in this book under the heading of the individual disease entities. For tumors, see p. 59; post-traumatic epilepsy, p. 55 and p. 531; degenerative diseases, p. 369; cerebrovascular diseases, p. 531. The *treatment* of generalized epilepsy is discussed on p. 532.

Status Epilepticus and Death Due to Epilepsy

Either primarily or secondarily generalized epilepsy may be complicated by *status epilepticus* (599d, 765c), which is defined as a succession of seizures occurring without any interruption in between, or without regaining of full, normal function in between. The seizures in status epilepticus are not necessarily generalized in all phases; there may be, for example, twitching in a single limb only. *Nonconvulsive status epilepticus*, without any visibly abnormal motor activity, can also occur. Status epilepticus is a life-threatening condition, as it produces central hyperthermia, aspiration, electrolyte disturbances, and hypoxic brain injury that may cause death. The mortality of status epilepticus varies from 5% to 20%, depending on its etiology. Its treatment is discussed on p. 543.

Mortality in the first 9 years after the onset of generalized epilepsy, in patients who continue to have seizures despite medication, is elevated by a factor of two to three in patients with symptomatic epilepsy, and by a factor of 1.6 in those with idiopathic epilepsy. Patients with symptomatic epilepsy who die usually do so as a result of the underlying disease. The more common causes of death related to epilepsy itself are (in order of decreasing frequency) refractory status epilepticus, death during a seizure, sudden, unexpected death, accidents, and suicide (181a).

It is thought that *sudden, unexpected death* in an epileptic patient may be due to a seizure-related cardiac arrhythmia, as these are sometimes seen during epileptic seizures (567b, 1027a). Patients with both epilepsy and heart disease need especially meticulous follow-up for optimization of seizure control.

■ Absence Seizures in Idiopathic Generalized Epilepsy ("Typical" Absence Seizures)

Grand mal seizures occur in adolescents and adults of any age; other types of generalized seizure are age-specific (711c). Table 7.**6** provides an overview of the epilepsy syndromes that predominantly affect children and adolescents.

Absence epilepsy is often designated "petit mal epilepsy of school age." Most authors use the term "petit mal" for all minor generalized seizures occurring between the ages of 1 and 13 years.

Clinical Features

In an absence seizure, the affected child suddenly stops whatever activity he or she was engaged in (including speaking), stares vacantly ahead for a period of impaired consciousness that usually lasts no more than a few seconds, and then resumes activity as before. Such absence seizures are sometimes mistaken for "daydreaming." The disorder affects girls more often than boys. The seizures

Table 7.**6**   Epilepsy syndromes that are found mainly or exclusively in children

Syndrome	Age group	Features	Remarks
West syndrome, propulsive petit mal, infantile spasms, salaam spasms	1st year of life	Rocking and nodding movements, twitching of the trunk, forward thrusting of the arms, seizures are very frequent	Often seen in brain-damaged, retarded children. Typical EEG finding: hypsar-rhythmia
Febrile seizures	0–5 years	Generalized seizures when febrile	Later development of true epilepsy is not uncommon
Myoclonic-astatic petit mal (Lennox-Gastaut syndrome)	0–8 years	Variable loss of muscle tone (nodding to collapse), very brief unconsciousness, frequent seizures	Usually in boys; seizures of this type often occur in association with tonic seizures
Typical absences	1–13 years	Unconsciousness lasts several seconds, falls are rare, minor motor phenomena are sometimes seen (picking at clothes), vacant stare, many times a day, precipitated by hyperventilation	Pyknolepsy (when absences are the sole manifestation); possibly seen together with grand mal seizures (mixed epilepsy); EEG typically shows 3 Hz spike-wave pattern
Juvenile myoclonus epilepsy (impulsive petit mal, Janz syndrome)	2nd decade into adulthood	Irregular rocking twitches, more frequent on awakening, no loss of consciousness	Later often combined with grand mal, usually grand mal on awakening
Epilepsy with grand mal seizures on awakening	6–35 years (usually in 2nd decade)	Grand mal seizures within 2 hours of awakening	May be combined with absence and myoclonic seizures
Benign focal epilepsy of childhood and adolescence	1st and 2nd decades	Focal twitching, usually during sleep; patient is conscious in seizures occurring when he/she is awake; 1/5 also have generalized seizures	Multiple subtypes; typical EEG change, biphasic centro-temporal spikes; good prognosis for spontaneous recovery

may be provoked by hyperventilation (a useful test in the doctor's office). Patients who only have absence seizures, and have no seizures of any other type, are said to suffer from pyknolepsy. Falls or major motor phenomena do not occur during absence seizures. So-called petit mal automatisms are common, however; these include movements of the mouth and tongue, picking at clothes, or other minor motor gestures.

Differential Diagnosis

Absence seizures must be distinguished from temporal lobe seizures (p. 524), psychogenic tic, or simple daydreaming. In general, absence seizures occur much more frequently than temporal lobe seizures (perhaps dozens of times per hour), and are usually of shorter duration.

Diagnostic Evaluation

The *neurological examination* reveals no abnormality. The *EEG* reveals an ictal 3–4 Hz "spike and wave" pattern that appears in primarily generalized fashion, in all leads, after previously normal baseline activity (Fig. 7.7). This EEG pattern is diagnostic of absence seizures and can be produced by hyperventilation in 90% of patients. Electroencephalographically recorded events that last less than 3 seconds are not associated with clinically evident absences. On rare occasion, analogous EEG changes are found in children with focal brain lesions; this implies that the child's brain is particularly susceptible to this type of abnormality.

Frequency

Absence epilepsy accounts for less than 10% of childhood epilepsy. About one-third of children with ab-

sence epilepsy have a family history of epilepsy. Thus, this form of epilepsy may be due, in part, to a genetically determined metabolic abnormality.

Prognosis

About one-quarter of patients spontaneously become free of seizures around the time of puberty. Others continue to have absence seizures exclusively, but more than half additionally develop grand mal seizures, which usually occur on awakening. *Mixed epilepsy,* with both petit mal and grand mal seizures, can also arise primarily rather than as a later development of absence epilepsy. Both seizure types are reflected in the EEG. For treatment, see p. 534.

■ Absence Status

A permanently abnormal EEG is the diagnostic feature of this condition, also known as petit mal status or status pyknolepticus. Affected patients appear to be confused, dazed, or in a dreamlike state; they react slowly and answer questions inappropriately, but can often act in a fairly reasonable way. Such states are also known to occur in adults; particularly in advanced age, de novo absence status is not uncommon, usually because of benzodiazepine or alcohol abuse.

■ Other Types of Epilepsy with Absence Seizures

Aside from absence epilepsy of early childhood or school age (pyknolepsy), absence seizures also occur in a number of other, rarer epilepsy syndromes:

- juvenile absence epilepsy,
- myoclonic-astatic epilepsy,
- juvenile myoclonus epilepsy,

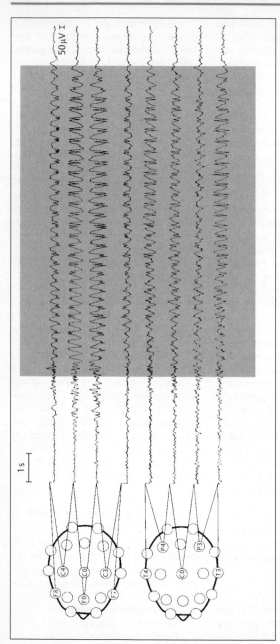

Fig. 7.7   **EEG in absence epilepsy.** Generalized 3–4 Hz spikes and waves on hyperventilation.

- epilepsy with myoclonic absences,
- Lennox-Gastaut syndrome,
- epilepsy with continuous spikes and waves during sleep.

Absence seizures in the context of symptomatic generalized epilepsy are called *atypical absence seizures.* These can arise in adults as well, particularly during benzodiazepine withdrawal.

■ West Syndrome (Infantile Spasms, Salaam Spasms, Propulsive Petit Mal)

This epilepsy syndrome appears in the first year of life and is apparently due to an age-specific reaction of the brain.

Etiology

West syndrome has highly varied causes, including developmental malformations of the brain, perinatal injury, congenital brain diseases, tuberous sclerosis, leukodystrophy, and others.

Clinical Features

The illness is clinically characterized by myoclonus or tonic spasms followed by rapid, jerky forward movements. Nodding of the head may be accompanied by a simultaneous thrust of the arms forward and sideways or by a sudden convulsion of the entire body, with flexion and elevation of the arms and flexion of the legs. These attacks can occur as many as 100 times an hour.

Diagnostic Evaluation

The characteristic *EEG* pattern of West syndrome consists of high-amplitude slow waves with sharp waves and spikes at varying locations (hypsarrhythmia).

Prognosis

The prognosis is poor. The mortality in West syndrome is ca. 25%. Only 20% or fewer of the surviving patients are more or less normal; half are severely retarded, and more than half suffer from persistent seizures of various types. Positive prognostic factors include the lack of a specific etiology, normal development up to the time of assessment, and the absence of other seizure types before the onset of infantile spasms. West syndrome has been reported to undergo a transition to myoclonic-astatic petit mal epilepsy (see below) in some cases.

Treatment

West syndrome is treated with a course of *ACTH* lasting several weeks and with *antiepileptic medication* (see Table 7.11).

■ Myoclonic-Astatic Petit Mal Epilepsy (Lennox-Gastaut Syndrome)

This syndrome is characterized by the combination of tonic seizures, drop attacks, and atypical absence seizures. It mainly affects boys aged 1–9 years (most commonly 1–3).

Etiology

Most cases are due to severe brain damage of some type. In as many as half of all patients, Lennox-Gastaut syndrome is the further progression of West syndrome.

Clinical Features

The seizures may be as minor as a brief nod of the head or may involve a collapse or violent fall to the ground. Falling may also be due to post-myoclonic hypotonia. Short seizures do not impair consciousness appreciably, but there may be brief absences or longer periods of confusion even in the absence of a fall. Tonic-clonic or purely clonic seizures are also present in three-quarters of cases. *Myoclonic-astatic status epilepticus* occurs in one-quarter of patients and is highly associated with the later development of dementia.

Diagnostic Evaluation
The *EEG* reveals a generalized, somewhat irregular spike-wave pattern at a frequency of about 2 Hz ("petit mal variant").

Treatment
See p. 532.

■ Juvenile Myoclonus Epilepsy (Impulsive Petit Mal Epilepsy, Janz Syndrome)
The hallmark of this disorder is bilateral myoclonus. The seizures usually begin in the second year of life and become less frequent thereafter. Myoclonic epilepsy is rare in adulthood.

Clinical Features
The seizures consist of brief, forceful, irregularly occurring twitches that may be single or multiple, independent or bilaterally symmetric and usually involve the neck, shoulders, and upper limbs. They are more common just after awakening and can be precipitated by sleep deprivation or by intense emotion, sudden fright, or a flickering light. Consciousness is preserved. More than half of all patients later develop grand mal seizures in addition, particularly in the morning on awakening. The neuro-

logical examination is normal, but personality disturbances are common.

Diagnostic Evaluation
The *ictal EEG* reveals multiple peaks interrupted by high-amplitude slow waves. This pattern is particularly prominent in photically induced seizures.

Treatment
Valproic acid is the medication of choice (p. 538).

■ Progressive Myoclonus Epilepsies
Progressive myoclonus epilepsy may dominate the clinical picture of Unverricht-Lundborg disease, Lafora disease, neuronal ceroid lipofuscinoses, or myoclonic epilepsy with ragged red fibers (MERRF; p. 905). These are hereditary diseases with an autosomal inheritance pattern, with the exception of MERRF, which is a mitochondrial disease. They are not to be confused with juvenile myoclonus epilepsy.

Etiology
The etiology of progressive myoclonus epilepsy is heterogeneous; it can be caused by storage diseases and by metabolic disorders. MERRF belongs to the group of mitochondrial encephalomyopathies (p. 905).

Pathologic Anatomy
Lafora disease is characterized by typical intracytoplasmic inclusions (Lafora bodies) in neurons, muscle cells, and hepatocytes. Purkinje cell degeneration is seen in Unverricht-Lundborg disease. For ceroid lipofuscinoses, see p. 290; for MERRF, see p. 908.

Clinical Features

This syndrome is characterized by grand mal seizures, progressive dementia, and myoclonus. The myoclonus is asymmetric and usually involves only portions of individual muscles or muscle groups and does not lead to large-scale movements. It is irregular rather than rhythmic and can be precipitated by voluntary movement or by sensory stimuli. Cerebellar ataxia develops later, and sometimes also pyramidal and extrapyramidal signs and visual loss. The illness progresses, leading to death.

■ Epilepsy with Grand Mal Seizures on Awakening

In this syndrome, more than 90% of the seizures occur "on awakening" – i.e., within 2 hours of awakening (by definition); in general, more than one-third of all grand mal seizures are of this type A positive family history is found in some 15% of patients with this syndrome. It begins between the ages of 6 and 35 years, usually in the second decade of life. The seizures are generalized tonic-clonic, and are not preceded by an aura. They may be precipitated by sleep deprivation and can occur in combination with absence or myoclonic seizures. The neurological examination is normal. The interictal EEG reveals generalized spike-wave complexes in 40–70% of cases.

Treatment

Some 80–90% of patients treated with valproic acid are free of seizures.

■ Epilepsy with Grand Mal Seizures during Sleep

In this syndrome, grand mal seizures occur mainly or exclusively during sleep (independently of the time of day or night).

Partial (Focal) Seizures

General Aspects

The clinical manifestations of a focal seizure correspond to the function of the region of brain involved. Partial seizures may have
- *simple manifestations*, such as focal twitching, localized paresthesiae, visual hallucinations, or subjective auras; or
- *complex manifestations*, such as twilight attacks, etc.

Any type of partial seizure may become secondarily generalized.

Etiology

Partial seizures are always due to a focal brain disturbance and are thus *symptomatic* (rather than idiopathic). Whenever partial seizures arise, the underlying pathologic process must be sought. It must also be emphasized, however, that seizures appearing to be of primarily generalized type may be symptomatic as well.

Localization of the Epileptogenic Focus

The clinical phenomenology at the onset of the partial seizure is the most important clue to the localization of the epileptogenic focus. The nature of the seizures should be determined precisely by questioning and by direct observation. The typical seizure semiology associated with epileptogenic foci in various regions

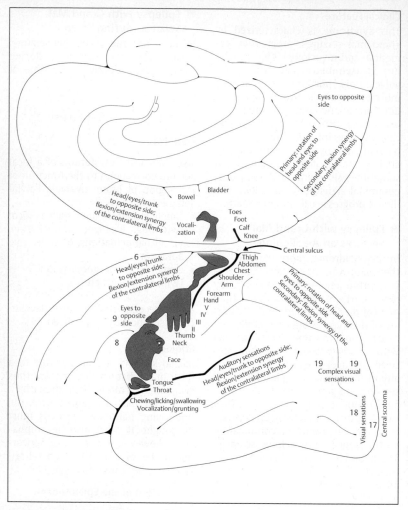

Fig. 7.**8** **Localization of focal epileptic seizures.** The type of attack depends on the site of the focal lesion (adapted from Foerster).

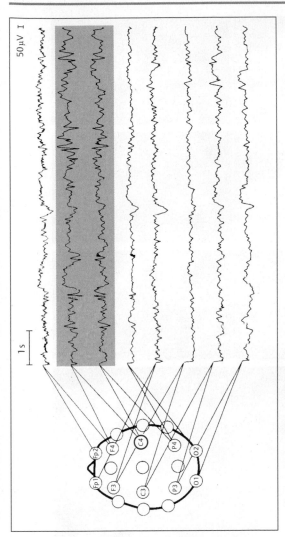

Fig. 7.9 **EEG during a focal epileptic seizure.**
Right central epileptogenic focus with spikes, sharp waves, and slow waves. Phase reversal at electrode C4.

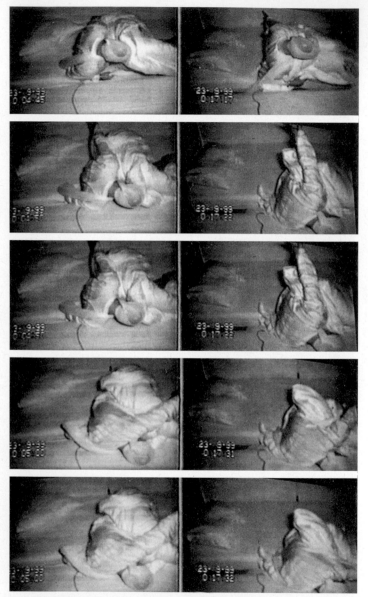

Fig. 7.**10 Infrared video images of a frontal lobe seizure with onset during sleep.**
The images on the left and right sides were taken during two different seizures. Note the parallel, stereotyped course of the two seizures.

of the brain is presented in Fig. 7.**8**. Unfortunately, the diagnostically all-important initial phase, before the seizure spreads and becomes generalized, may be very short and therefore hard to observe. In this situation, the EEG and video monitoring may afford further help in demonstrating focal seizure onset (Figs. 7.**9**, 7.**10**).

■ Simple Partial Seizures
■ Focal Motor and Sensory Epilepsy

Clinical Features

This form of epilepsy is clinically characterized by tonic spasms, clonic twitching, and/or paresthesiae limited to a particular region of the body. The more common sites of seizure onset are the hands and the face, as these are represented by a larger area of cortex than the lower limbs. The seizure may begin with either motor or sensory phenomena; frontal lobe seizures may begin with a tonic torsional movement of the head and trunk or a fencing posture. Other, rarer initial symptoms include sensations of light or visual hallucinations, if there is a focal lesion in the occipital lobe (see below). Simple partial seizures may last anywhere from a few seconds to a few minutes. Consciousness is preserved. Impairment of consciousness occurs only later, if at all, if the seizure spreads and becomes generalized.

Hemiparesis may be observed in the postictal period, for any of the following reasons:

- *Todd's postictal paralysis* is a phenomenon directly related to the seizure and is located on the same side as the focal event; it regresses within a few hours.
- *Persistent hemiparesis* may be due to epileptic activity continuing af-

ter the overt focal seizure has ended, sometimes recognizable as only a very fine clonic twitching of the affected limb.
- *Preexisting hemiparesis* in patients with focal lesions causing both hemiparesis and seizures – e.g., children with perinatal brain injury (HHE syndrome = hemiconvulsive hemiplegic epilepsy).
- *New hemiparesis* due to a new, acute lesion – e.g., infarction in the territory of the middle cerebral artery.

A partial seizure may begin with focal paresthesiae or *special sensory phenomena* if the responsible brain lesion is in a corresponding location; such phenomena include visual hallucinations, auditory sensations, and abnormal tastes and smells (see below, also Fig. 7.**9**). The initial seizure phenomenon, whether it is motor or sensory, may be followed by different focal phenomena (as in a Jacksonian motor seizure) or by secondary generalization to a grand mal seizure with loss of consciousness. *Focal status epilepticus*, with a rapid succession of focal seizures, can also occur. The *neurological examination* may reveal focal deficits in accordance with the focal nature of the disorder.

Diagnostic Evaluation

The *interictal EEG* may reveal epileptiform activity at the focus, slow waves, or, in many cases, no abnormal findings. *Ictal EEG* always reveals seizure activity at the focus (see Fig. 7.**9**).

■ Jacksonian Epilepsy

In a Jacksonian seizure, tonic or clonic motor activity usually begins in the fingers or hand, more rarely in the face or foot, and then spreads to neighboring parts of the body in succession (the "Jacksonian march"), finally involving the entire hemibody or giving rise to a grand mal seizure through secondary generalization.

■ Differential Diagnosis of Focal Seizures

The differential diagnosis of Jacksonian epilepsy includes migraine with aura (so-called *migraine accompagnée*, p. 811). This disorder usually affects patients who already have long-standing migraine. Accompanied migraine attacks almost always arise before age 50, almost always begin in the upper limb, and tend to spread over a period of minutes, rather than seconds as in Jacksonian epilepsy. Headache is present as a rule, and clonic twitching is almost never seen (again unlike Jacksonian epilepsy). Such attacks may appear on alternating sides in the same patient.

Focal spasms, twitching, or paresthesiae may be a manifestation of tetany. For tonic brainstem seizures, see p. 557. Repetitive, focal twitching in the face is seen in hemifacial spasm. Hemimasticatory spasm, which affects the masseter muscle, is a rarity (45) (p. 673). Psychogenic twitching is almost never focal, but rather practically always unsystematic and bilateral.

■ Epilepsia Partialis Continua (of Kozhevnikov)

In this disorder, clonic or myoclonic twitching persists in a limb or region of the body for hours or days, during sleep as well. The EEG reveals strictly focal epileptic discharges. Such seizures may arise many years after the causative brain lesion.

■ Rasmussen's Syndrome

This rare variety of chronic partial epilepsy mainly affects children. The focal seizures are accompanied by progressive neurologic deficits, and the EEG reveals multiple contralateral epileptogenic foci. MRI and histopathologic study reveal encephalitic changes; an autoimmune process can be demonstrated (antibodies against glutamate receptors). Plasmapheresis offers a chance of therapeutic benefit (729b).

■ Benign Partial Epilepsy of Childhood and Adolescence, Rolandic Epilepsy (1029c)

Clinical Features

These seizures are *age-dependent,* arising usually around age 10, and occur mainly during sleep. Those that occur during waking hours typically do not impair consciousness. The seizures usually begin with motor phenomena such as twitching of the face or oropharynx, more rarely with somatosensory or special sensory phenomena. Only about one-third of seizures become secondarily generalized. Twenty percent of the affected children or adolescents have only a single seizure, and only one-third have frequent seizures. Patients with this condition are usually neurologically normal and undergo normal cognitive and behavioral development.

Diagnostic Evaluation

The *EEG* almost always reveals unilateral, centrotemporal, biphasic spikes of high amplitude ("épilepsie à pointes rolandiques," rolandic spikes).

Differential Diagnosis

The differentiation of a single episode of rolandic epilepsy from a single focal seizure, when the EEG is normal, is probably no more than an arbitrary matter of nomenclature.

Prognosis

The prognosis is good. The seizures usually disappear during puberty, and the EEG becomes normal. A subgroup of patients with this disorder begin to experience seizures at the age of 5 years or earlier, have absence, myoclonic, and atonic seizures as well, and show continuous, generalized spike-wave activity on their sleep-EEG (711c); the seizures apparently stop spontaneously once these patients reach adulthood (243b). A further type of benign childhood epilepsy (the Panayiotopoulos type), which constitutes one of the occipital lobe epilepsy syndromes, has a similarly favorable course (166b). Children with this syndrome have partial seizures with ictal vomiting, ocular deviation, and, occasionally, loss of consciousness and convulsions, and their EEG reveals occipital lobe spikes.

▌Treatment▐

Treatment is not always required. *Sulthiame, carbamazepine,* and *valproate* are effective when needed (781a).

■ Adversive Seizures

Adversive seizures are caused by a focus lying in the precentral area of the

Table 7.7   Partial complex epilepsy: classification by site of origin

Site of origin, type of epilepsy	Subtype	Typical seizure type
Temporal lobe epilepsy	Medial temporal lobe	Complex focal seizures, epigastric aura
	Lateral temporal lobe	Complex focal seizures, auditory or vestibular aura
Frontal lobe epilepsy	Rolandic epilepsy	Simple focal seizures, mostly motor
	Supplementary motor area	Asymmetric tonic seizures, adversive seizures
	Cingulate gyrus	Absence-like complex focal seizures
	Frontopolar area	Complex focal seizures
	Dorsolateral area	Generalized tonic-clonic seizures
	Orbitofrontal area	Complex focal seizures
Parietal lobe epilepsy		Simple or complex focal seizures with sensory phenomena
Occipital lobe epilepsy		Simple or complex focal seizures, visual hallucinations

frontal lobe or in the supplementary motor area on the medial surface of the frontal lobe (see Fig. 7.**8**). They are clinically characterized by tonic deviation of the eyes, head, and (often) arm and shoulder to the side opposite the cortical focus. In some 10% of patients, however, the head turns to the side of the focus. Consciousness is preserved at first but may be lost secondarily if the seizure becomes generalized. A focus in the temporal, occipital, or parietal lobe may produce a seizure beginning with a sensory aura, in which consciousness is impaired before the adversive movements take place.

■ Complex Partial Seizures

This form of epilepsy, also called "focal epilepsy with complex partial seizures," is further subclassified according to the site of origin of seizures (Table 7.**7**). Some 60-70% of patients with complex partial seizures have a focus in the medial temporal lobe. The frontal lobe is the next most common site; parietal and occipital foci are rare.

■ Temporal Lobe Epilepsy

Medial temporal lobe epilepsy is common, while *lateral temporal lobe epilepsy* is rare.

Medial Temporal Lobe Epilepsy

The seizures originate in the amygdala-hippocampus complex, a portion of the limbic system. Earlier synonyms for this type of epilepsy were "psychomotor epilepsy" and "temporal lobe epilepsy" (not further specified). A current alternative name is "mesiobasal-limbic epilepsy." Twilight states, involving a clouding (but not total loss) of consciousness, are

the clinical hallmark of medial temporal lobe epilepsy.

Etiology and course. Seizures of this type are due to a lesion in the limbic system or the mediobasal portion of the temporal lobe. They may first appear in childhood, adolescence, or adulthood, but most commonly between the ages of 10 and 20. It is not uncommon for a patient who sustained from one or more febrile seizures in childhood to develop medial temporal lobe epilepsy in adolescence; in such cases, the underlying lesion is usually hippocampal sclerosis. Other causes include hamartoma, arteriovenous malformation, tumors such as astrocytoma and oligodendroglioma, and post-traumatic gliosis. Familial medial temporal lobe epilepsy can occur on a genetic basis.

Clinical features. The seizures typically consist of a twilight state that begins suddenly, lasts for a variable period from less than a minute to several hours, and then gradually subsides. Common auras heralding the seizure include a sensation of warmth or discomfort ascending from the stomach into the neck, nausea, olfactory and gustatory hallucinations, a dream-like state, anxiety, a feeling of familiarity (déjà vu) or unfamiliarity (jamais vu), followed by oral automatisms or grimacing, an arrest reaction, and a fixed, vacant stare. Consciousness is mildly impaired. The patient seems dazed. Hand automatisms, or a fixed posture of the contralateral hand, may appear. In a left-hemispheric seizure, the patient cannot follow commands, probably because of sensory aphasia. Verbal perseveration may also be found. The patient remains amnestic for the seizure.

Various complexes of symptoms and signs associated with medial temporal lobe seizures, to be described in detail in the following sections, are summarized in Table 7.**8**.

Sensory and perceptual disturbances. Disturbances of this type may appear by themselves or as auras heralding a seizure. They include dizziness, dysmorphopsia (macropsia, micropsia),

gustatory sensations, or usually unpleasant olfactory sensations (uncinate fits, see p. 624).

Autonomic phenomena. These may include palpitations, nausea, (rarely) vomiting, salivation or dry mouth, hunger, or the urge to urinate. Paroxysmal abdominal pain has also been described as a seizure equivalent, especially in children. Attacks of so-

Table 7.**8** Clinical manifestations of complex partial seizures (medial temporal lobe epilepsy)

Category	Manifestations	Remarks
Sensory and perceptual disturbances	Dizziness, dysmorphopsia (macropsia, micropsia, everything appears far away), gustatory sensations, malodorous olfactory sensations	Uncinate fits (p. 624)
Autonomic phenomena	Shortness of breath, palpitations, nausea, salivation, dry mouth, hunger, urge to urinate, abdominal sensations	Often, ascending sensation from stomach to throat
Behavioral and psychomotor manifestations	Traumatic experience, feeling of unreality, feeling of unfamiliarity (jamais vu), déjà vu, déjà vécu, unfounded anxiety or rage, hallucinations, twilight states	
Twilight states	Automatic, semi-organized, but inappropriate behavior – e.g., picking at clothes, senseless moving around of objects, etc. (twilight attacks); long-lasting, semi-organized complex behaviors that may even involve travel over a long distance (twilight states, *fugue épileptique*)	Amnesia for these states
Temporal syncope	Collapse, usually immediately following one of the above phenomena, typically with only brief unconsciousness	No sudden falling
Psychomotor status epilepticus	Very long persistence of the above phenomena, or repeated appearance with less than full recovery in between	Rare

called *abdominal epilepsy* last no more than a few minutes and are often accompanied by clouding, though not total loss, of consciousness. The EEG is almost always abnormal.

Motor phenomena. These consist of tonic-clonic twitching or, more frequently, complex motor behaviors such as the stereotyped repetition of a gesture, picking at clothes, and rubbing or wiping movements, then motor phenomena of a vegetative type such as abnormal breathing, chewing movements, sucking, lip-smacking, gagging, and swallowing, urination, etc. Any temporal lobe seizure can also become secondarily generalized to a grand mal seizure.

Behavioral and psychomotor manifestations. Diverse types of altered consciousness are encountered. Patients may experience an unreal, dreamlike state or have obsessive thoughts or a subjectively increased clarity of thinking. They may have a feeling that they have seen or experienced their present situation before, though this is actually not the case (déjà vu, déjà vécu). They may suffer from groundless anxiety, rage, or other emotions, or experience actual hallucinations that differ from those of schizophrenic psychosis only by their sudden appearance during a seizure.

Twilight states. These states are a very characteristic feature of "psychomotor epilepsy." The patient carries out complex activities in apparently organized fashion, while remaining conscious. These activities may be relatively brief and more or less well integrated into the behavioral context (*twilight attacks*). A twilight state may, however, last for hours or even days. The patient carries out highly complex activities – e.g., a long trip (*fugue épileptique*), which he or she cannot remember thereafter.

Temporal syncope. This term refers to brief loss of consciousness and collapse, without other motor manifestations, due to an epileptogenic focus in the temporal lobe. A further possible manifestation of temporal lobe epilepsy is *psychomotor status epilepticus.*

Neurological examination and diagnostic studies. There is usually no neurologic deficit, though the underlying focal pathologic process in the temporal lobe occasionally produces a deficit such as a contralateral upper homonymous quadrantanopsia. Very mild facial weakness, visible at the corner of the mouth contralateral to the focus, can be found in ca. 70% of patients. *MRI* often reveals an abnormal signal intensity in the hippocampus, together with hippocampal atrophy (made apparent by enlargement of the adjacent temporal horn). Rarer underlying lesions include hamartoma, arteriovenous malformation, tumor, gliosis, or tissue loss at the site of an old temporal lobe contusion.

The *EEG* is abnormal during wakefulness in only 30% of patients, during light or deep sleep in 70%. An epileptogenic focus in the anterior temporal lobe typically reveals itself through high θ and δ waves, as well as focal, sharp seizure potentials. Bitemporal foci are found in as many as 40% of cases of medically intractable temporal lobe epilepsy, possibly as the result of secondary epileptogenesis ("kindling") producing a so-called mirror focus. EEG recording during a seizure may be needed to determine which of the two foci is responsible for the seizures; in 25% of such patients, both foci produce seizures independently.

Lateral Temporal Lobe Epilepsy

Seizures of this type originate in the lateral temporal neocortex and often begin with an aura consisting of auditory or visual hallucinations, or dizziness. The aura is frequently followed by disorientation, protracted auditory hallucinations, movement of the head to one side, hand automatisms such as picking at clothes, leg automatisms, and (in the dominant hemisphere) aphasia.

Treatment
The first line of treatment for temporal lobe epilepsy is carbamazepine or valproate. Surgical treatment should be considered in medically intractable cases (p. 543).

■ Frontal Lobe Epilepsy (76d, 600a)

The manifestations of frontal lobe epilepsy are highly varied and depend on the site of the epileptogenic focus and the adjacent areas to which the epileptic discharge spreads. The seizure spectrum ranges from simple or complex partial seizures to secondarily generalized seizures. There are, however, several characteristic features that specifically suggest frontal lobe origin (Table 7.**9**, Fig. 7.**10**).

Frequency and Clinical Features

The seizures are brief (rarely longer than 1 minute), begin and end suddenly, and often occur in series of 20 to 50 seizures at a time, particularly during sleep. Auras are rare and nonspecific. The patient may report an unusual bodily sensation. Consciousness is usually only mildly impaired, if at all. An anxious facial expression is typical. Motor phenomena include

Table 7.**9** Frontal lobe seizures

Frequency	5–10% of all cases of epilepsy
Seizure types	Simple or complex partial seizures, often with secondary generalization; status epilepticus is frequent
Seizure frequency	Series of 20–50 seizures, often at night
Seizure duration	Brief, rarely longer than 1 minute, begin and end suddenly
Aura	Rare, nonspecific; peculiar bodily sensation
Impairment of consciousness	Usually no more than mild
Amnesia	None or incomplete
Automatisms	Marked, impressive: wild thrashing or rhythmic movements of the upper limbs/hands, pedaling movements of the feet, rocking of the hips, (rarely) genital manipulation
Typical motor phenomena	Vocalization, tonic-versive

vocalizations and tonic versive movements (adversive seizures, p. 523). Postural seizures are also typical, with a fencing posture of the arm contralateral to the focus. The motor automatisms may be grotesque or bizarre, leading to an erroneous impression of psychosis: flailing of the arms and hands, pedaling movements of the legs, rhythmic movements of the hips, or, rarely, genital manipulation.

There is incomplete amnesia, or none. Frontal lobe seizures often occur during sleep and have a marked tendency to generalization (> 90%). Status epilepticus is frequent. The following clinical phenomena may be seen, depending on the site of the focus (271):

- *Central motor seizures* are characterized by contralateral twitching, in a single limb at first, then spreading to adjacent areas in a Jacksonian march, sometimes to the entire contralateral hemibody.
- *Supplementary motor seizures* are characterized by stereotypical postures with tonic components – e.g., elevation and abduction of the contralateral and then the ipsilateral arm, possibly accompanied by high-frequency clonus.
- If the seizure originates in the *frontal eye fields,* there is versive movement of the eyes to the opposite side, possibly followed by movement of the head.
- If the seizure originates in *Broca's area,* there is iterative repetition of single syllables without impairment of consciousness or postictal amnesia. The patient is fully responsive immediately afterward.
- Seizures originating in the *premotor cortex* consist of complex movements such as rhythmic rocking or automatisms involving the arms, legs, or entire body, with partial clouding of consciousness. The patient tries to follow verbal commands given during the seizure but usually fails because of perseveration. Hypermotor seizures are also seen.
- A continuum of seizure types links the last-described type to *frontopolar, frontocingular and fronto-orbital seizures,* all of which are characterized by highly varied, perseverating automatisms that may appear psychogenic, and by an excess of movement (hypermotor state). The wide variety of seizure phenomena is due to the large number of directions in which the cortical seizure activity can spread.
- Seizure activity usually spreads to the limbic system, causing ictal clouding of consciousness and marked postictal disorientation.

Typical differences between frontal and temporal lobe seizures are listed in Table 7.**10**.

Frontal lobe seizures may seem bizarre to persons who observe them, and the patient's description of the (subjective) aura preceding the seizure may seem no less bizarre. It is thus not surprising, though unfortunate, that these seizures are often misdiagnosed as schizophrenia, depression, bipolar affective disorder, or another type of mental illness, or, if they occur during sleep, as nightmares, pavor nocturnus, or another type of parasomnia.

Table 7.**10**   Some characteristic differences between frontal and temporal lobe epilepsy

Feature	Frontal lobe seizures	Temporal lobe seizures
Aura	Rare, nonspecific	Common, often specific
Frequency	Many per day	Many per month
Initial signs	Anxiety, vocalization	Cessation of speaking/activity
Automatisms	Complex	Simple
Generalization	Common	Rare
Duration	10 60 s	1–3 min
Postictal phenomena	Minimal or none	Fatigue, confusion, agitation

Etiology

The causes of frontal lobe seizures are highly varied, including tumors, the late sequelae of head trauma and stroke, encephalitis, and genetic syndromes such as autosomal dominant nocturnal frontal lobe epilepsy (329b). The last-named disorder can be caused by any of at least three different ion-channel mutations.

Treatment

Carbamazepine and valproate constitute the first line of therapy. Surgical treatment may be beneficial for medically intractable seizures (p. 543).

■ Parietal and Occipital Lobe Epilepsy

Parietal lobe seizures usually consists of purely sensory disturbances, perhaps with a Jacksonian march, which may then develop into a motor seizure of the entire hemibody with conjugate deviation of the eyes and torsion of the trunk. Seizures in the speech area are manifest as receptive or expressive aphasia or speech arrest.

Occipital lobe seizures usually manifest themselves as elementary visual hallucinations or cortical blindness (p. 378). They are treated in the same way as other types of focal seizure (p. 540).

Differential Diagnosis of Complex Partial Seizures

Very brief complex partial seizures in children must be differentiated from *absence seizures.* The latter tend to occur much more frequently, generally last less than 15 seconds, and can be precipitated by hyperventilation. Complex partial seizures may be difficult to differentiate from severe *vegetative dystonia,* from *hyperventilation tetany* (p. 554), or from *psychogenic seizures.*

Complex partial seizures are also sometimes difficult to differentiate from β-*adrenergic hyperactivity,* which may express itself in tachycardia and chest pressure or in nervousness, shortness of breath, and tremulousness. Such attacks come on suddenly, perhaps several times per week, and last for minutes or hours. They can be eliminated by treatment with propranolol at a dose of 160 mg/day.

Complex partial seizures whose major feature is *anxiety* can be very difficult to distinguish from *panic attacks* (152), in which anxiety arises spontaneously and increases over a few minutes, often accompanied by shortness of breath, air hunger, palpitations, or dizziness.

Twilight attacks sometimes need to be differentiated from *hypovigilance due to narcolepsy;* twilight states occurring during the day, from *sleep apnea syndrome* (p. 569).

Special Seizure Types and Seizure Etiologies

■ Febrile Seizures

Clinical Features

Febrile seizures occur in children up to the age of 5 years in the setting of a febrile illness, usually an upper respiratory infection. They are usually generalized. A febrile seizure may later be followed by further seizures even in the absence of fever – i.e., it may be the first sign, or the initiating event, of epilepsy. Factors implying a good prognosis are the occurrence of a first febrile seizure between the ages of 6 and 18 months, no further febrile seizures from age 7 onward, duration less than 5 minutes, normal EEG 10 days later, absence of a neurologic deficit, a positive family history of febrile seizures, and the absence of birth-related or other brain injury. If all of these obtain, the chance that the patient will later develop seizures in the absence of fever is only about 10%.

▬ Treatment ▬

Acute event: Febrile seizures are treated acutely with diazepam per rectum. Patients with known febrile seizures can be treated prophylactically in this way whenever they develop a fever.

Chronic prophylaxis: Long-term preventive therapy, usually with phenobarbital or valproic acid, is indicated in all patients who have had three or more febrile seizures. It should be initiated after the second, or even the first, seizure if aggravating features are present, such as long duration of the seizure, a neurologic deficit, signs of brain damage, family history of epilepsy, or EEG changes indicating epilepsy.

■ Reflex Epilepsy

Reflex epilepsy consists of focal or generalized seizures (usually brief tonic-clonic seizures) that are induced by sensory stimuli, movements, or, rarely, complex activities such as reading or writing. The precipitating sensory stimuli are most commonly visual but may also be auditory (including musical), vestibular, gustatory, or olfactory.

In *photosensitive epilepsy,* which accounts for more than half of all cases, the seizures are induced by rapidly changing visual stimuli such as televised images, video games, sunlight reflected off the surface of a lake, or the play of light and shadows as the patient walks down the street.

Startle epilepsy is a rare form of reflex epilepsy that is often the result of perinatal brain damage. The seizures, induced by fright, may be focal or generalized; if focal, they usually affect a part of the body in which there is a fixed neurologic deficit. Treatment with carbamazepine is usually effective.

■ **Post-Traumatic Epilepsy**

Epileptic seizures arising after traumatic brain injury may be partial or primarily or secondarily generalized. Further, it is said that typical absence seizures can arise after traumatic brain injury, as can myoclonic-astatic petit mal epilepsy, though the latter claim has not been convincingly documented.

The manifestations of the seizures are determined by their site of origin in the brain. They are primarily generalized in more than 25% of cases, secondarily generalized in a further 65%, and purely focal in only 10%. Seizures may occur immediately after trauma; those occurring in the first week are called *early post-traumatic seizures*, while those occurring repeatedly thereafter are called *post-traumatic chronic epilepsy.*

The more severe the trauma, the more likely that epilepsy will develop. In open brain injuries, the probability of early seizures is 5%, and of chronic epilepsy 30–50%; the probability of chronic epilepsy is 15% after a depressed skull fracture and 5% after a brain contusion without a skull fracture or open injury. The first seizure occurs within 6 months of injury in almost half of all cases of post-traumatic epilepsy, within 2 years in 80%. Some 25–35% of patients with early post-traumatic seizures have seizures later as well.

Children can develop early post-traumatic seizures even after a mild brain injury. The more frequent these seizures are, the more likely that chronic epilepsy will develop.

Simple *concussion* does not predispose to epilepsy.

■ **Treatment** ■
Early post-traumatic seizures are treated with *phenytoin* (begun as an intravenous loading bolus), chronic post-traumatic epilepsy with carbamazepine or phenytoin. Half of all patients are free of seizures 5–10 years after the trauma, either with or without medication. Eight percent of cases of chronic post-traumatic epilepsy are medically intractable.

■ **Epilepsy after Stroke**
(153a, 516, 765b, 783a)

About 5% of patients with an acute stroke have seizures within 2 weeks; these are usually partial, rarely primarily or secondarily generalized. Seizures occur mainly in association with large cortical infarcts or hemorrhagic infarcts. Once the acute phase is past, the annual risk of a first seizure is 3–5% the first year after the stroke and 1–2% thereafter. Focal seizures in patients who have had a stroke are occasionally misinterpreted as a recurrent stroke. Furthermore, whenever seizures develop in the aftermath of a stroke, other possible causes should be ruled out.

■ **Treatment** ■
Recurrent seizures require *anticonvulsant therapy.*

■ **Epilepsy Due to Alcohol, Illicit Drugs, and Medications**

Alcohol. Alcohol consumption causes provoked seizures and chronic epilepsy in dose-dependent fashion

(575d). Alcohol-induced seizures may occur during a period of drunkenness or in the withdrawal phase. They are usually generalized, tonic-clonic seizures. Alcohol-withdrawal seizures, which usually occur 12 to 48 hours after the last drink, are associated with vegetative signs including sweating, disruption of the sleep-wake cycle, impaired attention, and increased startle response (p. 309). Alcohol abuse is also a common cause of status epilepticus.

> **Treatment**
>
> In the acute situation, *lorazepam* 2 mg i.v. significantly reduces the risk of further seizures (243a). Abstinence from alcohol is desirable as a long-term goal.

Illicit drugs and medications. *Illicit drugs* such as heroin and other opiates, cocaine, amphetamines, methylenedioxymetamphetamine (MDMA, "Ecstasy"), and phencyclidine exert manifold effects on the nervous system and can induce seizures (p. 313) that are usually generalized tonic-clonic. Many *medications* can also cause seizures, among them intravenous penicillin, lidocaine, tricyclic antidepressants, and neuroleptic agents. The chronic use of benzodiazepines or barbiturates elevates the risk of nonconvulsive status epilepticus, particularly in the medication withdrawal phase. *Radiological contrast substances,* particularly those given intrathecally for myelography, can also induce seizures or even status epilepticus.

Procedure after a First Seizure or Multiple Seizures (422a)

If the history and physical examination suggest the possibility of epilepsy in a patient who has had one or more seizures, the essential initial diagnostic studies are EEG and MRI. Depending on the clinical situation, serum metabolic tests and toxicologic studies may be indicated as well. A lumbar puncture should be performed if there is a question of meningitis or encephalitis. The EEG and MRI will reveal whether an epilepsy syndrome is present and whether there is a structural lesion in the brain. If either of these is the case, directed treatment can be provided.

If the ancillary studies yield negative results, the hypothesis of an epileptic event must be called in question and the differential diagnosis pursued. If there has only been a single seizure, further observation will likely clarify the situation. If the suspicion of epilepsy remains high, an EEG after sleep deprivation or a subacute EEG recording can be carried out.

Treatment of Epilepsy

Initiation of Treatment

Recurrent epileptic seizures require treatment both because untreated seizures can cause selective neural damage and because the epileptic patient is vulnerable to physical injury and social stigma. The goals of treatment are:

- freedom from seizures,
- social integration, and
- prevention of mental disorders,

while the side effects of antiepileptic medication are kept to a minimum. In a case where there has been only a single generalized clonic-tonic seizure, it must be decided on an individual basis whether long-term treatment is to be initiated. The risk of further seizures within 2 years ranges from 24% to 65%, depending on the cause of the seizure and on the associated EEG findings (90a). If there have already been two seizures, the risk of further seizures within 2 years rises to 70–80%; the next seizure will usually occur within 1 year (396b).

Elimination of Specific Causes

Identifiable causes of seizures should be eliminated whenever possible – e.g., a brain tumor or chronic alcoholism. Patients must also be instructed to avoid specific precipitating factors including sleep deprivation, alcohol abuse, flickering lights (in some cases), etc.

Choice of Medication

Before treatment is begun, the physician must define the type of seizure that is present, as different types respond to varying degrees to the different medications that are available. Suitable medications for each type of seizure are listed in Tables 7.**11** and 7.**12**:

- Medications that have been used for decades, with a known side-effect profile, and are relatively inexpensive: carbamazepine, clobazam, clonazepam, ethosuximide, nitrazepam, piracetam, phenobarbital, phenytoin, primidone, and valproic acid.
- Newer antiepileptic drugs that may have as yet unknown, rare and severe side effects: felbamate, gabapentin, lamotrigine, levetiracetam, oxcarbazepine, tiagabine, topiramate, vigabatrin, and zonisamide.

Principles of Antiepileptic Pharmacotherapy

The patient should take the prescribed medication(s) regularly in the dose(s) indicated and keep a protocol of any seizures that occur. Medications should be introduced at a low dose, which is then gradually increased to a typically effective dose, generally that recommended by the manufacturer. Excessively rapid dose elevation heightens the risk of adverse effects. Rapid loading to a therapeutic level is indicated only in cases of frequent seizures or status epilepticus.

Once a steady daily dose has been reached, it may be days or weeks, depending on the medication, before the serum drug level becomes constant. The physician must always bear this fact in mind when assessing the therapeutic benefit of a given dose. If seizure control is inadequate, the dose can be increased stepwise until therapeutic benefit is obtained or adverse effects appear. A change to another medication should be made only if the medication currently being given has been found ineffective or is not tolerated by the patient. Such changes must also be made in stepwise fashion; as a rule, the dose of the current, inadequately effective medication should be halved before the new medication is introduced. An antiepileptic medication may induce certain enzymes and thereby speed or slow the metabolism of other medications given concomitantly, altering their serum concentration; either the

Table 7.**11**   Epilepsy syndromes, seizure types, and their treatment

Seizure type, epilepsy syndrome	Clinical manifestations	Drug of 1st choice	Drugs of 2nd choice
Idiopathic generalized epilepsy	Generalized tonic-clinic seizures, grand mal on awakening, grand mal during sleep	Valproic acid	Phenobarbital, primidone, lamotrigine, topiramate
	Absence (petit mal)	Valproic acid, ethosuximide	Lamotrigine, clonazepam
	Myoclonic seizures	Valproic acid	Phenobarbital, primidone, lamotrigine, clonazepam, piracetam, zonisamide, acetazolamide
	Clonic, tonic, and atonic seizures	Valproic acid	Phenobarbital, primidone, lamotrigine, topiramate
	Light-induced seizures	Valproic acid	Lamotrigine, clonazepam
Symptomatic generalized epilepsy	Salaam spasms, infantile spasms, West syndrome	ACTH, corticosteroids, valproic acid	Vigabatrin,* clonazepam, nitrazepam
	Myoclonic-astatic petit mal (Lennox-Gastaut syndrome)	Valproic acid	Lamotrigine, topiramate, felbamate, ethosuximide, primidone, phenytoin
	Juvenile myoclonus epilepsy (impulsive petit mal, Janz syndrome)	Valproic acid	Lamotrigine, topiramate, phenobarbital, primidone, acetazolamide
Focal epilepsy	Simple or complex	Carbamazepine, oxcarbazepine, valproic acid, lamotrigine	Phenytoin, topiramate, tiagabine, clonazepam, zonisamide, gabapentin, felbamate
Unclassifiable epilepsy		Valproic acid	Carbamazepine, lamotrigine, clonazepam

* Possible side effect: retinal damage.

Table 7.**12** Antiepileptic drugs: their indications, dosage, therapeutic levels, side effects, and special considerations

Generic name (and proprietary name if available)	Indications	Contraindications	Average daily dose for adults	Average daily dose for children	Serum half-life	Therapeutic serum concentration	Relevant interactions	Side effects, interactions, and special considerations
Carbamazepine (Tegretol, Epitol)	Focal seizures, secondarily generalized seizures, unclassifiable seizures	Bradycardia, cardiac arrhythmia	800–1200 mg; 15–20 mg/kg in 1–2 doses	10–40 mg/kg in 1–2 doses	8–22 h	8–12 mg/L	Enzyme induction lessens effect of other medications	Dizziness, nausea, ataxia, rash, aplastic anemia, hepatitis, hyponatremia
Clobazam (Frisium)	Add-on therapy for focal and generalized seizures		10–40 mg in 2–3 doses	10–20 mg in 2–3 doses	20 h (desmethylclobazam, 50 h)	Clinically irrelevant	Cumulative sedation	Sedation, respiratory depression, withdrawal syndrome if suddenly discontinued
Clonazepam (Klonopin, Rivotril)	Add-on therapy for focal and generalized seizures, status epilepticus		2–4 mg in 2–3 doses	0.05–0.1 mg/kg, above 30 kg 1.5–3 mg, in 2–3 doses	20–50 h	Clinically irrelevant	Cumulative sedation	Sedation, respiratory depression, withdrawal syndrome if suddenly discontinued
Ethosuximide (Zarontin, Emeside)	Absence seizures		1200–1500 mg in 2–3 doses	20 mg/kg	60 h	100–120 mg/L	None	Nausea/vomiting, dizziness, hiccups, psychotic episodes
Felbamate (Felbatol)	Add-on therapy in Lennox-Gastaut syndrome, possibly also for refractory focal seizures		Up to 3600 mg in 2–3 doses	Up to 45 mg/kg	14–23 h	20–40 mg/L	Enzyme inhibition with rise in serum concentration of other antiepileptic drugs	Dizziness, nausea, weight loss, insomnia, psychotic reactions, aplastic anemia, hepatic failure, rash

Cont. →

Table **7.12**   (Cont.)

Generic name (and proprietary name if available)	Indications	Contraindications	Average daily dose for adults	Average daily dose for children	Serum half-life	Therapeutic serum concentration	Relevant interactions	Side effects, interactions, and special considerations
Gabapentin (Neurontin)	Focal seizures in adults		1800–3600 mg in 2–3 doses	30–40 mg/kg in 2–3 doses	5–7 h	> 2 mg/L; clinically irrelevant	None	Dizziness, ataxia, fatigue, headache, tremor, hyperactivity, aggressiveness
Lamotrigine (Lamictal)	Focal and primarily or secondarily generalized seizures; add-on therapy in Lennox-Gastaut syndrome		100–400 mg; half this amount if valproate is given simultaneously; in 1–3 doses	5–10 mg/kg	7 h (with valproate, 45–50 h)	1–4 mg/L; clinically irrelevant	None	Dizziness, headache, depression, psychotic reactions, rash, Stevens-Johnson syndrome, Lyell syndrome
Levetiracetam (Keppra)	Add-on therapy for focal and secondarily generalized seizures		1000–3000 mg	Data unavailable	7–10 h	Clinically irrelevant	None	Somnolence, confusion, asthenia, headache, infections
Nitrazepam (Mogadon, Nitrazadon)	Add-on therapy in West and Lennox-Gastaut syndromes		5–10 mg till age 1 y, then 10–15 mg for ages 2–14 y, in 3 doses		30 h	40 mg/L, clinically irrelevant	Cumulative sedation	Respiratory depression, hypersecretion in the airways

Cont. →

Table 7.**12** (*Cont.*)

Generic name (and proprietary name if available)	Indications	Contraindications	Average daily dose for adults	Average daily dose for children	Serum half-life	Therapeutic serum concentration	Relevant interactions	Side effects, interactions, and special considerations
Oxcarbazepine (Trileptal)	Focal seizures, secondarily generalized seizures, unclassifiable seizures	Bradycardia, cardiac arrhythmia	800–1600 mg in 2–3 doses	5–10 mg/kg in 2–3 doses	2 h; active metabolite (monohydroxy-carbamazepine) 9 h	Clinically irrelevant	Mild enzyme induction	Dizziness, nausea, ataxia, rash, aplastic anemia, hepatitis, hyponatremia
Piracetam (Nootropyl)	Cortical myoclonus		7.2–24 g in 2–4 doses	7.2–24 g in 2–4 doses	4–8 h	Clinically irrelevant	None known	Nervousness, irritability, tremor, depression, somnolence or insomnia
Phenobarbital (Luminal)	All types of seizures except absence	Barbiturate hypersensitivity	100–150 mg or 2–3 mg/kg in 1–2 doses	4–5 mg/kg in 1–2 doses	~100 h	15–40 mg/L	Enzyme induction lessens effect of other drugs	Somnolence, slowness, unsteady gait, rash, shoulder-arm syndrome, withdrawal syndrome, cognitive impairment
Phenytoin (Dilantin, Epanutin)	Focal and unclassifiable seizures	Progressive myoclonus epilepsy, generalized myoclonus epilepsy, absence seizures	250–300 mg or 4–6 mg/kg in 1–2 doses	5–8 mg/kg in 1–2 doses	22 h	10–20 mg/L; serum concentration rises exponentially as a function of dose	Enzyme induction lessens effect of other drugs	Dizziness, gait ataxia, gaze-evoked nystagmus, dysarthria, rarely extrapyramidal signs, rash, lymphadenopathy, gingival hyperplasia, acne, coarsening of facial features, osteoporosis

Cont. →

Table **7.12** (Cont.)

Generic name (and proprietary name if available)	Indications	Contraindications	Average daily dose for adults	Average daily dose for children	Serum half-life	Therapeutic serum concentration	Relevant interactions	Side effects, interactions, and special considerations
Primidone (Mysoline, Mylidone, Sertan)	All types other than absence	Barbiturate hypersensitivity	750–1000 mg or 10–20 mg/kg in 2–3 doses	10–30 mg/kg in 2–3 doses	Phenobarbital is the active metabolite (q.v.)	Phenobarbital is the active metabolite (q.v.)		Somnolence, slowing, unsteady gait, rash, shoulder-arm-syndrome, withdrawal syndrome, cognitive impairment
Tiagabine (Gabitril)	Add-on therapy for focal and secondarily generalized seizures		30–60 mg in 3 doses	In adolescents, 30–60 mg in 3 doses; no data for children under 12 y	5–13 h	Clinically irrelevant	None	Dizziness, asthenia, somnolence, (rare) constriction of visual fields
Topiramate (Topamax)	Add-on therapy for focal and secondarily generalized seizures; Lennox-Gastaut syndrome		200–600 mg in 2 doses		19–25 h	2–25 mg/L, clinically irrelevant	None	Dizziness, ataxia, headache, tremor, somnolence, difficulty concentrating, depression
Valproic acid (Depakene, Depakote, Depacon, Epival, Valprotate, Convulex)	All types	Hepatic disease (relative contraindication, caution required)	1200–1800 mg or 10–20 mg/kg	20–30 (up to 60) mg/kg	15–20 h	50–120 mg/L	Enzyme inhibition raises serum concentration of other drugs – e.g., lamotrigine	Nausea/vomiting, dizziness, tremor, acute hepatic failure weight gain

Cont. →

Table 7.**12**   *(Cont.)*

Generic name (and proprietary name if available)	Indications	Contraindications	Average daily dose for adults	Average daily dose for children	Serum half-life	Therapeutic serum concentration	Relevant interactions	Side effects, interactions, and special considerations
Vigabatrin (Sabril)	Drug of first choice in West syndrome due to tuberous sclerosis	Visual impairment (relative contraindication, caution required)	1000–3000 mg	Up to 100 mg/kg, adult dose for > 45 kg	5–7 h	Clinically irrelevant	None	Somnolence, dizziness, weight gain, depression, psychotic episodes, retinal degeneration
Zonisamide (Zonegran)	Add-on therapy for focal, tonic-clonic, and myoclonic seizures		400–600 mg in 2 doses			Clinically irrelevant	None	Somnolence, slowing, cognitive impairment, headache, ataxia, psychotic reactions, weight loss, kidney stones, Stevens-Johnson syndrome

medication originally given, the "add-on" medication, or both may act in this way. Thus monotherapy, if possible, is generally preferable, and combination therapy is used only when monotherapy has been found to be ineffective. Primary combination therapy is a reasonable option only in patients who suffer from several different types of seizure at once. Furthermore, there are favorable and unfavorable combinations of antiepileptic medications (Table 7.**13**). It usually seems best to combine medications that work by different mechanisms, though, admittedly, clinical studies have not yet proved this hypothesis (Table 7.**14**).

Once a particular regimen has been decided upon, it should be strictly adhered to. The dose should not be reduced until the patient has been free of seizures for 2 years or more.

Table 7.**13** Combination therapy: favorable, moderately favorable, and unfavorable combinations (after Schmidt and Elger)

Seizure type, epilepsy syndrome	Favorable combination	Moderately favorable combination	Unfavorable combination
Primarily generalized tonic-clonic seizures	Valproate with clonazepam	Valproate with lamotrigine, topiramate, or phenobarbital	
Absence seizures	Valproate with ethosuximide, clonazepam, or topiramate; lamotrigine with topiramate	Valproate with lamotrigine or felbamate	Valproate with phenobarbital, gabapentin, oxcarbazepine, tiagabine, vigabatrin or carbamazepine
Myoclonus	Valproate with clonazepam, piracetam, or zonisamide	Valproate with lamotrigine, phenobarbital, felbamate, or ethosuximide	Valproate with gabapentin, oxcarbazepine, vigabatrin, tiagabine, or carbamazepine
Focal and secondarily generalized seizures	Carbamazepine with clonazepam, gabapentin, lamotrigine, phenytoin, tiagabine, topiramate, vigabatrin, or zonisamide	Carbamazepine with felbamate, oxcarbazepine, phenobarbital, or valproate	
Unclassifiable seizures	Valproate with carbamazepine or clonazepam	Valproate with lamotrigine or topiramate; lamotrigine with topiramate	

Dosage and Serum Levels

Even though the serum concentrations of most antiepileptic drugs can now be easily measured, the correct dosage of each drug should still be determined by observation of its clinical effect on seizures. Typical therapeutic ranges are listed in Table 7.**12**, but it must be remembered that there is no fixed relation between the consumed dose, the serum level, and the clinical effect. Some patients, for example, become free of seizures even though the serum drug concentration lies below the quoted therapeutic range. Measurement of serum levels is appropriate in the following situations:

Table 7.**14**   Mechanism of action of antiepileptic drugs

Antiepileptic drug (generic name)	Mechanism of action
Carbamazepine	Na channel block
Clobazam	Enhancement of GABA-ergic inhibition
Clonazepam	Enhancement of GABA-ergic inhibition
Ethosuximide	Ca channel block
Felbamate	Enhancement of GABA-ergic inhibition, Na channel block
Gabapentin	Enhancement of GABA-ergic inhibition, Na channel block
Lamotrigine	Enhancement of GABA-ergic inhibition, Na channel block
Levetiracetam	Unknown
Nitrazepam	Enhancement of GABA-ergic inhibition
Oxcarbazepine	Na channel block
Piracetam	Unknown
Phenobarbital	Enhancement of GABA-ergic inhibition
Phenytoin	Na channel block
Primidone	Enhancement of GABA-ergic inhibition (and other mechanisms)
Tiagabine	Enhancement of GABA-ergic inhibition
Topiramate	Enhancement of GABA-ergic inhibition, Na channel block
Valproic acid	Enhancement of GABA-ergic inhibition (and other mechanisms)
Vigabatrin	Enhancement of GABA-ergic inhibition
Zonisamide	Na channel block (and other mechanisms)

- when the clinical effect is inadequate, and it is unclear whether the dose prescribed or actually consumed has produced a concentration in the usual therapeutic range;
- when toxic side effects are suspected;
- in combination therapy;
- when further elevation of an already high dose is considered;

- for medicolegal purposes, especially with regard to driving licenses.

The routine determination of serum drug concentrations, however, causes needless expense and yields no benefit. Slavish attention to "therapeutic levels," rather than to the frequency of seizures, sometimes stands in the way of effective treatment.

Table 7.**15**   Ten principles for the treatment of patients with epilepsy

1	Thorough patient education
2	Elimination of reversible causes of epilepsy: • Elimination of the etiology, if possible (e.g., meningioma) • Avoidance of precipitating factors (e.g., strobe lights) • Avoidance of other factors that promote seizures (alcohol, sleep deprivation)
3	Choice of a suitable medication for the particular seizure type (cf. Tables 7.**11**, 7.**12**)
4	Gradual increase of dose till seizure control is achieved (or unacceptable side effects arise)
5	Meticulous follow-up for possible complications, with especially close observation in the initial phase of treatment
6	Checking for compliance if medications appear to be ineffective – e.g., with serum levels
7	If therapy with the first agent tried is truly ineffective, stepwise change to another
8	Combination therapy if monotherapy fails (with at least two different agents)
9	Determination of serum levels when: • Poor compliance or a toxic effect is suspected • Drug interactions are suspected, particularly those involving enzyme induction • An already high dose is to be raised even further • Medicolegal questions arise, particularly with respect to driving
10	Guidelines for cessation of pharmacotherapy: • The patient should be free of seizures for at least 2 years before cessation • The EEG should be free of epileptiform activity • Traditionally, the medication is slowly tapered to off over several months (although the need for this has not been fully demonstrated) • The patient and family must be explicitly told that seizures may recur

General Lifestyle

The epileptic patient ought to be able to live as normally as possible. Clearly, however, he or she would be ill advised to work on a scaffolding or with machinery that may endanger the operator or others nearby, or to engage in sports such as mountain-climbing, unsupervised swimming, or windsurfing. In most countries, the patient may drive a car if there have been no seizures whatsoever for a defined period of time (generally 6 months to 2 years), the EEG does not show an epilepsy-specific pattern, and medications are taken regularly, if necessary. Needlessly harsh restrictions should be avoided. The principles of treatment of the epileptic patient are summarized in Table 7.**15**.

A *ketogenic diet* is a noninvasive method that can lower the frequency of seizures in certain cases (395a).

Epilepsy Surgery

Medically intractable epilepsy that can be reliably attributed to an identified epileptogenic focus in the brain can be treated by *neurosurgical resection* of the focus. The presurgical evaluation consists of subacute EEG recording for a prolonged period with si-

Table 7.**16**   Pharmacotherapy for generalized status epilepticus

1	Thiamine 100 mg, and 50% glucose 50 mL i.v.
2	Initial treatment with benzodiazepine: • Lorazepam 2–4 mg i.v. • Diazepam 10–20 mg i.v. • Clonazepam 1–2 mg i.v.
3	Repeat benzodiazepine injection in 3–5 min if necessary if seizure is ongoing
4	In all cases: • Phenytoin 750 mg as a slow i.v. bolus over 15–30 min, then 250–750 mg i.v. over the ensuing 12 h, then maintenance therapy with 300–400 mg/day or: • Valproic acid 900 mg as a slow i.v. bolus over 30 min, then 1500 mg i.v. over the ensuing 12 h, then maintenance therapy with 1200–1500 mg/d
5	If status epilepticus persists 30 min after phenytoin or valproic acid has been given: • Intubation and ventilation (if not yet done) • Thiopental 100–200 mg i.v. • Thiopental 50 mg i.v. boluses, repeatedly, until the EEG shows a burst-suppression pattern • Thiopental drip, 3–5 mg/kg/h (ca. 300 mg/h), for at least 12 h • After at least 12 h, trial cessation of thiopental or: • Propofol 1–2 mg/kg i.v. bolus, then 2–10 mg/kg/h *Note:* phenytoin or valproic acid should be continued while thiopental or propofol is given

multaneous video monitoring, high-resolution MRI, comprehensive neuropsychological testing, and sometimes magnetoencephalography (736b, 904a), recording through foramen ovale electrodes, depth electrodes, or subdural strip or grid electrodes, PET, SPECT, and/or selective angiography with a Wada test. The results of this presurgical battery of tests enable an estimation of the risks and benefits of surgery so that the decision can be made whether to operate.

The success rate of resective surgery for temporal lobe foci (either anterior temporal lobectomy or selective amygdalohippocampectomy) is ca. 60–70%, and for extratemporal neocortical foci ca. 45% (280a). Adolescents with frequent, medically refractory seizures originating in the temporal lobe should be evaluated early for neurosurgical treatment.

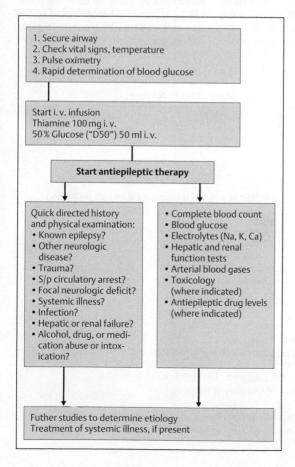

Fig. 7.**11   Procedure in status epilepticus** (adapted from Lowenstein and Alldredge).

1. Secure airway
2. Check vital signs, temperature
3. Pulse oximetry
4. Rapid determination of blood glucose

Start i. v. infusion
Thiamine 100 mg i. v.
50 % Glucose ("D50") 50 ml i. v.

Start antiepileptic therapy

Quick directed history and physical examination:
• Known epilepsy?
• Other neurologic disease?
• Trauma?
• S/p circulatory arrest?
• Focal neurologic deficit?
• Systemic illness?
• Infection?
• Hepatic or renal failure?
• Alcohol, drug, or medication abuse or intoxication?

• Complete blood count
• Blood glucose
• Electrolytes (Na, K, Ca)
• Hepatic and renal function tests
• Arterial blood gases
• Toxicology (where indicated)
• Antiepileptic drug levels (where indicated)

Futher studies to determine etiology
Treatment of systemic illness, if present

Resective surgery cannot be used to treat medically intractable seizures that are primarily generalized, or those that arise from a focus in a location where resection would carry an unacceptable risk. A method of treatment that is currently under discussion for such seizures is *chronic stimulation of the vagus nerve*. This is done with a surgically implanted system consisting of an electrode wrapped around the nerve and connected to an impulse generator that resembles a cardiac pacemaker. In one study, 30% of patients so treated had their seizure frequency reduced by at least half, as compared to 13% in a control group (936a).

Treatment of Status Epilepticus

Figure 7.**11** and Table 7.**16** summarize the major aspects of the treatment of status epilepticus.

Treatment

Grand mal status epilepticus:
This is a life-threatening condition requiring immediate treatment. The ongoing seizure activity should first be terminated with a bolus injection of benzodiazepine – e.g., diazepam 10–20 mg i.v. Phenytoin should be given next, either as one or two slow intravenous boluses of 250 mg, or as a single infusion of 750 mg i.v., perhaps followed by a further 250 mg i.m. An alternative to phenytoin is valproate, 900 mg i.v. over 30 minutes, followed by a further 1500 mg i.v. over the ensuing 12 hours. If these treatments fail to abort status epilepticus within 40 minutes, the patient must be intubated, artificially ventilated, and treated with thiopental or propofol.

Petit mal status epilepticus:
Petit mal status epilepticus responds both clinically and electrophysiologically to a slow intravenous bolus of clonazepam, at a dose of 2–4 mg in adults, 1–2 mg in school-age children, and 0.5–1.0 mg in infants.

Psychomotor status epilepticus:
This condition also responds to clonazepam. A typical dosage schedule for an adult would be 2 mg in a 250 mL i.v. bolus over 2 hours, q6h on the first day and q8h on the second day.

Side Effects of Antiepileptic Medication

The major side effects are listed in Table 7.**12**. They may arise "idiosyncratically" – i.e., in a non-dose-dependent fashion. This is particularly true of *acute allergic reactions and rashes*, and of *granulocytopenia*.
Most side effects, however, are dose-dependent. Thus, chronic intoxication can produce manifestations that disappear once the dose is lowered. The manifestations of phenytoin overdose, mainly ataxia, were described above on p. 305. Phenobarbital, diazepam, and clonazepam cause a disturbing fatigue, which fortunately tends to lessen or resolve within a few weeks. Carbamazepine may cause dizziness, particularly in elderly patients, and often causes hyponatremia. Phenobarbital, phenytoin, and carbamazepine lessen the effect of oral anticoagulants and oral contraceptives.

The rate of fetal malformations in the children of epileptic mothers has been found to be 4.2% if no antiepileptic medications are taken during pregnancy, and ca. 5% if they are taken, as compared to 2.5% in the children of nonepileptic parents. The apparent mild increase in risk associated with medication use may not be due to a teratogenic effect of the medications themselves, as their use is perhaps no more than a marker for more severe epilepsy. In any case, whether or not they take antiepileptic medication, epileptic women who might become pregnant should take an adequate amount of folic acid to prevent neural tube defects (124b).

Only a few of the numerous *drug interactions* complicating combination therapy for epilepsy can be mentioned here:

- Carbamazepine, primidone, and valproic acid lower the serum concentration of phenytoin.
- Phenytoin reduces the effect of carbamazepine.
- Valproic acid enhances the toxicity of phenytoin.

The effect of valproic acid is reduced by carbamazepine and enhanced by diazepam.

Secondary Medical Intractability or Increasing Seizure Frequency

In such cases, the diagnosis of the epilepsy syndrome and of the seizure type should be re-evaluated, and an underlying progressive lesion should be sought (227a). Current neuroimaging studies often enable the diagnosis of lesions that were invisible in the past (see Fig. 2.**12**). Thus, cases previously classified as cryptogenic epilepsy may turn out to be due to a structural lesion, and neurosurgical resection may become a newly viable option.

Possible metabolic causes should also be diligently sought. *Hypomagnesemia* and *recurrent hypoglycemia,* to name just two conditions, may cause seizures that fail to respond to antiepileptic medication but disappear once the metabolic abnormality is treated (716).

A previously effective treatment may also fail if the patient becomes noncompliant or makes a major change of lifestyle.

Finally, if the seizures have truly become resistant to the current mode of pharmacotherapy, the physician should review the medication regimen and optimize the dosages or change medications as necessary.

The patient's and the physician's expectations of treatment are often different and may need to be reconciled by a frank discussion. The physician, for example, may consider the treatment a success if a patient who previously had very frequent seizures now has only one partial complex seizure a month, with only mild side effects of medication. The patient, however, may remain unsatisfied, because his hope for a seizure-free state has not been realized. Such a state cannot always be achieved.

Prognosis

The prognosis of epilepsy depends on its cause. In general, idiopathic and cryptogenic seizures have a better prognosis than symptomatic ones. About half of all adolescents and adults who have suffered a single seizure go on to develop epilepsy (90a). Two-thirds of these patients can be rid of their seizures with a single antiepileptic medication. Of the remaining third of patients that fail to respond to monotherapy, 20–30% (i.e., 10% in absolute terms) become seizure-free with combination therapy. An additional seizure-free rate of perhaps 5% can be achieved with the addition of the newer antiepileptic medications. Thus, about 25% of all epileptics still have seizures 5 years after their first one, and are potential candidates for epilepsy surgery. Ten percent have one or more seizures per week, while 15% have rarer seizures.

As a rule, children have a better prognosis than adults. One-third to one-half of children with a first seizure go on to develop epilepsy (872a, 913c), but most of these will be seizure-free by the time they reach adulthood (877b). Those whose seizures do persist tend to have lower levels of educational achievement, a lower socioeconomic status, and an elevated risk of death compared with normal controls.

Episodic Disturbances of Consciousness, Syncope, and Other Nonepileptic Episodes

Overview:
Certain disorders sharing some of the features of epilepsy can be mistaken for it at times. These include episodic disturbances of consciousness, of more or less sudden onset, with or without falling; twitching and other repetitive motor phenomena; episodic sensations; falls; and combinations of the above.

The classes of disorders that enter into the differential diagnosis of epilepsy are listed in Table 7.**17**. Some of them are described in other chapters of this book. In our experience, the question of epilepsy arises most often when the patient suffers from episodic disturbances of consciousness associated with a loss of muscle tone and perhaps causing a fall. The possible causes of such disturbances, both epileptic and nonepileptic, are listed in Table 7.**18**.

Table 7.**17** Nonepileptic conditions in the differential diagnosis of epilepsy

1	**Disturbances of behavior and consciousness**
1.1	*With loss of consciousness*
	1.1.1 With fall
	• Syncope (see Tables 7.**18** and 7.**19**)
	• Hysterical seizures (p. 560)
	• Startle disease (p. 559)

(Cont.) →

Table 7.**17**   *(Cont.)*

1.1.2   Without fall
- Basilar migraine
- Psychogenic unconsciousness:
  - Sobbing syncope
- Sudden daytime sleep:
  - Sleep apnea syndrome (p. 569)
  - Narcolepsy-cataplexy syndrome (p. 565)
  - Kleine-Levin syndrome (p. 572)

1.2   *Without loss of consciousness*
- Dysphrenic migraine
- Panic attacks
- Intoxications:
  - Hypnotic agents
  - Illicit drugs
- Respiratory affect seizures
- Acute global amnesia

2   Falls without detectable disturbance of consciousness
- Cataplexy (isolated or in the narcolepsy-cataplexy syndrome) (p. 565)
- Cryptogenic drop attacks in women (p. 555)
- Falls due to Parkinson's disease
- Atonic brainstem seizures
- Drop attacks in vertebrobasilar insufficiency
- Drop attacks in odontoid subluxation and other craniocervical junction anomalies
- Vestibular cerebral syncope (Tumarkin syndrome)

3   Episodic motor phenomena
- Fasciculations
- Hyperekplexia
- Startle disease
- Migraine accompagnée
- Paroxysmal choreoathetosis (p. 557)
- Tonic brainstem seizures
- Respiratory affect seizures
- Tics
- Hemifacial spasm
- Hemimasticatory spasm
- Transient ischemic attacks (TIAs)

4   Episodic somatosensory phenomena
- Migraine accompagnée
- Transient ischemic attacks

5   Episodic special sensory phenomena
- Ophthalmic migraine
- Retinal migraine
- Metamorphopsia in migraine

Table 7.**18**   Etiologic classification of episodic disturbances of consciousness with syncopal character, and/or drop attacks

1	**Primary cerebral causes**

  1.1   *Epilepsy*

      1.1.1 Grand mal seizure

      1.1.2 Juvenile absence epilepsy
              Pure absence seizures
              Complex absence seizures

      1.1.3 Salaam spasms (West syndrome)

      1.1.4 Myoclonic-astatic seizures (Lennox-Gastaut syndrome)

      1.1.5 Bilateral epileptic myoclonus (myoclonic petit mal)

      1.1.6 Complex partial seizures, esp. temporal syncope

  1.2   *Nonepileptic primary cerebral causes*

      1.2.1 Narcolepsy-cataplexy syndrome

      1.2.2 Cryptogenic drop attacks in women

      1.2.3 Falls due to Parkinson's disease

      1.2.4 Vestibular cerebral syncope

      1.2.5 Other:
             – Atonic brainstem seizures
             – Brain tumor
             – Syringomyelia
             – Basilar impression
             – Malresorptive hydrocephalus
             – Toxic and metabolic disorders

2	**Cardiovascular causes**

  2.1   *Heart disease*

  2.2   *Extracardiac vascular disorders*

  2.3   *Vascular and cerebrovascular dysfunction*

  2.4   *Reflex circulatory syncope (neurocardiogenic syncope)*

  2.5   *Valsalva syncope*

3	**Psychogenic, or partially psychogenic, acute impairment of consciousness**

  3.1   *Attacks accompanied by abnormal breathing in childhood*

      3.1.1 Respiratory affect syncope:
             • Cyanotic
             • Noncyanotic

      3.1.2 Sobbing syncope

  3.2   *Hysterical (pseudo-)epilepsy*

  3.3   *Psychogenic pseudocoma*

  3.4   *Malingering*

Syncope and Drop Attacks (488a)

> **Definition:**
> Syncope and drop attacks are disorders consisting of very brief attacks in which the affected person slowly or suddenly collapses to the ground. These attacks may or may not be accompanied by a brief impairment of consciousness.

Syncope reflects a brief, transient functional disturbance of the brainstem centers regulating consciousness and muscle tone, particularly the reticular activating system (RAS) with its ascending and descending afferent projections.

Features distinguishing syncope from epilepsy include the very brief impairment of consciousness, the lack of twitching or automatisms, the immediate return to normal consciousness, and the lack of epilepsy-specific potentials in the EEG during the attack. The diagnostic distinction can, however, be very difficult to make in some cases, particularly when a syncopal attack is followed by a brief seizure with twitching and perhaps even urinary incontinence (so-called

Table 7.**19**   Syncope of cardiac origin (692b)

1 Heart disease without arrhythmia	2 Cardiac arrhythmia
1.1 *Left-ventricular outflow disturbance* • Aortic valvular stenosis • Status post aortic valve replacement • Hypertrophic obstructive cardiomyopathy • Myocardial dysfunction	2.1 *Bradyarrhythmia* • Third-degree atrioventricular block • Status post pacemaker implantation • Second-degree atrioventricular block • Chronic bi- or trifascicular block • Sick sinus syndrome • Other bradyarrhythmias
1.2 *Left-ventricular filling disturbance* • Left atrial thrombus or myxoma • Status post mitral valve replacement • Mitral stenosis • Mitral valve prolapse • Cardiac tamponade	2.2 *Tachyarrhythmia* • Paroxysmal supraventricular tachycardia • Paroxysmal ventricular tachycardia • Wolff-Parkinson-White syndrome • Prolonged QT syndrome, torsades des pointes • Atrial flutter and fibrillation
1.3 *Disturbances of the right heart chambers and pulmonary circulation* • Congenital malformations • Acute, massive pulmonary embolus • Chronic pulmonary hypertension	

convulsive syncope). A postictal elevation of the serum prolactin concentration can be seen in syncope as well as in epilepsy (726a) (see Table 7.**20**).

Syncope and Drop Attacks of Cardiovascular Origin

At least half of all cases of syncope evaluated on an inpatient service are found to be due to cardiovascular causes.

■ Cardiogenic Syncope

Cardiogenic syncope may be due to any of the causes listed in Table 7.**19**. Cardiac arrhythmia, the most common cause, produces an *Adams-Stokes attack* ca. 5–12 seconds after the disturbance of cardiac function begins (p. 151 and Fig. 2.**35**). The patient recovers completely only if normal cerebral perfusion is restored within 5 minutes. Patients with syncope of unknown origin must always be evaluated for a possible underlying cardiac disorder.

Cardiogenic syncope may also be produced by a disturbance of the reflex regulation of cardiac activity and blood pressure.

Reflex Circulatory Syncope

Various types of stimulus may precipitate excessive vagal activity that leads to bradycardia and/or vasomotor collapse, thus producing a seizure.

■ Vasovagal Syncope

Strong emotion (e.g., fright, revulsion, the sight of blood), pain, heat or cold can induce syncope in susceptible individuals. Once aware of their susceptibility, such persons often develop a fear of fainting that, in turn, reinforces the fainting tendency. Two-thirds of persons who experience va-

sovagal syncope will do so during an inclined table test (488a).

Treatment

β-*blockers* and *fludrocortisone* are effective in many cases.

■ Deglutition Syncope

Syncope during swallowing is most often a manifestation of glossopharyngeal neuralgia, but may also arise because of a local tumor or in the aftermath of radiation therapy. It is presumably due to misdirected (ephaptic) neural transmission, through which an unusually strong volley of afferent impulses is followed by an excessive vagal outflow.

Treatment

Carbamazepine is effective in some cases.

■ Carotid Sinus Syndrome
Pathophysiology

The normal carotid sinus reflex consists of a decrease in heart rate and peripheral vascular resistance in response to stimulation of the stretch receptors of the carotid sinus. The nerve of the carotid sinus and the glossopharyngeal nerve are the afferent arm of this reflex, the vagus and the sympathetic fibers its efferent arm. Hypersensitivity of the carotid sinus, which may occur in hypertension, diabetes, etc., leads to an exaggerated reflex bradycardia in response to local pressure or even merely turning the head or extending the neck. A decrease in heart rate by more than 50% or a fall of systolic blood pressure by more than 40 mmHg is considered abnormal.

Carotid sinus syndrome is subclassified into three types:
- cardio-inhibitory type,
- vasodepressor type,
- cerebral type (somewhat controversial).

Clinical Features

The typical patient is an elderly man, often suffering from one of the diseases mentioned above. The acute loss of consciousness is preceded by a brief period of dizziness or an uneasy feeling. The patient is unconscious for a few seconds only, or a few minutes in exceptional cases.

Diagnostic Evaluation

The risk factors and precipitating factors mentioned above should be specifically sought. The most important part of the evalution is the carotid sinus pressure test, which should be carried out with simultaneous ECG recording, and only on one side at a time. This test is not without risk. A syringe with atropine for injection should be at hand in case it becomes necessary, as well as an external cardiac pacemaker in patients at particular risk.

Treatment

Implantation of a *permanent pacemaker*. In carotid sinus syndrome of vasodepressor type, *surgical denervation* of one or both carotid sinuses.

■ Valsalva Syncope

Pathophysiology

Syncope in response to a Valsalva maneuver is a consequence of the acute rise in intrathoracic pressure. The elevated pressure is transmitted via the spinal veins to the spinal and intracranial cerebrospinal fluid, causing a rise in intracranial pressure (ICP). If the ICP exceeds the arterial blood pressure, cerebral perfusion ceases, as can be demonstrated by Doppler sonography; the transient finding is comparable to the permanent finding seen in death ("brain death"). If the intrathoracic pressure remains elevated for a few seconds – e.g., with prolonged coughing or laughing – the patient loses consciousness. The systemic blood pressure falls inappreciably (644). Once the patient is unconscious, the muscles relax, coughing ceases, and cerebral perfusion returns, so that consciousness is soon restored. In milder cases, coughing produces lightheadedness without syncope.

Similar pathogenetic mechanisms play a role in stretch syncope (see below).

Clinical Features

Valsalva syncope may be produced by various different mechanisms.

Cough syncope; laughing syncope (ictus laryngis, geloplexy). Patients suffering from these forms of syncope are typically short, stocky male smokers with chronic obstructive pulmonary disease. They faint after a severe coughing fit or a prolonged bout of laughter. Cough syncope accounts for only about 1% of all cases of syncope.

■ Reflex Syncope

▦ Micturition Syncope

Micturition syncope typically occurs when the sufferer awakens from sleep with a distended bladder and, still drowsy and perhaps under the effect of alcohol, stands up and immediately urinates. A sudden decrease in sympathetic vasoconstrictor tone leads to a drop in blood pressure and thus to collapse. The Valsalva maneuver at the onset of urination and the removal of the blood pressure-sustaining effect of the distended bladder also play their part to promote syncope. Micturition syncope accounts for about 5% of all cases of syncope and generally occurs in younger men, more rarely in polymorbid elderly patients of either sex.

■ Stretch Syncope

The pathophysiologic mechanisms outlined above are sometimes exploited by wayward schoolboys to provoke a syncopal attack. The procedure is as follows:

- First, intense hyperventilation, which produces hypercapnia and reflex constriction of the cerebral vasculature;
- then, sudden standing up from the original squatting position, causing orthostatic hypotension;
- then, a powerful Valsalva maneuver;
- and, finally (if necessary), the aid of a schoolmate, who further increases the intrathoracic pressure by squeezing the chest.

A syncopal attack ("fainting lark") ensues, before the eyes of the (usually horrified) schoolteacher.

■ Supine Hypotensive Syndrome

Pregnant women in the supine position may suffer from syncopal attacks because of compression of the inferior vena cava by the gravid uterus, resulting in impaired return of venous blood to the heart.

Syncope Due to Impaired Circulatory Regulation in the Standing Position

Pathophysiology

The failure of one or more circulatory regulating mechanisms may result in pooling of blood in the periphery when the individual stands up so that the pumping effect of the heart is inadequate to sustain the required level of perfusion to the brain. Such events most commonly occur in the standing position.

Clinical Features

The two major clinical forms are:

Idiopathic vasomotor collapse of adolescents. Most patients are adolescents who have undergone a rapid growth spurt. The precipitating factors include fatigue, emotional excitement, systemic illness, and heat. The patient first becomes dizzy, then sees darkness before his eyes, sweats profusely, and finally loses consciousness and falls to the ground, in a slow collapse rather than a heavy fall as in an epileptic seizure. The patient may remain partly aware of the environment, but is unable to react to it. There may be small, irregular movements or a tremor. Urinary incontinence rarely accompanies such attacks. Typical findings are pallor, a cold sweat, and wide, reactive pupils. Unconsciousness lasts for a few seconds to a few minutes; the patient recovers upon assuming a horizontal position. If, however, the patient is propped up in a chair or even stood upright by persons around him who are trying to help, *convulsive syncope* may result, with an epileptic seizure and urinary incontinence (as, indeed, in any other form of syncope). On regaining consciousness, the patient may be fully alert, or there may be a period of fatigue and exhaustion, but without the postictal confusion seen after primary epileptic seizures.

This disorder occurs mainly in school-age children, with peak occurrence at age 6 and again at age 11–12. It becomes less frequent with increasing age thereafter.

Orthostatic hypotension. Orthostatic hypotension, leading (when severe enough) to syncope, may result from any disorder impairing the normal regulation of blood pressure; prominent ones include hypovolemia, sodium deficiency, Addison's disease, hypothyroidism, autonomic denervation in diabetic polyneuropathy, Parkinson's disease, Shy-Drager syndrome, multisystem atrophy, and other dysautonomic disorders. It may also be iatrogenic, as an adverse effect of various medications such as diuretics, antihypertensive agents, tricyclic antidepressants, and others.

Syncope Due to Vascular Disease

Transient cerebral hypoperfusion particularly affecting the brainstem can occur in the aortic arch syndrome and other organic disorders of the cervicocranial blood vessels. Some of these disorders have been mentioned elsewhere in this book. For drop attacks in vertebrobasilar insufficiency, see p. 198; for subclavian steal syndrome, see p. 191.

Disturbances of Consciousness of Metabolic Origin

Some of the metabolic causes of impaired consciousness have already been discussed elsewhere: hypoglycemia (p. 313), electrolyte disorders, particularly hyponatremia (p. 335), hypothyroidism (p. 315), and hypoparathyroidism.

Tetany

Tetany is a clinical manifestation of hypocalcemia, which may, in turn, be due to a primary disorder of calcium metabolism, hyperparathyroidism (p. 318), or sprue, among other causes. Metabolic alkalosis and elevation of the serum phosphate concentration are part of the syndrome. In *normocalcemic tetany,* however, the phosphate concentration is always normal, and the accompanying alkalosis may be either metabolic (e.g., after administration of bicarbonate) or respiratory.

■ Hyperventilation Tetany

The tetanic attack often begins with vague anxiety and myalgia, followed by digital and oral paresthesiae and, most prominently, muscle contractions. The fingers are pressed together, the thumbs markedly adducted (*obstetrician's hand*), and the wrists and elbows flexed. The legs are extended, the feet plantar flexed and supinated, and the toes flexed (*carpopedal spasm*). The lips are pursed. Laryngeal spasm and stridor occur occasionally, as do spasm of the gastric cardia, bronchospasm, and vasospasm. The attacks, which last from less than a minute to several hours, may be very disturbing. Consciousness may be clouded in such a way that observers believe the patient to be unconscious, though the patient can usually perceive what is going on around him.

The *hyperventilation test* is a provocative diagnostic test that is considered positive if the patient's reported symptoms can be reproduced by 3 minutes of forced hyperventilation. The validity of this test in establishing the diagnosis of hyperventilation tetany has, however, been severely called into question by a recent, critical placebo controlled study (435a). In between attacks, latent tetany is evident in the form of mechanical irritability of major nerve trunks: tapping the main trunk of the facial nerve induces contraction of the facial musculature (*Chvostek's sign*), tapping the common peroneal nerve at the fibular head induces foot dorsiflexion and eversion (*Lust's sign*), and compression of the nerve trunks of the upper arm with a tourniquet induces the obstetrician's hand posture (*Trousseau's sign*).

Physical examination is otherwise normal. *Electromyography* may reveal repetitive discharges of motor units, usually in doublets or triplets, when one of the provocative maneuvers described above is performed. The tetanic syndrome must be distinguished from brainstem seizures. The diagnosis of hyperventilation tetany is clearly assigned too often.

Drop Attacks

Sudden, unprovoked falling ("drop attacks") may be the result of a sudden loss of consciousness of epileptic or nonepileptic origin, but may also occur with preserved or only momentarily impaired consciousness (see Table 7.**18**). For vertebrobasilar ischemia, see p. 198.

Falls in Parkinson's Disease

Akinesia in Parkinson's disease may hinder the rapid reflex muscle contractions that maintain the upright stance, so that the patient, having once lost his balance, falls unchecked to the ground. This may occur before other signs of the disease are evident.

Cryptogenic Drop Attacks in Women

These attacks (previously called menopausal drop attacks) tend to affect women between the ages of 40 and 60, though they begin at an earlier age in some patients. They appear sporadically and are not accompanied by an unambiguous loss of consciousness. The patient falls forward without warning and at lightning speed; she may injure herself, and bruised knees are common (whence the French term, "la maladie des genoux bleus"). The attacks occur only a few times a year and gradually decline in frequency over the years. Their cause is unknown.

Vestibular Cerebral Syncope (Tumarkin Syndrome)

In this syndrome, the patient falls to the ground as if struck by lightning, with body still straight. The falls are often on the same side. Simultaneously, or a fraction of a second earlier, a sudden, brief dizzy spell begins, in which the environment seems to tilt away. Such attacks may be induced by rapid head movements and other movements (see also p. 695, benign positional vertigo). Many patients have other vestibular symptoms as well. Likewise, *benign paroxysmal vertigo of childhood* lasts no more than a few seconds, causes sudden falls, and may recur up to several times a week.

Further Causes of Drop Attacks

Atonic brainstem seizures are described in the next section (p. 557). *Brain tumors,* too, may occasionally manifest with drop attacks (usually midline frontal tumors). *Syringobulbia, colloid cyst of the 3rd ventricle, Arnold-Chiari malformation,* and *basi-*

lar impression can also cause syncope. For drop attacks of cardiovascular origin, see above.

Some useful ancillary tests for the diagnostic evaluation of drop attacks are listed in Table 7.**20**.

Episodic Nonepileptic Motor Phenomena

Paroxysmal alterations of muscle tone and muscle contraction, such as dystonia, choreoathetosis, and hemiballism, are seen in a number of (usually hereditary) disorders. Such phenomena must be distinguished from epilepsy (520b).

Table 7.**20** Ancillary tests in the evaluation of falls and syncope

Test	Indication
EEG (standard) with photic stimulation and hyperventilation	Epilepsy
Subacute ECG recording (Holter monitoring, event recording)	Cardiac arrhythmia
ECG and echocardiography (transthoracic or transesophageal)	Myocardial or valvular heart disease
Carotid pressure test	Carotid sinus syndrome
Measurement of heart rate at rest, on standing, and with Valsalva maneuver	Disturbance of autonomic innervation of the heart
Tilt table test	Vasovagal syncope
Subacute EEG recording	Normal standard EEG with clinical suspicion of epilepsy
Video EEG monitoring	Seizure analysis in suspected or documented epilepsy; suspected psychogenic (pseudo-)seizures
Polysomnography	Narcolepsy-cataplexy syndrome, sleep apnea syndrome, other parasomnias
Postictal serum concentration of prolactin	Grand mal seizures

Brainstem Seizures

Pathogenesis

The pathogenesis of brainstem seizures is poorly understood, and there is thus some controversy over whether they should be considered a form of epilepsy.

Clinical Features

Brainstem seizures begin suddenly, often upon provocation by movement, change of position, or hyperventilation. The seizure itself typically involves a tonic, almost always painful contraction of the muscles of one side of the body; usually, the arm is flexed, and the leg hyperextended. Most seizures last less than a minute, and consciousness is preserved. There follows a refractory phase of variable length, during which the patient can perform with impunity the movements that usually precipitate a seizure. Seizures without any tonic muscle contraction but with paroxysmal *hemibody pain* are much rarer, as are localized *atonic states* – e.g., a sudden inability to open the eyes. There may be dozens of attacks each day.

Etiology

Such attacks may be due to multiple sclerosis, vascular lesions of the brainstem, tumors and infarcts of the basal ganglia, or unknown causes.

Physical Examination and Ancillary Tests

The neurological examination is usually normal except for evidence of the underlying disease, if known (e.g., multiple sclerosis). The EEG reveals no specific change, either during a seizure or in between seizures.

Differential Diagnosis

Similar-appearing entities include metabolic hyperventilation tetany and reflex epilepsy – e.g., in parasagittal brain tumors.

> **Treatment**
> Antiepileptic drugs, particularly carbamazepine and oxcarbazepine, are almost always effective.

Paroxysmal Choreoathetosis

This is another nonepileptic disorder that must be distinguished from true epilepsy (437a). It has both *idiopathic* and *familial* forms; the latter is autosomal dominant and becomes evident in childhood. The paroxysms may or may not be induced by movement (kinesiogenic vs. nonkinesiogenic forms). Genetic abnormalities producing this syndrome have been traced to chromosomes 2q and 16 (84d); these loci may encode an ion channel (684c).

Clinical Features

The paroxysmally appearing movements begin in the distal portions of the limbs and travel proximally, sometimes appearing in the entire body at once. They may be choreiform, ballistic, athetotic, dystonic, or mixed. Asymmetrical, and even unilateral, forms are found in addition to the usual generalized form. The attacks usually last no more than a few minutes; in kinesiogenic forms they may be shorter than a minute, while in nonkinesiogenic forms, they may exceptionally last for hours or even days. Consciousness is preserved, and each attack is followed by a refractory phase lasting several minutes. In paroxysmal kinesiogenic choreoathetosis

(225a), the attacks can be precipitated by sudden movement, especially after a period of rest, while, in nonkinesiogenic forms, they cannot; an *intermediate form* has also been described, as has an *exercise-induced form* (paroxysmal exercise-induced dystonia) in which a simple sudden movement is not enough, but physical exertion suffices to bring on an attack. This entity is sometimes combined with migraine (684c). A clinical continuum exists between attacks of these types and brainstem seizures. Such attacks may also be *symptomatic* – i.e., secondary to any of a number of conditions including phenytoin toxicity, Devic's syndrome (p. 484), multiple sclerosis (p. 470), birth asphyxia, hypoparathyroidism, hyperthyroidism, and hypoglycemia.

| Treatment |

As in brainstem seizures, *antiepileptic drugs* are effective, particularly *carbamazepine* and *oxcarbazepine*. Kinesiogenic forms respond markedly better to treatment.

Involuntary Movements and Extensor Spasms in Pontine Ischemia

Involuntary, sometimes boxing-like movements of the limbs and extensor spasms, without impairment of consciousness, may appear as an early sign of basilar artery thrombosis. They may be uni- or bilateral and are sometimes accompanied by laughing, crying, or urinary incontinence. These may be the same phenomena that were earlier described as "cerebellar fits" resulting from processes in the posterior fossa.

Episodic Disorders that are Partly or Wholly Psychogenic

In predisposed patients, emotional factors can precipitate acute physiologic events, such as vasovagal syncope. Such events can even occur in epidemic form among groups of (usually young) persons (127a). The disorders discussed in the following section are all partly or wholly psychogenic.

Emotionally Induced Attacks in Childhood

■ Respiratory Affect Spasms

Pathogenesis and Clinical Features

This age-specific disorder (also known as "screaming fits") usually appears in rebellious and highly active infants aged 6–18 months and wanes by about the age of 5 years. There are two clinical types:

- In *cyanotic affect spasms,* fright, anger, pain, or other situations provoke a bout of screaming and crying. The child suddenly stops breathing in the expiratory phase, becomes cyanotic, thrashes about or becomes rigid, and then starts breathing again 5–30 seconds later. The child occasionally becomes confused; true loss of consciousness or clonic twitching is rare. The pathogenetic mechanism is presumably similar to that of cough syncope (p. 552).
- In *noncyanotic affect spasms,* the event is precipitated by a sudden fright or fall. The screaming phase may be absent. Within a few seconds, the child becomes pale, flaccid, and unconscious. Rigor and myoclonus may follow. The pulse may temporarily cease as the result

of a massive vagal outflow, and cerebral ischemia may result.

Diagnostic Evaluation

The *EEG* remains free of epilepsy-specific potentials in both forms of affect spasm; θ activity appears during the attack itself as a result of hypoxia, and high-voltage δ activity during the ensuing period of unconsciousness.

Prognosis

The prognosis is favorable. Affect spasms are not related to epilepsy. Some patients go on to suffer from vasovagal syncope in later life.

■ Sobbing Syncope

Here, the attacks are precipitated by pain or emotion. The infant sobs for several minutes at a stretch, thereby breathing shallowly, moving air mainly in the dead space. The infant becomes cyanotic and consciousness is impaired. Full unconsciousness and muscle spasms are seen only occasionally. This condition is harmless.

■ Startle Disease

This term denotes not only an organic disorder involving exaggerated responsiveness to external stimuli (hyperekplexia, p. 272) but also another type of hyperreactivity induced by fright. The latter disorder occurs mainly in brain-damaged children. A few seconds after the frightening event, the child stands rigidly as if frozen, with an alarmed facial expression, then falls to the ground, usually backwards, with arms rigidly extended, lies immobile for a few seconds, and then immediately recovers, perhaps crying or with embarrassed laughter. This may happen several times a day.

This condition must be distinguished

from hyperekplexia, true reflex epilepsy, affect spasms, and a hysterical reaction.

Psychogenic Seizures Resembling Epilepsy ("Pseudoseizures")
(571a, 575g, 859a)

The terms "pseudoseizures" or "nonepileptic seizures" are acceptable nonjudgmental names for this condition. Such events occur in 10–20% of adults who are evaluated for intractable seizures (175a). The mean incidence of this condition in a Canadian province over a 4-year period was three per 100,000 persons (928a).

These attacks are of a demonstrative-appellative nature and always occur in the presence of an "audience" (544). Dramatic, irregular, unrestrained movements are characteristic. The attacks are recognizably non-epileptic, in that:

- their phenomenology is not that of true epileptic seizures;
- the "ictal" EEG is normal, and the "postictal" EEG is not slowed;
- the seizures do not become any more frequent when antiepileptic medication is withdrawn.

The diagnosis can be established with combined video-EEG monitoring (175a).

■ Psychogenic Pseudocoma

The patient appears to be sleeping, with normal pulse, blood pressure, and respiratory rate. The patient continues to swallow normally with the usual frequency, as the observer can note by watching the larynx. Passive eyelid opening is usually resisted, and the eyes, once opened, look at the examiner. An attempt to provoke the vestibulo-ocular reflex does not induce the doll's-eyes phenomenon, as in truly comatose patients; rather, the eyes remained fixed on a point in the distance, or they are moved in the same direction that the head is turned in, with overshoot. The neurological examination and the EEG are normal. (N.b., the EEG frequency is also normal in so-called α coma due to a brainstem lesion (p. 234).

■ Other Forms

On occasion, *eclamptic seizures* in pregnant women with arterial hypertension must be differentiated from epilepsy beginning during pregnancy. The distinction is important, as eclamptic seizures are best treated with magnesium sulfate, rather than with antiepileptic drugs (600).

Neurological Findings in the Unconscious Patient and in Psychogenic Pseudo-Neurological Conditions

Neurological Findings in the Unconscious Patient

The assessment of the unconscious patient proceeds along the lines indicated in Table 7.**21**. The Glasgow Coma Scale, with which the depth of coma is gauged, has already been presented above on p. 225. Even in comatose patients, it is often possible to find evidence of a particular type of neurologic deficit (e.g., hemiparesis due to a contralateral cerebral lesion). *Lack of meningismus* in a deeply comatose patient by no means excludes meningeal irritation (due to meningitis or subarachnoid hemorrhage, for example). *Unilateral facial weakness* may be discernible as an asymmetry of the patient's grimace in response to a painful stimulus. *Passive raising of the upper eyelid* meets with less resistance on the paretic side. The *corneal reflex,* if preserved, will be less intense on the paretic side. A paretic *leg* is more strongly externally rotated. *Passively elevated limbs* that are allowed to fall back onto the mattress do so more rapidly and loosely on the

paretic side. *Noxious stimuli* are warded off, if at all, then less promptly on the paretic side. Finally, *asymmetrical reflexes or pyramidal tract signs* may be noted. For the examination of ocular motility in the unconscious patient, see p. 225. The *EEG is always abnormal* in (organic) coma. There are diffuse abnormalities of cerebral electrical activity in all leads, consisting mainly of slow δ waves (1–3 Hz). Moreover, the EEG may reveal specific evidence of the *etiology* of coma – e.g.:

- epileptiform activity,
- focal slowing due to a mass lesion, or
  triphasic waves due to a metabolic disturbance.

The Neurological Examination in Psychogenic Pseudo-Neurological Conditions

Psychogenic (hysterical) disorders of sensation and movement (pseudohypesthesia, pseudoparesis) are typified by an incongruity between the supposed lack of function and the accompanying neurological findings, or by an inconsistency with known neuroanatomical facts.

Psychogenic sensory deficits. The spatial distribution of a psychogenic sensory deficit is not consistent with a central, radicular, or peripheral nerve lesion. Pseudodeficits in a limb may be in a circular band around the limb, while a pseudohemisensory deficit may stop well short of the midline. The supposed total anesthe-

sia and analgesia may contrast with a fully retained ability to examine an object by touch. If the differentiation between sharp and dull is tested with the patient's eyes closed, the patient may say "dull" to a sharp stimulus in the supposedly anesthetic area, or indeed say "I felt nothing" each time a stimulus of either type is delivered. Similarly, testing of the warm-cold distinction may produce incorrect answers with regard to the temperature, while simultaneously demonstrating intact touch perception. If the

Table 7.**21**   Alterations of consciousness (see also Table 2.**54**)

Designation	Features
Normal consciousness	Oriented to place, time, and person (self), answers questions promptly and appropriately, follows commands correctly
Drowsiness	Mostly awake, responds to questions and commands slowly but usually correctly (after repetition if necessary), moves in response to a sufficiently intense stimulus, mostly oriented and well-organized
Somnolence	Mostly asleep, arousable with a moderately intense stimulus, generally requires repetition of questions or commands, but then responds correctly, reacts slowly and after a delay but usually correctly
Stupor	Asleep unless awakened, can only be awakened with a strong (auditory) stimulus or perhaps only with a mechanical stimulus, cannot answer questions or follow commands or does so only after intense repetition, and then only incompletely
Coma	Unconscious, cannot be awakened, does not respond to a verbal or auditory stimulus, may respond to painful stimuli of graded intensities with specific (localizing) self-defense, nonlocalizing withdrawal of a limb, or abnormal flexion or extension responses, depending on the grade of coma (see also Table 2.**54**)
Confusion	Inappropriate spontaneous behavior and responses to questions and commands, deficient orientation to place, time, and/or person (self); the confused patient may be fully conscious, less than fully conscious, or agitated (see below)
Agitation	Motor unrest, inappropriate spontaneous behavior, cannot be quieted by verbal persuasion, more or less disoriented, does not follow commands appropriately

patient reports total anesthesia in individual fingers of one hand, the examiner should have the patient cross his hands behind his back and then retest, whereupon the patient with psychogenic anesthesia will often place the deficit in the "wrong" finger.

Psychogenic motor deficits. A psychogenic motor deficit – often monoplegia – is not accompanied by objective signs. In psychogenic paralysis, the muscles are often activated in saccadic fashion, as when a muscle is less than fully activated because of pain; if the patient does not complain of pain, this type of movement implies psychogenic submaximal effort. The muscle tone is not abnormally elevated (though it may be diminished), the reflexes are normal, and pyramidal tract signs are absent. If the standing patient is rapidly spun around the vertical body axis, a supposedly flaccid arm will be held rigidly to the body and prevented from swinging about. When the patient is lying down, the examiner can passively raise the supposedly paretic arm and then let go; it falls back, by gravity, onto the mattress. If the arm is brought up over the shoulder beforehand, it will fall next to the head if truly paretic, but, in pseudoparesis, usually finds its way back to the trunk. Such findings suffice to rule out an organic monoplegia; it must be pointed out, however, that the intrinsic muscle reflexes may be normal in the initial phase of central organic hemiplegia, as mentioned on p. 169. Psychogenic pseudoparesis is not accompanied by atrophy (except,

perhaps, a mild degree of atrophy due to disuse in long-standing pseudoparesis), the reflexes are normal and symmetric, and EMG and nerve conduction studies yield normal findings, ruling out an anterior horn or peripheral nerve lesion. The absence of a sensory deficit is another indication that there is probably no lesion of the spinal cord or peripheral nerve. N.b., tendon rupture, particularly of the long extensor tendons of the fingers, can be confused on occasion with psychogenic pseudoparesis.

Psychogenic gait impairment. This may be present even in the absence of psychogenic paresis (573). The gait disturbance is irregular and of fluctuating severity, usually consisting of various different types of "almost falling," manifested successively or in alternation. The patient typically walks slowly and hesitantly, the knees often partly give way, and the patient sometimes seems to be slipping on ice. The patient practically never falls, while the highly acrobatic movements that are executed "to keep from falling" in fact reveal that coordination is preserved.

Psychogenic unconsciousness. Such patients generally resist passive opening of the eyes and deliberately look away from the examiner once the eyes are opened. Testing of the oculocephalic reflex produces nystagmus or a geotropic gaze (i.e., directed toward the ground), and the eyes fail to drift back to their normal position along the vertical axis.

Sleep and Disturbances of Sleep

Sleep

> **Definition:**
> Sleep is a state of reduced motor activity and vigilance that alternates more or less regularly with wakefulness in higher animal species. It is accompanied by alterations in various bodily functions, particularly those controlled by the autonomic nervous system, as well as by changes in cerebral electrical activity.

Normal Sleep

Human beings sleep 7–8 hours a night on average (normal range, 4–11 hours). The wide variation in the amount of sleep different individuals need is largely genetically determined.

Anatomical Substrate and Pathophysiology of Sleep

The reticular formation of the midbrain contains a system of ascending nerve fibers that exerts an activating influence on wakefulness and muscle tone. Lesions at this level are responsible for abnormal sleep in encephalitis lethargica, a type of viral infection of the brain. The pineal hormone melatonin plays a role in the circadian regulation of sleep and interacts with specific receptors found almost exclusively on brain cells (though in highly variable locations depending on the species). Melatonin is involved in the pathophysiology of jet lag.

EEG Changes in Sleep

Sleep consists of five stages with distinct electroencephalographic characteristics.

- *Stages I and II* are known as "light sleep." Stage I is characterized by diffuse slowing of cerebral electrical activity and the appearance of θ rhythms, stage II by θ and δ rhythms and K complexes (slow rhythms of reversed polarity, mainly over the frontal lobes), as well as periods of high-frequency activity between 12 and 14 Hz.
- *Stages III and IV*, called "slow, deep sleep," are characterized by diffuse disorganization of potentials, with δ rhythms (2 Hz) with diffuse spread and a small amount of θ rhythm.
- In *stage V*, also called "paradoxical" or "rapid-eye-movement sleep" ("REM sleep"), the EEG resembles that of the waking phase, with a few interspersed θ and δ rhythms. Phenomena occurring during stage V sleep include rapid eye movements, a generalized decrease of muscle tone, and mild clonic twitching of the face and upper limbs. Seventy percent of the total duration of sleep is accounted for by slow sleep, and 25% by REM sleep. Five percent of the night is spent awake. A night's sleep is composed of four to six cycles of the five sleep stages described.

Sleep Disorders
(70b, 67a, 97e, 190a)

The disturbances of sleep include:
- difficulty falling asleep or staying asleep,
- abnormal daytime sleep, and
- special phenomena occurring during sleep.

Difficulty Falling Asleep

This is defined, for clinical purposes, as a latency of more than 30 minutes from going to bed to falling asleep. This type of disturbance may come about because:
- the individual is not tired enough, having arisen too late or gone to bed too early;
- disturbing influences, such as worry and anxiety, are present;
- the individual has consumed substances that maintain wakefulness; or
- an abnormal physical condition is present that impedes falling asleep, such as pain, hyperthyroidism, etc.

Patients should also be asked about specific phenomena that make it difficult to fall asleep, such as restless legs syndrome.

Difficulty Staying Asleep

An individual may have difficulty staying asleep because:
- he or she has already slept enough, or
- he or she is repeatedly awakened by external stimuli, bodily sensations (e.g., urinary urgency, perhaps as the result of diuretic use) or psychological factors (worry, depression).

Medications such as corticosteroids, thyroxine, diuretics, and many different antihypertensive agents, as well as actual *stimulants* such as coffee, tea, or alcohol, may also play a role.

■ Central Sleep Apnea Syndrome (see also p. 569)

Central sleep apnea syndrome, a rare disorder, may be the consequence of a neuromuscular disease or of a lesion of the medullary centers of respiration (e.g., after a stroke) (367a). It can be diagnosed by polysomnography. Sleep apnea syndrome is sometimes termed "Ondine's curse." (The allusion is to a legendary water nymph in a 19th century novel who condemned her former lover to stop breathing and die as soon as he fell asleep.)

Treatment

Central sleep apnea syndrome can be treated with *theophylline* but is more commonly treated with *artificial ventilation.*

Sleep in Old Age

Elderly individuals sleep differently in a number of respects:
- The elderly spend more time in bed, but sleep less, and more fitfully. Those aged 60–80 tend to sleep 6–6.5 hours a night.
- The elderly go to bed earlier but need more time to fall asleep, more than 30 minutes in 32% of women and 15% of men over 65.
- The elderly wake up more frequently and have greater difficulty falling asleep again. The average 65-year-old spends more than 1 hour awake during each night's "sleep." Many wake up earlier than

in younger years: 50% of 70-year-olds wake up before 7 a.m., 25% before 5 a.m.

- Sixty percent of men and 45% of women over 65 snore regularly. This leads to fatigue, inadequate rest, frequent falling asleep during the day, and abuse of hypnotic medications.

Sleep problems in the elderly are usually treated with sleep-hygienic measures.

Insomnia is a common accompaniment of *dementia* – e.g., due to Alzheimer's disease, as well as of Parkinson's disease. Structural lesions of the brain such as intraparenchymal hemorrhage, trauma, etc., can also cause refractory insomnia (70c). Dementia usually causes a disturbance of the sleep-wake cycle, resulting in daytime hypersomnia and occasional nighttime confusion (70a, 70b).

Hypersomnia

This term denotes abnormal daytime sleepiness. Occasional falling asleep during the day may be normal under conditions of fatigue. It also occurs increasingly with advancing age, particularly after eating or after consumption of alcohol. Certain diseases also cause hypersomnia, for example, myotonic dystrophy (761a).

Pronounced hypersomnia, however, is pathological. The various causes of morbid hypersomnia are described in this section and summarized in Table 7.**22**.

Narcolepsy-Cataplexy Syndrome

This syndrome accounts for 10–20% of all cases of hypersomnia (17b, 67a, 70b, 70d, 70e, 321b).

Etiology and Pathogenesis

Symptomatic forms of the narcolepsy-cataplexy syndrome are relatively rare (secondary to trauma, encephalitis, cerebrovascular disease, or multiple sclerosis); most cases are idiopathic. Narcolepsy (as well as hypersomnia) is familial in about one-third of cases, and has an autosomal dominant inheritance pattern. In a large group of narcoleptics considered in one study, 40% had at least one relative with unusual daytime somnolence, and 6% at least one relative with documented narcolepsy (367). Familial cataplexy has also been described. Ninety-five percent of narcoleptics are of the HLA-DR2 type. The syndrome is thought to be due to abnormal function of the vigilance centers of the midbrain and diencephalon. *Norrie's disease* is an X-linked recessive disorder of which cataplexy is one manifestation (along with optic atrophy, deafness, mental retardation, and dysmorphism). Monoamine oxidase deficiency has been found in persons with this disease; thus, the question arises whether such a deficiency plays a role in the pathogenesis of cataplexy in general (988a). Further study of this question is needed.

Epidemiology

This syndrome affects men much more frequently than women. Its overall prevalence is difficult to estimate because the diagnosis is often missed. It accounted for 0.6% of the senior author's neurological cases. Its prevalence was estimated at 0.06–0.1% in an American population-based study, but merely 0.026% in a Finnish study in which polysomnographic diagnostic criteria were used (440). The disease begins in ad-

Table **7.22**   Differential diagnosis of hypersomnia (after 70d and 70e)

Primary sleep disorders	Sleep apnea syndrome Chronic sleep deficiency Narcolepsy Restless legs syndrome (RLS) Periodic limb movements in sleep syndrome (PLMS) Idiopathic hypersomnia Parasomnias Insomnias Disturbances of the sleep-wake cycle (e.g., shift work, delayed sleep apnea syndrome)
Neurologic diseases	Focal lesions of the pons, midbrain, and diencephalon Hydrocephalus Neurodegenerative diseases Muscular dystrophies Encephalitis and meningitis Epilepsy Kleine-Levin syndrome
Toxic-metabolic encephalopathy	Medications (hypnotics, sedatives, stimulants, antihistamines; antivertiginous, antihypertensive, and antiparkinsonian drugs) Hepatic failure Renal failure Pulmonary diseases with hypercapnia
Mental illnesses	Depression with hypersomnia Psychosis Alcoholism
Endocrine diseases	Hypothyroidism Obesity Pituitary disorders Diabetes with hypo- or hyperglycemia

-escence but usually becomes distressing only when the patient reaches young adulthood and the demands of everyday life become more severe.

Clinical Features

Only about 10% of patients have all four of the cardinal signs of this syndrome:
- disturbances of vigilance,
- cataplectic attacks (affective loss of muscle tone),
- sleep disturbances ("waking attacks," sleep paralysis),
- hypnagogic hallucinations and other, rarer phenomena.

One or other of these signs dominates the clinical picture in most patients, while the remaining signs are absent or present only in milder form. Patients may not report their milder symptoms spontaneously and should be asked about them specifically.

Disturbances of vigilance. *Typical sleep attacks* occur even in well-rested patients in sleep-inducing situations (warmth, comfortable position, satiety, boredom). They cannot be voluntarily suppressed and usually last only 10–15 minutes, though they may exceptionally last an hour or more. The patient can be awaked normally during the sleep attack. Once the attack is over, the patient feels well rested. About half of all persons with narcolepsy also experience *partially hypovigilant states,* which are more frequent than sleep attacks in some patients. Examples of such states include a distressing "sleep drunkenness," a twilight state in which appropriate behavior is carried out automatically, or another type of twilight state in which the patient acts irrationally and is amnestic for the event afterward. Such states must be distinguished from similar states occurring in temporal lobe epilepsy.

Cataplexy. Cataplexy is characterized by a sudden loss of muscle tone. It occurs nearly exclusively in patients that also experience sleep attacks, though not in all such patients. Tone is suddenly lost in individual muscle groups or even in all muscles of the body at once; thus, there may be a sudden, flaccid drooping of an eyelid or the lower jaw, an arm may suddenly drop, or the patient may suddenly fall to the ground. The patient then briefly remains unable to move the affected part of the body, usually for less than 1 minute. Cataplexy may so completely dominate the clinical picture that patients will not report any disturbance of vigilance unless specifically asked. Cataplexy sometimes occurs as a reaction to emotion (hearty laughter, sudden fright); this is called *affective loss of muscle tone.* It may also occur in the absence of an emotional stimulus – e.g., on the as-

sumption of a specific posture or the performance of a specific movement. Consciousness is preserved during all such attacks.

Sleep disturbances. The patient's *nighttime sleep* is often disturbed. A characteristic problem that may appear either as the patient is falling asleep or during the awakening phase is *sleep paralysis* (sometimes termed "waking attacks"), a cataplectic state that occurs when the patient is half awake and is associated with a distressing feeling of helplessness. This state lasts a few seconds or a few minutes and ceases as soon as the patient is touched or spoken to. *Nightmares,* sometimes very disturbing ones, are another type of sleep disturbance affecting patients with the narcolepsy-cataplexy syndrome.

Rarer manifestations. These include *hypnagogic* hallucinations – i.e., hallucinations that occur as the patient is falling asleep; occasionally, true psychotic states; sleepwalking (somnambulism); and diplopia, either as a manifestation of sleep paralysis or something the patient notices as he fights to stay awake. It has been reported that migraine is more common in narcoleptic patients (200c).

Physical Examination and Diagnostic Testing

The neurological examination is normal except in the rare symptomatic cases. Patients are usually short and stocky, and often obese, with a low basal metabolic rate, vasolability and hypogenitalism. As for laboratory tests, demonstration of the HLA-DR2 type supports the diagnosis, as this type is present in 95 % of narcoleptics, but only 20 % of the general population. The demonstration of hypocretin deficiency is of as yet uncertain diagnostic significance (711a).

EEG is of major importance in the diagnosis of this syndrome. The EEG during wakefulness may be completely normal but often shows the typical signs of somnolence, even in patients who seem well rested. *Polygraphic recording,* with simultaneous registration of eye movements and muscle activity in the evening or at night, is more cumbersome, but also more informative. It reveals a very brief phase of falling asleep, followed by the onset of REM sleep within the first hour of sleep, and a frequent alternation between REM and deep sleep.

The major features of the narcolepsy-cataplexy syndrome and of sleep apnea syndrome are listed side by side in Table 7.**23**.

Table 7.**23** Distinguishing features of the narcolepsy-cataplexy and sleep apnea syndromes

Aspect	Narcolepsy-cataplexy	Sleep apnea
History	30–50% positive family history, onset usually in 2nd or 3rd decade of life	Negative family history, onset usually in middle or old age
Daytime sleep	Usually in sleep-promoting situations, patient feels rested afterward; there are also hypovigilant twilight states	Overwhelming need to sleep, not necessarily in sleep-promoting situations, patient does not feel rested afterward
Nighttime sleep	Often restless, nightmares, perhaps sleep paralysis, patients sometimes do not feel rested in the morning, no headache	Loud snoring, respiratory pauses lasting more than 10 s (hallmark), diminished O_2 saturation of the blood, occasionally angina pectoris during sleep, patients usually do not feel rested in the morning, headache
Other features	Cataplectic states, perhaps as loss of affective tone, hypnagogic hallucinations and automatic behavior, no dementia	No cataplexy, perhaps hypnagogic hallucinations and automatic behavior, perhaps (reversible) dementia
Clinical findings	Sometimes short, stocky build	Usually men, almost always obese, often hypertensive, occasionally anomaly of nasopharynx
Ancillary tests		
EEG	Often signs of somnolence, short sleep latency, early REM sleep, frequent alternation with non-REM sleep	Unremarkable
Other	HLA-DR2 constellation	No specific HLA type

Treatment

Disturbances of vigilance:
These do not always need treatment but can be treated effectively with methylphenidate 10–80 mg/d, phenmetrazine 25–75 mg/d, amphetamine 5–40 mg/d, mazindol 2–8 mg/d, or modafinil 200–400 mg/d (142a, 670a, 964b). The latter two are the drugs of choice.
Cataplexy/sleep disturbances/nightmares/hallucinations:
All of these manifestations respond to clomipramine 25–75 mg/d, imipramine 25–100 mg/d, or protriptyline 10–20 mg/d. Sleep attacks may be eliminated in some cases, but only temporarily, through beta-blockade with high doses of propranolol. On the other hand, it seems that both sleep attacks and cataplexy can be eliminated, with few side effects, with ı-tyrosine at a dose of 100 mg/kg body weight/day.

Sleep Apnea Syndrome
(624, 625, 964a)

Prevalence
This syndrome is said to affect about 1% of the population overall and as many as 10% of men in middle or old age.

Clinical Features
The affected patients are more commonly male than female, usually obese, and often hypertensive (748a). The typical manifestations of sleep apnea syndrome include:
- loud snoring,
- motor unrest during sleep,
- diminished arousability,

- respiratory pauses lasting up to 1 minute, followed by a jolt and then resumption of breathing.

The most common cause is intermittent obstruction of the upper airway during sleep (*obstructive sleep apnea syndrome*). *Central sleep apnea syndrome*, in which the muscles of respiration intermittently cease being active during sleep, is rarer (see above). Polygraphic recording during nighttime sleep reveals multiple phases of apnea lasting 10 seconds or more, in both REM and non-REM sleep, with a drop in the oxygen saturation of the blood. On awakening, patients do not feel well rested and often have a headache. During the day, they are tired, fall asleep repeatedly, engage in automatic behavior, have hypnagogic hallucinations, and may suffer from intellectual impairment, perhaps reaching the severity of a (reversible) dementia.
Sleep apnea syndrome may cause hypoxic optic neuropathy with a visual field defect that is reversible by CPAP therapy (671a). Motorcyclists with sleep apnea syndrome are much more likely to have an accident than others (435b). Children with sleep apnea syndrome should be evaluated for a possible acquired disorder affecting the autonomic nervous system.

Diagnostic Evaluation
The most important pieces of information in diagnosis are a description of the patient's sleep from his or her sleeping partner and the repeated demonstration of an inadequate oxygen saturation of the blood during the apnea phases. More than 15 episodes per hour of a drop in saturation by more than 4%, or a saturation below

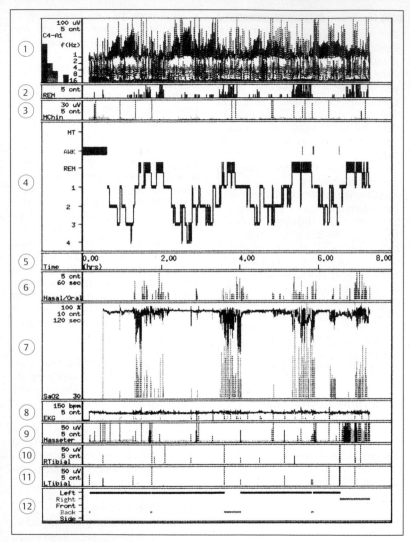

Fig. 7.**12**   **Polysomnography in a patient with REM-associated obstructive sleep apnea syndrome.**

90% for more than 1% of the entire period of measurement, indicate the presence of sleep apnea syndrome (365).

When the clinical suspicion of sleep apnea is high, the diagnosis can be definitively established by *polysomnography* (188, 321, 545). This technique was developed as an instrument for sleep research and can be used to investigate the cause of sleep disturbances (dyssomnias, parasomnias, sleep disturbances due to psychiatric, neurological, and general medical illness) as well as states of abnormal daytime fatigue and somnolence. It is performed in a dedicated sleep laboratory, in which the patient is allowed to sleep in a quiet, comfortable environment while be-

ing continuously monitored by infrared video cameras, and some or all of the following are recorded:
- EEG for determination of the sleep stage;
- an electro-oculogram (EOG) to monitor eye movements;
- an electromyogram (EMG) to monitor muscle activity (hypotonia and phasic movements during REM sleep, generalized movement during wakefulness and non-REM sleep); and
- ECG to monitor the heart rhythm.

The EMG is usually recorded through surface electrodes under the chin or on the limbs. The data are usually automatically analyzed and graphically represented as a *hypnogram*, on which the sleep stages and the various activities taking place in each stage can be easily read (Fig. 7.12). Additional parameters that are monitored in patients undergoing evaluation for apnea and hypopnea are air flow through the nose and mouth, respiratory movements, chest excursion, and changes in blood gases (O_2, CO_2). In some laboratories, the blood pressure is monitored as well.

Some sleep laboratories offer *home monitoring*, which has the advantage that the patient's sleep is less disturbed in the home environment and the test results are thus more reliable. A polysomnographic recording in a patient with obstructive sleep apnea syndrome is shown in Fig. 7.12.

◄ Abb. 7.12
1 EEG frequency analysis
2 REM sleep
3 Submental muscle activity, recorded through a surface electrode
4 Sleep stages: AWK = awake, REM = REM sleep, 1–4 = sleep stages 1 through 4
5 Time axis
6 Nasal/oral air flow and count (cnt) of episodes of apnea and hypopnea per minute
7 Transcutaneously measured O_2 saturation (upper curve) and frequency of drops in saturation by 4% or more (lower curve)
8 ECG (bpm = beats per minute) and count of episodes of tachycardia, bradycardia, or extrasystolic beats
9 Surface EMG (masseter)
10 Surface EMG (right tibialis anterior muscle)
11 Surface EMG (left tibialis anterior muscle)
12 Body position

Treatment

Sleep apnea syndrome is treated by highly diverse methods, including the *avoidance of sleep-inducing substances*; the *surgical correction of nasopharyngeal abnormalities*, if present; the fitting of a *retainer* to correct an overbite; and, most effective of all, nocturnal *continuous positive airway pressure (CPAP)*, in which the pressure is individually adjusted by means of an individually fitted nose or face mask.

Idiopathic Hypersomnia
(17b, 70b, 97e)

Clinical Features

Idiopathic hypersomnia is characterized by:

- prolonged nighttime sleep,
- delayed awakening, and
- more or less constant daytime somnolence.

Patients with this condition do not feel well rested after a daytime nap (unlike patients with narcolepsy).

Diagnostic Evaluation

There is no characteristic picture of this syndrome on polysomnography, nor are any specific laboratory findings known. This syndrome is about one-tenth as common as narcolepsy.

Treatment

Modafinil is effective against idiopathic hypersomnia as well.

Pickwickian Syndrome

This name (the reference is to a Dickens character) refers to episodic daytime somnolence (hypersomnia), confusion, and irregular breathing in an obese individual, sometimes accompanied by headache and papilledema.

Kleine-Levin(-Critchley) Syndrome

This rare disorder is of unknown etiology and seems to have a complex relationship to depression (1036). It is characterized by:

- intermittent episodes of disturbed sleep that may last several days at a time;
- vegetative disturbances, including periodically abnormal eating behavior (polyphagia, bulimia) and disturbed libido; and
- mental abnormalities, including confusion and agitation.

This syndrome affects pubertal and adolescent males above all; females are rarely affected. The episodes become shorter and less frequent over time, and the disorder generally resolves completely during the patient's twenties.

Diagnostic Evaluation

The neurologic examination is normal. The background rhythm of the EEG is slow during attacks. A diencephalic disturbance may be the cause.

Treatment

Successful treatment has been reported with *amphetamine*, *carbamazepine*, and *lithium*.

Fatal Familial Insomnia

This hereditary prion disease of autosomal dominant inheritance is described above on p. 124. There are also rare sporadic forms (829a).

Parasomnias

This term is used for a diverse collection of abnormal phenomena occurring during sleep or just before or after it (836a), of which the major types are listed in Table 7.**24**. *Sleep paralysis* also occurs in persons not suffering from the narcolepsy-catalepsy syndrome, often as a familial trait, and often when REM sleep is interfered with (nightlife, nighttime military maneuvers, etc.). *Somnambulism* (sleepwalking) occurs in about 17% of children and 4–10% of adults. Sleepwalking in the adult takes place during non-REM sleep and responds to clonazepam and certain other antiepileptic drugs (498). *Pavor nocturnus* is

rare, occurring in only 3% of children and 1% of adults.

Other Syndromes

It should not be forgotten that some 30% of persons with *epilepsy* have seizures mainly or exclusively at night. Nocturnal seizures may manifest with a shout or uncontrolled motor activity. Frontal lobe epilepsy with nighttime seizures is often difficult to distinguish from nocturnal paroxysmal dystonia. Patients (usually men) with *chronic REM behavior disorder*

Table 7.**24** Parasomnias

Sleep stage	Parasomnia
Wakefulness, falling asleep	Restless legs syndrome (RLS, p. 845)
Falling asleep and early sleep (stages I, II)	Myoclonus while falling asleep, sensory paroxysms Hypnagogic hallucinations Periodic leg movements (PLMS, p. 574) Bruxism Jactatio capitis Somniloquy (sleeptalking)
Mainly first half of night (non-REM stages III and IV, and arousal)	Somnambulism (sleepwalking) Pavor nocturnus
Mainly second half of night (REM sleep)	Nightmares REM behavioral disorder Cluster headache and hypnic headache (pp. 813 and 814) Painful erections Psychomotor seizures, frontal lobe seizures (p. 527)
Toward morning (neither REM nor non-REM sleep)	Cardiovascular symptoms Asthma
Arousal, awakening	Epilepsy upon awakening (p. 504) Hypnopompic hallucinations (REM sleep) Sleep drunkenness Sleep paralysis (REM sleep, also at onset of sleep) Nocturnal paroxysmal dystonia
Entire night	Enuresis (bedwetting) Calf cramps

act out their dreams – e.g., by shouting or running around; such disturbances may be a manifestation of a neurologic disease (occasionally the initial manifestation).

Night eating syndrome mainly affects women. Patients get up in the night and eat compulsively, often huge amounts of food, sometimes of a peculiar kind, usually in a half-awake state.

Restless legs syndrome (p. 845) and *periodic limb movements in sleep (PLMS)* often occur concomitantly and can seriously disturb the patient's (and partner's) sleep.

8   Polyradiculitis and Polyneuropathy

Overview:
Both of these conditions are characterized by the more or less simultaneous involvement of multiple peripheral nerve roots or trunks and manifest themselves in widespread sensory and motor deficits accompanied by loss of reflexes and muscle atrophy. Yet polyradiculitis and polyradiculopathy differ considerably in their specific clinical features and course, as will be discussed.

Polyradiculitis

Overview:
Guillain-Barré syndrome is an acute polyradiculitis that symmetrically affects the spinal nerve roots, and often the cranial nerve roots as well. It is occasionally preceded by an infectious illness. It presents with lower-motor-neuron-type weakness of acute, subacute, or slowly progressive onset that almost always begins in the lower extremities and then ascends to the rest of the body, accompanied by loss of tendon reflexes but often no more than minor sensory deficits. There may be no sensory deficit whatever (974c). The acute form may cause transient respiratory paralysis, necessitating artificial ventilation in an intensive care unit, but nonetheless carries a good prognosis. In contrast to Guillain-Barré syndrome, *atypical polyradiculitis,* of which there are several types, causes more slowly progressive and longer-lasting weakness that tends to recur and to leave a residual deficit. The prognosis is good in *Fisher syndrome,* a cranial polyradiculitis with ophthalmoplegia, ataxia, and areflexia. Autoimmune processes are important in the pathogenesis of all of these conditions.

Classic Acute Polyradiculitis (Guillain-Barré Syndrome, Landry-Guillain-Barré Syndrome) (901a, 968a)

This disorder, whose major features are briefly described above, was described in 1916 by Guillain, Barré, and Strohl (366).

Epidemiology

The disorder may strike at any age, including infancy; it affects males somewhat more frequently than females. Its incidence is 0.5–2 cases per 100,000 persons per year.

Clinical Features

In three-quarters of cases, the neurological signs are preceded by general medical symptoms of variable kinds, often due to an upper respiratory infection or gastrointestinal ailment. After a latency period of 2–4 days (in rare cases, 1 week or more) about half of all patients develop paresthesiae in the feet, and later in the hands as well. Only rare patients have pain, which may be present before any weakness develops. Weakness first appears in the legs at about the same time as the paresthesiae, or shortly thereafter, and progresses over one or more days to severe paresis or even quadriplegia ("Landry's ascending paralysis"). Weakness may ascend as far as the upper cervical level to paralyze the diaphragm (innervated by C4), causing respiratory insufficiency. Urinary and fecal incontinence are exceptional even when the weakness is severe.

Physical Examination

There is flaccid paresis with areflexia and, in severe and protracted cases,

muscle atrophy. Sensory function remains entirely intact in about 10% of patients, who neither complain of paresthesiae nor manifest a sensory deficit. The caudal cranial nerves are involved in about half of all patients, with resulting paralysis of swallowing and bilateral facial palsy (facial diplegia). Facial myokymia has also been described. Rare manifestations of central nervous system involvement, such as choreoathetotic movements, are presumably an expression of concurrent encephalitis.

The marked elevation of the CSF protein concentration (see below) occasionally leads to papilledema. There may also be general medical complications of disturbed respiratory function and prolonged immobility. Autonomic regulation is often impaired; there may be either orthostatic hypotension or hypertension, and there may be abnormal sweating. ECG changes reflecting cardiac involvement are seen in more than half of all patients; histologic study has revealed neuritis of the heart in such cases (291a). Urinary function is disturbed in about one-quarter of patients, without actual vesical paralysis (816b).

Ancillary Tests

CSF examination reveals the characteristic "albuminocytologic dissociation," i.e., an elevation of the protein concentration to as high as 3 g/L, while the cell count remains normal. This pattern may not arise till 2–3 weeks after the onset of weakness, but then remains evident for many weeks and resolves more slowly than the weakness does. The cell count is mildly elevated only in rare, exceptional cases; this finding should prompt a reconsideration of the diagnosis and a search for other causes.

Electrophysiologic studies reveal typical findings of demyelination. Slowed conduction, conduction block, and prolonged distal latency are found in more than 50% of cases when multiple nerves are examined, though occasionally not till the disease has been present for some time. Abnormal spontaneous activity (fibrillations, positive sharp waves) is rare and, if it appears in the first 4 weeks, signifies that the recovery will probably be incomplete, or at least delayed.

Course and Prognosis

In most patients, weakness gradually improves, in the reverse order of its appearance, until *complete recovery* is seen within a few weeks or, at most, months. In rare cases, however, maximal improvement is not seen until 2 or more years later. The overall *mortality* of the disease is largely a function of the quality of the nursing care provided, as well as the provision of artificial ventilation, if necessary. In our own patients (594a), the mortality was only 3%, and not a single patient died among the children who made up about 30% of our patient group.

Late follow-up reveals *residual deficits* in almost half of all patients, mainly absent reflexes and distal weakness in the lower extremities, but only 5–15% suffer any degree of impairment in everyday life. Residual deficits are more likely to be found when there has been a prolonged interval between the peak of weakness and the beginning of recovery, and also in cases where the weakness began suddenly after a prodromal gastrointestinal illness (737).

Pathologic Anatomy

Changes are found mainly where the ventral and dorsal roots join, but sometimes only in the ventral roots (which explains the cases of pure motor involvement). In other areas of the peripheral nervous system, too, there are zones of demyelination at those locations where lymphocytes and macrophages come in contact with the myelin sheaths. Axonal degeneration, seen in rare cases, generally indicates a poor prognosis, and may be regarded as the hallmark of a special form of the disease (291). Sural nerve biopsy reveals demyelination.

Etiology

The etiology of Guillain-Barré syndrome is probably heterogeneous; it seems to be a toxic or neuroallergic manifestation that may have many different causes. In most cases, the etiology cannot be determined; in others, the illness may be a consequence of a preceding infection such as infectious mononucleosis, *Mycoplasma* pneumonia, herpes zoster, or mumps. An elevated titer of complement binding antigen against cytomegalovirus is seen in one-third of cases, and herpes virus is found in others. A possible connection to influenza vaccination is the USA is currently under study.

Rare cases occur in the aftermath of a tick-borne infection with *Borrelia burgdorferi* (Lyme disease) or a febrile diarrheal illness due to *Campylobacter jejuni*. Antibodies to these organisms are more frequently demonstrable in patients with polyradiculitis than in normal controls. Some authors have reported a correlation between the severity of the initial illness and the occurrence of Guillain-Barré syndrome (782a), but this has not been confirmed by others (275, 989). Antibodies against *Campylobacter jejuni* may play a role in the generation of IgG-anti-GQ1b antibodies (1044b).

Cases following *Campylobacter jejuni* infection are more likely to involve axonal degeneration and thus to have a less favorable course. Polyradiculitis can also appear as a paraneoplastic syndrome, particularly in Hodgkin's disease. Familial cases, too, have been described. For polyradiculitis in HIV infection (188b), see p. 120.

Pathogenesis

Immunological processes play a major role. Anti-myelin antibodies are more commonly demonstrable in the serum and CSF of patients with polyradiculitis than in normal controls. Cell-mediated immunity is also important. Anti-GD1a antibodies are present only in cases with axonal degeneration (422c). Despite these suggestive findings, the pathogenetic mechanism has not yet been precisely identified.

Differential Diagnosis

Disorders with a similar clinical course include acute *peripheral polyneuropathy* of various causes, such as typhoid fever, porphyria, or acute poisoning (e.g., with triorthocresyl phosphate). *Acute sensory neuronopathy* may occur 4–12 days after treatment of an infection with penicillin.

Users of illicit drugs may develop a form of *wound botulism* that clinically resembles a polyradiculitis with purely motor cranial nerve deficits and flaccid quadriparesis (743b). The persons at risk are mainly those who inject heroin or cocaine subcutaneously or intramuscularly. Such persons may develop one or more purulent wounds in which *Clostridium botulinum* can multiply and elaborate its toxin, which blocks transmission at the neuromuscular junction. Impaired neuromuscular transmission can be demonstrated by electromyography, and the edrophonium chloride (Tensilon) test is often impressively positive (p. 924). In distinction to Guillain-Barré syndrome, however, there is neither blocked nerve conduction nor axonal involvement; in distinction to myasthenia gravis, there are no antibodies against the acetylcholine receptor. The demonstration of botulinum toxin in the patient's serum is diagnostic. This disease is treated by wound débridement and the administration of botulinum antitoxin (which is only effective if given early in the course of the disease), as well as symptomatic measures.

Infections involving the anterior horn ganglion cells may clinically mimic polyradiculitis, foremost among them acute anterior poliomyelitis (p. 909), above all in cases where pain is present from the outset, the initially high cell count declines after a few days, and the CSF protein concentration rises.

Polyradiculitis following a tick bite is discussed in the preceding and other sections (pp. 114 ff. and 613 ff.)

The *typical CSF pattern of albuminocytologic dissociation* can also create problems in differential diagnosis. The same pattern may be seen in chronic polyneuropathy, certain paraproteinemias, diabetes mellitus (p. 598 ff.), metaneoplastic syndromes (p. 320), and Refsum's disease (p. 290), as well as in *CSF inferior to a myelographic block* ("Froin syndrome") and in cases of *hypoliquorrhea*.

Table 8.1 provides an overview of the differential diagnosis of Guillain-Barré syndrome.

Table 8.1 Differential diagnosis of Guillain-Barré syndrome

Condition	Distinguishing characteristics for differential diagnosis	Remarks
Acute polyneuropathy	Sensorimotor deficits, more distal than proximal, appearing simultaneously in upper and lower limbs, axial musculature largely spared	E.g., in porphyria, acute poisoning, "critical illness neuropathy" in sepsis
Acute polyneuropathy after the administration of penicillin	Sensory disturbance of entire body surface appears in 4–12 days, with painful paresthesiae	Very rare
Infections affecting the anterior horn ganglion cells	Acute, purely motor paresis, occasionally focally distributed, nonascending, initial elevation of CSF cell count	Poliomyelitis, certain echoviruses and coxsackieviruses
Myasthenia gravis	Purely motor, exercise-induced weakness of fluctuating severity	Rarely acute
Acute myopathies	Purely motor paresis without sensory deficit	E.q., hyperthyroid myopathy, myopathy of acute myosin deficiency
Albuminocytologic dissociation of the CSF due to another disease (Table 2.21)	Possible causes: total obstruction to CSF flow by a mass in or adjacent to the spinal cord (with spinal cord transection syndrome and pyramidal tract signs); polyneuropathies – e.g., due to diabetes, metaneoplastic syndrome, Refsum's disease; hypoliquorrhea syndrome (headache, but no weakness)	

Treatment

Because the prognosis for spontaneous recovery is good, treatment is generally limited to supportive nursing care and meticulous prevention of complications. Prophylaxis against deep venous thrombosis and pulmonary embolism is of prime importance. Corticosteroids are generally not indicated.

Cases of chronic (inflammatory) recurrent polyradiculopathy are an exception (see below). Cases with unusually rapid progression and respiratory insufficiency (443a, 763a, 780b) should be treated with *plasmapheresis* or the intravenous administration of *immunoglobulins* at a dose of 0.4 mg/kg on five successive days, and possibly in a second, identical course 4 weeks later (968). Such treatment shortens both the stay in the intensive care unit and the overall hospital stay. A combination of the two methods yields no additional advantage (443a).

Atypical Polyradiculitis

The disorders discussed in this section are related to, but different from the more common acute polyradiculitis of Guillain-Barré type discussed above.

Chronic Inflammatory Recurrent Polyradiculoneuritis (125a, 967a)

This disorder is also commonly termed *chronic inflammatory demyelinating polyneuropathy (CIDP)*.

Clinical Features and Course

The clinical features and course of this disorder differ from those of Guillain-Barré syndrome in several respects. It may be chronic or stepwise progressive, or occur in acute attacks with remission in between, resembling a type of mononeuritis multiplex. A variant with subacute progression can be considered a special transitional form between CIDP and Guillain-Barré syndrome (443).

Pain is a very frequent accompaniment of this disorder. It characteristically produces asymmetric motor deficits and recurrent affection of the cranial nerves.

CIDP may be purely motor, purely sensory, or mixed. The purely motor form may be diagnosed electrophysiologically as a multifocal motor neuropathy (MMN) with conduction block (771a). A coarse and irregular tremor is also frequently seen, and seems to be associated with a higher likelihood of recurrence.

Pathogenesis

The pathogenesis of CIDP is likely to be heterogeneous (63). Abnormal immunoglobulins in the CSF and immunoglobulin deposits that can be seen on sural nerve biopsy indicate an autoimmune mechanism. Cases with monoclonal gammopathy have been seen, though this is more commonly associated with a chronic polyneuropathy. The Schwann cells are the likely point of autoimmune attack (422c). Similar mechanisms probably underlie motor polyneuropathy with multiple conduction block, a condition described elsewhere in this section.

Diagnostic Evaluation

As in Guillain-Barré syndrome, *areflexia* and *albuminocytologic dissociation in the CSF* are seen; the CSF protein concentration may be very high. *MRI* may reveal marked thickening of the nerve roots – e.g., in the cauda equina (832a). Though clinical signs of CNS involvement are rare and, if present, no more than mild, MRI and electrophysiologic measurement of central motor conduction reveal CNS involvement in far more cases (727). *Electrophysiologic studies* often document axonal involvement or reveal one or more conduction blocks in such patients.

Prognosis

CIDP is a serious illness from which 10% of patients die, 25% remain bed- or wheelchair-bound, and only about 60% can resume walking and return to work. The recurrence rate is 5–10%.

Treatment

CIDP is treated with a prolonged, combined course of *corticosteroids* and *immune suppressants*, specifically *cyclophosphamide* (63, 667a, 968c). *Plasmapheresis* and *intravenous immunoglobulin therapy* (see above) may also be necessary as the initial treatment steps (359b). Therapeutic success has also been achieved with *high-dose dexamethasone* (671c) and β-*interferon* (354,b, 621a).

Acute Motor Axonal Neuropathy (AMAN)

Motor deficits dominate the clinical picture in this rare acute condition. Patients often have high titers of IgG-anti-GD1a or anti-C3d antibodies (422c); many previously experienced a bout of *Campylobacter jejuni* infection (374a).

Acute Motor and Sensory Neuropathy (AMSN)

This disorder takes a course similar to that of AMAN, but marked sensory deficits are present as well.

Chronic Demyelinating Neuropathy with Persistent Conduction Block

This is a special form of CIDP (see above).

Clinical Features

This disorder is clinically characterized by asymmetric, more or less rapidly progressive weakness with muscle atrophy and sometimes fasciculations (it may thus need to be distinguished from ALS). Dysarthria and sensory deficits may also be present but are sometimes entirely absent. Individual reflexes are lost. This disorder has been described in combination with Sjögren's syndrome (968b).

Diagnostic Evaluation

Electroneurography reveals the site of conduction block. *Serology* reveals a high anti-G_{M1} titer.

Differential Diagnosis

This disorder must be distinguished from ALS.

■Treatment■

The treatment is the same as that of CIDP (see above).

Cranial Polyradiculitis and Fisher Syndrome

■ Cranial Polyradiculitis

Cranial polyradiculitis may be a component of an ascending polyradiculitis of Guillain-Barré type or the initial manifestation of a generalized polyradiculitis – e.g., in Lyme disease. Cranial polyradiculitis appearing in isolation may be accompanied by headache. It responds to treatment with penicillin and carries a good prognosis. It recurs rarely.

■ Fisher Syndrome

This condition (often called Miller Fisher syndrome in honor of its describer, the neurologist C. Miller Fisher) most commonly arises in male adolescents and is characterized by ophthalmoplegia with ataxia, areflexia, and sometimes pupillary involvement and facial palsy, along with an elevated CSF protein concentration. Neuro-ophthalmological findings such as Adie's pupil and the persistence of Bell's phenomenon despite the patient's inability to look up voluntarily imply additional involvement of central nervous structures by a concomitant brainstem encephalitis, which can be demonstrated by MRI (346, 758). Fisher syndrome is thus closely related to Bickerstaff's brainstem encephalitis.

The prognosis is generally good (379), but cases with respiratory paralysis have been described. Anti-GQ1b antibodies play a major role in pathogenesis (229c).

Polyradiculitis of the Cauda Equina (Elsberg Syndrome)

In 1913, Elsberg described a disease affecting the sacral nerve roots that progressed over the course of months or years (273), characterized by back pain, distal weakness, loss of reflexes in the lower extremities, sphincter disturbances, and urinary retention. Surgical exploration revealed inflammation of the cauda equina in the ab-sence of a mass lesion. A diagnosis of syphilis could be excluded. The patients recovered, but only over the course of several years.

We have seen similar cases, though usually of more rapid course, with elevated CSF protein concentration and cell count, and provisionally attributed them to borreliosis, as others have done as well (608, 687). The same syndrome has been reported to occur after genital herpes infection, with a good prognosis for recovery (336a, 359a, 575f, 972b, 982b, 1036a). HIV infection has been reported to cause not only peripheral neuropathy (331a), but also a purely motor lumbosacral radiculopathy (82). Such conditions must be diagnostically differentiated from a tumor or stenosis of the lumbar spinal canal (see p. 734).

▌Polyneuropathy (256, 602, 701)

Definition:

A *polyneuropathy* is a disorder affecting multiple peripheral nerves. There are many different types of polyneuropathy, which are due to a diverse range of (nonmechanical) causes (see Table 8.**4**), among them autoimmune processes, genetic disorders, toxic effects, metabolic disorders, infections, and other types of systemic disease. In general, polyneuropathy usually affects several peripheral nerves in more or less symmetric fashion. Different types of polyneuropathy may develop over the course of weeks, months, or years, in distinction to Guillain-Barré syndrome, whose progression is more rapid.

General Features

Clinical Manifestations

The major clinical features of polyneuropathy in general (regardless of etiology) are listed in Table 8.**2**.

Paresthesiae and sensory deficits. Polyneuropathy generally presents with paresthesiae and sensory deficits, usually beginning distally and symmetrically in the lower limbs. A stocking-and-glove distribution is characteristic. Particularly constant

Table 8.2 General clinical features of polyneuropathy

Category	Features
Initial symptoms	Usually paresthesiae, burning and/or "falling asleep," accompanied by hypesthesia, in the toes or soles of the feet
Sensory disturbances	First distally in the lower limbs, then perhaps also in the upper limbs, stocking-and-glove distribution, vibration sense practically always impaired or absent distally in the lower limbs, epicritic sensation (two-point discrimination, recognition of materials by touch) impaired in the fingertips
Motor deficits	Usually later than the sensory disturbances, beginning in the lower limbs, look for involvement of the intrinsic muscles of the dorsum of the foot; usually symmetric (except in mononeuritis multiplex, p. 607); affects foot dorsiflexors and upper limbs only later, most prominently the intrinsic muscles of the hand
Reflex abnormalities	Severe hypo- or areflexia; Achilles reflex disappears first
Trophic disturbances	Distal muscle atrophy, at first mainly of the tibialis anterior, later also interossei; sweating usually reduced, though sometimes increased at first; later, dry, smooth skin, ulcers (e.g., toe ulcers in diabetes), occasionally destruction of metatarsophalangeal joints
Tenderness to deep palpation	Peripheral nerve branches tender to deep palpation, particularly in the thigh

findings in polyneuropathy are distal loss of vibration sense and loss of epicritic sensation on the fingertips.

Motor deficits. These appear later than the sensory deficits, if at all, and are less common and less severe. They usually begin symmetrically in the lower limbs, mainly in the foot and toe dorsiflexors but also in the intrinsic muscles of the dorsum of the foot, perhaps later spreading to the hands. There may be atrophy of the tibialis anterior and interossei.

Loss of reflexes. This is practically an obligatory sign of polyneuropathy. The Achilles reflexes disappear first, followed by the quadriceps reflexes or the upper limb reflexes.

Trophic disturbances. These are unfailingly present and may be very impressive in some forms of polyneuropathy. For muscle atrophy, see above. Reduced sweating, a dry, smooth skin, trophic ulcers particularly on the soles of the feet (cf. especially diabetic polyneuropathy), and even dystrophic changes of the toes are the major manifestations of such disturbances.

Tenderness of peripheral nerves to deep pressure. This is a common finding, particularly in the calves.

Ataxia. Severe sensory loss is accompanied by ataxia, possibly creating the clinical picture of "polyneuropathic pseudotabes."

Ancillary Tests

Additional tests of various kinds are a major help in the diagnosis of polyneuropathy and the investigation of its etiology and are listed in Table 8.**3**.

Electromyography (needle electromyography). This technique demonstrates the presence of denervation even in the early stage of the disease.

Electroneurography. This technique is used to measure the sensory and motor conduction velocities of the peripheral nerves. Sensory conduction is impaired in a very early stage of the disease; motor conduction, too, may be very severely impaired even when nerve biopsy reveals no more than mild changes of the myelin sheaths. Testing the breadth of the distribution of conduction velocity across motor fibers enhances the sensitivity of the technique, providing objective evidence of additional types of polyneuropathy. This technique can also be used to distinguish polyneuropathy from polyradiculitis.

Muscle biopsy. Muscle biopsy may reveal the presence of neurogenic muscle atrophy, or of vasculitis, if present.

Nerve biopsy. Nerve biopsy can be used to distinguish axonal degeneration from demyelination, to demonstrate the deposition of extraneous material (e.g., amyloid), to demonstrate vasculitis, and to reveal the characteristic histologic appearance of various specific conditions (e.g., the onion-skin structure of the Schwann cells in hereditary sensorimotor neuropathy). Nerve biopsy may only be carried out on functionally unimportant nerves, thus practi-cally only on the sural nerve. It is indicated mainly in cases of chronic, asymmetric polyneuropathy, mononeuropathy multiplex, or thickening of the nerves of unknown etiology. Specimens are taken for both cross-sectional and longitudinal study under the light and electron microscopes for the demonstration of inflammatory changes, demyelination, vasculitis, amyloidosis, leprosy, sarcoidosis, and abnormal myelinating patterns. Nerve biopsy should be used sparingly in cases of symmetrical polyneuropathy, in which its diagnostic yield is low. Muscle and nerve biopsies can be complicated by local hematoma, wound dehiscence, and infection; thus, they should be carried out with strict aseptic technique, and the biopsied area should be properly bandaged and immobilized for at least 2 days afterward.

Lumbar puncture. Lumbar puncture aids only rarely in diagnosis. The findings are usually normal, though a nonspecific elevation of the CSF protein concentration may be found (e.g., in diabetic polyneuropathy, CIDP, or Refsum's disease).

General physical examination, general medical blood tests. A general medical work-up can often reveal the etiology of polyneuropathy.

Table 8.**3**   Useful additional tests for the etiologic diagnosis of polyneuropathy

Electrophysiology:
- Nerve conduction velocity (for confirmation of the diagnosis of polyneuropathy and differentiation of axonal from demyelinating forms)
- Somatosensory evoked potentials (to demonstrate posterior column involvement)
- Electromyography (for the differential diagnosis of neurogenic vs. myopathic weakness)

Erythrocyte sedimentation rate:
- Collagenoses
- Inflammatory processes
- Dys- and paraproteinemias
- Malignant neoplasia

Complete blood count:
- Inflammatory processes
- Lead poisoning (basophilic stippling)
- Leukoses
- Polycythemia

Blood sugar, glucose tolerance test:
- Diabetes

Blood urea nitrogen and creatinine:
- Uremia

Liver function tests:
- Hepatic disease
- Coagulopathy or anticoagulant-induced bleeding (PT, INR)
- Alcoholism

Thyroid function:
- Hypothyroidism

Serum levels of vitamin B_{12}, folic acid, thiamine, vitamin E:
- Malresorption
- Nutritional deficiency

Schilling test:
- (Partially treated) vitamin B_{12} deficiency

Uro- and coproporphyrins:
- Porphyria

Rheumatoid factor, antinuclear antibodies, circulating immune complexes:
- Rheumatoid arthritis
- Collagenoses

Phytanic acid:
- Refsum's disease in the differential diagnosis of HMSN

(Cont.) →

Table 8.**3**   *(Cont.)*

Serum electrophoresis:
- Collagenoses
- Dys- and paraproteinemias (M gradient?)

Gas chromatography:
- For the specific demonstration of toxins and heavy metals when suspected as the etiology of polyneuropathy

Microbial culture and serology:
- Infectious and parainfectious polyneuropathy

Bone marrow biopsy:
- Leukoses
- Myeloma
- Waldenström's macroglobulinemia

Lumbar puncture:
- Albuminocytologic dissociation in Guillain-Barré syndrome
- Total protein elevated in many types of polyneuropathy and in nerve root neurofibromas
- Pleocytosis: meningoradiculoneuritis (Garin-Bujadoux-Bannwarth)
- Tumor cells: carcinomatous meningitis, leukemia

Radiologic studies:
- Paraneoplastic (chest, colon, gastrointestinal tract; intravenous pyelography)
- Osteolytic and osteosclerotic myeloma (skull, spine)
- Lead (long-bone changes, lead line)

Endoscopy:
- Paraneoplastic

Scintigraphy:
- Skeletal metastases
- Myeloma

Nerve biopsy:
- Suspected vasculitis
- Special questions of formal and causal pathogenesis

Muscle biopsy:
- Suspected vasculitis
- Differential diagnosis of neurogenic vs. myopathic weakness

Hereditary polyneuropathy:
- Hereditary motor and sensory neuropathies (HMSN), cf. Table 8.**6**
- Neuropathy with tendency to pressure palsy
- In porphyria
- In primary amyloidosis

Table **8.4** The more common types of polyneuropathy

Polyneuropathy due to a metabolic disorder:
- In diabetes mellitus:
  - Symmetric, mainly distal type
  - Asymmetric, mainly proximal type
  - "Mononeuropathy"
  - Amyotrophy or myelopathy
- In uremia
- In hepatic cirrhosis
- In gout
- In hypothyroidism

Polyneuropathy due to improper or inadequate nutrition

Polyneuropathy due to vitamin B_{12} malabsorption

Polyneuropathy due to dys- or paraproteinemia

Polyneuropathy due to infectious disease:
- Leprosy
- Mumps
- Mononucleosis
- Typhoid and paratyphoid fever
- Typhus
- HIV infection
- Diphtheria
- Botulism
- After a tick bite (borreliosis, Lyme disease)

Polyneuropathy due to arterial disease:
- Polyarteritis nodosa
- Other collagenoses
- Atherosclerosis

Polyneuropathy due to sprue and other malabsorptive disorders

Polyneuropathy due to exogenous toxic substances:
- Ethanol
- Lead
- Arsenic
- Thallium
- Triaryl phosphate
- Solvents (e.g., carbon disulfide)
- Drug toxicity (isoniazid, thalidomide, nitrofurantoin, disulfiram)

Polyneuropathy of other causes:
- Serogenic
- Malignant neoplasia
- Sarcoidosis

Systematic Classification of Polyneuropathy

Polyneuropathy can be classified in various ways:
- acute vs. chronic course,
- by histopathologic features,
- axonal or myelin-sheath degeneration,
- by electrophysiological features,
- by etiology.

An etiologic classification would seem to make the most sense in clinical practice, and thus the more common types of polyneuropathy are classified by etiology in Table 8.**4**. The table is by no means complete and represents only one of the various, equally valid classification schemes.

Hereditary Polyneuropathy

Various types of polyneuropathy that may not become clinically evident until later in life are due to inborn errors of metabolism (not all of which have been fully characterized to date). Important clues to the etiological diagnosis may be derived from a meticulous recording of the family history, the investigation of close relatives if necessary, electrophysiologic testing, nerve biopsy, laboratory tests of metabolic function, and genetic analysis. The following major types of hereditary polyneuropathy are distinguished on the basis of their clinical and other features.

Hereditary Motor and Sensory Neuropathies (HMSN) (256)

HMSN IA, the most common subtype, is due to a mutation of the PMP22 gene on chromosome 17p11.2-12, while the more severe HMSN IB is

due to a mutation of the PO/MPZ gene on chromosome 1q22-23. Yet other mutations involving loci on chromosomes 3, 5, 7, 8, 9, and 11 and the X-chromosome cause changes in myelin proteins (79b, 903a). The subtypes of HMSN are listed in Table 8.**5** (44a).

The various subtypes can be diagnosed on the basis of their clinical manifestations, electrophysiologic findings, histologic characteristics on nerve biopsy, and, above all, genetic analysis (44a, 117a, 662a, 910c, 942b). These disorders are characterized by a progressive, symmetric polyneuropathy. Their subclassification according to the scheme proposed by Van Dyck, which has its share of arbitrary and problematic features, is summarized in Table 8.**6**. Only a few of the subtypes will be discussed in greater detail here.

■ HMSN Type IA (Charcot-Marie-Tooth Disease)

Genetics

HMSN type IA is caused by a 1.5 MB tandem duplication of a genetic locus on chromosome 17p11.2 or, less commonly, by a point mutation of the same locus, which contains the gene for peripheral myelin protein 22 (PMP22). The illness appears before age 20.

Clinical Features

The initial finding is a deformity of the foot that first appears in childhood, pes cavus in 70% of cases (Fig. 8.**1a**). Progressive atrophy of the calf muscles, mainly those innervated by the peroneal nerve, ensues. Weakness of dorsiflexion with relatively preserved plantar flexion is manifest as a steppage gait. The Achilles ten-

Table 8.5 Major features of hereditary motor and sensory neuropathies and other, similar hereditary neuropathies (reproduced with the kind permission of Dr. M. Auer-Grumbach, Neurological Clinic, University of Graz, Austria)

Type	Inheritance pattern	Gene locus/ Mutation	NCV (median n.)	Special features
HMSN type I				
• IA	AD	17p11.2/PMP22	< 38 m/s	Variant Roussy-Levy syndrome with tremor and ataxia
• IB	AD	1q22-q23/MPZ	9–11 m/s, variants > 38 m/s	Usually more severe than type IA, variant with pain, pupillary anomalies, and hearing loss
• IC	AD	?	< 38 m/s	
• I	AD, AR	10q21.1-q22.1/ EGR2	< 38 m/s	Phenotype like type I, congenital hypomyelination or Dejerine-Sottas syndrome
• IX	XD	Xq13.1/Cx32	25–35 m/s	Men more severely affected, often begins in the intrinsic hand muscles, knee-jerk reflexes preserved
HMSN type II				
• IIA	AD	1p35-36	Normal, > 38 m/s	Sensory deficits rare, lower limbs affected more than upper, pes planus
• IIB	AD	3q13-q22	Normal, > 38 m/s	Tendency toward plantar ulcers and amputation, moderate to marked sensory deficit, no pain, intrinsic muscle reflexes preserved
• IIC	AD	?	Normal, > 38 m/s	Accompanied by diaphragmatic and vocal cord weakness

(Cont.) →

Table 8.5   (Cont.)

Type	Inheritance pattern	Gene locus/ Mutation	NCV (median n.)	Special features
• IID	AD	7p14-15	Normal, > 38 m/s	Begins in intrinsic hand muscles
• IIE	AD	8p21/NF-L	38–52 m/s	Classic phenotype of CMT, variable sensory deficit; onset in 2nd or 3rd decade, questionable association with palmoplantar keratoses
HMSN type III				
• III	AR, AD	8q23-24/ PMP22, MPZ, EGR2	< 10 m/s	Severe phenotype, parents usually healthy, occasionally consanguinity
HMSN type IV				
• IVA	AR	8q13-q21	29 m/s	Described in Tunisia, consanguinity, unfavorable course
• IVB	AR	11q23/MTMR2	15–17 m/s	Facial muscles also involved
• IV	AR	5q23-q33	24 m/s	Described in Algeria, consanguinity, early marked kyphosis, unfavorable course
HMSN type LOM				
• L	AR	8q24/NDRG1	Normal, > 38 m/s	With deafness, occurs in Roma ("Gypsies"), consanguinity
HMSN type V				
• V	AD	?	Normal or mildly slowed	With spastic paraparesis

Table 8.**5** (Cont.)

Hereditary neuropathy with predisposition to pressure palsy

• HNPP	AD	17p11.2/PMP22	Mildly to moderately slowed	Pressure palsy after minimal trauma

Hereditary neuralgic amyotrophy

• HNA	AD	17q24-q25	Normal	Recurrent brachial plexus palsies, hypotelorism

Hereditary motor neuropathy

• HMN type II	AD	12q24	Normal or mildly slowed	No sensory deficit, mainly affects lower limbs
• HMN type V	AD	7p		Begins in intrinsic hand muscles, mainly abductor pollicis brevis and 1st dorsal interosseous m.; no sensory deficit, occasional pyramidal tract signs

Hereditary sensory neuropathy

• HSN type I	AD	9q22	Normal or mildly slowed	Dissociated sensory deficit, tendency toward plantar ulcers and amputation, lancinating pain

AD	Autosomal dominant	EGR2	Early growth response gene 2	NF-L	Neurofilament light gene
AR	Autosomal recessive	MPZ	Myelin protein 0	PMP22	Peripheral myelin protein 22
CMT	Charcot-Marie-Tooth disease	MTMR2	Myotubularin-related protein 2	XD	X-linked dominant
Cx32	Connexin 32	NDRG1	N-myo downstream regulated gene 1		

Table 8.**6**   Dyck's classification of the hereditary motor and sensory neuropathies (HMSN)

Type I (Charcot-Marie-Tooth disease)
- Autosomal dominant inheritance
- Onset in 2nd–4th decade
- Distal atrophy, beginning in the feet; pedal deformities
- Mild, mainly acral sensory deficits
- Marked slowing of nerve conduction velocity
- Peripheral nerves thickened and tough
- Sural nerve biopsy: axonal degeneration, de- and remyelination, onion-skin structures

Type II (neuronal type of peroneal muscle atrophy)
- Autosomal dominant inheritance
- Onset in 2nd–4th decade
- Distal atrophy in the feet and calves, hands less severely involved, pes cavus
- Mild, mainly acral sensory deficits
- Normal or mildly slowed nerve conduction velocity
- Peripheral nerves not thickened and of normal consistency
- Sural nerve biopsy: axonal degeneration, mild (secondary) segmental demyelination, no onion-skin structures

Type III (Dejerine-Sottas hypertrophic neuropathy)
- Autosomal recessive inheritance
- Onset in 1st decade
- Motor developmental delay, rapid progression, marked weakness in hands as well
- Marked, mainly distal sensory deficits
- Severely slowed nerve conduction velocity (slower than in type I)
- Peripheral nerves thickened, often also soft
- Sural nerve biopsy: hypomyelination, de- and remyelination, onion-skin structures, only thin myelinated fibers (no more than 4 μm in diameter), marked widening of endoneural interstitium
- Ceramide monohexoside sulfate accumulation in hepatic tissue (has been demonstrated in a few cases)

Type IV (hypertrophic neuropathy in Refsum's disease)
- Autosomal recessive inheritance
- Onset in 1st–3rd decade
- Retinitis pigmentosa, sensorimotor neuropathy, hearing loss, cardiac and cutaneous manifestations, skeletal deformities
- Markedly slowed nerve conduction velocity
- Sural nerve biopsy: axonal degeneration, segmental de- and reinnervation, onion-skin structures, lysosomal storage in Schwann cells
- Phytanic acid accumulation in various tissues, and in blood plasma

(Cont.) →

Table 8.**6**   *(Cont.)* →

Type V (with spastic paraparesis)
- Autosomal dominant inheritance
- Onset in 2nd decade or later
- Slow progression with spastic paraparesis but nearly normal life expectancy
- No sensory deficit, either subjectively or on clinical testing
- Normal or mildly slowed nerve conduction velocity
- Sural n. biopsy: marked diminution of myelinated fibers in a small number of patients

Type VI (with optic atrophy)
- Autosomal dominant or recessive inheritance
- Highly variable age of onset
- Progressive blindness, distal muscle atrophy
- Neurophysiologic findings unknown
- In rare cases, hypertrophic nerve changes

Type VII (with retinitis pigmentosa)
- Probably autosomal recessive inheritance
- Variable age of onset
- Distal muscle atrophy and weakness
- Mild distal sensory deficits
- Slowed nerve conduction velocity
- Biopsy findings not specified in available reports

don is lost at an early stage of the disease, and other deep tendon reflexes later follow. The atrophy and weakness of the calf muscles may progress over time, but the thigh muscles are hardly ever involved, so that the powerful thigh muscles contrast markedly with the wasted calf muscles ("stork legs," "inverted champagne-bottle sign") (Fig. 8.**1b**). The distal muscles of the upper extremities, particularly the intrinsic muscles of

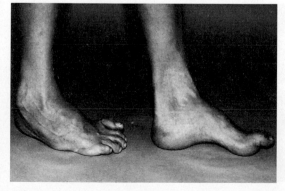

Fig. 8.**1a–c**   **Typical appearance of HMSN types I and II.**
a HMSN type I. Pes cavus in the varus position. The clawed appearance of the toes is produced by the greater strength of the deep flexors of the toes compared to the abnormally weak dorsiflexors.

the hands, may eventually be involved (Fig. 8.**1c**).

Only about one-quarter to half of all patients develop a distal sensory deficit to vibration and light touch, usually only later in the course of the disease. The examiner may be able to palpate thickened nerve trunks in the subcutaneous tissue, particularly in the neck. Rarely, there are other, accompanying neurologic abnormalities such as proximal muscle atrophy, nystagmus, posterior column signs, optic atrophy, pupillary anomalies, or essential tremor. Cases with pyramidal tract signs are separately designated as HMSN type V.

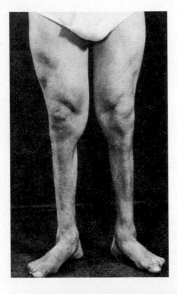

Abb. 8.**1**
b HMSN type I. Typical "stork legs." The marked atrophy of the calf muscles contrasts with the normal bulk of the relatively preserved quadriceps femoris muscle.

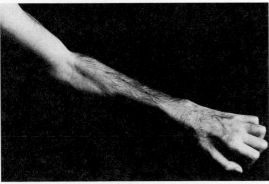

c HMSN type II. Atrophy of the distal forearm muscles and of the intrinsic muscles of the hand (from C. Meier, W. Tackmann, *Fortschr Neurol Psychiatr* 1982; 50: 349–65).

Diagnostic Evaluation

Electroneurography is of basic importance. The nerve conduction velocity is markedly diminished in all cases, sometimes even before the appearance of symptoms in persons with a positive family history.

Nerve biopsy reveals widening of the endoneural interstitium, signs of chronic segmental denervation and regeneration, onion-skin-like Schwann cells, and axonal degeneration.

Muscle biopsy reveals signs of neurogenic atrophy and, frequently, an accompanying myopathy.

Course

This disorder generally progresses very slowly. The patients are often remarkably free of impairment and can work even into old age.

■ HMSN Type IB

This autosomal dominant disorder is due to a mutation of the PO-MPZ gene on chromosome 1q22-23. It is more severe than type IA. Proximal muscle atrophy and pes planus are often present. The sensory deficit is also more pronounced than in type IA. The illness often appears before age 10; it is occasionally accompanied by other neurologic abnormalities such as hearing loss, pupillary anomalies, pain, etc. Electrophysiologic studies may reveal no more than a modest slowing of nerve conduction velocity.

■ HMSN Type II

This neuronal type of peroneal muscle atrophy is a disorder of autosomal dominant inheritance whose clinical features closely resemble those of neural hypertrophic neuropathy (see below), though its onset is somewhat

later and the hands are less severely involved. The peripheral nerve trunks are not palpably thickened, and the nerve conduction velocity is only mildly slowed. Electromyographic study reveals evidence of involvement of the anterior horn ganglion cells. Nerve biopsy reveals similar, though less extensive, changes to those seen in Type I.

A comparison of the electrophysiologic and histologic findings in HMSN types I and II suggests that these are two independent diseases that are separately inherited. Autosomal recessive forms that begin in early childhood and progress rapidly thereafter have also been described.

■ HMSN Type III

Genetics

This disorder, also called Dejerine-Sottas hypertrophic neuropathy, is of autosomal recessive inheritance.

Clinical Features

The clinical manifestations resemble those of HMSN type I but generally appear earlier, impairing the child's motor development. The motor deficit is more severe and more rapidly progressive, in proximal as well as distal muscles. The reflexes are absent, the peripheral nerves (including major trunks) are markedly thickened, and the spinal nerve roots may be so thickened as to cause spinal cord compression.

Diagnostic Evaluation

The *CSF protein concentration* is often elevated. The *motor conduction velocity* is more severely slowed than in HMSN type I, and *nerve biopsy* reveals a large number of onion-skin structures (abnormal Schwann cells). Sural nerve biopsy and liver biopsy reveal abnormal quantities of cerebrosides and sulfatides in the tissue. The disorder is probably caused by an inborn error in the metabolism of ceramine hexoside and ceramide hexoside sulfate.

■ **Hereditary Motor Neuropathy, Hereditary Sensory Neuropathy, Hereditary Neuralgic Amyotrophy**

See Table 8.5.

■ **Hereditary Neuropathy with Predisposition to Pressure Palsies (HNPP, Tomaculous Neuropathy)**

Genetics

This autosomal dominant disorder is due to a mutation in chromosome 17p11 (611, 740b).

Clinical Features

Affected individuals develop recurrent pressure palsies of individual peripheral nerves or of the brachial plexus. These may arise after even light pressure and can regress fully afterward. Writer's cramp and hand dystonia have been reported in some cases of this disorder (913a), paresthesiae, myoclonus, and fasciculations in others (28b).

Diagnostic Evaluation

Electrophysiologic study reveals the characteristic marked slowing of conduction velocity in peripheral nerves, even in those that are clinically uninvolved. Histologic examination shows a sausage-like ("tomaculous") internodal swelling of myelin sheaths, combined with segmental demyelination.

Polyneuropathy in acute hepatic porphyria

Genetics

Porphyria is a genetic disorder of autosomal dominant inheritance.

Pathophysiology

The underlying genetic defect of pyrrole metabolism, a partial deficiency of uroporphyrinogen synthetase, leads to accumulation of δ-aminolevulinic acid, porphobilinogen, and uro- and coproporphyrins, which are excreted in the urine. A change in the color of the urine after exposure to light, due to the light-induced transformation of the colorless leuko-form to the reddish-brown uro- and coproporphyrins, may suggest the diagnosis. Alternatively, urinary porphobilinogen can be demonstrated with Ehrlich's urobilinogen reagent.

Pathologic Anatomy

Sporadic myelin loss in peripheral nerves with axonal preservation is occasionally accompanied by secondary (retrograde) ganglion cell loss in the central nervous system, as well as foci of vascular change.

Clinical Features (123)

The disorder classically manifests itself in intermittent *acute abdominal attacks* (colic, constipation, vomiting), accompanied by high blood pressure, which may be induced by the administration of barbiturates. The major *neurologic manifestations,* which appear more or less simultaneously with the abdominal attacks, include signs of CNS involvement such as delirium, psychosis, seizures, impairment of consciousness, central blindness, and other focal ischemic phenomena.

Within a few days of the onset of the disease, polyneuropathy becomes clinically evident, either in the form of mononeuritis multiplex (p. 607) or as a severe, mainly motor polyneuropathy or polyradiculopathy causing a rapidly progressive, ascending, flaccid quadriplegia. A sensory deficit is hardly ever present, though pain and paresthesiae may be felt in the paralyzed limbs.

The spatial distribution of the motor neuropathy is often unusual, particularly at its onset. Thus, it may begin in the upper limbs and affect mainly the proximal muscle groups. Cranial nerve palsies, transient blindness due to vasospasm of the retinal arteries, and fluctuating central nervous manifestations are also occasionally seen. The autonomic nervous manifestations of porphyria include tachycardia, arterial hypertension, constipation, and sometimes bladder dysfunction. Agitation, hallucinations, impairment of consciousness, bizarre, hysteriform mental changes, and epileptic seizures can also occur.

Diagnostic Evaluation

The *CSF* is usually normal. Albuminocytologic dissociation is seen in rare cases.

Prognosis

The prognosis is poor. As many as one-third of patients eventually die during an acute attack of porphyria, generally because of brainstem involvement leading to respiratory paralysis.

Treatment

Adenosine-5-monophosphate (AMP) and hematin have been found to be of therapeutic value. Patients should meticulously avoid taking barbiturates, which can induce attacks of porphyria.

Polyneuropathy in Primary Amyloidosis

Genetics

Primary amyloidosis is an uncommon disorder. Most cases are familial, of autosomal dominant inheritance; the remainder are sporadic.

Clinical Features

Some 15% of patients have neurologic manifestations, of which *chronic polyneuropathy* is the most prominent. It becomes evident at some time between the ages of 10 and 60, most often between 20 and 30, more commonly in men than in women. Distal parestheslae and a sensory deficit in the calves (often dissociated) are the initial symptoms, followed by progressive, mainly distal weakness and muscle atrophy, which may be asymmetrical at first. There are often signs of autonomic dysfunction as well, including autonomic hypotension, abnormalities of sweating, impotence, and trophic ulcers.

Gastrointestinal manifestations such as diarrhea or constipation are present in nearly every case, and hoarseness, cardiac and renal manifestations, and opacification of the vitreous body are common. The disease continues to progress for many years.

Diagnostic Evaluation

The diagnosis is established by *biopsy* of the gingiva, rectal mucosa, muscle, or peripheral nerve.

Giant Axon Polyneuropathy

This autosomal recessive disorder manifests itself in childhood with a severe, slowly progressive polyneuropathy and later affects the central nervous system as well. Nerve biopsy reveals segmental axonal swelling due to an accumulation of neurofilaments. Affected children have kinky hair.

Polyneuropathy Due to Metabolic Disorders

Diabetic Polyneuropathies
(422b, 602, 791)

Frequency

The frequency of neurological complications in diabetes mellitus has been variably estimated in published reports; the more carefully the patients are examined, the more deficits are found. If reflex abnormalities and minor sensory disturbances are counted, 20–40% of diabetics in an otherwise unselected patient group will be found to have a neurologic deficit. Diabetic neuropathy most commonly arises between the ages of 60 and 70, when the patient has had overt diabetes for 5–10 years. In about 10% of cases, however, it is the diagnostic work-up for peripheral neuropathy that leads to the discovery of diabetes. Men and women are equally affected.

Pathogenesis and Clinical Features

The disturbance of glucose metabolism affects the peripheral nerves both indirectly, through pathologic changes in the blood vessels supplying them, and directly. Neurologic deficits of sudden onset are best explained as being due to suddenly impaired perfusion through the vasa nervorum. In patients with diabetic neuropathy, the walls of the vasa nervorum are hyalinized and contain deposits of abnormal material; these changes are significantly less common in diabetics without neuropathy, and in nondiabetics (343). They can be seen even before the onset of neuropathy, and their extent is correlated with the severity of the neuropathy.

The fact that the sensory nerve fibers are often affected early in the course of diabetic neuropathy, with resulting paresthesiae, pain, and areflexia, speaks for a direct effect of altered glucose metabolism rather than an ischemic effect, because these thin, poorly myelinated fibers are relatively resistant to ischemia. Similarly, the many *reversible* manifestations of diabetic neuropathy (e.g., pareses of the extraocular muscles) are likely to be of metabolic rather than ischemic origin. Nonetheless, there is no clear correlation between the severity of the metabolic disturbance and that of the neurologic manifestations, which may appear even in cases of mild or well-treated diabetes.

It is important to realize that neuropathy can develop even in latent preclinical diabetes, which can be diagnosed only by an abnormal glucose tolerance test. Nonetheless, measurement of the motor conduction velocity in the peripheral nerves of diabetic patients has revealed a correlation between the degree of slowing and the elevation of the blood glucose concentration. Neuropathy also tends to improve, or at least stop progressing, once the patient's blood glucose is under optimal therapeutic control. Parenthetically, we note here that not only hyperglycemia, but also *recur-*

rent hypoglycemia due to insulinoma can cause a motor polyneuropathy (or perhaps chronic injury to the anterior horn ganglion cells).

The frequency of the individual signs and symptoms of diabetic neuropathy in a group of 200 patients is shown graphically in Fig. 8.**2**. Distal paresthesiae and sensory deficits are the most common clinical findings. Contrary to the prevailing belief among many clinicians, the pain of diabetic neuropathy is frequently proximal (near the trunk), and more commonly uni- than bilateral. The extent to which the various signs and symptoms are expressed in the individual patient is highly variable, but one can nonetheless group certain patterns of clinical presentation into *characteristic syndromes,* whose features are summarized in Table 8.**7**.

Diagnostic Evaluation

Electroneurography reveals slowed conduction in motor nerve fibers, even in cases where the abnormality is still too mild to cause clinically evident weakness.

The *CSF,* too, is often abnormal. The CSF protein concentration may be elevated in diabetic patients even in the absence of clinically evident peripheral neuropathy. Some two-thirds of diabetics have an abnormally high total protein concentration, with values ranging as high as 400 mg/dL. The cell count is always normal; thus, there is an albuminocytologic dissociation in such cases. As expected, the CSF glucose concentration is high in 75% of cases.

Sensorimotor Diabetic Polyneuropathy

Symmetric, predominantly distal diabetic polyneuropathy is the most common neurologic complication of diabetes.

Mild form. The milder clinical form is usually seen in patients with type II diabetes, who complain of symmetrical paresthesiae and burning sensations in the lower limbs, and rarely in the upper limbs as well. The Achilles reflexes are practically always absent, and sometimes other deep tendon reflexes as well. Vibration sense is usually impaired distally, while position sense is less frequently impaired. Motor deficits, when present, are generally mild.

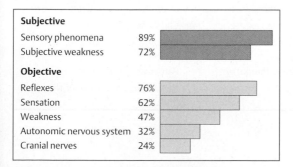

Subjective	
Sensory phenomena	89%
Subjective weakness	72%
Objective	
Reflexes	76%
Sensation	62%
Weakness	47%
Autonomic nervous system	32%
Cranial nerves	24%

Fig. 8.**2** Neurologic deficits in 200 diabetic patients (from A. Bischoff, *Die diabetische Neuropathie,* Stuttgart: Thieme, 1963).

Table 8.**7**   Effects of diabetes mellitus on the nervous system

Site	Manifestation	Special features
Central nervous system	Cerebrovascular accident Spinal cord ischemia	
Peripheral nervous system	Polyneuropathy:	
	• Sensorimotor	Distal, perhaps painful, symmetric, gradually worsening paresthesiae or burning pain in the feet, absent Achilles reflexes, diminished vibration sense, hyperesthesia in a stocking distribution, occasionally dorsiflexor weakness, occasionally toe ulcers and joint destruction
	• Proximal asymmetric	Mainly affects lumbar plexus or femoral nerve, unilateral, acute, painful, weakness of hip flexors and quadriceps m., diminished knee-jerk reflexes, positive reverse Lasègue sign, hypesthesia in femoral n. distribution, occas. similar findings in upper limb, spontaneous improvement possible (as in mononeuropathy, see below)
	Mononeuropathy: • CN III (most common)	Painful, affects only extraocular muscles, regresses within a few months
	• Other peripheral nerve	E.g., thoracic nerves with abdominal muscle weakness
Autonomic nervous system	Bladder dysfunction	Sphincter disturbance, atonic flaccid bladder
	Impotence	In younger male patients
	Diarrhea	Chiefly at night
	Necrobiosis lipoidica	Polycyclic cutaneous atrophy in women
	Osteoarthropathy	Particularly in the toes
	Ulcers	Particularly on the sole of the foot

Severe form. Severe sensorimotor diabetic polyneuropathy typically affects younger patients with poorly controlled type I diabetes. The symptoms arise gradually in the lower limbs, sometimes more on one side than the other. In the *hyperalgesic variant,* there may be extremely severe burning and dysesthesia, particularly at night; the patient may be unable to tolerate contact with the bedclothes and may seek relief by changing position or, less commonly, by lying still. Cold, too, often induces pain. The distal sensory deficit is always severe, and there may be ataxia as well, which is sometimes (though rarely) so severe as to produce the clinical picture of *diabetic pseudotabes.* The intrinsic muscle reflexes are almost always abnormal, and weakness may also be detectable. The weakness may lead to a steppage gait or to difficulty climbing a staircase.

Proximal, Asymmetric Diabetic Polyneuropathy

This form is much rarer than the distal form just described. The distribution of the deficits implies involvement of multiple nerve roots on one side, or of a nerve plexus. The symptoms arise suddenly, often with very intense pain that worsens at night, usually proximal rather than distal, and far more often in the lower than in the upper limbs. "Sciatica" is often the initial diagnosis. Weakness becomes evident simultaneously, and muscle atrophy somewhat later; patients often have trouble climbing a staircase or rising from a chair. Individual muscles of the trunk may also be weak – e.g., a single abdominal muscle, causing a flaccid protrusion of the abdomen on one side.

This type of diabetic neuropathy commonly involves the distribution of the femoral nerve; in such cases, the reverse Lasègue sign is positive (pain on hyperextension of the hip joint). The quadriceps reflex is usually absent, and there may be evidence of a distal polyneuropathy. The latter finding is, however, not obligatory; there may be no sensory deficit whatsoever.

This syndrome is presumably due to plexus ischemia. While asymmetric, proximal polyneuropathy is more common in poorly controlled diabetes, it can also arise in patients with clinically occult diabetes, in the absence of glycosuria. It tends to improve spontaneously over time. The clinician should be on guard against mistaking femoral neuropathy for an upper lumbar radiculopathy.

Symmetric Proximal Weakness

There is an entire spectrum of transitional forms between the acute, unilateral polyneuropathy described above and a symmetric, slowly progressive weakness involving both lower limbs and the pelvic girdle, without any discernible sensory deficit. The latter syndrome is termed *diabetic amyotrophy* (Bruns-Garland syndrome). It is doubtful whether this really constitutes a separate disease entity (64).

The weakness often becomes evident on one side at first, and on the other side after a variable interval of days to months. The weakness may progress either steadily or in stepwise fashion thereafter, and there may also be a transition from one type of progression to the other. The cause is presumably a combination of metabolic and vascular involvement of the peripheral nerves.

Both types of proximal diabetic neuropathy have a favorable prognosis for spontaneous recovery. Recovery is less likely, however, in cases involving chronic hypoxic-ischemic injury of the anterior horn ganglion cells. Fasciculations are seen in such cases, which are comparable in their clinical course to ischemic forms of spinal muscular atrophy or amyotrophic lateral sclerosis (p. 434).

Diabetic Mononeuropathy

Mononeuropathy in diabetes is the result of mechanical irritation of a nerve that is unusually vulnerable to injury because of the underlying metabolic abnormality, or else the result of infarction of a nerve trunk. Evidence in favor of the hypothesis of a local, mechanical nerve injury comes from the observation that electrophysiologic testing may reveal no abnormality other than in the single nerve that is affected. In such cases, the particular local cause of mechanical irritation should be sought (e.g., carpal tunnel syndrome).

Cranial Nerve Palsies in Diabetes

Palsies affecting the extraocular muscles. These are seen in approximately 0.5% of diabetics. The oculomotor and abducens nerves are affected at about equal frequency, the trochlear nerve only rarely. Weakness of the muscle(s) supplied by the affected nerve is of acute onset and often accompanied by orbital pain, which may be very intense. Oculomotor nerve palsies of diabetic origin, unlike those of other causes, spare pupillary motility. Diabetic palsies of the extraocular muscles are usually unilateral, but may also be bilateral in rare cases (generally at different times, rather than simultaneous). These palsies may be the initial clinical manifestation of diabetes. They usually regress spontaneously in 2–3 months.

Pupillary dysfunction. Pupillary motility is disturbed in 10–20% of diabetics. Anisocoria and an abnormally slow light response are the most common abnormalities. A true Argyll Robertson pupil, with an absent light response but a preserved near response, is a rare finding. If seen in diabetes, it is usually unilateral; in syphilis, it is typically bilateral.

Other cranial nerve palsies. Palsies of other cranial nerves are rare in diabetes. Their causal connection to diabetes is difficult to establish. Cases of dysfunction of cranial nerves I, II, VII, and VIII in diabetes have been reported.

Autonomic Dysfunction in Diabetes

Autonomic disturbances in diabetes are usually, though not always, accompanied by other neurologic deficits. Such disturbances include:

Bladder dysfunction. There may be either *sphincter insufficiency,* leading to incontinence, or *bladder atonia,* leading to large residual volumes in the absence of a painful sensation of fullness.

Diarrhea. The patient may suffer from bouts of diarrhea, occurring especially at night.

Sexual dysfunction. One-fourth of male diabetics suffer from impotence or retrograde ejaculation.

Other autonomic disturbances. The diabetic patient may suffer from *tachycardia, orthostatic hypotension, pedal edema,* and *lack of sweating,* particularly in areas of hypesthesia. *Necrobiosis lipoidica diabeticorum* is a focal, painless, polycyclically delimited, reddish-green cutaneous atrophy that is more common in women and is probably specific to diabetes. It should not be confused with local changes of fatty tissue at the site of insulin injections (*lipodystrophy*). *Diabetic arthropathy and osteopathy* are seen practically exclusively in the lower limbs. Imaging studies reveal osteolytic foci and areas of joint destruction, particularly in the tibiotarsal and tarsometatarsal joints, rarely more distally. As a rule, these osseous processes are painless, as are the stubborn *perforating ulcers* of the soles of the feet. The *skin* of the soles is usually markedly thin, smooth, and dry.

Disturbances of the Central Nervous System in Diabetics

These disturbances will be briefly mentioned here for completeness. The possible occurrence of diabetic myelopathy has already been hinted at above, but remains a controversial issue. The histopathologic changes that have been described in the anterior horn ganglion cells may, in fact, be retrograde changes secondary to peripheral neuropathy. Cases of amyotrophic lateral sclerosis in diabetics have been reported, but a more than random association between these two diseases has not been documented.

There is no question, however, that diabetic angiopathy leads to a greater incidence of *cerebrovascular accidents* among diabetics than in the general population. *Seizures,* too, can occur during hypoglycemic coma. In one study, 7% of a group of young, insulin-dependent diabetics had such seizures, and one-fifth of these went on develop true epilepsy in the aftermath of prolonged hypoglycemic crises.

Treatment of diabetic polyneuropathy

The most important component of treatment is *optimal glycemic control.* Reduction of the patient's blood glucose has been found to result in improvement of a number of the above syndromes, including proximal asymmetric neuropathy and palsies of the extraocular muscles, but not others. The paresthesiae and burning pain of severe symmetric polyneuropathy do not regress with improved glycemic control and may be long-lasting and severe. They can be treated with *anticonvulsants* – e.g., *carbamazepine,* or with *gabapentin* (48a). *Thioctic acid* has also been used. The centrally active, nonnarcotic analgesic *tramadol* is also effective (385a). The most effective treatment of all seems to be *clomipramine in combination with small doses of neuroleptics* (882a). Other proposed treatments for diabetic neuropathy include *B group vitamins, cessation of smoking, vasodilators,* and *sedatives.* Some patients gain some degree of relief from the topical application of *capsaicin ointment* to the dysesthetic areas.

Uremic Polyneuropathy

Polyneuropathy is sometimes a complication of chronic renal failure. One-quarter of all nephrodialysis patients have signs and symptoms of polyneuropathy. In addition, the arteriovenous fistula that is created for the purpose of dialysis may lead to local ischemic neuropathy of the median nerve (carpal tunnel syndrome).

Polyneuropathy in Hepatic Cirrhosis

Primary biliary cirrhosis is a rare cause of polyneuropathy. A purely sensory neuropathy may manifest itself before the hepatic disease does.

Polyneuropathy in Gout

Polyneuropathy is a rare complication of gout that responds to normalization of the uric acid level. Other neurologic manifestations are more common (carpal tunnel syndrome, ulnar neuropathy, spinal root compression, or even spinal cord compression).

Polyneuropathy Due to Improper or Inadequate Nutrition

These disorders are uncommon in the developed countries. An exclusively vegetarian diet without due regard to nutrition may lead to *vitamin B_{12} deficiency*, resulting in funicular myelosis with a neuropathic component. *Thiamine (vitamin B_1) deficiency* produces neuropathy as a component of beriberi, *niacin deficiency* as a component of pellagra along with other manifestations (dermatosis, diarrhea, agitation, psycho-organic syndrome). *Vitamin E malabsorption,* due to chronic cholestasis or other causes, produces polyneuropathy as well as ophthalmoplegia, ptosis, paresis, nystagmus, and pyramidal tract signs.

The pathogenesis of polyneuropathy in such cases is complex; aside from the vitamin deficiency, concomitant *protein deficiency* and other factors seem to be important.

Nutritional deficiency is also a major contributing cause of the neurologic complications of alcoholism (p. 609).

Neuropathy due to nutritional deficiency may in rare cases persist for years, or even decades, after correction of the deficiency itself. Thus, decades after the end of the Second World War, 5.5% of a group of former prisoners of war in the Far East still suffered from burning feet as a manifestation of peripheral neuropathy, as well as optic atrophy and hearing loss. Epidemic polyneuropathy may affect entire nations as the result of a chronic nutritional deficiency of B vitamins (especially thiamine) or sulfur-containing amino acids (793).

Polyneuropathy Due to Vitamin B_{12} Malabsorption

Polyneuropathy of this type was mentioned above in the discussion of funicular myelosis (p. 441). Careful clinical and neurophysiologic examination reveals evidence of peripheral neuropathy in two-thirds of patients with as yet untreated pernicious anemia. *Thiamine deficiency* is usually simultaneously present. *Folic acid deficiency,* too, can cause polyneuropathy, sometimes in combination with funicular myelosis.

Autoimmune Polyneuropathy

Pathogenesis

Polyneuropathy can be caused by either *dysproteinemias* or *paraproteinemias*. *Multiple (or solitary) myeloma* can cause local compression of a nerve or the spinal cord, or, by a humoral mechanism, a progressive and painful polyneuropathy with either purely motor or sensorimotor manifestations, mainly in the lower limbs. The polyneuropathy usually becomes evident before the myeloma is discovered and responds well to radiotherapy of the myeloma, but less well to chemotherapy.

Amyloid deposition in the interstitium of peripheral nerve is seen in some, but not all, such cases. The pathogenetic mechanism of polyneuropathy in myeloma and other *monoclonal gammopathy* is thought to be an autoimmune attack by immunoglobulin molecules on components of peripheral nerve, such as myelin-associated glycoprotein (MAG). Nonetheless, administration of anti-MAG antibodies to experimental animals has thus far not been found to produce peripheral neuropathy.

Histopathology

Demyelination, degeneration of myelin lamellae, and Schwann cell reactions are seen under the electron microscope. Endothelial changes causing widespread obliteration of the vasa nervorum in some cases are presumably contributing factors for the polyneuropathy.

Clinical Features

Polyneuropathy of this type is usually a chronically progressive and mixed sensory and motor polyneuropathy. Stepwise progression is rare, and purely sensory neuropathy is also rare. The manifestations are most severe distally in the lower limbs. Tremor is frequent, pain not uncommon. *Paraprotein-associated polyneuropathy* (IgM, IgG, or IgA) has essentially the same clinical picture (1038). Benign, anti-myelin-associated IgM gammopathy (271a, 568a), a special type of monoclonal gammopathy, occurs mainly in elderly men and produces a mainly sensory polyneuropathy. A characteristic histologic finding is widening of the space between adjacent myelin lamellae.

Treatment

Autoimmune polyneuropathy usually progresses slowly. Only a minority of cases respond to *corticosteroids, cytostatic agents, plasmapheresis,* or *immunoglobulin therapy* (271a), while many respond to the purine analog *fludarabine* (1028c).

POEMS

Solitary myeloma is associated with a particular syndrome designated as POEMS, in which polyneuropathy is combined with organomegaly (e.g., hepatosplenomegaly), endocrine disturbances, monoclonal gammopathy, and skin changes such as hyperpigmentation and cyanosis. Radiotherapy of the myeloma leads to regression of the disease manifestations.

Polyneuropathy may also complicate *Waldenström's macroglobulinemia*. The pathogenic mechanism is thought to involve occlusion of the smaller vasa nervorum due to macroglobulin-induced erythrocyte "sludging," as well as a competitive effect of the neoplastic process on the nervous system with respect to the demand for cocarboxylase.

Polyneuropathy Due to Infectious Disease

These polyneuropathies often develop acutely, sometimes only after resolution of the causative infectious illness.

Diphtheria

Polyneuropathy may appear after diphtheria has resolved, or after a case of unrecognized diphtheria. The more severe diphtheria is, the more likely it is to produce polyneuropathy; cases with polyneuropathy not uncommonly involve the myocardium as well. As a rule, palatal weakness is the first sign of polyneuropathy to appear, usually between the 5th and 12th day of the illness. Other cranial nerve palsies follow; weakness of accommodation is a characteristic finding. These initial manifestations resolve in 1–2 weeks.

Later, however, in a second phase of the disease, a sensorimotor polyneuropathy of the limbs may arise. By this time, the acute infectious process has resolved and the patient is afebrile and feels well. The manifestations of this second phase begin to regress within one to three weeks of their appearance and eventually disappear completely.

Mumps

Mumps may cause polyneuropathy as well as myelitis or encephalitis (p. 100). The disorder may manifest itself in cranial nerve deficits (e.g., sudden deafness), plexus neuritis, or ascending polyradiculoneuritis (p. 576) with elevation of the CSF protein concentration.

Other Infectious Diseases

Mononucleosis has already been mentioned as a cause of polyradiculoneuritis (p. 577). *Typhoid and paratyphoid fever, typhus, syphilis,* and *leprosy* can also cause polyneuropathy. The polyneuropathy of leprosy is the only one that can truly be called a polyneuritis – i.e., an inflammatory affection of the peripheral nerves. For *botulism*, see p. 455.

Polyneuropathy Due to Arterial Disease

Arterial inflammation in the collagenoses and, to a lesser extent, in rheumatoid arthritis can affect either the central or the peripheral nervous system. Peripheral nervous system involvement is manifest as *mononeuritis multiplex.* At first, ischemic damage affects a single nerve trunk. Later, further nerve trunks are involved, so that, at length, the clinical picture of a polyneuropathy results.

Polyarteritis Nodosa

Pathogenesis

Fibrinous exudation, damage to the tunica media of small arteries and arterioles, and inflammatory infiltration of vessel walls lead to intravascular thrombosis and thus to ischemic lesions of the nervous system and other organs.

Clinical Features

The *general manifestations* of the underlying disease are fever spikes, fatigue, arthralgia, cardiac disturbances, renal failure, skin rash, anemia, and often an elevated erythrocyte sedimentation rate. Neurologic manifestations are the first sign of the illness in about one-half of all cases. Those affecting the CNS were already described on p. 324. Polyneuropathy, however, is much more frequently seen.

Mononeuritis multiplex, as described at the beginning of this section, is typical in polyarteritis nodosa. Nerve trunks in the lower limbs are usually affected first; paresthesiae or pain appear initially, rapidly followed by paresis. As more and more nerve trunks become affected, more and more muscles become paretic, and the cumulative weakness increases. Yet half of all cases of polyneuropathy in polyarteritis nodosa are more or less symmetric and progressive from the outset. Peripheral cranial nerve palsies are sometimes the most prominent feature (Cogan syndrome, p. 325).

We have seen sciatica as the initial presentation of polyarteritis nodosa. In such cases, the diagnosis can only be established by careful examination for other signs of the disease, and by nerve and/or muscle biopsy.

Treatment and prognosis

Steroids may effect a temporary improvement, and cyclophosphamide may improve the long-term prognosis.

Other (Necrotizing) Arteritides and Arteriopathies

Other disorders affecting the arteries can cause polyneuropathy in analogous fashion to polyarteritis nodosa.

■ Rheumatoid Arthritis

Two forms of polyneuropathy have been described in rheumatoid arthritis:

Mononeuritis multiplex. Mononeuritis multiplex frequently occurs when rheumatoid arthritis is accompanied by a necrotizing arteritis clinically and histologically resembling that of polyarteritis nodosa (it affects other organs in addition, yet carries a somewhat better prognosis). Corticosteroid therapy appears to promote the development of mononeuritis multiplex and should be cautiously changed to another medication if this problem should arise.

Symmetric, mainly distal polyneuropathy. This second form of polyneuropathy in rheumatoid arthritis progresses slowly and is occasionally accompanied by nonnecrotizing arteritis.

■ Systemic Lupus Erythematosus

The neurologic complications of lupus more commonly affect the central than the peripheral nervous system (p. 327), but a chronic, progressive, demyelinating sensorimotor neuropathy can occur, sometimes with autonomic dysfunction as well. Mononeuritis multiplex is also possible.

■ Sjögren's Syndrome

This disease is characterized by keratoconjunctivitis sicca, rhinitis sicca, parotid swelling, and rheumatic joint pain. There may be both CNS deficits and polyneuropathy, often sensory with marked ataxia, sometimes with cranial nerve deficits. Primary myopathy also occurs (see pp. 327 and 909).

■ **Churg-Strauss Syndrome**

Patients with asthma and allergic vasomotor rhinitis may develop a form of necrotizing arteritis with eosinophilia affecting the internal organs and causing mononeuritis multiplex (612). The arteritis responds to steroids.

■ **Scleroderma**

Polyneuropathy is seen in this disease, too, and indeed paresthesiae may be among its initial symptoms. Myopathy with the histological features of polymyositis is also seen, in rare cases.

■ **Wegener's Granulomatosis**

See p. 326.

■ **Thrombotic Microangiopathy**

This disease, described above on p. 194, is also mainly associated with polyneuropathy.

■ **Polycythemia Vera**

Polyneuropathy is a rare complication of this disorder. For other neurologic complications, see p. 344.

■ **Atherosclerosis**

Atherosclerosis, too, can lead to polyneuropathy. Experimental vascular occlusion produces focal changes, first in the myelin sheaths and then in the axons; regenerative processes begin to function in 10 days. Atherosclerosis can cause sudden or more or less rapidly progressive deficits of individual peripheral nerves or of portions of nerve plexuses. We have seen isolated brachial and lumbar plexus pareses as well as true sciatic pareses. Deficits of this type remain confined to the site at which they arose and do not spread to become an actual polyneuropathy.

Migrating sensory neuropathy, a condition originally described by Wartenberg, is probably also of vascular origin. Transient pain and sensory deficits appear in attacks in the distribution of multiple peripheral sensory nerve branches.

Peripheral nerve trunks can be secondarily damaged by compression and ischemia in *compartment syndromes* due to ischemic necrosis of muscle. In *Volkmann's contracture,* ischemic necrosis of the flexor muscles of the hand and the long flexors of the fingers is accompanied by a usually reversible lesion of the median nerve (in about 2/3 of cases) and/or the ulnar nerve (less common). The *tibialis anterior syndrome* (p. 794) may transiently involve the deep peroneal nerve.

■ **Chronic Hypoxemia**

As mentioned above (p. 773), an arteriovenous fistula surgically created to facilitate hemodialysis can cause carpal tunnel syndrome by producing focal ischemia of the median nerve. Generalized polyneuropathy, too, can be caused by hypoxemia: distal, sensorimotor polyneuropathy was found in one-fifth of a group of patients with long-standing hypoxemia due to chronic obstructive pulmonary disease (759). Its severity was correlated with that of the lung disease.

Polyneuropathy Due to Sprue and Other Malabsorptive Disorders

Nontropical Sprue

This disease of adults, also termed celiac disease or idiopathic steatorrhea, is characterized by fatty stools, a poor nutritional state with thin body habitus, and anemia. Its most common neurologic complication is polyneuropathy. There may be accompanying funicular myelosis and cerebellar signs, as well as myopathy due to vitamin D deficiency and osteomalacia and tetany due to hypocalcemia. The neurologic manifestations may precede the gastrointestinal symptoms. Not all cases respond to vitamin B_{12} treatment; a gluten-free diet or antibiotics may be necessary (gastrointestinal flora, see p. 441).

Extensive Small-Bowel Resection

Patients in whom a long segment of small bowel has been resected can develop vitamin E deficiency, which can, in turn, cause a complex neurologic syndrome. Muscle symptoms (p. 917) are accompanied by ataxia, oculomotor disturbances, and glossal atrophy and fasciculations, as well as sensory disturbances and hyper- or areflexia. Abetalipoproteinemia causes vitamin E deficiency even more commonly than small-bowel resection or chronic cholestasis.

Treatment
The signs and symptoms can be improved, or at least stabilized, with vitamin E at a dose of 200 mg/ kg daily.

Impaired Gastric Emptying

A mainly sensory neuropathy may arise as a complication of impaired gastric emptying, which has a number of possible causes, including surgical narrowing of the gastric outlet by banding or gastroplasty for the treatment of morbid obesity. The neuropathy may be combined with Wernicke-Korsakoff encephalopathy (179b).

Polyneuropathy Due to Exogenous Toxic Substances

This etiologic category accounts for more cases of polyneuropathy than any other, about one-quarter of the total. The toxic agents include substances consumed for pleasure, medications, industrial toxins, and other substances. Only the more important ones will be discussed in what follows.

Chronic Alcoholism

Pathophysiology (p. 307)

The harmful effect of alcohol on the human organism is in relation to the total amount consumed. Thus, the risk of hepatic cirrhosis rises three-fold if daily ethanol consumption is increased from 20 to 40 g, 600-fold if it is increased to 140 g. The individual's susceptibility to alcohol-induced damage is affected by genetically determined variation in alcohol dehydrogenase and aldehyde dehydrogenase activity (there is interethnic variation in these factors as well). A mild elevation of the acetaldehyde concentration may indicate a genetic defect of both types of dehydrogenase that raises the patient's risk of toxicity from chronic alcohol consumption. Disulfiram (Antabuse) is an aldehyde dehydrogenase inhibitor. Aside from the toxic effects of ethanol and acetaldehyde, poor nutrition is a further contributory factor toward neurologic dysfunction in practically all alcoholics.

Effects of Alcohol on the Nervous System

The effects of alcohol on the nervous system are summarized in Table 2.**79**. We will not discuss the psychopathological phenomena any further here. For epilepsy, see p. 309; Wernicke's encephalopathy, p. 310; cerebellar ataxia, p. 310; myopathy, p. 917; amblyopia, p. 625.

■ **Polyneuropathy**

Clinical Features

The most prominent symptoms are intense, neuralgic pain, mainly in the lower extremities, occasionally accompanied by muscle cramps, mainly at night. Muscle weakness is a rarer initial complaint. Alcoholic polyneuropathy is generally slowly progressive and long-lasting, but there is also an acute axonal form (1031b).

Physical examination reveals diminished or absent deep tendon reflexes; in half of all patients, both Achilles reflexes are absent. Impaired proprioception, hypesthesia in a stocking distribution, and primarily dorsiflexor weakness are found. Pressure on the calf is often painful. A slow tremor of the leg (ca. 3 Hz) is frequently seen, and a brainstem auditory evoked potential study reveals prolonged latencies. Electroneurography reveals delayed conduction of motor action potentials, particularly in the peroneal nerve.

Involvement of the autonomic nervous system leads to a disturbance of sweating, including increased sweating on the soles of the feet; trophic disturbances; impaired regulation of blood pressure; hyperthermia; hoarseness; and impotence. Both electrophysiologic and structural (biopsy) studies of the sural nerve reveal mainly axonal degeneration in both myelinated and unmyelinated fibers.

Lead Poisoning

See p. 302.

Arsenic Poisoning

Clinical Features

The most common cause of arsenic poisoning is the ingestion of certain types of insecticide, though an overdose of certain arsenic-containing medications can also be responsible. One to two weeks after the ingestion of arsenic, a neuropathy appears, with intense dysesthesia, muscle tenderness, and distal weakness. Diarrhea, skin changes with pigment abnormalities, hair loss, and white striations of the fingernails, called Mees lines (*not* pathognomonic), also appear. Encephalopathy and myelopathy are rare.

The polyneuropathy reaches a clinical peak at about 4 weeks, though electrophysiologic testing shows that the nerve conduction delay continues to progress for at least 3 months.

Prognosis

The prognosis is poor, in that recovery is often incomplete, and burning dysesthesia of the foot may persist for years.

▌**Treatment**▌

Chelators should be given, if possible, before the signs of polyneuropathy develop.

Thallium Poisoning

An odorless, tasteless salt of the heavy metal thallium is found in rat poison. Thallium poisoning has the same clinical manifestations as arsenic poisoning. Histopathologic study reveals axonal degeneration.

Triaryl Phosphate Poisoning

Cause

This type of poisoning is mainly caused by ingestion of certain industrial oils used for extraction and lubrication. Triaryl phosphate is also used in the extraction of apiol (an abortifacient) from parsley. Mass poisoning with triaryl phosphate can occur through the misuse of industrial oils as cooking oil.

Pathologic Anatomy

Even in the early phase of the disorder, pathologic study reveals axoplasmic changes as well as alterations in the CNS and in muscle.

Clinical Features

Soon after ingestion of contaminated food, the patient generally experiences *nausea and diarrhea.* Next comes a clinically silent latency period lasting 1–5 weeks, followed by a *prodromal phase,* with mild fever and flu-like and gastrointestinal symptoms. Finally, 10–38 days after the ingestion, the *paralytic phase* begins. Flaccid, usually symmetrical weakness appears in the toes and then spreads to the feet within a few hours, and to the fingers and hands a few days later. The weakness is maximally severe by 8–10 days from its onset, by which time it involves the proximal muscle groups as well. The deep tendon reflexes are absent, sensation is impaired in a stocking distribution, and muscle atrophy is found. The *further course* is variable. Sometimes, the deficits just described regress in the ensuing period. In other

cases, however, spasticity and pyramidal tract signs appear and then slowly progress. Almost one-third of affected adults have exaggerated quadriceps reflexes by 1 year from the ingestion. In the late phase, spasticity may dominate the clinical picture.

Medications

■ Thalidomide

Clinical Features

This formerly used hypnotic caused clinical symptoms of polyneuropathy after a few weeks of use, even at the normally prescribed doses.

Symptoms. Paresthesiae (mainly in the toes), neuralgic pain, and weakness were the more prominent symptoms. The paresthesiae became more severe at night in the warmth of the bedclothes; their character was sometimes reminiscent of causalgia.

Signs. Hypesthesia in a stocking-and-glove distribution and (nearly always) absence of the Achilles reflexes could be found. Thalidomide neuropathy was thus a mainly sensory polyneuropathy.

Prognosis

The manifestations of thalidomide neuropathy tended to persist for a long time, even many years after cessation of the drug.

■ Isoniazid

Clinical Features

Polyneuropathy generally appears only when the dose exceeds 15 mg/kg daily. At such high doses, more than

50% of patients develop polyneuropathy. Children, however, can usually tolerate high doses.

Symptoms. Around 6–8 weeks after treatment with isoniazid is begun, patients complain of paresthesiae and "falling asleep" in their feet and toes. These sensations gradually worsen, spread to the hands, and become painful.

Signs. Neurologic examination reveals a severe, distal, predominantly sensory polyneuropathy accompanied by vasomotor dysfunction. Psychosis and other signs of CNS dysfunction may arise.

Pathophysiology
Isoniazid impairs the functioning of the nervous system by interfering with pyridoxine metabolism.

> ████ **Treatment** ████████
> Isoniazid polyneuropathy can be *prevented* by the simultaneous administration of *pyridoxine*, 50–100 mg/day. Once isoniazid polyneuropathy has arisen, it should be treated by cessation of the drug or reduction of its dose, and the injection of 200–400 mg of pyridoxine daily.

■ **Nitrofurantoin**
This medication, used to treat urinary tract infections, can cause polyneuropathy even in the usually prescribed doses if renal failure is present. The severity and prognosis of the neurologic manifestations is directly related to the degree of renal failure. In patients with marked renal failure, nitrofurantoin can produce a severe, irreversible sensorimotor

polyneuropathy 1–2 weeks after the start of treatment.

■ **Other Medications**
Meprobamate, hydralazine, and *disulfiram* are rarer causes of polyneuropathy. Alcoholics who take disulfiram in high doses can develop fulminant, severe polyneuropathy. *Vincristine* can induce polyneuropathy, in addition to hair loss and constipation. Severe polyneuropathy has also been described with *lithium* and the thyrostatic agent *carbimazole. Pyridoxine abuse* can cause a type of sensory polyneuropathy whose dominant feature is ataxia.

Other Toxic Polyneuropathies

In the early 1980s, an epidemic of toxic polyneuropathy occurred in Spain, due to the consumption of *olive oil* contaminated with a substance that was never definitively identified. Three-quarters of persons who consumed the oil developed neurologic symptoms 4–8 weeks later, and eventually this figure rose to 92%. There was an axonal neuropathy with myalgia, cramps, weakness, areflexia, muscle atrophy, and sensory disturbances. Many patients were still disabled 12 months later.

A number of solvents, including *trichloroethylene* and *carbon disulfide,* can cause a mainly sensory polyneuropathy. Likewise, recreational sniffing of the industrial solvent *n-hexane* (found in glue) causes polyneuropathy.

Finally, polyneuropathy can result from exposure to *acrylamide* and from *carbon monoxide* poisoning.

Polyneuropathy of Other Causes

Serogenic Polyneuropathy

Serogenic polyneuropathy most commonly follows prophylactic tetanus immunization, always as a component of a generalized serum disease, usually 4–12 days after the injection. It may appear in localized form, either in the shoulder (resembling neuralgic shoulder amyotrophy, p. 765) or at other sites (e.g., peroneal nerve palsy), or it may be a generalized, acute polyradiculoneuropathy causing quadriparesis, and sometimes cranial nerve palsies as well.

Proximal Motor Neuropathy with Multifocal Conduction Block

Clinical Features

This disorder is clinically characterized by chronically progressive, asymmetric, at first purely motor paresis, accompanied by fasciculations, pain or cramps, and sometimes myokymia (129, 580, 742). The intrinsic muscle reflexes are diminished or absent (125). Weakness worsens over months or years and is progressively disabling. It is not always easy to establish the necessary differential diagnosis of this disorder from spinal muscular atrophy and amyotrophic lateral sclerosis.

Diagnosis

Electroneurography yields the diagnostically essential finding of mainly proximal, segmental conduction block in multiple peripheral nerve trunks. High titers of anti-G_{M1} antibody can often be measured.

▰▰▰ Treatment ▰▰▰
Patients in whom atrophy is still mild benefit especially well from intravenous immunoglobulin therapy.

Meningopolyneuritis after a Tick Bite (Borreliosis)

Epidemiology

This illness is transmitted by the bite of a tick, usually *Ixodes ricinus,* and rarely by other insects. We are not concerned here with viral early summer meningoencephalitis (p. 101), but rather with a disease caused by the spirochete *Borrelia burgdorferi* with peak incidence in the summer and fall, mainly in areas in which there are many ticks bearing the spirochete.

Nomenclature

This disorder is known under various names: *erythema chronicum migrans disease* after the characteristic skin lesion (see below), *Lyme disease* after a town in Connecticut in which a number of cases were described, *meningopolyneuritis,* and *Garin-Bujadoux-Bannwarth syndrome.*

Clinical Features (330)

In many but not all cases, a ring-shaped skin rash called *erythema chronicum migrans* appears immediately at the site of the tick bite and slowly expands in the ensuing days or weeks. A few weeks later, the patient experiences *intense pain,* usually at the site of the bite. Later, polyneuropathy or polyradiculopathy develops, often asymmetrically, sometimes accompanied by *facial palsy* (which is often bilateral) (377).

The distribution of weakness is highly variable. The clinical picture may be of a painful, localized neuropathy or radiculopathy, a painful polyradiculitis of Guillain-Barré type, or cranial polyradiculitis.

These neurologic manifestations are almost always accompanied by an elevation of both the CSF protein concentration and the CSF cell count (up to ca. 400 cells/μL), justifying use of the term *lymphocytic meningoradiculitis*. The disease may involve other organs to produce *monoarthritic pain* as well as *cardiac and hepatic disease*, findings typical of Lyme disease as originally described in the USA and subsequently found in Europe. The CNS manifestations of neuroborreliosis were already described on p. 114.

Diagnostic Evaluation

The typical clinical manifestations are preceded by a known tick bite in only half of all patients; likewise, the skin rash is found in only half of all patients. The CSF changes described above are always present in the acute stage. In nearly every case, antibodies against *Borrelia burgdorferi* can be found, and the IgM titer is high. Yet about 10% of the normal population also bears antibodies against *Borrelia burgdorferi*.

Prognosis

The manifestations generally improve spontaneously, but only after a protracted course.

> **Treatment**
>
> *Penicillin and tetracycline,* used effectively against Lyme disease outside the nervous system, are also effective against *Borrelia* meningoradiculitis.

Tick Paralysis

Subacute paralysis with loss of reflexes 4–14 days after a tick bite is a different clinical entity. The weakness either remains confined to a single limb or else rapidly progresses to involve all of the muscles on both sides. The cause is a disturbance of conduction in peripheral nerve and/or a disturbance of neuromuscular transmission, similar to botulism.

Polyneuropathy Due to Malignant Neoplasia

Even in the absence of metastases, cancer can cause various metaneoplastic manifestations. CNS involvement, including cerebellar involvement (p. 321), and myopathy (p. 910) are discussed elsewhere in this book.

Clinical Features

Sensory polyneuropathy (of Denny-Brown) is the most common type. Radiating pain, paresthesiae, and sensory loss first appear distally on the limbs (calves, feet, hands). Marked proprioceptive impairment results in ataxia. Muscle tone is diminished and the deep tendon reflexes are absent, though there is minimal or no weakness.

The same clinical syndrome sometimes develops in patients without malignant disease. On the other hand, some patients with cancer develop a different syndrome, namely mononeuritis multiplex secondary to a vasculitis that is practically limited to the nervous system. This occurs particularly often in lymphoma.

Pathologic Anatomy and Pathophysiology

Degenerative changes are found in the spinal ganglia, the posterior roots, the posterior columns, and the peripheral nerves. The pathogenesis of this disorder is not well understood. Although it is most commonly due to bronchial carcinoma, it may also be due to other carcinomatous and noncarcinomatous tumors – e.g., Hodgkin's lymphoma.

Prognosis

This disorder usually progresses rapidly. In rare cases, the neurologic deficits regress after the causative tumor is resected.

Sarcoidosis

Sarcoid granulomas may be embedded in single or multiple peripheral nerves. Involvement of multiple nerves produces the clinical picture of subacute, generalized polyneuropathy (326).

Hypothyroidism

Pathologic Anatomy

Hypothyroidism causes axonal degeneration.

Clinical Features

Hypothyroidism produces not only the already described CNS disturbances (p. 315) and myopathy (p. 914), but also a symmetric, predominantly distal polyneuropathy. Its prevalence among hypothyroid patients varies from 15% to 60% depending on the criteria used to define it. It is characterized by unpleasant paresthesiae in the limbs, myalgia particularly in the calves, lancinating pain in the feet, and objectifiable distal sensory loss. The weakness of which many patients complain is usually due to concomitant myopathy.

Treatment
Like the other neurologic manifestations of hypothyroidism, polyneuropathy responds well to the administration of thyroid hormone.

Thalassemia

One-third of patients with thalassemia major suffer from polyneuropathy, mostly in mild form. Its onset is usually in the 2nd decade. It is characterized by paresthesiae, a mild motor deficit, and (in some cases) hyporeflexia and can be demonstrated electrophysiologically (740).

Chronic Idiopathic Ataxic Polyneuropathy

This is a purely sensory neuropathy that progresses over many years and ultimately becomes disabling. It is characterized by distal paresthesiae, severe proprioceptive deficits, ataxia, and areflexia (205). Many patients have a monoclonal gammopathy. The pathogenesis is not understood, and the disease responds neither to cortisone nor to immune suppression.

Cortisone-Dependent Polyneuropathy

In rare cases, a polyneuropathy of unknown etiology may be markedly cortisone-dependent: the signs and symptoms are relatively well controlled for as long as the medication is maintained, but become much worse as soon as it is discontinued. Thus, a trial of cortisone is worthwhile in cases of polyneuropathy whose etiology remains undetermined after thorough evaluation.

Chronic Cryptogenic Sensory Neuropathy

This diagnosis of exclusion, which can only be assigned when all sensory polyneuropathies of known cause have been ruled out, accounted for 23% of all cases of polyneuropathy in a large series (1033a). The disorder affects the elderly and has purely sensory manifestations, beginning in the feet, consisting of paresthesiae and, in three-quarters of all cases, intense pain. Burning feet are common (424c). The ENG and EMG are abnormal. The disorder progresses very slowly and is not disabling.

Hypereosinophilic Syndrome

Polyneuropathy is the most common neurologic abnormality in this disorder, whose hallmark is a constantly elevated number of eosinophils in the blood (172a). It responds to corticosteroids in most but not all cases.

Tropical Neuropathies

The following types of peripheral neuropathy are found mainly or exclusively in the tropical and subtropical zones (937b).

Infectious forms. Both lepromatous and tuberculoid *leprosy* can produce polyneuropathy. The examiner should look for thickened nerve trunks in the cubital groove and behind the ear, and for the anesthetic, anhidrotic, hypopigmented spots on the skin. *Brucellosis* and *leptospirosis* are also associated with polyneuropathy. For *HIV-associated polyneuropathy,* see p. 120. Neuropathy in *trypanosomiasis* affects mainly the autonomic fibers of the bowel and esophagus.

Biological toxins. Neuropathy can be caused by *cyanide* from cassava, *ciguatoxin* from tropical fishes, and many other biological toxins.

Nutritional deficiency. *Beriberi, pellagra,* and other nutritional deficiencies are among the causes of polyneuropathy in the tropics. Likewise, *multiple vitamin deficiency* is probably the cause of the so-called Strachan syndrome, in which prisoners of war typically develop neuropathy with ataxia. A *protein-poor diet* in children impairs the development of the peripheral nervous system, resulting in hypotonia and hyporeflexia (179a).

Critical Illness Neuropathy

Clinical Features

This sensorimotor neuropathy arises acutely in patients suffering from a very severe illness of some type (369a, 555a, 701a), often in combination with myopathy (p. 917). It is manifested by flaccid paresis ranging to quadriplegia and areflexia. Difficulty weaning the patient off artificial ventilation may be the first sign of this condition. Most patients developing this condition have been in intensive care for many days and have been treated with paralytic agents and corticosteroids.

Diagnosis

Histologic examination reveals a marked, distal, noninflammatory axonal neuropathy. Electrophysiologic testing reveals a diminished or absent motor response.

Prognosis

The prognosis of the neuropathy *per se* is good.

9   Diseases Affecting the Cranial Nerves

Overview:

The cranial nerves mediate the afferent conduction of somatosensory and special sensory information and the efferent conduction of impulses driving the motor and autonomic functions in the head and face. Of the 12 pairs of cranial "nerves," the first two are not peripheral nerves at all, but rather tracts of the CNS that are conveyed to an outlying position during embryonic development. The functioning of CN III–XII may be disturbed either by lesions of the corresponding brainstem nuclei, or by lesions of the nerves themselves as they course from the brainstem to their end organs. In the former case, but not in the latter, the neurologic examination usually reveals CNS deficits in addition to the specific cranial nerve deficit. The signs and symptoms of a cranial nerve deficit are determined, of course, by the functions subserved by that particular nerve. Table 9.1 provides an overview of the cranial nerves, their function, and techniques for examining them. Fig. 9.1 shows the brainstem nuclei of CN III–XII. In what follows, the methods of distinguishing nuclear lesions in the brainstem from lesions of the peripheral trunks of the cranial nerves will be carefully considered. Fig. 9.2 shows the anatomical relationships of the exiting cranial nerves at the base of the brain, and Fig. 9.3 shows them in relation to the skull base. These relationships are important to understand, because, in many cases, the topography of a mass lesion will determine the pattern of cranial nerve deficits that it produces.

Table 9.1 Function and clinical examination of the cranial nerves

Cranial nerves	Function	Examining techniques	Remarks
I Olfactory nerve	Olfaction	Test ability to smell coffee, cloves, peppermint, etc.	Irritants (e.g., ammonia) excite CN V rather than CN I; test to rule out factitious anosmia or local mucosal changes
II Optic nerve	Conducts visual impulses from the retina	Visual acuity, inspection of the nerve head by ophthalmoscopy, digital or mechanized visual field testing	Visual field defects may also result from lesions further along the visual pathway
III Oculomotor nerve	Innervates levator palpebrae muscle, superior, inferior, and medial recti, pupillary sphincter, and ciliary muscle	Axis of primary gaze, ocular pursuit in all directions, pupillary reflexes (light and convergence)	CN III palsies must be differentiated from nuclear and supranuclear ophthalmoplegia and from pupillary dysfunction due to CN II lesions or myasthenia
IV Trochlear nerve	Innervates superior oblique muscle (adducts and depresses eye)	Ocular pursuit	Look for head tilt
V Trigeminal nerve	Innervates muscles of mastication; sensation on the face, eye, tongue, and part of the nasopharynx	Jaw opening (deviates to paralyzed side), bite (palpation of temporalis and masseter muscles), sensation to light touch and pinprick, corneal reflexes	The corneal reflex is also impaired by lesions of CN VII and by central sensory disturbances
VI Abducens nerve	Innervates lateral rectus muscle (abducts eye)	Horizontal ocular pursuit	CN VI palsies must be differentiated from nuclear and supranuclear ophthalmoplegia and myasthenia

(Cont.) →

Table 9.1 (Cont.)

Cranial nerves	Function	Examining techniques	Remarks
VII Facial nerve	Innervates muscles of facial expression, lacrimal and salivary glands; subserves taste on the anterior two-thirds of the tongue	Wrinkling of forehead, pressing eyes shut, flaring nostrils, whistling, smiling, Schirmer lacrimation test, taste test	CN VII palsy must be differentiated from central facial palsy
VIII Vestibulocochlear nerve	Hearing, equilibrium	Whispered numbers, tuning fork tests (Weber, Rinne), nystagmus, tests of balance (Romberg, standing on one foot, Unterberger, Babinski-Weil walking test)	Disturbances of the vestibular portion of CN VII must be differentiated from central disorders of equilibrium
IX, X Glossopharyngeal and vagus nerves	Innervate the muscles of the soft palate, pharynx, and larynx (through the recurrent laryngeal nerve); sensory innervation of the soft palate, pharynx, tonsillar fossa, inner ear; innervate the parotid gland; subserve taste on the posterior third of the tongue	Swallowing, gag reflex (palatal symmetry, displacement of the posterior pharyngeal wall away from the paralyzed side), hoarseness, sensation on pharyngeal mucosa (comparison of the two sides)	
XI Accessory nerve	Innervates sternocleidomastoid muscle and upper portion of trapezius muscle	Head turning against resistance is weak to side opposite sternocleidomastoid weakness; shoulder shrug against resistance is weak on side of trapezius weakness, which also causes shoulder drop and scapular tilt	
XII Hypoglossal nerve	Innervates tongue musculature	Glossal atrophy (wrinkled mucosa, irregularly puckered margin), deviation of protruded tongue to paralyzed side	Tongue deviation to the paralyzed side is also seen in central paresis, but only in the acute phase (soon compensated)

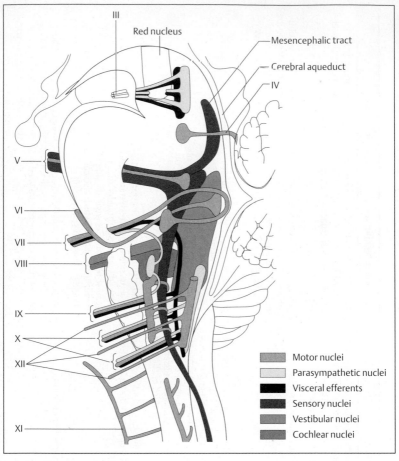

Fig. 9.**1**   **The cranial nerves and their brainstem nuclei** (adapted from Braus and Elze).

III	Oculomotor nerve	VIII	Vestibulocochlear nerve
IV	Trochlear nerve	IX	Glossopharyngeal nerve
V	Trigeminal nerve	X	Vagus nerve
VI	Abducens nerve	XI	Accessory nerve
VII	Facial nerve	XII	Hypoglossal nerve

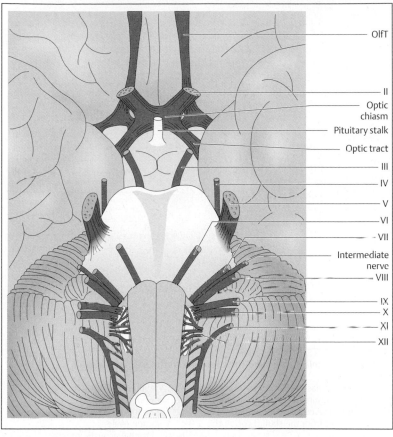

Fig. 9.2 **The cranial nerves and their relation to the base of the brain.**

OlfT	Olfactory tract	VII	Facial nerve
II	Optic nerve	VIII	Vestibulocochlear nerve
III	Oculomotor nerve	IX	Glossopharyngeal nerve
IV	Trochlear nerve	X	Vagus nerve
V	Trigeminal nerve	XI	Accessory nerve
VI	Abducens nerve	XII	Hypoglossal nerve

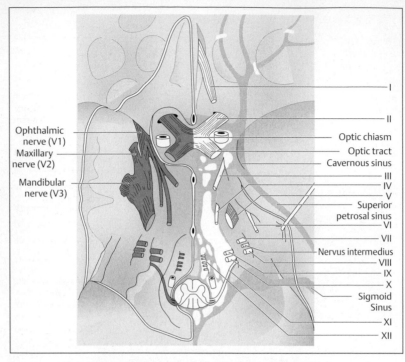

Fig. 9.**3**   **The cranial nerves and their relation to the base of the skull.**

The dura mater has been removed on the left side of the figure; on the right side, the dural venous sinuses are shadowed. Cranial nerves I–XII exit from the skull through the following openings:
I Cribriform plate
II Optic canal

III, IV, VI Superior orbital fissure
V/1 Superior orbital fissure
V/2 Foramen rotundum
V/3 Foramen ovale
VII, VIII Internal acoustic meatus
(= porus acusticus)
IX, X, XI Jugular foramen
XII Hypoglossal canal

I Olfactory nerve
II Optic nerve
III Oculomotor nerve
IV Trochlear nerve
V Trigeminal nerve
VI Abducens nerve

VII Facial nerve
VIII Vestibulocochlear nerve
IX Glossopharyngeal nerve
X Vagus nerve
XI Accessory nerve
XII Hypoglossal nerve

Disturbances of Olfaction (447a)

Anatomy

The axons constituting the olfactory nerve arise in the 10–20 million receptor cells embedded in the olfactory mucosa and pass through the cribriform plate to the olfactory bulb. The first neuron of the olfactory pathway terminates here, making a synapse onto the dendrites of a mitral cell (second neuron); the mitral cells, in turn, projects via the olfactory tract and olfactory striae to the amygdala and other temporal areas. Olfactory perception can only occur when the substance to be smelled is dissolved in the layer of fluid covering the olfactory epithelium.

Terminology

Subtotal impairment of the sense of smell is called *hyposmia* and is of little or no relevance in neurology. *Parosmia* is the faulty recognition of smells, *cacosmia* the abnormal perception of unpleasant odors (with or without an actual substrate being smelled). In this section, we will discuss only *anosmia*, the total absence of the sense of smell.

Anosmia

Anosmia may be due to *disorders of the nose*, such as rhinitis sicca; unilateral anosmia may be due to lack of ventilation of one side of the nose. *Nonrhinogenic anosmia* is occasionally the sole manifestation of an *olfactory groove meningioma*, but is most commonly due to *head trauma* (243c). The mechanism may be either tearing of the olfactory nerve as it crosses the cribriform plate, or a con-

tusion of the olfactory bulb. Post-traumatic anosmia usually goes unnoticed till several weeks or months after the injury. Secondary meningeal scarring may perhaps play a role. The longer the duration of post-traumatic amnesia, the more likely that post-traumatic anosmia will develop. Anosmia resolves spontaneously in one-third of cases, generally within a year. *Viral influenza* impairs the sense of smell in three-quarters of cases, causing anosmia in as many as one-third; among the anosmic patients, only two-thirds recover their sense of smell in 6–12 months, but usually only incompletely. As after head trauma, parosmia and cacosmia may remain. Similar phenomena occur more rarely after minor upper respiratory infections, or without any identifiable cause at all. Olfactory disturbances may also be a side effect of medication (300a).

Rare causes of anosmia include Paget's disease and diabetes mellitus. Hyposmia after laryngectomy has been described. Intermittent disturbances of smell and taste have been described in sarcoidosis (p. 329). Hyposmia and anosmia may occur in Parkinson's disease and Alzheimer's disease (153b, 447a, 863a). Anosmia due to aplasia of the olfactory bulb is a component of Kallmann syndrome (hypogonadotropic hypogonadism with eunuchoid habitus, delayed puberty, and color blindness in some cases).
Impairment of the sense of taste (ageusia) often accompanies anosmia (243c), usually as an indirect effect, indicating the importance of smell in taste perception. True ageusia may be caused by the local effect of a toxic

substance on the glossal mucosa (e.g., after wetting the tip of a pen with one's tongue). Transient ageusia may also follow the oral ingestion of medications such as penicillamine, ʟ-dopa, phenytoin (1046a), clopidogrel (352b), phenindione, the thyrostatic agent thiamazole, and the H_2-blocker ranitidine (along with headache and cough), as well as the coronary vasodilator oxyfedrine. Zinc deficiency, as may occur after histidine therapy for scleroderma, can cause ageusia and anosmia in addition to mental disturbances and cerebellar dysfunction. Ageusia can occur after tonsillectomy, or suddenly in the antiphospholipid antibody syndrome (414a). Hypogeusia has been described in diabetes mellitus, Sheehan's syndrome, and hypothyroidism. Disturbances of the sense of taste are not uncommon in the elderly or in persons suffering from arteritis; a disturbance of taste combined with burning of the tongue may be an early symptom of the polymyalgia rheumatica/giant cell arteritis complex. Intermittent distur-

bances of smell and taste in sarcoidosis have already been mentioned. Unilateral ageusia on the anterior two-thirds of the tongue is a classic sign of facial nerve palsy (p. 673).

True Combined Anosmia and Ageusia

This condition is rarely found in the aftermath of head trauma (which may also cause isolated ageusia, in exceptional cases). It is due to contusional injury of a portion of the diencephalon in the wall of the third ventricle.

Cacosmia

Spontaneous, episodic, unpleasant olfactory sensations may be due to irritation of the olfactory bulb, the amygdala, or the uncus. When they constitute the aura before an epileptic seizure (uncinate fits), they imply a pathological process in the anterobasal portion of the temporal lobe (p. 525).

Visual Disturbances of Neurologic Origin

Only the more common neuro-ophthalmologic syndromes will be discussed here.

Loss of Vision
Sudden, Unilateral Loss of Vision

Vision may be suddenly lost on one side because of a *traumatic fracture* involving the optic canal (best seen on thin-slice CT with bone windows). *Amaurosis fugax* is a manifestation of *carotid stenosis or occlusion*. Atherosclerotic changes in the arterioles

supplying the optic nerve cause *ischemic optic neuropathy* or *malacia of the optic nerve*, either of which can produce *pseudopapilledema*. *Sudden hypotension or hemorrhage* can trigger loss of vision, as can *temporal arteritis* (p. 816).
Papilledema is sometimes associated with gradually progressive visual loss over weeks or months, at other times with *amblyopic attacks* with transient blindness. Blindness may persist after such an attack. Among the many *ocular causes* of visual loss, we will only

mention *retinal detachment* (usually due to myopia), *preretinal hemorrhage* as an accompaniment of subarachnoid hemorrhage (Terson syndrome, p. 217), and *central venous thrombosis.*

Acute central retinal artery occlusion can be successfully treated by selective thrombolysis performed in the neuroradiology suite by catheterization of the ophthalmic artery.

Sudden, Bilateral Loss of Vision

This is rarely the result of *bilateral retinal ischemia* – e.g., in aortic arch syndrome, but more commonly of *bilateral ischemia of the occipital lobes* due to basilar insufficiency. A characteristic prodrome consists of loss of color vision, hemianopic episodes, the relative preservation of central vision, and, sometimes, the denial of a visual disturbance despite obvious, severe impairment. Sudden normalization of elevated intracranial pressure by the insertion of a *shunt for hydrocephalus* occasionally causes immediate, irreversible blindness, presumably because of optic nerve ischemia. *Intracranial masses* can cause episodic visual disturbances even in the absence of papilledema (generally by compression of the posterior cerebral artery in the tentorial notch, producing occipital lobe ischemia).

Rapid or Gradual Loss of Vision in One or Both Eyes

These events have many causes. *Retrobulbar neuritis* and *papillitis* cause visual loss within a few days, with recovery within a few weeks in most cases. Simultaneous bilateral retrobulbar neuritis can occur. *Ischemic optic neuropathy* sometimes causes gradual rather than sudden visual loss. Recurrent hypoxia is the likely cause of the partially reversible visual field defects seen in patients with sleep apnea syndrome (671a).

Hemorrhagic anemia, usually due to gastrointestinal bleeding in men and pelvic bleeding in women, may impair vision within hours or days, usually in both eyes; about 10% of patients are blinded in one eye. There is often a visual field defect with symmetric loss of the lower half of the field. The prognosis is poor. *Toxic causes* include methanol poisoning and tobacco-alcohol amblyopia. The latter causes bilateral visual loss with an early inability to tell red from green. Vitamin B_{12} deficiency plays an important contributory role, as was the case in an epidemic of optic neuropathy with polyneuropathy that was reported in Cuba in the 1990s (935). For SMON, see p. 485.

Optic nerve compression by a mass (tumor, carotid aneurysm) causes gradual loss of visual acuity, a visual field defect, and optic atrophy. *Optic glioma* (more common in children, especially girls) causes gradual visual loss. CT and MRI establish the diagnosis (direct visualization of the enlarged optic nerve, widening of the optic canal). Exophthalmos may be present.

Visual Field Defects and Perceptual Disturbances

Techniques of Examination

Coarse testing of the visual fields, in the doctor's office or at the hospital bedside, is performed with finger movements (Fig. 9.**4**). *Perimetry* (measurement of the visual field) (350) is the most important of the various technical aids available for more detailed testing. Dynamic (Goldmann) perimetry is distinct from static, computerized perimetry. In the former, test objects of various sizes are brought from the periphery toward the center of the visual field until the patient reports seeing them. The visual field can then be mapped as a set of isopter curves, one for each test object (Fig. 9.**5**). In the latter (e.g., with the Octopus), the brightness of a stationary light source is increased until the patient sees it. The visual field is mapped numerically, on a gray scale, or as a three-dimensional visual field surface corresponding to the measured threshold intensities (Fig. 9.**6**).

Topographic Classification of Visual Field Defects

Various visual field defects of localizing significance are depicted schematically in Fig. 9.**7**. From such defects, and in consideration of the accompanying historical data and physical findings, the clinician may be able to infer the etiology of the problem. Notably, incomplete or even complete *homonymous hemianopsia*

is sometimes unnoticed by the patient.

Special Phenomena

"Visual neglect," also called *extinction* or, less appropriately, inattention hemianopsia, involves the failure to perceive a stimulus on one side during bilateral presentation, even though the same stimulus can be perceived on that side when presented unilaterally. This is a characteristic finding in lesions of the parietal lobe on the nondominant (usually right) side.

The *Riddoch phenomenon* is the ability to perceive moving stimuli in a portion of the visual field where static stimuli cannot be perceived. It is a good prognostic sign for recovery in hemianopsia.

Palinopsia, or visual perseveration, occurs in patients with right temporo-occipital lesions. Images displayed to the patient are seen for longer than they are displayed, or are seen again after an interval, despite the absence of the original stimulus. The illusory image is incorporated into the current visual environment.

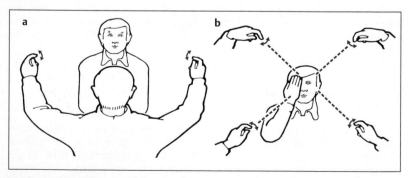

Fig. 9.**4a, b**   **Digital visual field testing.**
a Simultaneous bilateral testing to check for inattention hemianopsia (visual neglect).
b Testing of one eye at a time.

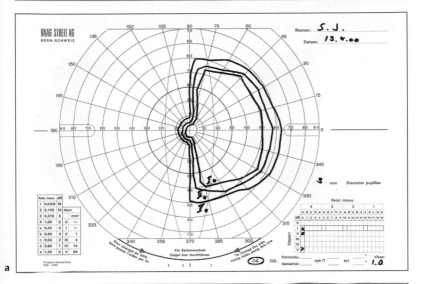

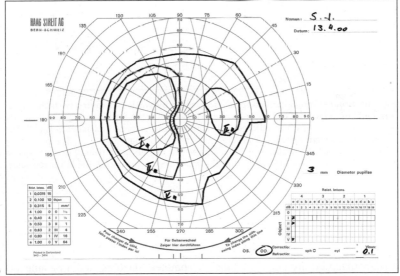

Fig. 9.**5a, b** **A visual field defect as revealed by kinetic Goldmann perimetry.** Bitemporal hemianopsia due to compression of the optic chiasm by a pituitary tumor. **a** In the left eye, the hemianopsia is complete, though the macula is spared. **b** In the right eye, the hemianopsia is less marked in the periphery, but the macula is involved. In accordance with the pattern of macular involvement, the visual acuity is normal in the left eye and diminished in the right eye. OD = right eye, OS = left eye.

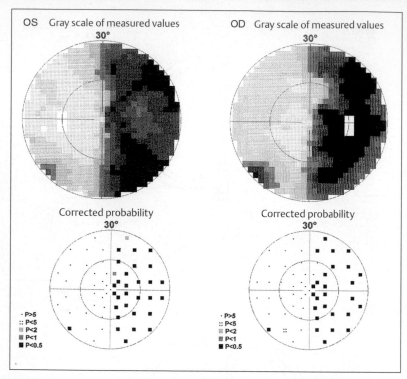

Fig. 9.**6**   **Homonymous hemianopsia as revealed by static perimetry with the Octopus.** Right homonymous hemianopsia due to infarction in the territory of the left posterior cerebral artery. Sensitivity to differences in light intensity is measured in decibels (dB). The measured values are depicted on a gray scale and as probability values. The probability symbols represent the chance of finding a particular degree of (impaired) performance in a normal subject of the same age; thus, the worse the performance, the lower the value. OD = right eye, OS = left eye.

Metamorphopsias are perceptual disturbances in which objects appear to be abnormally shaped (*dysmorphopsias*) or of abnormal size, either smaller than they really are (*micropsia*) or larger (*macropsia*). Such phenomena are encountered in partial complex seizures and migraine attacks. *Tilting of the visual image*, or even an upside-down image, can result from parieto-occipital lesions sparing the optic radiation (791c). *Visual hallucinations* are by no means restricted to schizophrenic patients.

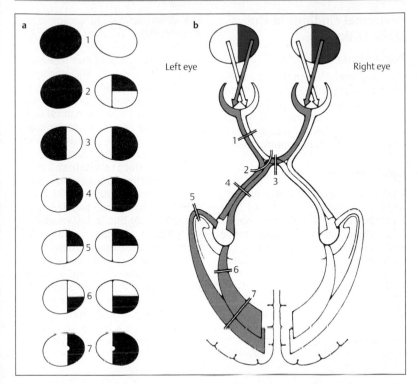

Fig. 9.**7 Visual field defects caused by lesions at various sites along the visual pathway.**

They may be due to local processes in the third-order visual cortex and be present in the aural phase of an epileptic seizure, or constitute the seizure itself. *Bonnet syndrome* consists of visual hallucinations without any identifiable anatomical substrate in persons who are otherwise psychologically normal (932a).

Unilateral occipital lobe lesions, typically ischemic, that spare the central portion of the calcarine fissure cause hemianopsia with a preserved *temporal crescent* (remnant of the visual field in the far temporal area belonging to the contralateral eye).

Chiasm syndromes are discussed on p. 64.

Abnormal Findings in the Optic Disks

Papilledema

The differential diagnosis of papilledema (Table 9.**2**) includes inflammatory papillitis, vascular papillitis due to arterial hypertension, and various other entities. Fluorescence angiography is a useful aid in doubtful cases.

Optic Atrophy

The extent of optic atrophy, if present, need not parallel that of visual loss. The following causes must be considered: optic glioma or optic nerve compression by a mass, trauma to the optic nerve, end-stage retrobulbar neuritis (temporal pallor), end-stage papilledema, syphilis, and Leber's familial optic neuropathy (affects men only). The last-named condition is due to a point mutation in mitochondrial DNA and is thus transmitted by maternal inheritance. MRI occasionally demonstrates an accompanying abnormality in the brain (745) (p. 905).

Optic atrophy, sometimes bilateral, is seen in *turricephaly. Radiotherapy* in the chiasmatic region can cause bilateral optic atrophy. *Opticochiasmatic arachnoiditis*, i.e., a mechanical lesion of the optic nerve caused by arachnoid adhesions, is probably too frequently diagnosed. *Foster-Kennedy syndrome*, which results from a tumor in the anterior cranial fossa, consists of compressive optic atrophy on the side of the tumor and papilledema on the other side due to intracranial hypertension. Chronic vitamin deficiency can cause optic atrophy ("Cuba neuropathy"), as can *poisoning* with various substances, including methanol, the combination of alcohol and tobacco, and medications such as ethambutol (see p. 301). Optic neuropathy can also be a feature of *endocrine ophthalmopathy* in hyperthyroidism.

▌ Oculomotor Disturbances (84, 130, 347, 571, 668)

Overview:

Eye movements enable us to fixate on and follow a moving visual target. They are initiated in the frontal and posterior eye fields of the cerebral cortex, whose principal projection passes to the paramedian pontine reticular formation (PPRF). The PPRF, in turn, directly controls horizontal gaze movements, and indirectly controls vertical gaze movements as well by way of its projection, through the medial longitudinal fasciculus (MLF), to the midbrain reticular formation. Vestibular and cerebellar connections also play an important role in the control of eye movement. Lesions of any kind affecting the supranuclear structures controlling eye movement cause horizontal or vertical gaze paresis or internuclear ophthalmoplegia (INO). It is important to distinguish supranuclear from nuclear and infranuclear disturbances affecting CN III, IV, and VI, which are of highly varied etiology. Finally, myasthenia gravis, myopathy, and intraorbital processes can impair ocular motility and cause diplopia.

Table 9.2 Differential diagnosis of papilledema

Condition	Appearance of fundus	Visual acuity	Visual field	Other signs and symptoms	Causes	Unilateral or bilateral
Papilledema	Blurred margins, disk enlarged and prominent, engorged veins, occasionally splinter hemorrhages in or near the disk, retina otherwise normal	Usually remains normal for a long time	Blind spot enlarged	Brief amblyopic attacks	Brain tumor in 75% of cases; venous thrombosis, other causes of intracranial hypertension	Almost always bilateral
Hypertensive retinopathy	Disk findings as above, but also: vascular changes involving the entire retina, with AV crossing, variations in caliber, silver wiring of arteries, yellowish-white exudates, hemorrhages far out in the periphery	Sometimes diminished	Normal	Symptoms of hypertension (may resemble those of brain tumor!), high blood pressure, renal signs	Essential hypertension, renal disease	Almost always bilateral

(Cont.) →

Table 9.2 (Cont.)

Condition	Appearance of fundus	Visual acuity	Visual field	Other signs and symptoms	Causes	Unilateral or bilateral
Central retinal vein thrombosis	Disk blurred, edematous, and prominent, veins massively engorged, corkscrew appearance, hemorrhages reaching far out into the periphery, sometimes confluent	Rapid, though not abrupt decline	Variable	Pain in the eye	Hypercoagulable states	Usually unilateral
Papillitis	Often not distinguishable from papilledema by ophthalmoscopy; disk less prominent, veins less engorged	Marked loss of visual acuity within a few days, recovery in one or more weeks	Early central and paracentral scotoma, occasionally sector-shaped peripheral scotoma	Pain in the region of the eye, especially. with eye movement, which sometimes also induces flashes of light	Focal infection? multiple sclerosis	Almost always unilateral at first, may spread to other side within a few weeks
Retrobulbar neuritis	Like papillitis, but disk findings normal					

(Cont.) →

Table 9.2 (Cont.)

Drusen	Enlarged, prominent, blurred margins, yellow discoloration of disk; veins normal, no hemorrhage. If drusen are superficial, the disk has a glistening, granular appearance	Normal	Occasional mild defects	None	Congenital deposition of hyaline material (often hereditary)	Usually bilateral
Persistent myelinated fibers	Snow-white, fluffy myelinated fibers extending from the disk toward the periphery, disk otherwise normal	Normal	Normal	Sometimes in the retina as well, independently of the disk	Congenital disorder	Bilateral in 20%
Pseudopapilledema (pseudoneuritis)	Optic nerve fibers raised, disk prominent and enlarged, gray-white turbid color without hyperemia. Veins may be tortuous, but not engorged	Normal	Normal	Often hypermetropic	Congenital overgrowth of glial tissue, occasionally familial	Either unilateral or bilateral

The Neuroanatomical Basis of Ocular Motility

The infranuclear structures subserving eye movement are depicted in Fig. 9.**8**, and the functions of the individual extraocular muscles in Fig. 9.**9** and 9.**10**. Table 9.**3** summarizes the principal and subsidiary functions of each extraocular muscle. Supranuclear control mechanisms are depicted schematically in Fig. 9.**13**.

The nuclear complex of the oculomotor nerve is found in the midbrain ventrolateral to the aqueduct. The axons emerging from it travel ventrally through the midbrain in close relation to the red nucleus and the superior cerebellar peduncle. They lie immediately medial to the pyramidal pathway just before their exit from the brainstem into the interpeduncular fossa as the *oculomotor nerve* (CN III). The nerve then traverses the subarachnoid space of the posterior fossa, past the petrous apex and in proximity to the posterior communicating artery, to reach the cavernous sinus. From its lateral position in the cavernous sinus, it passes through the superior orbital fissure into the orbit to supply the pupillary sphincter, the superior, inferior, and medial rectus muscles, and the inferior oblique muscle.

The trochlear nucleus lies dorsal and caudal to the nuclear complex of the oculomotor nerve. Its fibers exit the dorsal surface of the midbrain to form the *trochlear nerve* (CN IV), which

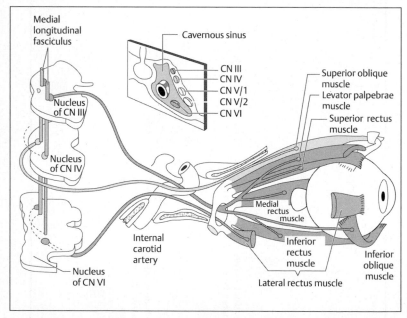

Fig. 9.**8**   **Nerves subserving eye movements and the muscles they innervate.**

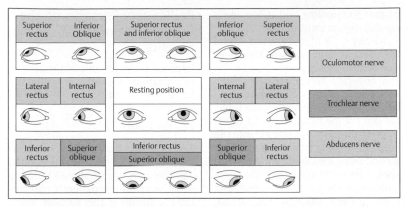

Fig. 9.**9 Diagram of the function of the extraocular muscles** (adapted from Hering). Hering's diagram indicates the direction of gaze in which the principal function of each extraocular muscle is most purely expressed. Other ocular muscles are first activated to reach this position of maximum function.

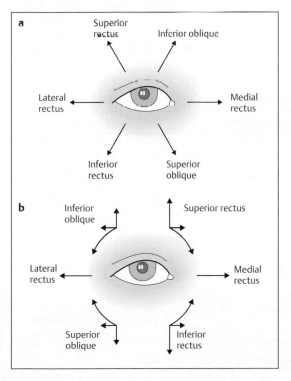

Fig. 9.**10a, b Principal and subsidiary functions of the extraocular muscles** (after Brandt and Büchele). For explanations, cf. Table 9.**3**.

crosses the midline and then travels around the brainstem and in close proximity to CN III to reach the orbital apex and its target muscle, the superior oblique muscle.

The *abducens nerve* originates from its nucleus in the dorsal portion of the pons, which lies within the internal genu of the facial nerve. Its fibers traverse the pons and emerge into the prepontine subarachnoid space, then ascend along the clivus to the petrous apex, pass under the petroclinoid ligament into the cavernous sinus, and then proceed through the orbital apex to the lateral rectus muscle.

Preliminary Remarks on the Examination of Ocular Motility

Important components of the clinical examination of ocular motility are listed in Table 9.**4**.

Eye Position

The examiner first looks at the position of the two eyes. The reflection of a distant light source should be in the same place on the patient's two corneas, confirming the parallel alignment of the two visual axes. It is best for the examiner to have the light source between his or her own eyes. If the positions of the light reflexes are different, then a *manifest strabismus* is present (*tropia*: divergent position = exotropia, convergent position = esotropia). If the eyes are parallel, the *cover test* is performed, in

Table 9.**3**   Principal and subsidiary functions of the extraocular muscles (after Stern et al.)

Muscle	Principal function	Subsidiary function
Superior rectus	Elevates the abducted eye. No effect on adducted eye	Adduction and internal rotation. Internal rotation is enhanced if the eye is adducted. Also elevates upper lid
Inferior oblique	Elevates the adducted eye. No effect on abducted eye	Abduction and external rotation. External rotation is enhanced if the eye is abducted
Inferior rectus	Depresses the abducted eye. No effect on adducted eye	Adduction and external rotation. External rotation is enhanced if the eye is adducted. Also depresses lower lid
Superior oblique	Depresses the adducted eye. No effect on abducted eye	Abduction and internal rotation. Internal rotation is enhanced if the eye is abducted
Medial rectus	Adducts the eye	None
Lateral rectus	Abducts the eye	None

Table 9.**4** Important components of the examination of ocular motility

| Spontaneous position of eyes |
| Spontaneous movements of eyes |
| Ocular pursuit movements |
| Eccentric gaze |
| Diplopia |
| Saccades |
| Optokinetic nystagmus |
| Oculovestibular reflex |

which first one eye and then the other is covered while the patient stares at the light source. In the normal situation, neither eye moves during the test. If one or the other eye corrects its position when uncovered, then a *latent strabismus* is present (*phoria*: exo- and esophoria, analogous to exo- and esotropia).

Spontaneous Eye Movements

The examiner should then observe spontaneous eye movements during fixation and also when fixation is prevented with Frenzel goggles (p. 646). Abnormal phenomena that may be seen include spontaneous vestibular nystagmus, congenital fixation nystagmus and opsoclonus (pp. 651 and 652).

Testing of Ocular Pursuit and Eccentric Gaze

The patient's head is held steady while he or she follows the examiner's finger to the left, right, left above and below, and right above and

below. If the eye movements are visibly abnormal (p. 640), or if the patient complains of *diplopia*, further tests are performed.

The functions of the individual extraocular muscles are detailed in Figs. 9.**9** and 9.**10** and in Table 9.**3**. For example, in the initial straight-ahead resting position of gaze, the right superior rectus muscle adducts and internally rotates the eye. Its elevating effect is minimal in this position and comes into play only when the eye is abducted by other muscles (lateral rectus, inferior and superior oblique muscles).

Paralytic strabismus. Paralytic strabismus is that due to paralysis of one or more extraocular muscles. The affected muscle can be identified as follows:

- Diplopia is worst when the patient looks in the direction of gaze subserved by the affected muscle. Thus, if the two images lie farthest apart when the patient looks to the left, the paralyzed muscle is either the left lateral rectus or the right medial rectus. The image from the bad eye ("false image") is projected toward the periphery in relation to that from the good eye ("true image").
- If the examiner now covers one eye or the other, the patient can report whether the more central or peripheral image disappears. If the central image disappears, the covered eye must be the good eye; if the peripheral image disappears, the covered eye must be the bad eye (i.e., the one in which an extraocular muscle is paralyzed).
- The technique may be further refined with the use of a colored glass before one eye and with lin-

ear light sources to be held horizontally or vertically, accordingly as the diplopia is vertical or horizontal (cf. Maddox cross, p. 640).

- Terminology: diplopia is said to be *uncrossed* when the images from the right and left eyes lie to the right and left, respectively, and crossed when they lie to the left and right. For example, in left abducens palsy, the left eye fails to follow an object moved to the left of the patient's visual field. The object therefore lies lateral to the visual axis of the left eye, and its image is projected laterally – i.e., to

the left – so the diplopia is uncrossed (Fig. 9.**11**).

- *Vertical diplopia* is due to paralysis either of a rectus muscle or of an oblique muscle. If the distance between the two images is greatest when the patient looks to the side of the affected eye, then a rectus muscle paralysis is present; if the distance between the two images is greatest when the patient looks away from the affected eye, then an oblique muscle paresis is present.

The positions of the eyes in palsies of CN III, IV, and VI are shown in

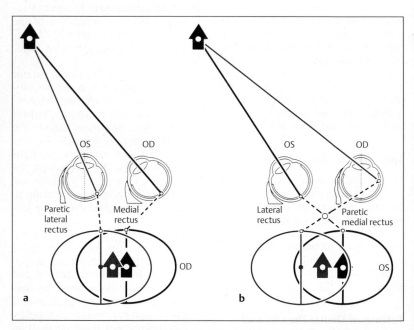

Fig. 9.**11a, b** **Crossed and uncrossed diplopia: mechanism and clinical significance.** Diplopia that is worst on left gaze may be due to either left lateral rectus palsy or right medial rectus palsy. It is uncrossed in the former case, crossed in the latter, as shown. OD = right eye, OS = left eye.
a Left lateral rectus palsy. Outer image from affected (left) eye. Uncrossed diplopia.
b Right medial rectus palsy. Outer image from affected (right) eye. Crossed diplopia.

Figs. 9.**18**–9.**20**. When the deviation between the two eyes is very large, the patient may no longer see double.

Concomitant strabismus. In this condition, the extraocular muscles of each eye function normally when the eye is tested independently, but strabismus emerges when they are tested together. The underlying problem cannot be paralysis of an extraocular muscle; the deviation of the two visual axes must have another cause. Concomitant strabismus can be demonstrated by the *cover test:*

- The examiner asks the patient to keep both eyes open and covers one of the patient's eyes.
- The patient is then asked to fixate on an object (either an object in the distance or, preferably, the examiner's nose).
- The examiner now simultaneously uncovers the covered eye and covers the previously uncovered eye. If the newly uncovered eye shifts its position, a concomitant strabismus is present.

This type of strabismus is rarely due to an acquired paresis, but is much more commonly due to a congenital imbalance of the oculomotor apparatus, often in association with visual impairment (amblyopia) that is either congenital or acquired in early childhood.

Gaze paresis (conjugate extraocular muscle paresis). Gaze paresis is a limitation of movement of both eyes in a particular direction. It does not cause diplopia. The underlying lesion is supranuclear – i.e., above the level of the brainstem nuclei of CN III, IV, and VI. Gaze paresis is discussed further on p. 648.

Other abnormal eye movements. The testing of eccentric gaze may reveal abnormal eye movements of other types, most commonly *gaze nystagmus* (p. 643), sometimes *upbeat* or *downbeat nystagmus* (p. 651).

Saccades. These can be tested by having the patient alternately fixate the examiner's extended index fingers, held wide apart, either horizontally or vertically.

Optokinetic nystagmus. This is best tested with an optokinetic drum. Saccadic disturbances are usually seen in combination with disturbances of optokinetic nystagmus.

Other disturbances. Clinically significant disturbances of ocular motility arise in system atrophies, cerebellar and monohemispheric cerebral lesions, and intoxications. The oculovestibular reflex and the oculovestibular reflex suppression test (nystagmus suppression test) are described on p. 646.

Ancillary Tests in Oculomotor Disturbances

Oculography, Electronystagmography, Fundus Photography

Oculography is useful for the documentation and analysis of eye movements. Eye movements cause corneal-retinal potential fluctuations of intensity proportional to the amplitude of movement, which can be detected through surface electrodes located near the orbit (53). Alternatives include the infrared reflection method and the search coil technique (656) (Fig. 9.**12**).

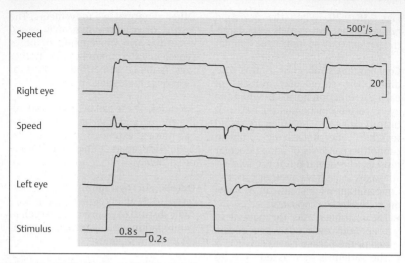

Fig. 9.12   Oculography with infrared reflection method.
The right eye adducts more slowly than the left in horizontal saccades, but the speed of saccades on abduction is normal bilaterally.

Electronystagmography is oculography used for the investigation of the vestibular system and vestibular disturbances. After initial calibration of the system, it is used to test static and dynamic gaze, saccades, pursuit, the oculovestibular reflex and its suppression, optokinetic responses, and positional nystagmus, and caloric testing with warm and cold water is performed separately in each ear. In some laboratories, the patient is spun in a swivel chair while the vestibular response is measured.

Oculo- and electronystagmography are useful for the documentation and quantification of normal and pathological conditions of the oculomotor and vestibular systems. Most pathological conditions can be detected qualitatively by clinical examination, with the aid of Frenzel goggles if necessary (p. 646). *Fundus photogra-*

phy is used to document and analyze rotatory movement of the eye.

Maddox Cross, Hess Screen, Lancaster Red-Green Test

These tests are used to document and longitudinally assess the vertical and horizontal components of subjective diplopia due to neuro- and myogenic extraocular muscle palsy. Binocular fusion is rendered impossible by the wearing of goggles with one red lens and one green lens. The patient must then superimpose a linear light source on a screen onto one shown by the examiner. The test is carried out in all nine cardinal positions of gaze. In diplopia, the red and green images lie farthest apart when the patient looks in the direction of function of the paralyzed muscle.

General Principles of Ocular Motility (84, 156, 157, 214, 407, 408, 409, 762a)

In this section, we will discuss the principal types of eye movement.

Rapid Movements (Saccades, Rapid Phase of Nystagmus)

Rapid eye movements can be voluntary or involuntary. *Saccades* serve to fix an object on the fovea and are either voluntary or a reflex response to visual, tactile, or auditory stimuli. *The rapid phase of nystagmus* returns the eyes to their original position after a deviation in response to an optokinetic or vestibular stimulus. Rapid eye movements serve to direct the eyes to a visual object along the shortest possible path; they are conjugate – i.e., both eyes move by the same angle, in the same direction, and with the same angular velocity. Their speed varies from 50°/s for microsaccades to 700°/s for large saccades.

The anatomic basis of rapid eye movements is depicted schematically in Fig. 9.**13**. The *paramedian pontine reticular formation (PPRF)* in the dorsal portion of the pons is of central importance. It contains the burst neurons, projecting to the nuclei of CN III, IV, and VI, that are essential for *rapid horizontal eye movements*. It receives afferent input from the *frontal eye field* (Brodmann area 8 in the middle frontal gyrus) and from the posterior (parietal) eye field by way of tracts that descend in the anterior limb of the internal capsule and the cerebral peduncle and then cross the midline at midbrain level. The frontal eye field itself receives afferent input from the supplementary motor, occipital, and parietal cortex.

The critical structure for vertical eye movements is the *rostral interstitial nucleus of the medial longitudinal fasciculus (riMLF, also called the Büttner-Ennever nucleus),* located in the rostral portion of the midbrain. The riMLF probably receives some direct input from the frontal eye fields, but in any case its activity is largely controlled by impulses from the PPRF.

The *superior colliculi* receive afferent input from the posterior and frontal eye fields both directly and indirectly by way of the basal ganglia (caudate nucleus, substantia nigra). They play an important role in both voluntary and reflex saccades. Voluntary saccades are initiated in the frontal eye field, which is also responsible for remembered saccades that serve to fixate an object, and for their suppression.

Slow Movements (Pursuit, Slow Phase of Nystagmus)

The eyes must be kept fixated on the target of vision even when the body, the head, or the target itself is in motion. The pursuit system serves to stabilize the image of the visual target on the retina. Pursuit movements are much slower than saccades, with speed typically ranging from 30 to 50°/s, and maximum speed ca. 100°/s. The part of the brain ultimately responsible for slow eye movements is the *visual cortex* of the occipital lobe. In the rhesus monkey, the visual cortex has been shown to project to the middle temporal visual area (MT), the medial superior temporal visual area (MST), and the adjacent parietal cortex (253). The MST sends projections to the contralateral dorsolateral pontine nuclei (DLPN) and to the floccu-

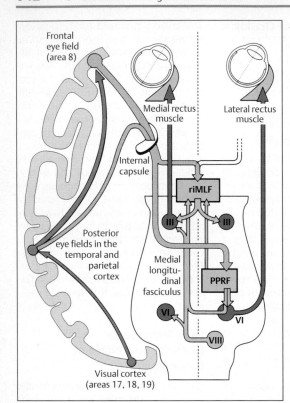

Fig. 9.**13   The neuro-anatomic basis of eye movements.**

Schematic depiction of the anatomic structures responsible for horizontal and (shown only in part) vertical eye movements. The pathway for movement of the eyes to the right runs from the left hemisphere to the right PPRF, and thence by way of the abducens nucleus and nerve to the right lateral rectus muscle, and simultaneously by way of interneurons in the medial longitudinal fasciculus (MLF) and the oculomotor nucleus and nerve to the left medial rectus muscle. Gaze paresis may thus be caused by a lesion of the hemisphere, the PPRF, or the abducens nucleus. MLF lesions cause an isolated weakness of the medial rectus muscle of one side on attempted contralat-eral gaze, though not on convergence (internuclear ophthalmoplegia, INO), while lesions of the abducens nucleus or nerve cause lateral rectus palsy. Purely vertical eye movements are generated by both hemispheres in concert. The riMLF is the supranuclear brainstem center for vertical gaze. It is subject to the influence of both the cerebral cortex and the PPRF. Gaze can be initiated not only by the cortex, but also by the vestibular system.

PPRF Paramedian pontine reticular for-mation
riMLF Rostral interstitial nucleus of the medial longitudinal fasciculus

lus, paraflocculus, and vermis (499). The flocculus, in turn, projects to the ipsilateral vestibular nuclei, which then project to the nuclei of CN III, IV, and VI.

Disturbances of the pursuit system manifest themselves clinically in *saccadic pursuit movements* and, if the saccade system is simultaneously impaired, in *gaze paresis*. Saccadic pursuit movements are not smooth and at a constant speed, as in normal pursuit, but are rather composed of, or interrupted by, rapid jerking movements.

Vergence

Vergence is the movement of the two eyes in opposite directions (convergence, toward each other; divergence, away from each other). Vergence movements are necessary for the fixation of objects at varying distances from the eyes; convergence is accompanied by accommodation of the lens so that the retinal image remains sharp. Vergence movements can also compensate to some degree for nonparallelism of the visual axes and for binocular disparity.

Rotation (133, 133b, 133c)

Rotation of the eyes about the visual axis ("cyclorotation") occurs as an optokinetic response to a rotating target or as a reflex compensation for rotation of the head or body, subserved by the vestibular system. The otoliths and the vertical semicircular canals play an important role in the latter process. Persistent abnormal cyclorotation can only be detected by fundus photography. It is, however, frequently accompanied by a clinically evident vertical skew deviation,

which may be specifically described as hyper- or hypotropia, or simply and unambiguously as "left-over-right deviation" or "right-over-left deviation."

Lesions of the vestibular cortex or of the vestibular thalamic nuclei alter the subjective vertical axis, perhaps shifting it a few degrees away from the true vertical axis. Lesions affecting the brainstem or labyrinthine structures that mediate the oculovestibular reflex alter not only the subjective vertical axis, but also the rotational position of the head. Pontomesencephalic lesions cause a contralateral head tilt, peripheral or pontomedullary lesions an ipsilateral head tilt. Thus, if the patient has a left-sided pontomesencephalic lesion, then the head is tilted to the right, and the examiner notes a left-over-right skew deviation of the eyes. Fundus photography reveals counterclockwise rotation. On the other hand, if the patient has a left-sided peripheral or pontomedullary lesion, then the head is tilted to the left, and the examiner notes a right-over-left skew deviation of the eyes. Fundus photography reveals clockwise rotation (Fig. 9.**14**).

Nystagmus and its Suppression (410)

Nystagmus is defined as a periodic, repetitive eye movement consisting of a slow movement in one direction followed by a rapid movement in the opposite direction. The major types of nystagmus are listed in Table 9.**5**. Conventionally, the direction of nystagmus is defined as that of the fast phase (e.g., in rightward nystagmus, the fast phase is to the right). Optokinetic and vestibular nystagmus are present in the normal individual.

Optokinetic nystagmus (OKN). OKN is produced by fixation on an object that is moving relatively to the observer (classic example: telephone poles as viewed by a passenger riding past in a train). The image of the object is stabilized on the retina by a pursuit movement (maximum angular velocity ca. 50°/s). As soon as the eye reaches an angular displacement of a certain magnitude, it returns, with a saccade, to its original position, to fixate anew and resume pursuit movement. OKN can be tested with a rotating striped drum or with a moving, patterned piece of material – e.g., measuring tape or a specially designed OKN tape. Asymmetry of OKN with movement to the left and right is the most important finding for clinical diagnosis. OKN ceases or becomes irregular if the stimulus moves too rapidly, or if the patient is inattentive.

Vestibular nystagmus. Vestibular nystagmus is generated by angular acceleration of the head, which excites the organs of the semicircular canals (labyrinth). Its physiological basis is the oculovestibular reflex (570).

- *Oculovestibular reflex:* This is a bi- and trisynaptic reflex whose neural pathway originates in the labyrinth and ends in cranial nerves III, IV, and VI. The mediating synapses are found in the vestibular nuclei and in the archicerebellum (flocculus). Teleologically speaking, any movement of the head must be accompanied by a movement of the eyes in the opposite direction so that the image of the visual target can be held stable on the retina. The pursuit system suffices to achieve this goal if the movement is slow enough, but most head movements are too rapid and would thus "overshoot" the ocular correction if there were not some other mechanism in place. Thus, it is the oculovestibular reflex that makes it possible, for example, to read a newspaper while walking or riding a bus, despite the continual, rapid head movements produced by

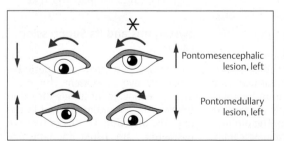

Fig. 9.**14 Diagram of head and eye position accompanying a left pontomesencephalic or pontomedullary lesion.**

A left pontomesencephalic lesion causes a left-over-right skew deviation with counterclockwise rotation of the eyes (ocular skew torsion). The head is tilted away from the side of the lesion – i.e., to the right. In contrast, a left pontomedullary lesion causes a right-over-left skew deviation with clockwise rotation of the eyes. The head is tilted toward the side of the lesion – i.e., to the left (adapted from Brandt and Dieterich 1993).

Table 9.**5** Major physiologic and pathologic types of nystagmus (adapted from Henn).

Type of nystagmus	Physiologic	Pathologic	Remarks
Optokinetic nystagmus	Symmetrically present	Asymmetric, dissociated, slowed, or absent	In hemispheric lesions, contralateral OKN is slowed; in pontine lesions, ipsilateral OKN is slowed
Vestibular nystagmus	Symmetrically present	Asymmetric, dissociated, or absent	
Spontaneous vestibular nystagmus	Up to 5°/s is normal in the dark only; absent in light	Present in light	Central or peripheral lesion
Gaze-evoked nystagmus	Absent	Always pathological	Defined as nystagmus in binocular visual field; lesion always central
End-gaze nystagmus	Symmetric	Asymmetric or dissociated	Defined as nystagmus in monocular visual field
Positional nystagmus		Always pathological	See p. 695
Congenital pendular nystagmus		Always abnormal, but does not indicate disease	Differential diagnosis: acquired pendular nystagmus

these activities. A short time after any angular acceleration of the head (typical latency, ca. 15 ms), the eyes reflexively move in the opposite direction, so that foveal fixation is maintained even at angular velocities greater than the fastest possible pursuit movement. The oculovestibular reflex functions in all three dimensions, whether the head is rotated in the sagittal plane, as if to say "yes" (pitch), in the horizontal plane, as if to say "no" (yaw), or in the coronal plane (roll). One can easily observe and test on oneself the difference between the relatively slow pursuit system and the relatively fast oculovestibular reflex. If one moves a book or newspaper rapidly back and forth before one's eyes, the writing becomes blurred; but, if one instead shakes one's head to produce relative movement of roughly the same angular velocity, the writing can be read effortlessly. In the first case, the fixation system and the pursuit system are activated; in the second case, the fixation system and the oculovestibular reflex.

- *Oculocephalic reflex:* This reflex functions similarly to, but more slowly than, the oculovestibular reflex. It is triggered by cervical, rather than vestibular, afferents and is of clinical significance in the examination of the comatose patient (p. 653, eye movements and coma).

Suppression of vestibular nystagmus by visual fixation. The normally occurring, physiological suppression of vestibular nystagmus by visual fixation makes it difficult to test clinically. Prevention of fixation by strongly positive lenses before the eyes (Frenzel goggles) makes vestibular nystagmus visible. One may test it qualitatively (present or absent) by rotating the patient *en bloc*, while he or she wears Frenzel goggles, in a swivel chair (a regular office chair, or one specially designed for this test). Passive turning generally brings out detectable nystagmus. More commonly, however, vestibular nystagmus is tested by lavage of the external auditory canal with warm or cold water and recorded by electronystagmography (see above).

Suppression of the oculovestibular reflex. If one wishes to test the *suppression* of the oculovestibular reflex by fixation, one can perform a simple *nystagmus suppression test*, as in Fig. 9.**15**. The patient extends the arms, fixates on his or her own thumbs, and is rotated rapidly back and forth, en bloc, by the examiner. Normal individuals will have no nystagmus whatsoever. Any nystagmus that may arise indicates the presence of a central lesion, usually in the cerebellum or its connections.

Oscillopsia. Oscillopsia is the (pathological) illusion that an object is moving back and forth even though it is actually stationary. The major diagnostic dichotomy is between spontaneous oscillopsia and oscillopsia with head movement.

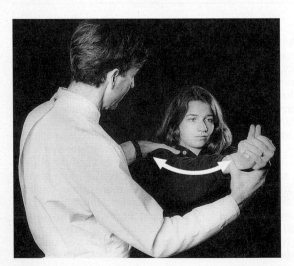

Fig. 9.**15 Nystagmus suppression test.** The patient extends her arms and fixates on her thumbs while being turned en bloc. Vestibular nystagmus induced by the rotation is normally fully suppressed by fixation and is pathological if seen.

- *Spontaneous oscillopsia:* This is a product of spontaneous vestibular nystagmus. When the patient tries to fixate on a visual target, it appears blurred and seems to move in the direction opposite the slow phase of nystagmus.

- *Oscillopsia with head movement:* By definition, this appears only when the patient's head is moving – e.g., during walking. It implies a disturbance of the oculovestibular reflex. Either the reflex cannot be activated (p. 706), or it cannot be suppressed by fixation. The latter is the case in cerebellar dysfunction: the eye movements either under- or overshoot the head movements for which they are supposed to compensate.

Cerebellar System

The cerebellum – in particular, the dorsal portion of the vermis, the fastigial nucleus, and the nodulus, flocculus, and paraflocculus – plays an important role in the control of eye movements. It ensures the stabilization of the visual image on the retina by maintaining gaze in the correct direction and finely tuning the necessary pursuit movements. Furthermore, it controls the duration and speed of saccades (and thus their amplitude). If the cerebellar maintenance of gaze is impaired, *gaze deviation nystagmus* results – a type of nystagmus that beats in the direction of gaze (Fig. 9.**16** and Table 9.**5**).

Supranuclear Disturbances of Eye Movement

Supranuclear disturbances, by definition, are those resulting from a lesion above the level of the cranial nerve

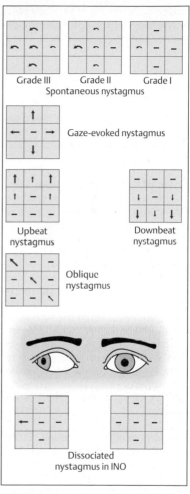

Fig. 9.**16 Types of nystagmus.** Spontaneous nystagmus may result from a central or peripheral lesion. Gaze-evoked nystagmus, upbeat, downbeat, and oblique nystagmus, dissociated nystagmus, and other types differing from those depicted here are usually of central origin. For positional nystagmus, cf. Fig. 9.**29**, p. 696.

INO Internuclear ophthalmoplegia

nuclei (569a) (cf. Fig. 9.**13**). *Gaze palsy* is weakness of the conjugate movement of the eyes in a particular direction.

Horizontal Gaze Palsy

Horizontal gaze palsy, a weakness of leftward or rightward gaze, is due to a lesion in either the contralateral hemisphere or the ipsilateral side of the pons.

Lesion of the frontal eye field. These lesions initially abolish all saccades to the opposite side, usually in association with contralateral hemiparesis. The eyes can no longer cross the midline to the side of the hemiparesis, because the impulses from the healthy, contralateral hemisphere, which push the eyes to the side of the lesion, predominate. Thus, there is conjugate deviation to the side of the lesion ("the patient with a hemispheric lesion looks toward the lesion"). This type of gaze paresis resolves within a few days of an ischemic stroke or cerebral hemorrhage as long as the other hemisphere is undamaged.

Posterior hemispheric lesion. Posterior hemispheric lesions impair pursuit movements to the opposite side, usually in association with contralateral homonymous hemianopsia (762). Clinical examination reveals *saccadic pursuit movements* and *impairment of optokinetic nystagmus.* Saccadic pursuit by itself is a nonspecific finding; it occurs normally in the setting of inattentiveness, somnolence, sedative use, or old age, as well as in diffuse cerebral processes of many different kinds.

Lesion of the PPRF (cf. Fig. 9.**13**). The last supranuclear neurons in the pathway for horizontal saccades are found in the PPRF. Thus, PPRF lesions, unlike hemispheric lesions, tend to cause long-lasting or permanent gaze paresis. The gaze paresis is ipsilateral to the lesion ("the patient with a pontine lesion looks away from the lesion").

Lesion of the abducens nucleus. Lesions of the abducens nucleus have the same effect on gaze as those of the PPRF, because the abducens nucleus contains not only the motor neurons that innervate the ipsilateral lateral rectus muscle, but also the axons of PPRF neurons, on their way to the contralateral medial longitudinal fasciculus. The contralateral medial rectus muscle is thereby involved. Thus, a lesion of the right abducens nucleus causes a right gaze palsy in which neither the right nor the left eye can look to the right. (See also internuclear ophthalmoplegia, p. 649).

Differentiation of PPRF and abducens nucleus lesions. PPRF lesions spare the oculovestibular connections via the MLF, but nuclear lesions do not. Thus, the gaze paresis can be overcome by vestibular stimulation in PPRF lesions, but not in nuclear lesions.

Isolated bilateral horizontal gaze palsy due to bilateral PPRF or abducens nucleus lesions. This rare phenomenon is usually a component of "locked-in syndrome," in addition to quadriplegia and swallowing paralysis. Locked-in syndrome is usually the result of pontine infarction due to basilar artery thrombosis (p. 171).

Vertical Gaze Palsy (84, 157)

Vertical gaze palsy is the inability to look up or down. If a vertical gaze palsy is present, but horizontal gaze is intact to the left and right, *the lesion is always in the midbrain;* more specifically, it must involve the riMLF nucleus (Büttner-Ennever nucleus) or its connections. The lesion involves either the riMLF of both sides, or the riMLF of one side and the fibers of the posterior commissure. Bilateral rostral midbrain lesions generally also damage the reticular formation with its ascending projections, producing coma (see p. 221 and, for eye movements in comatose patients, p. 653). Vertical gaze palsy is usually for both upward and downward gaze, though pretectal lesions may produce only an upward gaze palsy. Isolated downward gaze palsy is a rarity, produced by two separate, small lesions in the riMLF (157). Vertical eye movements induced by the vestibular system are not affected by riMLF lesions.

An acute PPRF lesion can produce, in addition to the horizontal gaze palsy (see above), a *transient vertical gaze palsy* that recovers rapidly, usually leaving residual vertical gaze deviation nystagmus and slowing of vertical saccades.

Internuclear Ophthalmoplegia (694)

The clinical picture of internuclear ophthalmoplegia (INO) consists of partial or total *inability of one eye to adduct on attempted lateral gaze, combined with nystagmus of the other, abducting eye.* Adduction is normally intact in both eyes with convergence movements, which demonstrates that the medial rectus muscle of the nonadducting eye is not, in fact, paralyzed. Vertical skew deviation may also be present, and bilateral INO is usually accompanied by vertical gaze deviation nystagmus. Not all patients with INO complain of diplopia. If the impairment of adduction is only partial, it may still be recognizable in the form of slowness of large-amplitude horizontal saccades in the affected, adducting eye as compared to the opposite, abducting eye (cf. Fig. 9.**12**). INO is due to a lesion of the medial longitudinal fasciculus (MLF) (Fig. 9.**17**). This vertically oriented brainstem tract contains the projection subserving horizontal gaze that runs from the abducens nucleus of one side to the oculomotor nucleus of the other (specifically, to the subnucleus controlling the medial rectus muscle). The vestibular nucleus also sends a projection to the MLF, which thus mediates impulses for saccadic, pursuit, and oculovestibular reflex movements as well. The MLF crosses the midline a short distance above its origin from the abducens nucleus; this explains why, for example, a right MLF lesion generally impairs adduction of the right eye on attempted leftward gaze – i.e., produces right internuclear ophthalmoplegia.

INO is usually due to *multiple sclerosis* in younger patients, particularly when bilateral, and usually of *vascular* origin in the elderly. In principle, however, any pathologic process affecting the MLF can cause INO.

One-and-a-Half Syndrome

This descriptive name designates the syndrome produced by a lesion that involves both the PPRF (or the abducens nucleus) and the MLF (Fig. 9.**17**). It consists of both an ipsilateral hori-

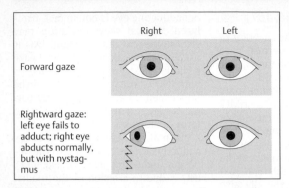

Fig. 9.**17** **Internuclear ophthalmoplegia** (INO). A left INO is depicted. The forward gaze is normal, as is the leftward gaze. On rightward gaze, the left eye fails to adduct, and nystagmus is seen in the abducted right eye.

zontal gaze palsy ("1") and an INO on attempted contralateral gaze ("1/2"). The only horizontal eye movement that still occurs on attempted lateral gaze is abduction of the eye contralateral to the lesion.

Oculomotor Disturbances Due to Cerebellar Dysfunction

The cerebellum is responsible not only for the coordination of bodily movements, but also for the motor control of gaze and for head-eye coordination. The maintenance of gaze, the fine control of ocular pursuit, and the temporal and spatial precision of saccades all critically depend on normal cerebellar function. Nearly all cerebellar lesions impair oculomotor function in addition to bodily motor function (Table 9.**6**). These types of disturbances, however, are not specific to lesions in the cerebellum itself, as they may also be produced by lesions of the cerebellar afferents or efferents in the brainstem. Symmetric disturbances are usually of toxic or metabolic origin (including drug intoxication), while asymmetric disturbances are more often due to a structural lesion.

Complex Supranuclear Disturbances

Ocular apraxia. Ocular apraxia is the inability to perform voluntary saccades, while reflex saccades are preserved. Patients with *congenital* ocular apraxia (*Cogan's syndrome*, which mainly affects boys) are unable to use a voluntary saccade to bring the image of an object, such as the start of a line of text, into the center of the visual field. Instead, they rapidly turn the head until the desired image is projected onto the macula, then slowly bring the head back to resting position, while the image is held stable by ocular pursuit. *Acquired forms* can arise, for example, from extensive bilateral infarction of the frontal and posterior eye fields.

Congenital nystagmus. Congenital nystagmus is usually characterized by pendulum-like, horizontal, conjugate eye movements. The oscillation of the eyes is sinusoidal, sometimes with a superimposed, exponentially accelerating movement resembling a saccade. Congenital nystagmus worsens with attention, visual fixation, and (usually) when the eye is out of pri-

Table 9.**6** Oculomotor disturbances due to cerebellar dysfunction

Saccadic pursuit
Gaze-evoked nystagmus
Diminished optokinetic nystagmus
Dysmetric saccades (under- and over-shoot)
Inability to suppress the oculovestibular reflex by fixation
Overshooting oculovestibular reflex
Special types of nystagmus, such as: • Upbeat nystagmus • Downbeat nystagmus • Rebound nystagmus • Periodically alternating nystagmus • Acquired pendular nystagmus • Central positional nystagmus, etc.
Skew deviation (with head tilt)
Unilateral cerebellar lesions cause nystagmus to the ipsilateral side (as in spontaneous vestibular nystagmus)

mary position, and improves with convergence. The optokinetic response is often in the wrong direction – i.e., the same direction in which the pattern is moving ("inverted pursuit"). The differential diagnosis of congenital pendular nystagmus includes acquired forms that may be seen in oculopalatal myoclonus, Whipple's disease, stroke, multiple sclerosis, and monocular blindness.

Latent fixation nystagmus. This entity, also called *manifest latent nystagmus,* is also congenital. It is always accompanied by strabismus, occurs only on monocular fixation, and beats in the direction of the fixating (uncovered) eye. It is often discovered incidentally during ophthalmoscopy.

Dissociated nystagmus. Nystagmus that beats with a different amplitude, speed, or direction in the two eyes is called dissociated nystagmus.

Downbeat nystagmus (376) (see Fig. 9.**16**.) Nystagmus that beats downward when the eye is in primary position is called downbeat nystagmus. It is most prominent when the patient gazes to one side and slightly below primary position. The patients complains of oscillopsia. Downbeat nystagmus is caused by anomalies of the craniocervical junction, spinocerebellar degeneration, and many other types of pathology affecting the caudal brainstem.

Upbeat nystagmus (52) (see Fig. 9.**16**.) This type of nystagmus beats upward when the eye is in primary position and, like downbeat nystagmus, usually produces oscillopsia. It may worsen on lateral gaze. It is caused by lesions of the anterior vermis or of the brainstem.

Convergence-retraction nystagmus (503). This type of nystagmus consists of saccades in opposite directions in the two eyes, resulting in jerky, alternating convergence and retraction. It is caused by midbrain processes involving the posterior commissure. It is generally accompanied by upward gaze paresis and other midbrain oculomotor signs.

Periodically alternating nystagmus. In this entity, nystagmus (usually horizontal) periodically reverses its direction approximately every 2 minutes. It may be congenital or acquired, often as the result of a cerebellar lesion.

Macro-square-wave jerks. As the name implies, these are involuntary saccades away from, and then back to, the point of fixation. They are typically a sign of cerebellar disease.

See-saw nystagmus. This entity consists of conjugate rotation of the eyes during which the internally rotating eye is elevated and the externally rotating eye is depressed. The movement periodically changes direction, giving the eyes a see-saw appearance. It is either congenital or the product of a midbrain or diencephalic lesion.

Opsoclonus. Rapid, conjugate saccades without any intervening fixation are termed *ocular flutter* when they occur only in the horizontal plane and *opsoclonus* when they are multidirectional. Opsoclonus occurs as a paraneoplastic phenomenon as well as in neuroblastoma, encephalitis, and intoxications (p. 321).

Ocular myoclonus. The pendulum-like eye movements of ocular myoclonus are accompanied by myoclonus in other muscles as well – e.g., the palatal muscles (so-called "palatal nystagmus," actually myoclonus) and the muscles of the tongue, face, pharynx, larynx, and diaphragm. The underlying lesion interrupts, at some point, the regulatory circuit formed by the red nucleus, the ipsilateral inferior olive, and the contralateral cerebellar dentate nucleus.

Myokymia of the superior oblique muscle. This may arise spontaneously, in the aftermath of a trochlear nerve palsy, or as a consequence of multiple sclerosis. The episodes of high-frequency monocular nystagmus with diplopia and oscillopsia may regress spontaneously or persist for years.

Brown syndrome. This entity is of mechanical rather than neurological origin. Oblique diplopia occurs intermittently because the tendon of the superior oblique muscle briefly sticks in the trochlea (671). Brown syndrome is to be distinguished from myokymia of the superior oblique muscle.

Other abnormal eye movements. Further clinically relevant types of nystagmus and oculomotor phenomena occurring in comatose patients are described, in the relevant chapters, on pp. 221 and 653.

Some Diseases in which Oculomotor Disturbances are Prominent

Progressive Supranuclear Palsy

Downward gaze palsy as the initial sign may enable very early diagnosis of this hypokinetic extrapyramidal disorder (p. 253). In later stages of the disease, gaze is impaired in all directions.

> **Treatment**
>
> Dopaminergic agonists may alleviate the signs and symptoms of this disease in its early stage.

Parkinson's Disease

A number of nonspecific oculomotor disturbances are found in Parkinson's disease, among them infrequent blinking, hypometric saccades, saccadic pursuit, and impaired suppression of the oculovestibular reflex.

Treatment

The oculomotor disturbances of Parkinson's disease generally improve under treatment with l-dopa or dopaminergic agonists.

Whipple's Disease

Oculomasticatory myorhythmia or gaze paresis can be a prominent manifestation of Whipple's disease (p. 273).

Cerebral Metabolic Disturbances and Wernicke's Encephalopathy

Abnormal eye movements may point to the correct diagnosis in cerebral metabolic disturbances of various types and in Wernicke's encephalopathy (p. 310).

Diseases that Mimic Supranuclear Disturbances of Eye Movement

Cranial polyradiculitis, Fisher syndrome, and basilar meningitis should always be considered in the differential diagnosis of gaze palsy. If pupillomotor dysfunction is present in addition to external ophthalmoplegia, botulism should also be considered. Myasthenia can cause fluctuating abnormalities of eye movements, often accompanied by ptosis, and can be mistaken on occasion for supranuclear ophthalmoplegia. Progressive external ophthalmoplegia is characteristic of Kearns-Sayre syndrome and other mitochondrial encephalomyopathies.

Eye Movements in the Comatose Patient

Coma disables fixation and thus abolishes all pursuit movements and, normally, all saccades and nystagmus as well. Gaze deviation in a comatose patient often indicates an ipsilateral hemispheric lesion or a contralateral pontine lesion. Epileptic seizures can cause intermittent nystagmus and tonic gaze deviation to the side opposite the epileptogenic focus.

Slow, pendulum-like ("roving") eye movements generally accompany the superficial stages of coma and have no special pathologic significance. Other spontaneous movements, such as ocular bobbing and ping-pong gaze, are always abnormal.

Ocular bobbing. This consists of rapid downward deviation of both eyes followed by a slow return to primary position. Reflex eye movements are usually not elicitable in this situation. Ocular bobbing generally implies a severe pontine injury.

Reverse bobbing, ocular dipping. These terms signify a movement similar to ocular bobbing, but in the opposite direction.

Periodically alternating gaze deviation in the horizontal plane (ping-pong gaze). The direction of gaze changes every few seconds. This is seen in diffuse, bilateral cortical injury.

Testing of eye movements. Only reflex eye movements can be tested in the comatose patient, namely, the oculovestibular and oculocephalic reflexes (cf. Fig. 2.**69**). Note that these terms are usual in English, though, strictly speaking, "vestibulo-ocular" and "cephalo-ocular" would be more correct. The testing of these two reflexes permits inferences to be drawn about the function of various structures in the midbrain, pons, and medulla (Fig. 2.**69**). The oculocephalic reflex should only be tested after the examiner has made sure that the patient has not suffered a traumatic fracture or subluxation of the cervical spine.

- *Oculocephalic reflex:* This reflex is tested first. With the comatose patient in the supine position, the examiner grasps the head with both hands, holds the eyelids open with his thumbs, and rotates the head sideways (i.e., in the horizontal plane = yaw). The eyes normally move passively in the same direction as the head at first, but then drift back to the vertical position (reflex present). An abnormal response consists of lack of movement of the eyes relative to the orbits (reflex absent). The next step is to incline the head forward and backward (rotation in the sagittal plane = pitch). Here, too, the eyes should move in an opposite direction, to find the vertical position (doll's-eyes phenomenon), if the brainstem is intact. In midbrain lesions, the oculocephalic reflex can be used to elicit horizontal but not vertical eye movements, or, in some cases, only a downward vertical movement. In pontine lesions, the reflex components are abnormal or absent in both directions. Disjugate movement may indicate a supranuclear, or infranuclear disturbance – e.g., INO or abducens palsy.
- *Oculovestibular reflex:* If the oculocephalic reflex is absent, the oculovestibular reflex should be tested with caloric stimulation, as it can often be elicited even when the oculocephalic reflex cannot (683). In an awake patient, irrigation of the external ear canal with *cold* water causes nystagmus to the *opposite* side, while irrigation with *warm* water causes nystagmus to the *same* side. In a comatose patient, the fast (saccadic) phase of nystagmus is absent, and thus irrigation of the ear canal causes *tonic eye deviation* in the same direction as the *slow phase* of nystagmus in the awake patient: cold water – same side, warm water – opposite side. To test midbrain function, vertical movements can be elicited with bilateral simultaneous caloric irrigation. Bilateral cold water irrigation produces downward deviation, while bilateral hot water irrigation produces upward deviation.

Lesions of the Cranial Nerves Subserving Eye Movement and their Brainstem Nuclei (811, 814)

Lesions of cranial nerves III, IV and VI always produce paralytic strabismus; lesions of the corresponding brainstem nuclei often do as well.

Oculomotor Nerve Palsy

Clinical Features

A complete infranuclear oculomotor nerve palsy is characterized by *both external and internal ophthalmoplegia* (Fig. 9.**18**).

External ophthalmoplegia in this case is paralysis of all of the extraocular muscles innervated by CN III (i.e., the superior, inferior, and middle recti, the inferior oblique muscle, as well as

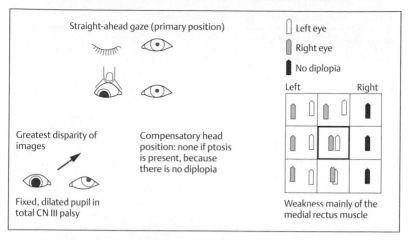

Fig. 9.**18 Right oculomotor nerve palsy.**
Note the position of the eyes and the positions of the two visual images (diplopia).

the levator palpebrae superioris muscle, causing ptosis), while internal ophthalmoplegia is paralysis of the pupillary sphincter and of the ciliary muscle, visible as a mydriatic pupil that reacts neither to light nor to convergence. Because the functions of the lateral rectus and superior oblique muscles remain intact, the paretic eye is deviated outward and downward, and cannot be elevated above the horizontal. The ptotic eyelid covers the pupil of the affected eye; the patient thus does not complain of diplopia unless the lid is passively elevated, in which case diplopia is worst on upward gaze to the side opposite the palsy. Oculomotor nerve palsy may affect only some components of the oculomotor nerve, and thus internal and external ophthalmoplegia may be found in various different combinations. Occasionally, mild exophthalmos is seen, reflecting loss of the normal, mild retraction of

the bulb by the combined action of the rectus muscles, which leaves the forward pull of the superior oblique muscle unopposed.

Localization (Table 9.7)

A *nuclear oculomotor palsy* generally presents with the same findings described above and, in addition, a supranuclear disturbance of vertical gaze. If unilateral oculomotor palsy is seen in combination with weakness of the contralateral superior rectus muscle and bilateral ptosis, or if ptosis is absent in bilateral oculomotor palsy, a lesion of the nuclear zone should be suspected. Bilateral, total oculomotor palsy or isolated partial muscle palsies may also be of nuclear origin.

A *fascicular oculomotor palsy* may cause internal or external ophthalmoplegia, or both. It can usually be diagnosed on the basis of accompanying midbrain signs, such as contra-

Table 9.**7**   Localization and etiology of oculomotor palsy

Site of lesion	Clinical features	Etiology
Nuclear	Oculomotor palsy, bilateral vertical gaze palsy, bilateral ptosis	Infarct, hemorrhage, trauma, tumor, multiple sclerosis, inflammation, congenital hypoplasia
Fascicular	Oculomotor palsy, contralateral hemiparesis, ataxia or rubral tremor (differential diagnosis: transtentorial herniation)	Infarct, hemorrhage, multiple sclerosis
Subarachnoid space	Isolated oculomotor palsy	Aneurysm (posterior communicating artery, rarely basilar artery or other arteries), basilar meningitis, cranial polyradiculitis, intracranial hypertension, trauma, neurosurgical complication, tumor of the oculomotor nerve, transtentorial herniation
Cavernous sinus, superior orbital fissure, or orbit	Oculomotor palsy accompanied by dysfunction of CN IV, V/1, and VI in varying combinations	Aneurysm (internal carotid artery), carotid-cavernous fistula, thrombosis of the cavernous sinus, parasellar tumor or pituitary tumor with parasellar extension, sphenoid sinusitis, Tolosa-Hunt syndrome, herpes zoster
Orbital apex	Oculomotor palsy accompanied by dysfunction of CN II, IV, V/1, and VI in varying combinations	See lists of causes above and below (cavernous sinus, orbit)
Orbit	Superior ramus: ptosis and superior rectus palsy	Trauma, orbital tumor, orbital pseudotumor, infection, mucocele
	Inferior ramus: palsy of inferior and medial recti and inferior oblique muscle	Trauma, orbital tumor, orbital pseudotumor, infection, mucocele
No localizing significance	Isolated external ophthalmoplegia (i.e., pupillary sparing)	Diabetes, hypertension, arteritis, migraine

lateral hemiparesis, rubral tremor, or ataxia (cf. Table 2.**42**).

A lesion of the oculomotor nerve as it traverses the *subarachnoid space,* or in the *tentorial notch,* usually affects the nerve in isolation, while lesions in the *cavernous sinus* or *superior orbital fissure* often additionally affect the nearby trochlear, ophthalmic, and abducens nerves.

Orbital apex syndrome consists of the signs of oculomotor nerve palsy in addition to a visual disturbance due to optic nerve involvement, and perhaps also papilledema or optic disk atrophy. The oculomotor nerve divides within the cavernous sinus into superior and inferior rami, which may be individually affected, particularly within the orbit. The superior ramus innervates the superior rectus and levator palpebrae muscles, while the inferior ramus innervates the pupil, the ciliary body, the inferior and medial recti, and the inferior oblique muscle.

Etiology (Table 9.7)

As a rule, compressive oculomotor nerve palsy produces first internal, then external ophthalmoplegia. In oculomotor nerve palsy of diabetic or vascular origin, the pupil may be spared (isolated external ophthalmoplegia) (933), and pain is usually present as well. Yet the converse does not hold: sparing of the pupil does not rule out a compressive origin of oculomotor nerve palsy (696).

Certain causes of oculomotor nerve palsy that were common decades ago, such as sphenoidal or ethmoidal sinusitis and mucocele, are now rare but should not be forgotten in the differential diagnosis.

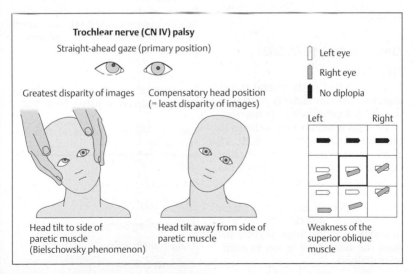

Fig. 9.**19 Right trochlear nerve palsy.**
Note the head posture, the position of the eyes, and the positions of the two visual images (diplopia).

Trochlear Nerve Palsy
(985, 1043)

Clinical Features

Trochlear nerve palsy is characterized by loss of function of the superior oblique muscle, impairing depression of the adducted eye and internal rotation of the abducted eye (Fig. 9.**19**). Vertical diplopia with slightly tilted images is the result; diplopia is worst on downward gaze, as during reading or climbing stairs. The diplopia can be reduced or eliminated by tilting the head to the side opposite the palsy and bowing the head slightly. The patient may assume this position spontaneously and unconsciously (ocular torticollis). Tilting the head to the side of the palsy brings out the diplopia (Bielschowsky phenomenon).

Causes

The common causes of trochlear nerve palsy (811, 814, 985) are listed in Table 9.**8**.

Abducens Palsy (328, 502)

Clinical Features

Loss of function of the lateral rectus muscle causes an inability to abduct the affected eye, resulting in horizontal diplopia when the patient looks to the side of the lesion (Fig. 9.**20**; cf. also Fig. 9.**11**). The images are parallel and horizontally displaced. When the patient looks straight ahead, the affected eye is mildly adducted because of the unopposed tone of the intact medial rectus muscle. The patient therefore turns his head slightly toward the side of the lesion to minimize diplopia.

Localization

Nuclear abducens palsy causes gaze paresis to the side of the lesion, as discussed above (p. 648), often accompanied by an infranuclear facial palsy. Abducens palsy due to a *fascicular lesion in the brainstem* is generally accompanied by other brainstem signs, such as contralateral hemiparesis or ipsilateral trigeminal signs. Lesions affecting the abducens nerve along its course in the *subarachnoid space* from the pons to the petrous apex usually cause isolated abducens palsy, but there may be accompanying deficits of other cranial nerves – e.g., in the syndrome of the cerebellopontine angle or in cranial polyradiculitis. A lesion at the *petrous apex* can affect both the abducens nerve and the trigeminal nerve (*Gradenigo's syndrome*). Lesions lying more distally along the course of the nerve (in the *cavernous sinus, superior orbital fissure,* or *orbit*) usually affect other nearby nerves as well (cf. discussion in the above section on oculomotor palsy).

Etiology

The spectrum of causes is similar to that of oculomotor palsy (Table 9.**9**).

Table 9.**8** Common causes of trochlear nerve palsy

Trauma
Midbrain hemorrhage
Multiple sclerosis
Ischemic neuropathy
Diabetic neuropathy
Congenital aplasia
Lesions of the cavernous sinus and orbit (see Table 9.**7**)

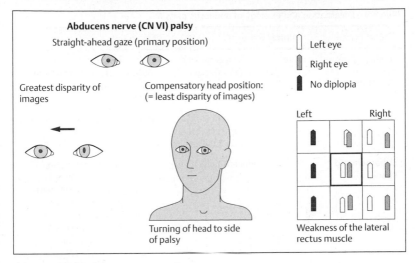

Fig. 9.**20** **Right abducens nerve palsy.**
Note the head posture, the position of the eyes and the positions of the two visual images (diplopia).

Combined Deficits of the Cranial Nerves Subserving Eye Movement

Oculomotor nerve palsy puts the eye in a mildly abducted position. Looking downward from this position induces internal rotation of the eye, which, however, is absent if there is a superimposed trochlear nerve palsy. If the abducens nerve is affected, too, then the eye cannot be abducted.

■ Simultaneous Palsies of Multiple Cranial Nerves Subserving Eye Movement

Such processes have a broad differential diagnosis. If the cranial nerves *on one side only* are affected, the cause is usually a local process in the cavernous sinus, superior orbital fissure, or orbital apex. Such processes usually also involve the first division of the trigeminal nerve (the ophthalmic

nerve). If the cranial nerves are affected *on both sides*, the cause may be:

- cranial polyradiculitis,
- basilar meningitis,
- clivus chordoma,
- sphenoid and nasopharyngeal carcinoma infiltrating the skull base,
- sellar tumor with lateral extension,
- bilateral cavernous sinus thrombosis.

Bilateral palsies of the cranial nerves subserving eye movement can be mistaken for nuclear and supranuclear oculomotor disorders. They must also be differentiated from endocrine ophthalmopathy (p. 661), myasthenia gravis (p. 918), Kearns-Sayre syndrome (p. 904), and ocular myositis.
Ancillary tests that may be of diagnostic value, depending on the suspected diagnosis, include CSF examination, CT, MRI, electrophysiologic

Table 9.**9**   Localization and etiology of abducens palsy

Site of lesion	Clinical features	Etiology
Nuclear, pontine paramedian reticular formation	Gaze palsy, often combined with peripheral or nuclear facial palsy	Infarct, hemorrhage, tumor, multiple sclerosis, inflammation, trauma, congenital aplasia
Fascicular	Abducens palsy with contralateral hemiparesis, occasionally also trigeminal deficit	Infarct, hemorrhage, multiple sclerosis
Subarachnoid space	Isolated abducens palsy	Intracranial hypertension, hypoliquorrhea syndrome, aneurysm (AICA, PICA, basilar artery), subarachnoid hemorrhage, basilar meningitis, cranial polyradiculitis, trauma, neurosurgical complication, tumor of the abducens nerve, clivus tumor
Petrous apex, petrous bone	Deficits of CN V and VI, sometimes also VII and VIII	Extradural inflammation in otitis media
Cavernous sinus, superior orbital fissure	Abducens palsy accompanied by dysfunction of CN III, IV, and V/1 in varying combinations	Aneurysm (internal carotid a.), carotid-cavernous fistula, thrombosis of the cavernous sinus, parasellar tumor or pituitary tumor with parasellar extension, sphenoid sinusitis, Tolosa-Hunt syndrome, herpes zoster
Orbital apex	Abducens palsy accompanied by dysfunction of CN III, IV, and V/1 in varying combinations	See lists of causes above and below (cavernous sinus, orbit)
Orbit	Isolated lateral rectus palsy or combined with other deficits	Trauma, orbital tumor, orbital pseudotumor, endocrine ophthalmopathy, infection, mucocele
No localizing significance	Isolated lateral rectus palsy	Diabetes, hypertension, arteritis, migraine

testing, and an edrophonium (Tensilon) test.

■ Painful Ophthalmoplegia

This is usually the result of a process in the cavernous sinus or superior orbital fissure (cf. Tables 9.**7**, 9.**9**). Aneurysms of the posterior communicating artery or of the basilar artery can compress the oculomotor nerve and simultaneously cause pain. The ischemic oculomotor palsy of diabetes, hypertension or arteritis can also be very painful.

■ Tolosa-Hunt Syndrome (897)

This is a special form of painful ophthalmoplegia that may additionally involve pupillomotor function, the first and sometimes second division of the trigeminal nerve, and (rarely) the facial nerve. It is due to granulomatous inflammation of the cavernous sinus. The pain responds well to steroid therapy (this may be considered a diagnostic test). This diagnosis can only be made by exclusion.

Treatment
Tolosa-Hunt syndrome responds to treatment with cortisone.

■ Intraorbital Masses

Intraorbital masses disturb ocular motility mechanically. They are characterized by displacement of the globe, with or without exophthalmos, and by impaired passive mobility of the globe. Exophthalmos may increase when the patient lies down or performs a Valsalva maneuver if a retrobulbar varix or cavernoma is present. A varix can also become thrombosed. Carotid-cavernous fistulae cause pulsatile exophthalmos. *Orbital pseudotumor* consists of exophthalmos and ophthalmoplegia due to an intraorbital inflammatory process causing myositis of the extraocular muscles.

Further Causes of Infranuclear Palsies of the Cranial Nerves Subserving Eye Movement, and of Diplopia

■ Brown's Tendon Sheath Syndrome

Diplopia on upward gaze (49) is caused in this syndrome by a thickening of the superior oblique tendon, or by pathology in the bony trochlea, resulting in impairment of the normally frictionless sliding of the tendon within the trochlea. A mechanical restriction of eye elevation results, which can be demonstrated with a forced duction test. This syndrome is usually congenital; most acquired cases are post-traumatic.

■ Endocrine Ophthalmopathy (245)

Endocrine ophthalmopathy may arise in the presence or absence of hyperthyroidism. Edema, infiltration, hypertrophy, and fibrosis affect some or all of the extraocular muscles, most commonly the inferior and medial recti. Diplopia is the initial symptom, typically on upward gaze if the inferior rectus is infiltrated, because the thickened muscle impedes elevation of the globe. Ophthalmoplegia may be total in severe cases, and optic neuropathy can also occur.

Anomalous Innervation of the Extraocular Muscles

Various congenital and acquired anomalies of the innervation of the extraocular muscles can cause abnormal eye movements.

■ Marcus Gunn Phenomenon ("Winking Jaw")
Ptosis at rest disappears when the patient opens or moves the jaw.

■ Pseudo-Graefe's Sign
In recovering oculomotor nerve palsy, downward gaze is accompanied by elevation of the eyelid. The term also refers to a sign of myotonia, in which the eyelid remains in an elevated position when the patient looks up and then down.

■ Duane's Retraction Syndrome
In this syndrome (type I), weakness of abduction is accompanied by involuntary retraction of the globe and narrowing of the palpebral fissure on adduction of the involved eye. Electromyography reveals simultaneous contraction of the medial and lateral recti. There are similar syndromes involving weakness of adduction (type II) or of both abduction and adduction (type III).

■ Möbius Syndrome
This is a congenital, usually bilateral facial and abducens (or gaze) palsy combined with esotropia and, occasionally, other deficits as well. Electromyography or muscle biopsy of the limbs reveals evidence of peripheral neuropathy.

Ptosis (508, 921)

The upper eyelid is elevated by two muscles, the levator palpebrae superioris muscle (innervated by CN III) and the superior tarsal muscle of Müller (sympathetic innervation).

The lid normally covers the upper margin of the iris, but no part of the pupil; in ptosis, by definition, part or all of the pupil is covered. As already seen in Table 4.**3**, ptosis may be
- neurogenic,
- synaptogenic,
- myogenic,
- desmogenic, or
- mechanical.

The clinical evaluation of ptosis requires attention to pupil size and reactivity, eye movements, uni- or bilaterality of ptosis, and any associated neurologic findings.

Neurogenic Ptosis and its Differential Diagnosis
Neurogenic ptosis may be due either to an oculomotor nerve palsy (p. 654) or to a sympathetic lesion. In the latter, ptosis is a component of Horner's syndrome, whose full expression consists of ptosis, miosis, enophthalmos, and anhidrosis of the face on the same side (p. 458). Sympathetic lesions, however, usually produce only mild ptosis, hardly ever covering the pupil, while the pupil in oculomotor nerve palsy may be entirely covered by the ptotic eyelid.

The following observations are useful in the differential diagnosis of mild ptosis:
- *Ptosis due to sympathetic denervation* is easiest to recognize when the patient looks slightly downward and disappears when the patient looks upward.
- *Ptosis due to oculomotor nerve palsy* is most severe when the patient looks slightly upward.
- *Congenital ptosis* is often accompanied by synkinesia with other eye muscles. Activation of other mus-

cles may either induce ptosis (as in Duane syndrome) or abolish it (as in the Marcus Gunn phenomenon).

- *Other types of neurogenic ptosis* include narrowing of the palpebral fissure due to blepharospasm (p. 267) or hemifacial spasm (p. 678), and synkinesia due to anomalous regeneration of the facial nerve after a facial nerve palsy (p. 673).

Synaptogenic Ptosis

The most common cause is *myasthenia gravis* (p. 918), which causes ptosis with or without accompanying weakness of the extraocular or other muscles. As the patient maintains upward gaze for a prolonged period, the eyelid gradually droops downward (Simpson test). Edrophonium (Tensilon) improves the ptosis. *Botulism* causes synaptogenic ptosis in addition to disturbances of accommodation, ocular motility, and swallowing (p. 455).

Myogenic Ptosis

Myopathy usually causes bilateral, slowly progressive ptosis along with other characteristic clinical signs.

Mechanical Ptosis

Mechanical ptosis is not accompanied by any disturbance of pupillary or ocular motility. It is usually unilateral, except in the elderly. So-called *senile ptosis* is often due to dehiscence of the aponeurosis of the levator palpebrae muscle, which can be repaired surgically. In younger individuals, isolated ptosis may be caused by chronic irritation from contact lenses (508).

Local changes of the globe and orbit can also cause ptosis.

Treatment of Oculomotor Disorders

Oculomotor disorders are generally treated according to their etiology. Diplopia and nystagmus can also be treated with symptomatic measures to reduce double vision and oscillopsia.

Diplopia

Treatment

Diplopia can be eliminated with an *eye patch* or *spectacles with an opaque glass on one side.* If the angular disparity is small, *prisms* may bring the two images back into fusion. If diplopia is not due to a progressive illness, the underlying strabismus can also be corrected *surgically.*

Nystagmus (571)

Treatment

If nystagmus causes distressing oscillopsia and vegetative symptoms such as nausea, antivertiginous medication can be tried. Some types of nystagmus can be suppressed with *baclofen, trihexyphenidyl, valproic acid, carbamazepine,* or other *centrally active agents.*

Some types of congenital nystagmus can be alleviated with visual aids that simultaneously improve visual acuity. Botulinum toxin is occasionally useful in the treatment of nystagmus and strabismus.

Pupillary Disorders

Anatomy and Clinical Examination of the Pupils

The anatomic basis of pupillary motility is described on p. 452 and 453 and depicted in Fig. 4.2. The reader is assumed to be familiar with the clinical examination of the pupils.

Abnormal Size and Shape of the Pupils

Pupillary ectopia is not uncommon; the ectopic pupil is usually displaced upward and outward, often in association with lens ectopy and other abnormalities of the globe. *Abnormally shaped (oval, rectangular) pupils* may be due to partial aniridia (absence of part of the iris) or acquired posterior synechiae, or indeed to partial atrophy of the iris – e.g., in tabes.

Inequality in size of the right and left pupils is called *anisocoria*. It may be a harmless congenital trait (physiological or "central" anisocoria), in which case the difference is rarely larger than 1 mm, may change sides or fluctuate in size over the course of the day, and is more pronounced in dim light, as in Horner syndrome (p. 458). Rarely, pupils that are equal in dim light become unequal when one pupil is illuminated because the illuminated pupil constricts more than the other one. This is not necessarily of pathological significance. Anisocoria is seen in ciliary ganglionitis (p. 665) and Horner's syndrome (p. 458), is a component of compressive oculomotor nerve palsy (p. 654), may be present in pupillotonia (see below), and may be an early sign of pupillary dysfunction in syphilis (see below).

Anisocoria is more pronounced in bright light in oculomotor nerve palsy, ciliary ganglionitis, and Adie's pupil.

Bilateral abnormality of the size of the pupils may be due to a locally or systemically administered drug (atropine, morphine, pilocarpine), while a unilateral abnormality may be due to unilateral local application of a drug, e.g., atropine or scopolamine in ointments or plasters taken to combat seasickness.

Abnormalities of Pupillary Reactivity

Local abnormalities of the eye. These should be excluded (posterior synechiae, glaucoma).

Amaurotic pupil. The amaurotic pupil is of normal width and has a consensual but not a direct light response; thus, when both eyes are open, no abnormality is seen. The pupil of the blind eye dilates when the seeing eye is covered.

Oculomotor nerve lesions. A dilated pupil that constricts neither in response to illumination (direct or consensual) nor on convergence may be the first sign of an oculomotor nerve lesion while ocular motility is still normal.

Marcus Gunn pupil (afferent pupillary defect). This phenomenon is a less extreme version of that seen in a fully amaurotic pupil and may be evident, for example, in the aftermath of (healed) retrobulbar neuritis. The pupil on the involved side dilates when the intact eye is covered to a greater extent than the pupil of the intact eye dilates when the involved eye is covered.

Argyll Robertson pupil. This finding is usually bilateral. The pupils are small, often misshapen, and react to convergence but not to light. Syphilis is the most common cause (though this can also cause fixed and dilated pupils). A small, nonreactive pupil is seen in diabetes as well, but then usually only on one side (p. 602).

Adie's pupil (pupillotonia). This finding is usually unilateral. The pupil is somewhat dilated and reacts only after prolonged illumination, but more rapidly to convergence. Slow, tonic dilatation afterward is characteristic. The pupillary finding is often, though not always, accompanied by the absence of certain reflexes in Adie's syndrome, which mostly affects women; there may also be a chronic cough (517a). It is thought that this condition may be the expression of a process in the midbrain and/or diencephalon, perhaps of an inflammatory nature. Another hypothesis is that it represents anomalous reinnervation of the pupillary sphincter in the aftermath of a lesion of the ciliary ganglion (see below). Alternatively, it may be due to a herpes simplex virus infection (786).

Mild chronic irritation of the oculomotor nerve. This may be caused by a saccular aneurysm, a tumor, or any other kind of slowly growing mass or inflammatory process. The clinical picture may resemble that of Adie's pupil.

Acute ciliary ganglionitis. This condition usually arises within a few days of an infectious illness, and sometimes after orbital trauma. It is characterized by a dilated pupil that reacts neither to light nor to convergence. Transient accommodation disturbance with difficulty reading is also present at first. The pupillary anomaly persists, in the absence of any oculomotor disturbance (which distinguishes this entity from a third nerve palsy).

Hippus. The normal, spontaneous rhythmic dilatation and constriction of the pupil is too small in amplitude to be seen with the naked eye; an exaggeration of this phenomenon so that it becomes visible is called *hippus* (374b). Its significance is unclear; it is presumably related, in some way, to pupillotonia. It can be seen in incipient cataract, multiple sclerosis, and meningitis, and in the aftermath of a (resolved) oculomotor nerve palsy. It can also be an incidental finding in normal persons.

Rare pupillary abnormalities. The pupils may be fixed and dilated because of *medications* (homatropine ointment) or toxic effects (botulism, diphtheria, Wernicke's encephalopathy, etc.). Transient unilateral mydriasis may also occur in *migraine*, as may transient miosis, which is also typical of cluster headache. For nonreactive pupils in acute pandysautonomia, see p. 454.

Strongly pinching the upper border of the trapezius muscle normally induces dilatation of both pupils (*ciliospinal reflex*). Absence of this reflex implies a lesion somewhere along the reflex arc – i.e., in the somatosensory afferents from the shoulder area, in the brainstem, or in the descending and ascending sympathetic path-

	Initial position		Direct illumination	Contralateral illumintion	Conver-gence	Characteristic features
	Right	Left				
Normal	●	●	• | •	• | •	• | •	
Amaurotic fixed pupil	●	●	● | ●	• | •	• | •	Blind in right eye, normal reaction to atropine and physostigmine
Oculomotor nerve lesion (and ciliary ganglionitis)	●	•	● | •	● | •	● | •	Ocular motility disturbed only in oculomotor nerve lesion; constriction in response to miotic agent
Adie's pupil (pupillotonia)	●	•	● | •	● | •	• | •	Normal ocular motility, tonic dilatation after convergence reaction, normal response to mydriatic agents
Argyll Robertson pupil	‐	‐	‐ | ‐	‐ | ‐	‐ | ‐	Pupils often misshapen, no response to weak mydriatic agents, enhanced constriction with physostigmine, mild dilatation with atropine
Early optic nerve lesion (afferent pupillary defect)	●	●	• | •	• | •	• | •	
Local atropine effect	●	•	● | •	● | •	● | •	Normal ocular motility, no contriction in response to miotic agents, no constriction with physostigmine
Systemic atropine effect	●	●	● | ●	● | ●	● | ●	No change with physostigmine
Diencephalic lesion	•	•	• | •	• | •	• | •	Narrow, reacive
Midbrain lesion	●	●	● | ●	● | ●	● | ●	Fixed in midposition
Pontine lesion	•	•	• | •	• | •	• | •	Fixed pinpoint pupils

Fig. 9.**21** **Abnormalities of the pupillary reflexes (right side abnormal).**

way terminating in the ciliospinal center.

Synopsis. The features of the major pupillary disorders are listed in Table 9.**10** and depicted schematically in Fig. 9.**21**. Figure 9.**22** contains a flowchart for the diagnostic evaluation of anisocoria.

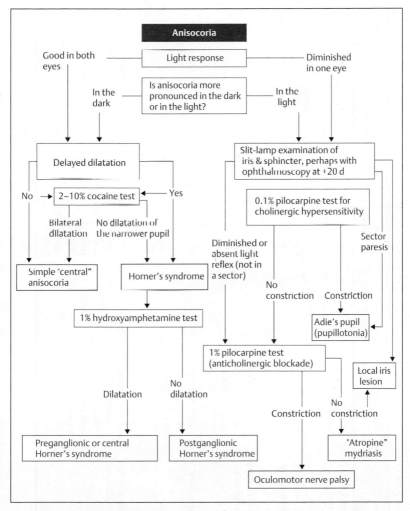

Fig. 9.**22** **Diagnostic flowchart for anisocoria** (adapted from Thompson et al.)

Table 9.**10**   Pupillary disorders (right pupil abnormal) (see also Fig. 9.**21**)

Condition	Features	Without illumination	Direct illumination	Illumination of other eye	On convergence	Response to test drugs
Amaurotic fixed pupil	Blind, disk may be white	R = L	Both fixed	Both constrict	Both constrict	Normal reaction to atropine and physostigmine
Oculomotor nerve palsy	Sees; ocular motility usually abnormal	R >> L	R fixed, L constricts	R fixed, L constricts	R fixed, L constricts	Constriction in response to miotic agents
Acute ciliary ganglionitis	Normal ocular motility, otherwise as in oculomotor nerve palsy					
Synechiae	Normal ocular motility, pupil may be misshapen	R may be < L	R fixed, L constricts	R fixed, L constricts	R fixed, L constricts	Dilates in response to mydriatic agents; synechiae become visible
Adie's pupil (pupillotonia)	80% unilateral; slow increase of "visual acuity" as test pattern nears, because of increasing accommodation	R > L	R at first fixed, constricts after prolonged and intense illumination, then slow (tonic) dilatation; L constricts	R fixed, L constricts	Both constrict; thereafter tonic dilation on R	Normal response to mydriatic agents

(*Cont.*) →

Table 9.**10** (Cont.)

Condition	Features	Without illumination	Direct illumination	Illumination of other eye	On convergence	Response to test drugs
Argyll Robertson pupil	Pupils usually both narrow, often misshapen	R < L	Both essentially fixed	Both essentially fixed	Both constrict marked y	No response to weak mydriatic agents, enhanced constriction with physostigmine, mild dilatation with atropine
Atropine effect	Accommodation abolished for 10–14 days	R >> L	R fixed, L constricts	R fixed, L constricts	R fixed, L constricts	No constriction in response to physostigmine

Trigeminal Disturbances

Anatomy and Clinical Examination
The reader is assumed to be familiar with the clinical examination of the trigeminal nerve. Its anatomy is illustrated in Figs. 9.**23** and 9.**24**. A disturbance of trigeminal nerve function or of a reflex in which the trigeminal nerve participates can be objectified and quantified by examination of the corneal blink and masseteric reflexes and by electrophysiologic testing.

Clinical Features
Lesions of individual divisions of the trigeminal nerve. These may be due to skull fracture, meningitis, tumor, sarcoidosis (122a) or aneurysm. Trigeminal deficits appear in isolation in trigeminal nerve schwannoma, or in combination with other cranial nerve deficits in the syndrome of the cerebellopontine angle. Processes in the cavernous sinus region – e.g., thrombosis or Raeder's syndrome – can involve the first and second divisions as well as cranial nerves III, IV, and VI. They usually also cause exophthalmos and lid edema. The mental nerve is often involved by metastatic cancer at the skull base or in the jaw (see below). Occasionally, the superior or inferior alveolar nerve sustains permanent damage during a dental procedure, either from the procedure itself (usually tooth extraction, particularly of a wisdom tooth) or from the needle used to inject the local anesthetic.

Lesions in the nuclear complex of the trigeminal nerve, and in the central trigeminal pathways in the pons and medulla. These may be caused by ischemia or by tumor, encephalitis, multiple sclerosis, or syringomyelia/syringobulbia. They can be differentiated from peripheral lesions of the trigeminal nerve by neuroimaging, particularly MRI. The associated abnormality of the blink reflex differs characteristically from that of infranuclear lesions, in that the R1 component is absent on the affected side (23a).

Paresthesiae in the trigeminal nerve distribution. These may be due to cranial polyneuritis (p. 581) or poisoning with trichlorethylene or other chlorinated acetylenes. It is unclear, however, whether these toxins exert a primary deleterious effect or reactivate a latent herpes virus infection (172). Trigeminal paresthesiae (sometimes painful) not uncommonly accompany the onset of (peripheral) facial nerve palsy; this combination is perhaps explained by a common blood supply of the two nerves. Yet trigeminal paresthesiae can also arise as an isolated symptom, without pain, weakness, or abnormality of taste, usually in the maxillary or mandibular division. They may regress within weeks, though a sensory deficit remains in some cases. Persistent paresthesiae and pain on one or both sides, sometimes restricted to two divisions of the trigeminal nerve, may appear early in the course of certain collagenoses, primarily scleroderma. An isolated sensory deficit in the mental nerve distribution ("numb chin syndrome") is often the expression of a malignant tumor spreading along the skull base or the meninges (598). Burning of the tongue may be caused by iron deficiency, vitamin B$_{12}$ deficiency, or the use of colistin or sumatriptan nasal spray. It also occurs

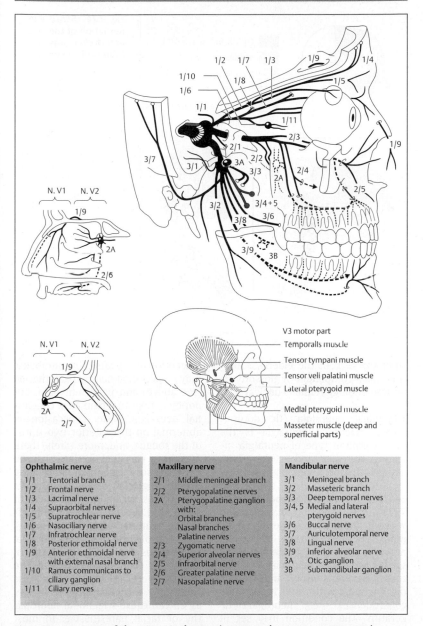

Ophthalmic nerve

1/1	Tentorial branch
1/2	Frontal nerve
1/3	Lacrimal nerve
1/4	Supraorbital nerves
1/5	Supratrochlear nerve
1/6	Nasociliary nerve
1/7	Infratrochlear nerve
1/8	Posterior ethmoidal nerve
1/9	Anterior ethmoidal nerve with external nasal branch
1/10	Ramus communicans to ciliary ganglion
1/11	Ciliary nerves

Maxillary nerve

2/1	Middle meningeal branch
2/2	Pterygopalatine nerves
2A	Pterygopalatine ganglion with:
	Orbital branches
	Nasal branches
	Palatine nerves
2/3	Zygomatic nerve
2/4	Superior alveolar nerves
2/5	Infraorbital nerve
2/6	Greater palatine nerve
2/7	Nasopalatine nerve

Mandibular nerve

3/1	Meningeal branch
3/2	Masseteric branch
3/3	Deep temporal nerves
3/4, 5	Medial and lateral pterygoid nerves
3/6	Buccal nerve
3/7	Auriculotemporal nerve
3/8	Lingual nerve
3/9	inferior alveolar nerve
3A	Otic ganglion
3B	Submandibular ganglion

Fig. 9.**23** **Anatomy of the trigeminal nerve (motor and sensory components).**

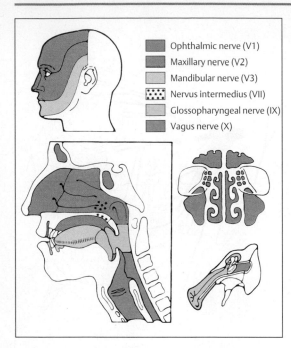

Fig. 9.**24   Sensory innervation of the face and the mucous membranes of the head.**

Ophthalmic nerve (V1)
Maxillary nerve (V2)
Mandibular nerve (V3)
Nervus intermedius (VII)
Glossopharyngeal nerve (IX)
Vagus nerve (X)

spontaneously in the elderly, sometimes as a component of glossodynia (whose etiology remains unclear).

Trigeminal neuralgia (tic douloureux). Trigeminal neuralgia is the most common type of neuralgia affecting the face and is described, along with other types, on p. 821.

Sensory trigeminal neuropathy (747a, 797a). This condition may develop without any known cause in one or more divisions of the trigeminal nerve, in rare cases bilaterally. Sensory trigeminal neuropathy often causes severe sensory and trophic dysfunction, with the predictable consequences – e.g., neuroparalytic keratitis. The condition may set in suddenly and last for days, months, or

(exceptionally) years. The numbness may be accompanied by paresthesiae (see above) and persistent pain, but not by paroxysmal pain as in trigeminal neuralgia. Taste is occasionally abnormal on the anterior two-thirds of the tongue, and, more rarely, there may be a transient ipsilateral facial palsy. Sensory trigeminal neuropathy usually regresses spontaneously. In some cases, an underlying illness of some kind becomes evident only after the neuropathy has disappeared – e.g., multiple sclerosis, syringobulbia, a cavernous sinus process, a fusiform aneurysm or dolichoectasia of the basilar artery, or scleroderma. Less commonly, a cervical process as low as C5 can cause trigeminal neuropathy or facial paresthesiae. In most cases, however, the symptoms remain an isolated and unexplained phenomenon, and are presumably the expression of a viral mononeuritis ascending from the periphery.

Trigeminal motor phenomena. Among the various motor phenomena associated with the trigeminal nerve, we will mention *hemimasticatory spasm* here. This condition involves involuntary contraction of the muscles of mastication on one side, leading to powerful closure of the jaw. Some cases are associated with hemiatrophy of the face.

Treatment

Hemimasticatory spasm responds well to *carbamazepine* and, if necessary, to local injection of *botulinum toxin* (45).

Facial Nerve Disturbances

Anatomy and Clinical Examination
The anatomy of the facial nerve is depicted in Fig. 9.**25**. It is assumed that the reader is already familiar with the relevant clinical examination techniques.

Symptoms and Signs of Peripheral Facial Nerve Palsy
These can be largely deduced from the anatomical facts illustrated in Fig. 9.**25**. The major findings are:
- paresis of the muscles of facial expression,
- hyperacusis,
- diminished lacrimation and salivation, and
- diminished taste on the anterior two-thirds of the tongue.

The last three functions named are contained in the portion of the facial nerve called the nervus intermedius up to the level of the geniculate ganglion. Total peripheral facial nerve palsy involves all branches of the nerve on one side, and complete closure of the eye is no longer possible.

Central facial palsy. In central facial palsy (which can no longer be correctly termed a "facial nerve palsy," as the nerve is intact) the muscles of the forehead are less affected than those of the face below the eyes, because the rostral portion of the facial nerve nucleus receives innervation from the motor cortex of both hemispheres and the forehead muscles generally contract synergistically with those of the opposite side (Fig. 9.**26**). Central facial palsy never makes eye closure impossible, though it may become weak.

Cryptogenic Peripheral Facial Nerve Palsy (13)

Incidence and Epidemiology
Three-quarters of cases of peripheral facial nerve palsy are cryptogenic (Bell's palsy). The incidence of this disorder is ca. 25 per 100,000 persons per year (496). It affects men and women equally, and can occur at any age, though most commonly in middle age. Familial clustering has been observed.

Pathogenesis
Much evidence suggests that Bell's palsy is a kind of cranial neuritis that

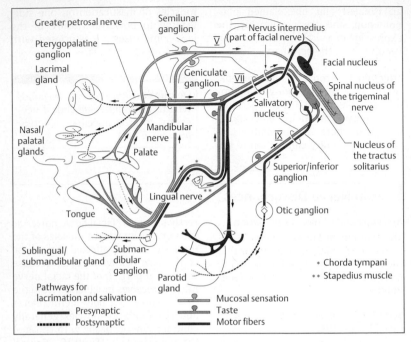

Fig. 9.**25**   **Anatomy of the facial nerve.**

affects the facial nerve more severely than any other, but not exclusively. Most cases are probably due to an as yet unidentified type of viral infection (the CSF cell count is often elevated). A possible causative role for the herpes simplex virus has been postulated and seems to be supported by the analysis of a very large series of patients from a specialized clinic. Other cases may be due to ischemia of the nerve as it passes through the facial canal (canal of Fallopius). There seem to be an abnormally large number of diabetics and prediabetics (i.e., persons with impaired glucose tolerance) among patients with Bell's palsy; in one study, the percentage was 66%. The older the patient, the more likely to be diabetic or prediabetic.

There also seems to be an association with malignant hypertension: a study of a group of patients with this condition revealed peripheral facial palsy in 4% of 90 adults, and in 20% of 35 children.

Surgical observations and intraoperative electrophysiologic testing of the exposed nerve trunks have confirmed that the nerve is edematous even as close to the brainstem as the internal acoustic meatus, and that the site of conduction block is immediately distal to the entrance to the facial canal – i.e., proximal to the geniculate ganglion.

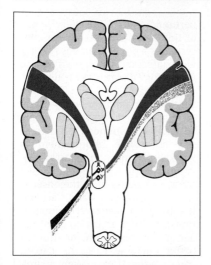

Fig. 9.**26 Bilateral corticobulbar innervation of the rostral portion of the facial nucleus.** In central facial palsy, the upper portion of the face remains unparalyzed, because the upper portion of the facial nucleus receives innervation from both cerebral hemispheres.

Clinical Features

Unilateral weakness of all facial muscles innervated by the facial nerve usually develops within a few hours, or over 1–3 days at most. The weakness is of variable severity and need not be a complete paralysis. It is often already at its maximum extent when first noticed by the patient on arising in the morning. Usually no precipitating factor can be identified. The patient's general condition is unimpaired.

Clinical examination reveals paresis of all muscles of facial expression on one side, and often also diminished taste on the anterior two-thirds of the tongue on that side. A careful search

not uncommonly reveals evidence of involvement of other cranial nerves as well. About half of all patients complain of paresthesiae (sometimes painful) in the trigeminal area, and pain behind the ear on the affected side is particularly common. These symptoms begin either simultaneously with the weakness, or just before it. The glossopharyngeal and vagus nerves and, less commonly, the upper cervical segments may be involved as well.

In some cases, the signs and symptoms regress fully within 4–6 weeks. In others, however, improvement does not begin till 3–6 months have elapsed, and is even then incomplete. The long-term result is good in about 80% of cases, and poor, with distressing residual deficits, in only about 5–8%.

Course and Prognosis

Unfavorable prognostic factors include:

- advanced age,
- hyperacusis,
- disturbance of taste,
- severe paralysis at onset and
- electrophysiological evidence of denervation.

Residual deficits. Careful examination at long-term follow-up reveals residual deficits in more than a few patients, including mild contracture of the facial muscles at rest and, most prominently, synergistic mass contraction due to faulty reinnervation. Thus, in some patients, an attempt to show the teeth is accompanied by involuntary lid closure; or else, when the patient puffs his cheeks, the originally paretic cheek contracts when the lips are closed and is thus not as fully inflated as the other cheek. The "crocodile tears" phenomenon (abnormal lacrimation while eating) is rare; it is caused by a faulty reinnervation in which fibers originally destined for the salivary gland instead terminate in the lacrimal gland.

Ipsilateral and contralateral recurrence. Bell's palsy recurs on the same or opposite side in 10% of patients. These cases are associated with electrophysiologic evidence of marked denervation and thus may have a worse prognosis.

Ancillary Tests

Additional tests are rarely necessary to confirm the diagnosis of this classic clinical entity. *Electrophysiologic studies* are useful to define the degree of paresis more precisely and, above all, to document reinnervation even in its early stage. The *CSF* is abnormal in only about 10% of cryptogenic cases, but much more commonly in cases due to herpes zoster oticus (Ramsay Hunt syndrome, see below), and invariably in the HIV-associated form (529a). *Magnetic stimulation of the motor cortex* can be used to activate the facial nerve, enabling electrophysiologic differentiation of lesions within and proximal to the canal of the facial nerve (Fallopian canal) (349) (cf. Fig. 5.**5**).

Treatment

Bell's palsy is usually treated with *prednisone*. Once the diagnosis is established, and as long as there is no contraindication, adult patients are given 60 mg daily for 4 days, then a tapering dose that is reduced by 5 mg every other day, all the way to zero in a little over three weeks. There is a difference of expert opinion over the effectiveness of this treatment. Because of concern over a possible herpes simplex virus infection, valaciclovir is also given for 10 days at a dose of 1000 mg t.i.d.

Surgical decompression (by an otologist) is controversial. Some specialists recommend it if there is still no visible improvement of weakness, and no electromyographically detectable muscle activity, 3–4 weeks after the onset of the disease (or even earlier, according to the newest recommendations). There is as yet no clear evidence that this treatment affords a better outcome than the natural course of the disease. Many neurologists, ourselves included, have stopped recommending this procedure.

Bilateral Facial Nerve Palsy

Though facial nerve palsy recurs in about 7% of cases, simultaneous bilateral facial nerve palsy is only about one one-hundredth as common as unilateral facial nerve palsy. Perhaps half of all such cases have a benign prognosis no different from that of the unilateral cryptogenic form. The remaining cases are due to meningeal or central tumors, infection (sometimes HIV) (1044a), or other, rarer causes.

Melkersson-Rosenthal Syndrome (335)

Clinical Features

This illness consists of the clinical triad of peripheral facial nerve palsy (no different from that of Bell's palsy), facial swelling, and a plicated tongue (as in Miescher's granulomatous cheilitis). Recurrences and bilateral facial palsies are particularly common. Melkersson-Rosenthal syndrome is due to a multifocal granulomatous angiitis that may involve other cranial nerves and cause mono- or polyneuropathy, plexus lesions, psychosis, or encephalomyelitis. The prognosis for spontaneous recovery is good.

Treatment

Treatment should be started early with *prednisone*, 1 mg/kg daily, and *valaciclovir*, 100 mg t.i.d. for 10 days.

Other Causes of Peripheral Facial Nerve Palsy

■ Head Trauma

Some 3% of patients who sustain head trauma develop delayed facial palsy, always in conjunction with bleeding from the ear. Among patients with *basilar skull fractures,* about half of those with transverse fractures of the petrous pyramid develop facial palsy, and 10–30% of those with longitudinal fractures. Seventy percent of early palsies and 90% of delayed palsies regress spontaneously.

The prognosis for recovery is worst in patients with transverse fractures, and best in those with delayed palsy after a longitudinal fracture (arising 1–20 days after the injury because of edema or slowly expanding hematoma). Operative decompression is indicated in early paralysis due to either a transverse or a longitudinal fracture, as well as in delayed paralysis due to a longitudinal fracture if electromyography reveals total denervation.

■ Post-Infectious Facial Nerve Palsy

The usual cause is *herpes zoster oticus,* which accounts for some 15% of peripheral facial nerve palsies. Vesicles should therefore be looked for in every case, particularly on the pinna and on the palate. *Ramsay Hunt syndrome* consists of peripheral facial nerve palsy and neuralgic pain after a herpes zoster infection of the geniculate ganglion (p. 824). The CSF is often abnormal in these cases (529a). *Zoster colli,* too, can cause peripheral facial nerve palsy. *Other neurotropic viruses* rarely cause either nuclear or peripheral facial palsies, which may be seen accompanying other manifestations of poliomyelitis, echovirus and coxsackievirus infections, tickborne radiculomyelomeningoencephalitis (p. 114), etc.

■ Other Types of Facial Palsy

Middle ear processes (purulent otitis, tumors such as glomus tumor) can cause facial palsy along with hearing loss and other local signs. Among *intracranial tumors,* those in the cerebellopontine angle (e.g., acoustic neuroma) often cause peripheral facial nerve palsy. *Guillain-Barré syndrome* (p. 575) often causes bilateral facial palsy; if facial palsy is the first sign of polyradiculitis, *borreliosis* may be the cause. *Sarcoidosis* can cause bilateral facial palsy in association with the parotid swelling and ocular manifestations of *Heerfordt syndrome* (p. 329). *Basilar (infectious) meningitis* and *lymphomatous or carcinomatous meningitis* (p. 104) can also cause facial palsy, usually along with other cranial nerve deficits. Several cases of peripheral facial palsy, usually bilateral and associated with trismus, have been described in *tetanus*, especially cephalic tetanus. *Pressure at the edge of the mandible*, produced, for example, by the anesthesiologist's Esmarch handgrip or by surgical procedures in the vicinity (such as carotid endarterectomy), can cause a pressure palsy of the *marginal mandibular branch of the facial nerve*, with weakness of the perioral muscles. Sparing of the frontal and orbital branches of the nerve may lead to the erroneous diagnosis of central facial palsy. *Congenital absence (aplasia) of the depressor anguli oris muscle* is evident in infants and toddlers only when they cry and is almost always on the left side. Finally, congenital facial palsy is a component of *Möbius syndrome* and is often bilateral in such cases (*facial diplegia*).

Disturbances of Taste (300a)

Taste is impaired on the anterior two-thirds of the tongue when the chorda tympani is involved by a facial nerve lesion – e.g., in Bell's palsy. Lingual nerve lesions can impair taste in the same way. Glossopharyngeal nerve lesions impair taste on the posterior third of the tongue; the deficit may be bilateral, as after tonsillectomy (241, 246).

Hemifacial Spasm

Clinical Features

The hallmark of hemifacial spasm is an involuntary, synchronous, sudden, tonic contraction of all muscles innervated by the facial nerve on one side of the face, lasting several seconds and repeating itself at irregular intervals, as frequently as several times per minute. Spasms can sometimes be induced by particular voluntary movements but generally occur without apparent provocation. This condition usually arises in middle age and has no tendency to regress spontaneously. It often persists without change for months or years.

Pathogenesis

A minority of cases of hemifacial spasm arise in the setting of a previous (healed) peripheral facial palsy. In other, rare cases, an anomaly of the craniocervical junction (p. 43) or an intracranial process compressing the root of the facial nerve may cause this syndrome. A vascular loop is sometimes found to be compressing the nerve in the cerebellopontine angle; the loop is usually a segment of the superior or the anterior inferior cerebellar artery.
Persistent hemifacial spasm is sometimes a sign of brainstem glioma.

Treatment

Hemifacial spasm can be abolished, in about 80% of cases, by a *neurosurgical procedure* in which the cerebellopontine angle is explored and a piece of inert material is inserted between the facial nerve and a compressing vascular loop, if present (*"microvascular decompression"*), or the nerve is merely freed from surrounding structures *("neurolysis")*. Such procedures carry a small risk of ipsilateral deafness and of technical complications such as CSF leak and meningitis. *Partial extracranial division or compression of the facial nerve trunk* was previously performed to treat hemifacial spasm, particularly by otologists, but always caused partial facial weakness and was only temporarily effective. This procedure should no longer be performed. *Botulinum toxin injections* may bring symptomatic relief.

Facial Myokymia

Clinical Features

This condition is characterized by continuous wavelike contractions of individual muscles on one side of the face.

Causes

Facial myokymia is often due to multiple sclerosis or tumors of the brainstem (in which case there is accompanying facial weakness).

Facial Tic

Tics are sudden, involuntary contractions of the facial musculature, of variable location, usually in nervous individuals. *Blepharospasm* (p. 267) is a particular form that is often the oligo-symptomatic manifestation of an organic extrapyramidal disorder. Facial tic is sometimes the initial sign of a more generalized tic disease, such as Gilles de la Tourette syndrome.

Progressive Facial Hemiatrophy

Clinical Features

This occasionally congenital type of facial atrophy often begins with "saber-cut atrophy" in the midline of the face and forehead and progresses to involve bone and cartilage, as well as the brain. It is often accompanied by ipsilateral Horner's syndrome and oculomotor disturbances, as well as by contralateral Jacksonian or generalized seizures.

Differential Diagnosis

This disorder must be differentiated from other types of facial asymmetry – e.g., caput obstipum musculare. *Bilateral facial atrophy* may be simulated by hypotrophy of the fat pad of Bichat. True bilateral atrophy of the facial musculature has been described after β-blocker use and exposure to cold and is presumably due to peripheral vasoconstriction.

Disturbances of the Vestibulocochlear Nerve (Statoacoustic Nerve, Auditory Nerve)
(52, 57, 133, 837, 838, 912)

Overview:
CN VIII mediates hearing through its cochlear portion and equilibrium through its vestibular portion. Dysfunction of this nerve thus leads to hearing loss, tinnitus, dysequilibrium, and vertigo. This section deals with the disease entities that can affect this nerve and the clinical diagnostic approach to patients suffering from these problems. An understanding of ocular motility, as discussed above, is a prerequisite for the clinical assessment of vertigo (p. 630).

Anatomy

The cochlear portion of the 8th cranial nerve conducts auditory impulses arising from the cochlea, while its vestibular portion conducts impulses relating to position and movement arising from the semicircular canals. All of these impulses travel to the brainstem (Fig. 9.**27**).

Testing of Hearing

The neurologist tests hearing
- to detect partial or total hearing loss (deafness), and
- to differentiate conductive from sensorineural hearing loss.

First, the examiner determines *at what distance the patient can hear regular and whispered speech with each ear,* while hearing in the other ear is prevented by back-and-forth movement of the examiner's or another person's finger in the external ear canal. If hearing loss is found, *otoscopy* should be performed. The two well-known *tuning fork tests* are used to determine whether hearing loss is of conductive or sensorineural origin:

- In the *Weber test,* a vibrating tuning fork is placed in the middle of the forehead. Patients with hearing loss will localize the sound to the deficient ear if the hearing loss is conductive, to the good ear if it is sensorineural.
- The *Rinne test* is based on the fact that air conduction of sound normally yields better hearing than bone conduction. The tuning fork is first placed on the mastoid process; then, as soon as it is no longer heard, it is held in front of the ear. A normal individual will hear it in front of the ear roughly twice as long as on the bone (normal Rinne test). In conductive hearing loss, the sound conducted through the air is heard very briefly, or not at all (abnormal Rinne test). Sensorineural hearing loss is not detected by the Rinne test, as air and bone conduction are equally impaired.

The characteristics of the two types of hearing loss are listed in Table 9.**11**. Total deafness in an ear is always sensorineural and cannot be due to a disturbance of the conductive apparatus alone (e.g., otitis media). A unilateral

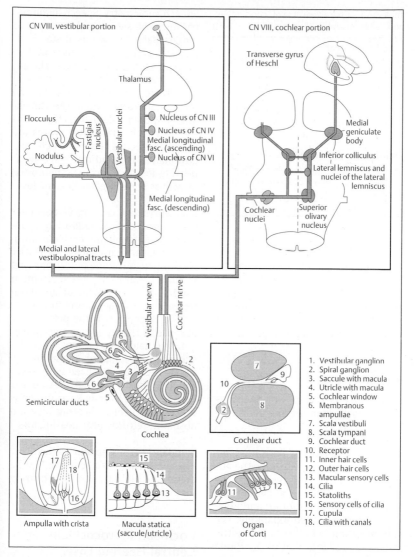

CN VIII, vestibular portion

Thalamus

Flocculus

Nodulus

Fastigial nucleus

Vestibular nuclei

Nucleus of CN III
Nucleus of CN IV
Medial longitudinal fasc. (ascending)
Nucleus of CN VI

Medial longitudinal fasc. (descending)

Medial and lateral vestibulospinal tracts

CN VIII, cochlear portion

Transverse gyrus of Heschl

Medial geniculate body

Inferior colliculus

Lateral lemniscus and nuclei of the lateral lemniscus

Cochlear nuclei

Superior olivary nucleus

Vestibular nerve

Cochlear nerve

Semicircular ducts

Cochlea

Cochlear duct

Ampulla with crista

Macula statica (saccule/utricle)

Organ of Corti

1. Vestibular ganglion
2. Spiral ganglion
3. Saccule with macula
4. Utricle with macula
5. Cochlear window
6. Membranous ampullae
7. Scala vestibuli
8. Scala tympani
9. Cochlear duct
10. Receptor
11. Inner hair cells
12. Outer hair cells
13. Macular sensory cells
14. Cilia
15. Statoliths
16. Sensory cells of cilia
17. Cupula
18. Cilia with canals

Fig. 9.**27** **Anatomy of the inner ear and vestibulocochlear nerve (CN VIII).**

Table 9.**11**   Characteristics of conductive and sensorineural hearing loss

Conductive hearing loss:
- Hearing diminished, but never totally absent
- Weber test: sound localizes to bad ear
- Rinne test: abnormal (air-conducted sound heard only briefly, or not at all)

Sensorineural hearing loss:
- Hearing diminished or totally absent
- Weber test: sound localizes to good ear
- Rinne test: normal

lesion of the cerebral hemisphere or brainstem hardly ever impairs hearing, as the cochleocortical pathway projects bilaterally. Deafness due to simultaneous, bilateral lesions of the auditory cortices on both sides is extremely rare.

Audiometry

Audiometry is a means of quantitative assessment of hearing and hearing disorders.

Pure-tone audiometry. Pure-tone audiometry is used to determine the auditory threshold – i.e., the lowest intensity of sound that the patient can still hear. Thresholds for air and bone conduction are tested separately. The interpretation of the audiometric curves is similar to that of the Rinne test. The curves are nearly superimposable in the normal situation and in sensorineural nearing loss, while air conduction is worse than bone conduction in conductive hearing loss.

Speech audiometry. Speech audiometry tests the subject's ability to hear monosyllabic test words at standardized intensities. Hearing loss can then be expressed as a percentage. The auditory thresholds for pure tones and speech are normally separated by no more than 70 dB (where the threshold for speech is defined as the intensity at which 50% of test words are heard correctly). Poor speech discrimination is found in retrocochlear hearing loss (e.g., acoustic neuroma) as well as in nonorganic hearing loss.

Suprathreshold auditory tests/Fowler test. *Suprathreshold auditory tests* are used to differentiate cochlear from retrocochlear hearing loss. The *Fowler test,* in which volume perception and volume balance are tested, is often used in the assessment of unilateral hearing loss. The most important finding of this test is the presence or absence of the *recruitment phenomenon:* it is said to be present when the subjective volume of sound in the two ears can be equalized with lower sound intensity in the affected ear than in the normal ear. Recruitment is present in cochlear hearing loss and absent in retrocochlear hearing loss.

Tympanometry/stapedius reflex. These tests may also be helpful in the diagnostic localization of hearing loss.

Cochlear, Retrocochlear, or Central Hearing Loss?

It is not possible to distinguish cochlear from retrocochlear (i.e., auditory nerve) hearing loss by clinical examination alone; further testing is required, either the audiometric tests described above, or auditory evoked potentials. Central hearing loss can usually be recognized by the presence of accompanying neurologic deficits of other kinds and is hardly ever the patient's most prominent symptom. The reason for this lies in the anatomy of the auditory pathway. The peripheral auditory neurons divide, shortly after entering the brainstem, into branches to the ventral and dorsal cochlear nuclei, which then, in turn, project to the ipsi- and contralateral transverse temporal gyri by way of at least three further neurons. Bilateral representation all along the central pathway has the consequence that unilateral lesions do not cause clinically relevant hearing loss.

When bilateral lesions are present in the brainstem or thalamus, the patient generally has severe enough deficits of other kinds that it becomes difficult or impossible to assess for hearing loss. The auditory evoked potentials may be abnormal in such situations (p. 473). Temporal cortical lesions, too, impair hearing only when they are bilateral (p. 377).

Diseases Causing Hearing Loss

Etiology and Clinical Features

The diagnosis and treatment of conductive hearing loss is within the purview of the otologist. The neurologist, on the other hand, is often called on to assess sensorineural hearing loss, with a view to both localization (cochlear, retrocochlear, central) and etiology. Children who become deaf before learning to speak can never learn to speak correctly; they pronounce consonants with exaggerated emphasis, vowels hardly at all. This condition is called deaf-mutism. Table 9.**12** contains a list of diseases causing prominent cochlear or retrocochlear hearing loss, sometimes in combination with vestibular and other neurologic signs and symptoms. Hardness of hearing is often genetic (1028a).

Hearing loss is common, affecting 10% of all 60-year-olds and half of all 80-year-olds. It is often a polygenic inherited trait, but a number of single genes have recently been identified, a mutation in any one of which can cause monogenic hearing loss or deafness. These genes are all designated DFN (for deafness), and more specifically as DFNA for autosomal dominant, DFNB for autosomal recessive, and DFNX for X-linked recessive deafness. Mitochondrial gene mutations can also cause deafness, in isolation or as part of a syndrome. The protein products of these genes include ion channels, connexins, transcription factors, structural proteins of the cochlea, and mitochondrial proteins. Connexins are membrane proteins. Connexin mutations are the most common cause of monogenic hearing loss – e.g., mutation of the connexin-32 gene in X-linked Charcot-Marie-Tooth syndrome (p. 588).

Differential Diagnosis

Important considerations for differential diagnosis are:
- the age of onset of hearing loss,
- the rapidity of onset,
- uni- or bilaterality,
- cochlear or retrocochlear type,
- combination with vestibular or other neurologic signs and symptoms.

Table 9.12   Diseases causing prominent hearing loss

Category	Disease	Hearing loss	Dysequilibrium	Brainstem or other neurologic signs	Remarks
Hereditary congenital malformations of the inner ear (900)	Isolated hereditary deafness	+	–	–	80% autosomal recessive, 15% autosomal dominant, 5% X-linked
	Mondini syndrome	+	+	–	Malformation of the bony and membranous labyrinth, often perilymph fistula, mutation of the pendrin gene in Pendred syndrome, also goiter
	Alport syndrome	+	–	–	X-linked recessive disorder of amino acid metabolism, hematuria, renal failure, deformation of lens (lenticonus)
	Klein-Waardenburg syndrome	+	+	–	Autosomal dominant, wide root of nose, narrow palpebral fissure, hyperplasia of medial portions of eyebrows, heterochromia of the iris, unpigmented streaks in hair
	Usher syndrome	+	(+)	(–)	Autosomal recessive, slowly progressive retinitis pigmentosa beginning in childhood, myosin-7A gene mutation
	Laurence-Moon-Bardet-Biedl syndrome	+	–	+	Obesity, short stature, feeble-mindedness, polydactyly, retinitis pigmentosa

Table 9.12 (Cont.)

Mitochondrial encephalomyopathies	(+)	(+)	(+)	Hearing loss may be the sole or most prominent sign of mitochondrial mutations, as in MERRF, MELAS, Kearns-Sayre syndrome, or DAD (deafness and diabetes) syndrome
Nonhereditary congenital malformations of the inner ear				
Thalidomide dysplasia	+	+	(+)	Limb deformities
Rubella embryopathy	+	(+)	+	Cataract, cardiac anomaly, microcephaly
Hyperbilirubinemia (kernicterus)	+	–	+	Athetosis, gaze palsy, tooth enamel dysplasia
Perinatal asphyxia	+	–	+	
Cretinism	+	–	+	Often feeble-mindedness and short stature
Congenital syphilis	+	–	+	
Toxoplasmosis	+	–	+	
Infections				
Viral: herpes zoster oticus, mumps, measles, mononucleosis, HIV, and other neurotropic viruses	+	(+)	+	For herpes zoster oticus (Ramsay Hunt syndrome), see pp. 677 and 824.

(Cont.)→

Table 9.12   (Cont.)

Category	Disease	Hearing loss	Dysequilibrium	Brainstem or other neurologic signs	Remarks
	Bacterial meningitis	+	(–)	(+)	Hearing loss is one of the more common late sequelae, esp. in childhood
	Chronic (basilar) meningitis	+	+	+	For etiologies, cf. Table 2.29
	Intracranial complications of otitis media and malignant otitis	+	+	+	Deafness combined with caudal cranial nerve deficits, usually in diabetics
	Chronic otitis media, cholesteatoma	+	+	–	Only conductive hearing loss at first, later sensorineural hearing loss and dizziness with positive fistula sign, seen on otoscopy
	Syphilis, borreliosis	+	(+)	+	
Polyneuropathies combined with hearing loss	Refsum's disease	+	(–)	+	Polyneuropathy, retinitis pigmentosa, and hearing loss
	Hereditary neuropathy (Charcot-Marie-Tooth)	+	–	+	Connexin-32 gene mutation
Tumors	Acoustic neuroma	+	+	(+)	Cerebellopontine angle syndrome with large neuromas, usually unilateral, but bilateral in neurofibromatosis II

Table 9.**12**   (Cont.)

	Glomus tumor	+	(+)	–	Conductive hearing loss and pulsatile tinnitus at first, later sensorineural hearing loss and vestibular signs with invasion of the labyrinth, visible by otoscopy
	Paraneoplastic	+	(+)	+	E.g., in paraneoplastic cerebellar degeneration
Cerebrovascular disorders	Infarct in the territory of the labyrinthine artery	+	+	–	The labyrinthine artery is usually a branch of AICA, less commonly of the basilar or vertebral artery. It divides into the common cochlear and anterior vestibular arteries.
	Migraine	+	+	+	
Autoimmune disorders	Collagen diseases, Cogan syndrome (983), isolated involvement of the labyrinth	+	+	(+)	Cf. CNS collagen diseases, interstitial keratit's in Cogan syndrome
	Susac syndrome (925)	+	+	+	Cerebral and retinal microangiopathy with hearing loss and multifocal neurologic signs, as in multiple sclerosis
Trauma	Transverse fracture of petrous bone	+	+	+	Tinnitus is typical; other neurologic symptoms, if any, are due to accompanying brain contusion
	Labyrinthine contusion	+	+	–	Commonly bilateral, may progress

(Cont.)→

Table 9.12 (Cont.)

Category	Disease	Hearing loss	Dysequilibrium	Brainstem or other neurologic signs	Remarks
	Acoustic trauma or chronic exposure to noise	+	–	–	Symmetrical; a drop in the audiogram at 4000 Hz is typical
	Barotrauma	+	+	–	Possible rupture of the round or oval window; flying, diving, weightlifting
Toxic/iatrogenic	Industrial toxins, cytostatic agents (bleomycin, vincristine), furosemide, quinine, salicylates, aminoglycosides	+	(+)	(–)	Usually bilateral; if there is a bilateral vestibular deficit, the patient complains of oscillopsia depending on the position of the head – e.g., while walking; the deficits often persist after cessation of the medication that caused them
Specific ear diseases	Ménière's disease	+	+	–	Typically with tinnitus, attacks of vestibulopathy with hearing loss
	Lermoyez syndrome	+	+	–	As in Ménière's disease, but hearing improves during attacks
	Otosclerosis	+	+	–	Bilateral in 75%, conductive hearing loss is most prominent sign, but there may be a mixed conductive and sensorineural hearing loss together with vestibular signs

Table 9.**12** Diseases causing prominent hearing loss

	Acute hearing loss	+	(+)	–	Often accompanied by tinnitus, etiology not known with certainty
	Paget's disease, fibrous dysplasia, osteopetrosis, osteogenesis imperfecta	+	+	(+)	Often only conductive hearing loss at first, later often mixed conductive and sensorineural hearing loss with vestibular signs; in Paget's disease, other cranial nerves may also be affected – e.g., hemifacial spasm, trigeminal neuralgia
	Perilymph fistula	+	+	–	May present with purely vestibular or purely auditory symptoms, positive fistula test in 50%, there may be acoustically evoked dizziness (Tullio phenomenon)
Miscellaneous	Superficial hemosiderosis of the CNS	+	(+)	+	Progressive hearing loss and ataxia, loss of signal from meninges in MRI; rule out recurrent subarachnoid hemorrhage; treat source of bleeding if found

+ Always present
(+) Often present
(–) Rarely present
– Absent

Ancillary Tests in the Diagnostic Evaluation of Hearing Loss

Fine-section CT of the petrous bone. This technique enables visualization of changes in the middle and inner ear and the internal acoustic meatus and is helpful in the diagnosis of malformations, bony erosion, and fistulae accompanying otitis, tumors, fractures, and other primary diseases of bone.

MRI and CT. *MRI*, perhaps with surface coils over the petrous bone instead of the usual head coil, enables visualization of the soft tissues of the middle and inner ear, the cranial nerves, the meninges, the brainstem, and the cerebellum. It reveals tumors and fistulae well. Superficial hemosiderosis of the CNS can be detected in the living patient only with MRI. As a rule of thumb, the imaging study of choice is *CT* for cochlear hearing loss, MRI for retrocochlear hearing loss.

Lumbar puncture. Lumbar puncture is indicated when there is suspicion of a meningitic process or meningeal spread of neoplasia affecting CN VIII and other cranial nerves.

Molecular genetics. If monogenic hereditary hearing loss is suspected (as an isolated manifestation or as part of a syndrome), a search for one of the known genetic defects can be carried out.

Tinnitus and Other Abnormal Sounds (57, 950)

> **Definition:**
>
> *Tinnitus* is a regular noise heard practically all the time in one or both ears and perceived by the patient as being diffusely localized throughout the head. Patients refer to it variously as ringing, buzzing, humming, hissing, whistling, and so forth. Tinnitus heard only by the patient is subjective tinnitus; if the examiner can hear it as well (usually through the stethoscope), it is *objective tinnitus*. Subjective tinnitus is usually nonpulsatile, while objective tinnitus is usually pulsatile and heard with every heartbeat.

Nonpulsatile Tinnitus

Pathogenesis

Tinnitus may be the result of a disturbance in practically any part of the auditory apparatus – the external auditory canal, the middle or inner ear, the auditory nerve, the central auditory pathway, or the auditory cortex. Cochlear injury is by far the most common cause. Patients with tinnitus usually have impaired hearing as well: audiometry reveals hearing loss in 92%.

Etiology

The same diseases that cause hearing loss (Table 9.**12**) also cause tinnitus. The etiology is often acoustic trauma, presbyacusis, or medication effect rather than a disease state.

| Treatment |

The treatment of tinnitus depends on its etiology. Tinnitus due to cochlear lesions accounts for a large percentage of cases and is, unfortunately, not treatable. Nonetheless, a very disturbing tinnitus can be made more bearable by a *masking noise*, and any associated hearing loss can be treated with a *hearing aid*.

Pulsatile Tinnitus (991a)

Etiology and Clinical Features

Pulsatile tinnitus differs from nonpulsatile tinnitus in both etiology and pathogenesis. It is a vascular noise that either originates in the petrous bone or is loud enough to be conducted through it to the auditory apparatus. Diseases that can cause prominent pulsatile tinnitus are listed in Table 9.13.

Table 9.**13**   Diseases that can cause prominent pulsatile tinnitus

Carotid dissection
Fibromuscular dysplasia
High-lying carotid stenosis due to atheromatous plaque
Arteriovenous malformation
Retromastoid dural fistula
Carotid-cavernous fistula
Glomus tumor (glomus jugulare, glomus tympanicum)
Tumor in or near petrous bone
Infection in or near petrous bone
Intracranial hypertension
Pseudotumor cerebri

Diagnostic Evaluation

The evaluation of pulsatile tinnitus begins with an *MRI scan of the head* and *neurovascular ultrasonography*, followed by *selective cerebral angiography*. If the MRI and ultrasound study are normal, a dural fistula must be especially carefully sought by angiography. If the angiogram is normal, a *lumbar puncture* may provide additional useful information (pressure? inflammation?).

| Treatment |

The treatment is determined by the etiology. It usually consists of an *interventional neuroradiological or neurosurgical procedure*.

Vertigo (52, 131, 133)

Pathophysiology

The *symptoms* of vestibular disturbances are:

- vertigo,
- dysequilibrium,
- gait impairment, and
- falls.

The most important *objective sign* of a vestibular disturbance is *nystagmus*, a rhythmic, rapid, jerky movement of both eyes (almost always in the same direction). Nystagmus can be classified by its intensity and by the circumstances in which it arises. If it arises only on far lateral gaze, it is termed *end-gaze nystagmus;* symmetrical end-gaze nystagmus is a normal finding. It can only be termed *gaze-evoked nystagmus* if it is also present when the bulb is in the binocular visual field. In some patients, nystagmus can only be induced by repeated shaking of the head, or by putting the head in a particular posi-

Table 9.**14**   Differentiation of peripheral and central vestibular disturbances

Test	Peripheral (lesion on the right)	Central
Nystagmus	Rapid component to the left	May be vertical, rotatory, or dissociated (i.e., only detectable in one eye in particular positions); may be accompanied by other brainstem signs
Excitability of labyrinth	Diminished or none on right	Normal
Other	• Romberg test: fall to right • Walking a straight line: deviation to right • Unterberger stepping test: more than 45% turn to right after 40 steps • Arm position test: deviation to right • Bárány pointing test: past-pointing to right	These tests yield variable and often mutually inconsistent findings with respect to laterality and direction (so-called "dysharmonie vestibulaire")

tion (cf. positional nystagmus, p. 695). The various types of nystagmus and their localizing significance are described on p. 643.

The features that distinguish *central* from *peripheral* vestibular disorders are important to know and are summarized in Table 9.**14**.

Various *tests of stance and gait* are useful in the demonstration of vestibular disturbances (and other types of disturbances causing dysequilibrium), particularly the *Unterberger step test* and the *Babinski-Weil walking test*. In the *Bárány pointing test* (see Fig. 9.**31**), the patient extends his arms and points with his index fingers to the examiner's index fingers. He is then asked to close his eyes and advance his index fingers straight forward to touch the examiner's fingers. In the presence of a vestibular lesion,

the patient's fingers deviate to the side of the lesion.

The brain has multiple sources of information that help it to maintain the body's balance and orientation in space (Figs. 9.**27**, 9.**28**): the vestibular apparatus, the visual system, and the proprioceptive system (in which impulses from the peripheral nerves are relayed to the spinal cord and upward to the cerebellum. If one of these systems should cease to function, the body can remain in balance, but if two or all three cease to function, dysequilibrium arises. Patients experience this as unsteady gait, subjective imbalance, and vertigo.

Information from the vestibular, visual, and proprioceptive systems converges in the central nervous system, where it is integrated and determines the motor response that regulates muscle tone and body posture. A major role is played by reciprocal connections between the visual and vestibular systems and by motor control of the eyes and head, which depends on the normal functioning of the cerebellum and cerebral cortex (see also ocular motility, p. 634). If all of the information converging on the CNS is consistent with prior experience, it is processed without reaching the level of consciousness, and the individual remains unaware of it. If, however, information arrives that is inconsistent with prior experience, an unpleasant sensation generally arises, namely, vertigo. (This is an outline of the so-called *mismatch hypothesis*.) If this sensation persists, the individual feels unwell and begins to suffer from other vegetative phenomena such as nausea, diaphoresis, salivation, or vomiting.

Physiologic vertigo. Individual experience has trained the brain of each of us to expect a certain amount of shift in the retinal image of the environment when we take a step forward. If we stand on top of a mountain or skyscraper, the retinal image of the now very distant objects around us shifts much less than we are accustomed to when we move. As a result, we become nervous or dizzy (*height dizziness, acrophobia*). This is one example of normal, physiologic vertigo; another is *motion sickness*, with its variants *carsickness* and *seasickness*, in which unusual movement of the body creates a conflict between visual and vestibular input, and thereby produces vertigo.

Pathological vertigo. Temporary or persistent, functional or structural impairment of the vestibular, visual, or proprioceptive systems or of the central integrative mechanism also causes "mismatch" and, therefore, pathological vertigo. The diagnostic evaluation of vertigo has two purposes: localizing its site of origin and determining its etiology.

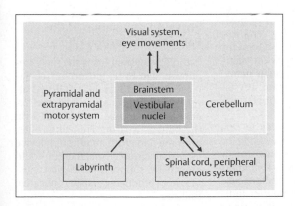

Fig. 9.**28 Maintenance of balance by integration of information from multiple channels.**

Clinical History

The patient's spontaneous description of vertigo is rarely precise enough to yield useful information for diagnosis. Thus, the clinician must know what specific questions to ask to bring the diagnostic process further. The most important points to be clarified are listed in Table 9.**15**.

Historical Clues to Differential Diagnosis

The subjective quality of vertigo may already constitute strong evidence for or against a vestibular disturbance. Directional sensations such as rotation, a "carousel" feeling, lateropulsion, or a feeling of being lifted are more likely to be due to a vestibular lesion than such sensations as reeling, staggering, dazedness, quasidrunkenness, lightheadedness, darkness before one's eyes, or a feeling of emptiness.

The duration of vertigo may point to a particular group of possible etiologies. An attack duration of a few seconds is typical for all forms of positional vertigo, minutes for vertebrobasilar TIA or migraine, hours for Ménière's disease, and days for vestibulopathies such as vestibular neuritis or labyrinthine infarction. Persistent vertigo is rarely of vestibular origin.

Positional vertigo occurs only in certain positions of the head or body, or only during certain changes of position. Concomitant *auditory symptoms* indicate a peripheral vestibular etiology, while *visual abnormalities* indicate cortical pathology (in the case of diminished visual acuity or a field defect) or a brainstem process (in the case of diplopia).

Accompanying *vegetative disturbances* point to a peripheral vestibular origin for vertigo, as such disturbances are generally only mild in central vestibular or nonvestibular vertigo.

Gait unsteadiness due to polyneuropathy or posterior column disease may be perceived by the patient as vertigo. This symptom worsens when the eyes are closed or in the dark, just as in the rarer case of a bilateral vestibular deficit. Characteristic of the latter is a perception of the environment as being in motion – dancing or sliding away (*oscillopsia*, cf. p. 646).

Psychogenic vertigo, of which the most common type is phobic postural vertigo, should be suspected in patients with obsessive-compulsive or hysterical personality traits combined with anxiety or *phobias* (agoraphobia, fear of falling, fear of death), and in patients complaining of *situation-dependent vertiginous attacks* (e.g., only on bridges or on staircases, while driving on the highway, etc.).

Physical Examination of the Patient with Vertigo (298e)

Pathologic nystagmus is the most important sign to be looked for (cf. Tables 9.**5** and 9.**13**, and Fig. 9.**16**). As already mentioned on p. 643, the examination must be carried out with the patient wearing Frenzel goggles, or in the dark with an infrared device for visualization. Visual fixation could otherwise suppress vestibular nystagmus, producing falsely negative findings.

Spontaneous vestibular nystagmus. This is characterized by a horizontal beat with a small torsional compo-

Table 9.**15** Questions for history-taking in a patient complaining of dizziness

Circumstances in which dizziness first arose?
Quality of dizziness?
Episodic or continuous?
Single or multiple episodes?
Duration of episode (seconds, minutes, hours, days)?
In what bodily position(s) is dizziness worst?
Do particular changes of position induce dizziness (bending forward, lying down, turning in bed, looking up or down)?
Auditory symptoms such as tinnitus, hearing loss, ear pain or pressure?
Visual symptoms (blurring, diplopia, phosphenes)?
Oscillopsia, spontaneous or induced by particular head positions?
Effect of darkness or closing eyes on dizziness?
Autonomic symptoms (nausea, vomiting, diaphoresis)?
Situational dizziness (in a department store, in a crowd, on a staircase)?
Neurologic symptoms, such as dysphagia, dysarthria, sensory disturbances on the face or body, or weakness of the face, arm, or leg?
History of migraine?
Medications?

nent (see Fig. 9.**16**). It is provoked by gaze in the direction of the beat. It can be graded in terms of severity (Alexander grades I, II, and III). An attempt should also be made to pro-voke vestibular nystagmus by maneuvers such as shaking the head; any nystagmus produced in this way is abnormal and should be considered a form of perhaps very mild spontaneous vestibular nystagmus. Finally, the examiner should look for other forms of nystagmus, such as *gaze-evoked, upbeat, downbeat, purely horizontal,* or *diagonal nystagmus,* and note whether the beat is conjugate or dissociated.

Positional nystagmus. Nystagmus may arise only *when the head is in certain positions;* as a typical example, when the head is positioned with the right ear down, there may be a nonfatigable, left-beating nystagmus. Note the rule of thumb that positional nystagmus of this type beats toward the higher ear, or, in equivalent terms, away from the ground – it is "ageotropic."

Positioning nystagmus. On the other hand, nystagmus may be present only transiently after a *shift of position* (cf. the above discussion of positional vertigo, p. 694). Nystagmus of this type must be sought with the Hallpike maneuver, illustrated in Fig. 9.**29**. The patient is shifted from the sitting position to the supine position with the head 30° downward and to the left or right. Nystagmus typically appears after a latency of a few seconds, increases in intensity over a few seconds, then diminishes and disappears. The patient simultaneously experiences intense rotatory vertigo, perhaps accompanied by nausea. The nystagmus is mainly rotatory, clockwise when the head is down and to the left and counterclockwise when the head is down and to the right. If the patient looks toward the floor, the nystagmus becomes purely rotatory; if the patient looks at his own nose (away from the floor), it beats upward. This type of positioning nystagmus generally fatigues rapidly and can often be elicited only if the patient is allowed to rest for a while before the test is performed.

Further Tests

- The normal suppression of vestibular nystagmus by visual fixation can be checked with the *nystagmus suppression test* (p. 643; see Fig. 9.**15**).
- *Elicitation of vestibular nystagmus.* Vestibular nystagmus is normally symmetrically elicitable and visible to the examiner when the patient,

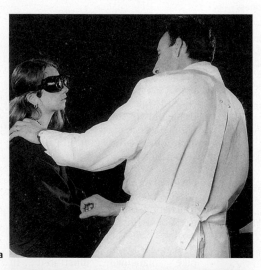

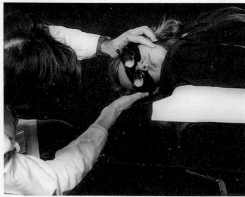

Fig. 9.**29a–e   Positioning vertigo and nystagmus.** The patient, wearing Frenzel goggles, is rapidly moved from the sitting position (**a**) to the supine position with the head hanging down and to the right (**b**) or left (**c**). Positioning vertigo manifests itself in counterclockwise rotating nystagmus when the head is down and to the right (**d**), clockwise rotating nystagmus when the head is down and to the left (**e**). The nystagmus may beat vertically if the subject looks away from the floor. The intensity of nystagmus and vertigo first increases and then decreases within a few seconds.

wearing Frenzel goggles, is rotated back and forth on a swivel chair. This test is not very sensitive, but any asymmetry or absence of nystagmus indicates uni- or bilateral vestibular pathology.

- *Caloric vestibular testing* provides a more sensitive indication of a vestibular deficit. The patient lies with the body and head rotated 30° from the supine position, or else sits upright with the head tilted back 60°. If the left ear canal is then irrigated with 100–200 mL of water at room temperature, or 5–10 mL of ice water, horizontal nystagmus normally appears, beating to the right. The patient points to the left on the Bárány pointing test (see below) and tends to fall to the left. Vertigo and nausea are simultaneously induced. Irrigation with warm water (44 °C) produces the opposite effects. Absence of these reactions indicates that the labyrinth is unexcitable or that its connection to the brainstem is interrupted. Tympanic perforation should always

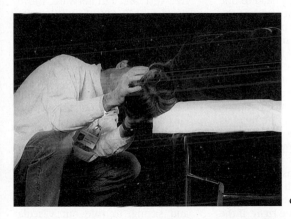

Fig. 9.**29c–e**

c

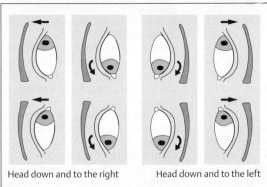

Head down and to the right   Head down and to the left

d, e

be ruled out by otoscopy before caloric testing is performed.

- *Electronystagmography* allows standardized evaluation of differences between the caloric responses of the right and left ears. It is even more informative when combined with the use of a computer-controlled swivel chair.

- The *head thrust maneuver* (Halmagyi-Curthoys test) (376a) is used to test the oculovestibular reflex in the horizontal plane and is thus a test of the horizontal semicircular canal. The examiner rapidly turns the patient's head to one side while the patient looks at the examiner's nose. The patient's eyes should remain fixed on the examiner's nose the entire time, including while the head is turning, because the oculovestibular reflex is very fast (p. 653). If the labyrinth is partially or totally dysfunctional, the eyes go along with the head as it is rotated, and, as soon as the head comes to a stop, a saccade brings the eyes back into fixation on the examiner's nose (Fig. 9.**30**). If the *right* labyrinth is dysfunctional, the saccade is to the left after a head thrust to the *right*; if the *left* labyrinth is dysfunctional, the saccade is to the right after a head thrust to the *left*.

- *Walking with the eyes closed* in the presence of a vestibular deficit results in the appearance (or worsening) of gait unsteadiness or a constant deviation to one side. The patient is asked to walk toward the examiner from a distance of 5 m. This test is performed three times in succession. If there is an asymmetry of vestibular tone, the patient's gait will consistently deviate to one side. Care should be taken to eliminate brightness cues that the patient might see even with the eyes closed (e.g., the examiner should not stand in front of the window on a sunny day).

- *Positional and pointing tests* (Fig. 9.**31**) and *Unterberger's stepping test* can also reveal deviation to one side. In the Unterberger test, the patient walks in place for 1–3 minutes. Rotation or change of position is no more than slight in the normal situation, but marked if there is an asymmetry of vestibular tone. Threshold values for a positive test are 1 m forward movement and 40–60° of rotation after 50 steps.

- The *Babinski-Weil walking test* is analogous to the above. The patient closes his eyes and walks repeatedly two steps forward and two steps backward; any rotation or linear displacement implies a vestibular deficit.

- *Otoscopy* and a *complete neurological and general physical examination* complete the work-up. The examiner should remember to measure the blood pressure in both arms, and with the patient lying and sitting, to rule out vascular presyncope due to orthostatic hypotension or subclavian steal syndrome (p. 554).

- Patients with oscillopsia depending on head position or whose vertigo worsens in the dark should undergo caloric vestibular testing, as described above.

- A *fistula test* should be performed whenever a *perilymph fistula* is suspected, as well as routinely in chronic otitis. Digital pressure on the tragus suffices, in some cases, to provoke the symptoms; in other cases, a pressure wave of graded in-

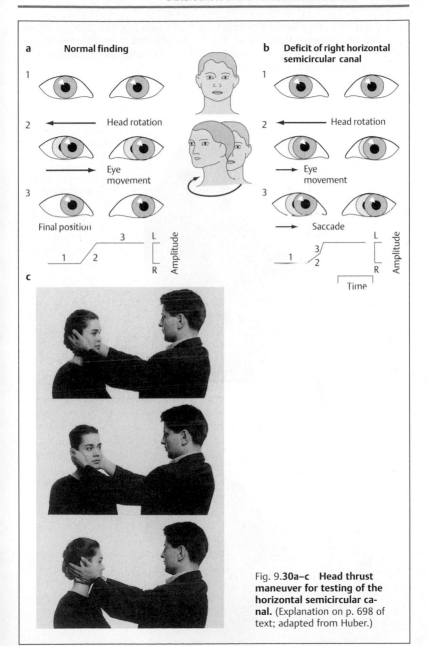

a Normal finding

1

2 ← Head rotation

→ Eye movement

3

Final position

1 2 3 L R Amplitude

b Deficit of right horizontal semicircular canal

1

2 ← Head rotation

→ Eye movement

3 → Saccade

1 3 2 L R Amplitude

Time

c

Fig. 9.**30a–c Head thrust maneuver for testing of the horizontal semicircular canal.** (Explanation on p. 698 of text; adapted from Huber.)

tensity can be created in the external ear canal by stepwise inflation of a *Politzer balloon.* A positive test is associated with the appearance of *Hen-* *nebert's sign* (vertigo and nystagmus to the affected side). This test detects fistulae of the lateral semicircular canal (912).

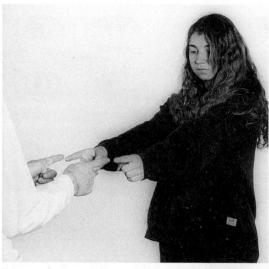

Fig. 9.**31a, b   Modified Bárány pointing test.**
a The patient points with her extended index fingers to the examiner's index fingers.
b The patient closes her eyes. Deviation to one side or the other indicates asymmetry of vestibular tone.

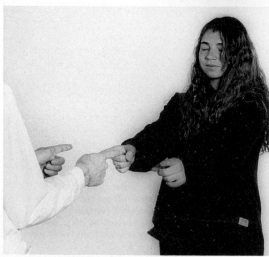

Differential Diagnosis

A complete history and physical examination usually enables the differentiation of vestibular from nonvestibular vertigo, and the classification of vestibular vertigo as central or peripheral. Details are given in Table 9.16.

Ancillary Tests

Electronystagmography is useful for the objective documentation of oculomotor disturbances of vestibular origin. It enables the quantitative assessment of abnormal findings but nonetheless does not obviate the need for clinical examination. In par-

Table 9.16 Differentiation of peripheral vestibular, central vestibular, and nonvestibular vertigo

Symptoms and signs	Type of vertigo		
	Peripheral vestibular (labyrinth, nerve)	Central vestibular	Nonvestibular
Nausea, vomiting, diaphoresis	Marked	Mild	Mild
Intensity of vertigo	Marked	Mild	Mild
Quality of vertigo	Directional	Moderately directional	Nondirectional
Nystagmus	Spontaneous vestibular nystagmus to opposite side	Spontaneous vestibular nystagmus	Nonvestibular nystagmus or no nystagmus
Hearing loss, tinnitus	Usually present	Usually absent	None
Romberg test, straight-line walk, Unterberger stepping test, Bárány pointing test	Deviation to affected side	Deviation, not always consistently in one direction, not always to affected side	No directional deviation
Head thrust test (Halmagyi test)	Returning saccade after head thrust to affected side	Returning saccade often evident	Normal
Caloric excitability	Diminished on the affected side	Usually normal	Normal
Effect of darkness or eye closure on vertigo or gait unsteadiness	Usually no effect; worsening in bilateral labyrinthine lesions	Usually no effect	Worsening if proprioception is impaired
Other neurologic deficits	Unusual	Usually present	The neurological examination may be normal or abnormal

ticular, positioning nystagmus is more readily detected clinically than by electronystagmography. Other ancillary tests are of analogous usefulness in vestibular as in auditory dysfunction – for *imaging studies* and *lumbar puncture,* see above (p. 77).

Treatment of Vertigo

Vertigo is treated according to its etiology, as discussed below.

> **Treatment**
>
> Nonspecific vertigo, particularly in the elderly, may be relieved to some extent by *cinnarizine, calcium antagonists* such as flunarizine, or *co-dergocrine. Physical therapy* and *ball games* may also be useful means of vestibular training.

Diseases Causing Prominent Vertigo

Acute Vestibular Dysfunction

Commonly used synonyms for the syndrome of acute vestibular dysfunction are "vestibular neuritis," "acute vestibulopathy," and "labyrinthitis" or (if hearing is also affected) "cochleolabyrinthitis."

Pathogenesis

The same clinical syndrome is produced by any acute, unilateral vestibular disturbance, be it of vascular, infectious, or neoplastic origin. A small number of autopsy studies support the hypothesis that the cause is usually infectious. Further evidence comes from the epidemic appearance of this syndrome and from the fact that it mainly affects middle-aged adults without significant vascular risk factors. Neurophysiological investigation reveals an asymmetry of vestibular tone, in which the vestibular neurons on one side fail to discharge spontaneously.

Clinical Features

Typical features include:
- acute rotatory vertigo,
- a tendency to fall to the side of the affected ear,
- vegetative symptoms (nausea, vomiting, diaphoresis).

Movement of the head worsens the symptoms to such a degree that patients initially cannot get out of bed. Abnormal auditory sensations or hearing loss are exceptional (unlike in Ménière's disease). Examination reveals horizontal spontaneous nystagmus with a rotatory component, rightward and counterclockwise or leftward and clockwise (see Fig. 9.**16**). The nystagmus beats away from the side of the lesion and can be suppressed by visual fixation or enhanced by lying with the affected ear down. Ocular pursuit movements and saccades are normal. The caloric response is diminished or absent on the affected side.

Course and Prognosis

The initial vertigo subsides within a few days. The patient can often get out of bed on the first day, within a few days at most. At this point, grade I or II nystagmus and deviation can still be found on positional testing, with the Unterberger test, and when the patient walks with eyes closed, but the patient is less nauseated and has stopped vomiting. A few days later, all that remains of the initial symptoms is a mild unsteadiness of stance and gait, particularly when the head is suddenly moved. At this point, nystagmus can usually be elicited by head shaking. All clinical symptoms resolve 1–6 weeks after their onset. Most patients experience vestibular neuritis only once, but single or multiple recurrences in the ensuing years are not unusual. The resolution of symptoms may be due either to recovery of the temporarily affected vestibular organ, or to central compensation for a permanent peripheral deficit.

Ancillary Tests

No further testing is required if the symptoms are sufficiently characteristic, but may be indicated if atypical features are found in the clinical history or physical examination, or if the symptoms persist.

Differential Diagnosis

Acute vestibular dysfunction has various causes.

Ménière's disease causes attacks that last for hours and are accompanied by hearing loss and tinnitus. Circulatory disturbances may cause transient or permanent *ischemia* of the labyrinth, brainstem, or cerebellum (p. 172).

A *cerebellar hemispheric infarct* is usually accompanied by clinically evident ataxia on the side of the lesion (which is not found in a vestibular deficit). Likewise, *brainstem infarcts* produce vestibular as well as other neurologic deficits.

Tumors (acoustic neuroma, meningioma, glomus tumor, etc., p. 68) usually cause slowly progressive vertigo.

Trauma is usually evident from the clinical history (e.g., petrous fracture). Isolated acute attacks of vertigo can occur in *migraine* (p. 805).

Otitis media, whose clinical hallmark is conductive hearing loss, may ex-

tend to other pneumatized portions of the petrous bone (otomastoiditis) and secondarily cause vestibular dysfunction. A mixed vestibulocochlear deficit is usually found in such cases. In *malignant otitis,* the infection spreads into the subarachnoid space and affects other cranial nerves as well.

Specific infections, such as mumps and measles, can cause both vestibular and auditory deficits, and syphilis, borreliosis, and tuberculosis usually affect other cranial nerves as well. Herpes zoster oticus usually causes facial nerve palsy and vesicles on the palatal arch and external auditory canal (Ramsay Hunt syndrome, pp. 677 and 824).

Cogan syndrome is characterized by the combination of interstitial keratitis with sudden hearing loss and vestibular dysfunction (983). While the keratitis heals relatively quickly, the auditory and vestibular deficits persist. The disease usually affects the labyrinth on both sides and is typically accompanied by aortitis. An autoimmune pathogenesis is presumed.

Treatment

Antivertiginous and antiemetic medications are given in the acute phase, among them antihistamines (e.g., promethazine), phenothiazines (e.g., thiethylperazine), benzodiazepines, and neuroleptics such as dihydrobenzperidol or scopolamine.

These medications may need to be given intramuscularly, intravenously, or per rectum, rather than orally. Once the patient has stopped vomiting, the medications should be discontinued as soon as possible, so that the vestibular compensation will not be delayed or prevented.

If the patient can tolerate them, *ocular fixation exercises* should be performed, as well as head turning and *static* and *dynamic equilibrium exercises*. Ball games are a form of dynamic equilibrium exercise.

The underlying cause should be treated, as far as possible.

Ménière's Disease

Tinnitus, hearing loss, and vertigo typify this disease, which most commonly affects men and women between the ages of 30 and 60.

Pathogenesis

Ménière's disease is due to *endolymphatic hydrops*. The membranes separating endolymph from perilymph rupture at irregular intervals, causing an abrupt rise in the potassium concentration of the endolymph, which, in turn, impairs neuronal function until the physiologic concentration is restored. Endolymphatic hydrops may be idiopathic or a late complication of a labyrinthine disease of some kind, such as Mondini's inner ear dysplasia, viral, bacterial, or spirochetal infection, or petrous fractures. An autoimmune mechanism has also been postulated.

Clinical Features

A typical attack consists of:
- a sensation of pressure and fullness in the ear,
- hearing loss,
- tinnitus, and
- severe rotatory vertigo.

In most patients, the pressure sensation, hearing loss, and tinnitus precede the vertigo in the manner of an aura, but are nonetheless most severe during the attack itself. The hearing loss at first mainly involves the high-frequency range, but can spread to the entire frequency spectrum after repeated attacks. Vertigo is usually so severe that the patient cannot stand up or walk, and it is accompanied by nausea, vomiting, and diaphoresis. Other clinical features are those of acute vestibular dysfunction, as described above. Attacks resolve within a few hours, though the patient may remain mildly vertiginous and feel mildly unwell for several days thereafter.

Lermoyez syndrome. In this variant of Ménière's disease, hearing improves during the attacks of vertigo, but the pathogenesis, clinical features, and treatment are otherwise typical.

Course and Prognosis

There are, at first, no symptoms in between attacks. The attacks repeat every few weeks or months. Once a few of them have occurred, most patients develop tinnitus and slowly progressive hearing loss, at first for low frequencies, and then for higher frequencies as well. Labyrinthine atrophy is the presumed cause. In some patients, the hearing loss progresses to complete deafness, and vestibular function can be lost as well. Bilateral disease is not uncommon (133) and is seen in 15% of cases after 2 years, and in 30–60% after 10–20 years. Nonetheless, the course is generally benign, in that 80% of cases remit spontaneously in 5–10 years.

Diagnosis

The diagnosis of Ménière's disease is based on the clinical triad described above. The administration of hyperosmolar substances, such as glycerin and urea, may transiently improve hearing, which supports the diagnosis. There is no other specific test for the disease.

Treatment

The acute attacks are self-limited. As in the syndrome of acute vestibular dysfunction, they can be treated symptomatically with *antivertiginous* and *antiemetic agents*. The goal of interval therapy is a reduction in the frequency of the attacks, so that hearing can be preserved. *Betahistine* has been shown to be effective for this purpose (667).

Some patients benefit from a *low-sodium diet* (1–2 g/day for at least 2 months, longer if effective).

Surgical treatment may be indicated in carefully selected, medically intractable cases, though it should be borne in mind that the disease is often self-limiting, and also that it may later affect the other side in 30–60% of cases. *Selective vestibular neurectomy* can be performed in patients with preserved hearing, *labyrinthectomy* in those that are already deaf in the affected ear.

Pharmacologic destruction of the vestibular apparatus is a less invasive treatment that can be of benefit in some cases. Vestibulotoxic aminoglycosides such as streptomycin or gentamicin are used.

Transverse Fracture of the Petrous Bone

These fractures cause acute, complete vestibular dysfunction with rotatory vertigo, vomiting, inability to stand, deafness with or without tinnitus, facial nerve palsy, and, in about half of all patients, otorhinoliquorrhea. Otoscopy reveals a dark discoloration of the eardrum due to an accumulation of blood behind it. There is marked spontaneous vestibular nystagmus, and the traumatized ear is deaf. The Weber test is lateralized to the opposite side. Antibiotics are often given to prevent labyrinthitis and early and late post-traumatic meningitis.

Perilymph Fistula

This condition arises from a rupture of the oval or round window or through erosion of the bony semicircular canal by an osteolytic process. It may present clinically in a variety of ways, including:
- purely vestibular vertigo,
- purely cochlear hearing loss,
- tinnitus,
- or a combination of the above.

Vertigo is the most common symptom, generally in the form of episodic rotatory or positional vertigo. The diagnosis is based on the clinical history, or, less commonly, on the detection of an osteolytic process (such as chronic otitis with cholesteatoma).

Particular entities to be borne in mind during history-taking include head trauma, barotrauma (flying, diving), Valsalva maneuvers (e.g., during coughing, blowing the nose, or weight-lifting), or surgical procedures on the stapes. The fistula test is usually positive (p. 698).

Tullio's phenomenon is also demonstrable in many cases: loud acoustic stimuli (90 dB or above) induce vestibular manifestations such as vertigo, nystagmus, oscillopsia, and vestibulospinal dysfunction. Most fistulae heal spontaneously with bedrest with slight elevation of the head, but a few require surgical repair.

Bilateral Vestibular Dysfunction (55)

The typical symptoms of bilateral vestibular dysfunction are:
- gait unsteadiness that worsens when the eyes are closed, on uneven ground, or in the dark; and
- oscillopsia depending on head position (e.g., bobbing of the horizon when the patient walks).

On clinical examination, the head thrust test is abnormal bilaterally, and caloric testing reveals diminished or absent excitability of the vestibular apparatus bilaterally.

Bilateral vestibular dysfunction can arise either with or without hearing loss. It can be caused by any disease or condition that affects both labyrinths or both vestibular nerves simultaneously, including:
- ototoxic medications (streptomycin, gentamicin),
- bilateral Ménière's disease,
- residual deficits after meningitis or labyrinthitis,
- bilateral (sequential) vestibular neuritis,
- autoimmune and idiopathic vestibular neuropathy,
- neurofibromatosis II.

> **Treatment**
>
> *Physiotherapeutic exercises* are performed to train head movement in all three dimensions. Such exercises promote the strengthening of nonvestibular – i.e., oculocephalic and proprioceptive compensatory mechanisms, with resulting improvement of stance and gait.

Positional and Positioning Vertigo

The terms "positional vertigo" and "positioning vertigo" refer to any type of vertigo that arises only when the head is in a certain position, or only with certain movements of the head. Positional and positioning vertigo have diverse causes.

The most common type of positioning vertigo – indeed, of vertigo in general – is *benign paroxysmal positioning vertigo*, or BPPV (see below).

Central positional nystagmus typically arises as soon as the head is positioned to lie on one side, does not fatigue, and beats toward the upper ear – i.e., to the left ear when the patient is lying on the right side, and vice versa. (Other types of beat may also be encountered.) There is often little or no accompanying vertigo. The lesion is always in the brainstem or vestibulocerebellum and may be of any type. *Downbeat nystagmus,* too, may be worst with certain positions of the head, typically when the patient is supine and the head hangs down (p. 651).

Another type of central positional nystagmus arises only with certain movements of the head and is characterized by rotatory vertigo with nystagmus, truncal ataxia, and usually the inability to walk. The lesion is most commonly in the roof of the fourth ventricle, generally a tumor or hemorrhage of the fourth ventricle or vermis.

In the healing phase of acute vestibulopathy, too, vertigo may be present only when the labyrinth is stressed – i.e., only with certain head movements.

Benign Paroxysmal Positioning Vertigo (BPPV) (Cupulolithiasis, Canalolithiasis) (237, 856)

This disorder consists of transient, severe vertigo induced by changes in the position of the head. It affects persons of any age, women somewhat more commonly than men.

Pathogenesis

For anatomic reasons, detritus, such as particles shed by the otolith membrane, tends to land in the posterior semicircular canal. It may be caught on the cupula (cupulolithiasis) or float freely in the endolymph (canalolithiasis). Excessive loading of the cupula in the first case, or the increase in the overall specific gravity of the endolymph in the second case (which is much more common), leads to an excessive post-rotatory response when the head is turned in the plane of the posterior semicircular canal of the affected ear.

Etiology

Paroxysmal positioning vertigo may be a sequela of head trauma, viral neurolabyrinthitis, or, in rarer cases, other processes affecting the labyrinth. In most cases, however, no specific etiology or precipitating event can be identified.

Clinical Features

Vertigo typically arises when the patient turns in bed, lies down, sits up, stands up, bends over, or looks upward. Attacks of vertigo often occur when the patient attempts to pick an object up off the floor or from a high or low shelf. Severe rotational vertigo mostly lasts no more than a few seconds, never more than a minute, though the accompanying vegetative phenomena, such as queasiness, may last longer. Patients are often so distressed by the first attack that they seek medical help immediately. On examination, the *Hallpike maneuver* (best performed with Frenzel goggles) produces a *mainly rotatory nystagmus* that is counterclockwise when the head hangs downward and to the right, clockwise when it hangs downward and to the left (cf. Fig. 9.**29**). If the patient looks away from the floor (i.e., toward his own nose), the nystagmus may beat purely vertically. When the patient sits up again, nystagmus occurs in the downbeating direction. Both on lying down and on sitting up, it occurs with a latency of one or more seconds, rapidly reaches peak intensity, then declines and disappears over a further 10–40 seconds. Vertigo takes a parallel time course. The nystagmus and vertigo are more severe when the patient is positioned on the side of the affected labyrinth. They become less pronounced on repeated testing (habituation), eventually becoming unelicitable unless the patient is given a brief rest between tests.

Diagnostic Evaluation

The diagnosis is based solely on the clinical history and physical examination. Ignorance of this condition among physicians sometimes leads to the performance of unnecessary CT and MRI scans, Doppler ultrasonography, and various cardiologic studies.

Differential Diagnosis

Positional and positioning vertigo, as we have seen, may also be a sign of *perilymph fistula* or *Ménière's disease,* as well as of *labyrinthine atelectasis* or a *central lesion*. Precise observation of the clinical manifestations generally enables a clear-cut differentiation of BPPV from other causes of positional and positioning vertigo. Neurovascular compression syndromes have also been reported to cause "disabling positional vertigo," but this entity is, in our opinion, poorly definable at best.

Specific positioning maneuvers (the Semont and Epley maneuvers) can be used to flush the detritus out of the posterior semicircular canal and relieve vertigo immediately (132, 282a). The patient himself can also bring about relief, though not immediately, by repeatedly putting himself in the position that induces vertigo (*Brandt-Daroff maneuver*). Patients initially disinclined to use the last-named method can be persuaded of its usefulness by a test-run in the doctor's office. In our experience, the Epley maneuver is the best of the three, with a success rate above 90% (Fig. 9.**32**).

Canalolithiasis of the horizontal semicircular canal. This entity is analogous to the more common disorder just described, which affects the posterior semicircular canal (54, 572). It is characterized by positioning vertigo and horizontal nystagmus that arise when the patient turns from the supine to the lateral decubitus position.

Canalolithiasis of the anterior semicircular canal is even rarer than that of the horizontal semicircular canal. The anterior canal lies in the same plane as the contralateral posterior canal. The symptoms of anterior canalolithiasis therefore resemble those of the more common posterior canalolithia-

sis. If the left side is involved (for example), vertigo is induced when the patient lies down with the head turned to the right. The nystagmus is down-beating and torsional, and then beats upwards when the patient sits up again. This type of canalolithiasis, like the other types, can be treated with specific positioning maneuvers.

Central Vertigo

Central (vestibular or nonvestibular) vertigo is usually accompanied by some form of oculomotor disturbance, as mentioned on p. 630. The findings in such patients include strabismus, diplopia, central nystagmus, impairment of head-eye coordination and the oculovestibular reflex, oscillopsia, ataxia, and other brainstem and cerebellar signs.

Vertebrobasilar insufficiency can produce shorter or longer attacks of either peripheral or central vertigo (p. 198).

Vestibular epilepsy, a rare central cause of vertigo, is due to a temporal or parietal lesion (490). Focal discharges in the posterior portion of the superior temporal gyrus (primary vestibular cortex) or in the intraparietal gyrus (vestibular association cortex) generate vertigo, which can be either a nonspecific feeling or a sensation of turning, leaning, or falling to one side. Nystagmus may be present or absent. These patients usually also suffer from complex partial and grand mal seizures, of which vertigo may be the aura.

Migraine and Vertigo (p. 804)

Vertigo may be the expression of migraine (so-called "vestibular migraine"). This condition is easy to diagnose when vertigo appears as an aura preceding a typical headache, with or without other accompanying manifestations of basilar migraine.

The diagnosis is much more difficult when the vertigo occurs without headache, as is the case in *benign, recurrent vertigo in adulthood* (675). This disorder, which affects persons suffering from migraine, consists of recurrent attacks of vertigo and dysequilibrium lasting minutes to hours and sometimes accompanied by nausea, spontaneous nystagmus, and positional vertigo, but no other vestibular or neurologic manifestations. The clinical examination is normal in between attacks.

Benign, recurrent vertigo in childhood is another disorder that can be considered to be a migraine equivalent. It affects children between the ages of 1 and 4 years (rarely older). The attacks last seconds to minutes and consist of disabling vertigo and ataxia, nystagmus, nausea, vomiting, sweating, and pallor, without headache, and without impairment of consciousness. In many cases, these attacks are replaced by another form of migraine as the patient grows older.

Treatment

Prophylactic treatment, such as is used to prevent migraine headache, is often beneficial in patients suffering from vertigo as a migraine equivalent, or from recurrent vertigo of indeterminate etiology.

Medications and Vertigo (133)

The list of medications that can cause vertigo is long, and the pathogenetic mechanisms are varied. Medications can induce vertigo by way of cerebellar dysfunction, oculomotor disturbances, positional vertigo and nystagmus, direct effects on the labyrinth, or systemic cardiovascular effects.

Visually Induced Vertigo

Vertigo can be induced by a sudden change of refraction, as after a change of spectacle prescription, or a switch to bifocal lenses or special spectacles after cataract extraction. Vertigo can also be induced by diplopia or extraocular muscle palsies that impair stabilization of the visual image on the retina when the head is moving. A visual field defect can impair visual perception of movement of the body relative to the environment; acute visual field defects can thus cause visual-vestibular "mismatch," and hence vertigo.

Visual hallucinations can also cause vertigo, as can *tilted* and *inverted vision*, types of visual illusion produced by lesions of the occipital lobes and cerebellar hemispheres, probably through a vestibular mechanism.

Cervical Vertigo

Patients with spontaneous or posttraumatic neck pain often complain of nonspecific vertigo (dizziness), perhaps because of abnormal afferent input from cervical levels.

Vertigo Due to Impaired Proprioception

Spinal cord lesions that involve the posterior columns (p. 441) and polyneuropathies (p. 581) may produce vertigo, or simply unsteadiness of stance and gait, as their principal symptom because of impaired proprioception. These problems worsen

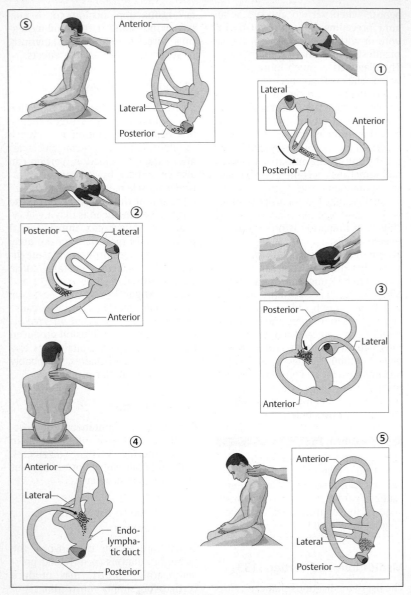

Fig. 9.**32** **The Epley maneuver for the treatment of benign paroxysmal positioning vertigo due to canalolithiasis (shown for a patient whose left posterior semicircular canal is affected).**

when visual input is removed – i.e., in the dark or when the patient's eyes are closed.

Psychogenic and Phobic Postural Vertigo (133)

Vertigo in patients suffering from anxiety, depression, hysteria or psychosis, or in the aftermath of (bodily) trauma, may lack an organic basis or an objective correlate on neuro-otologic examination. Generally, however, at least some organic component can be identified – e.g., a transient post-traumatic otolithic dysfunction that assumes a life of its own as a later, psychogenic development.

Acrophobia and *agoraphobia* are types of psychogenic vertigo. Affected individuals feel unsteady and out of balance, and may suffer panic attacks, when they find themselves on a (possibly very mild) elevation, or in a wide open space or public square.

Phobic postural vertigo is practically always associated with specific situations – e.g., walking across a bridge, driving a car, empty spaces, department stores, restaurants, theaters. These situations induce unsteadiness of stance and gait, without any objective correlate. Any mode of physical support, even a relatively flimsy one such as leaning against a wall or on the armrest of a chair, may suffice to restore a sense of security. Patients

with this condition are usually gripped by a fear of falling and hurting themselves. Such fears may result in full-blown panic attacks, and anticipatory anxiety with regard to such situations can finally result in a conditioned reflex that markedly limit the patient's ability to participate in and enjoy life.

Cardiovascular, Endocrine, Metabolic, and Hematopoietic Diseases Causing Vertigo

Any hemodynamic disturbance that impairs circulation in the brain, or any metabolic disturbance that limits its energy supply, can cause prominent vertigo in the absence of any positive findings on neuro-otologic examination.

Vertigo is a frequent manifestation of *orthostatic hypotension*, generally occurring when the patient rises from a lying or sitting position, or after prolonged standing. This type of vertigo is accompanied by tinnitus, darkness before the eyes, diaphoresis, yawning, and dyspnea.

The other types of vertigo in this class are independent of bodily position. *Cardiac arrhythmia* produces brief dazedness and darkness before the eyes or more severe manifestations up to and including Adams-Stokes attacks with loss of consciousness. In *vasovagal reactions*, vertigo is asso-

◀ Fig. 9.**32**
S The patient sits on the examining table.
1 The patient is rapidly shifted to the supine position with the head hanging 30° downward and 45° to the affected side.
2 The head is rotated to the unaffected side.
3 The head and body together are further rotated to the unaffected side until the body is in the lateral decubitus

position and the head looks toward the floor.
4 The patient sits up by raising the trunk laterally, keeping the head turned to the side.
5 The head is inclined.
Any one of these steps can induce vertigo. There should thus be a pause of 20–30 seconds between steps, or as long as it takes for vertigo to subside.

ciated with hypotonia and bradycardia. Vertigo due to *elevated intrathoracic pressure* – e.g., during coughing – is due to the resulting intracranial hypertension and transient cerebral hypoperfusion (644). Vertigo due to *arterial hypertension* is usually accompanied by headache. Nonspecific vertigo is also a major complaint of many patients with *vegetative dystonia* and *hyperventilation tetany*; such patients also commonly suffer from a fainting tendency, depression, and headaches. Vertigo due to *endocrine disorders* is generally accompanied by fatigue, lethargy, fainting tendency, and hypoglycemia. Finally, *anemia, hyperviscosity syndromes, electrolyte disturbances, vitamin B_{12} deficiency,* and other diseases may also lie behind nonspecific vertigo with negative neuro-otologic findings.

▌ Glossopharyngeal and Vagus Nerve Dysfunction

Anatomy and Examining Techniques
The reader is assumed to be familiar with the anatomy and examining techniques of CN IX and X.

Clinical Features
Lesions of the ninth and tenth cranial nerves cause dysphagia and hoarseness. Examination reveals a sensory deficit on the palatal arch and posterior pharyngeal wall of the affected side, unilateral vocal fold paresis (visible by laryngoscopy), and the "curtain sign," in which the response to a gag stimulus consists of a pulling of the palatal arch and posterior pharyngeal wall to the unaffected side (Fig. 9.**33**).

Causes
Nuclear pareses. Dysfunction of the brainstem nuclei of cranial nerves IX and X is seen in syndromes of medullary dysfunction caused by vascular disorders, tumors, encephalitis, or multiple sclerosis.

Nerve trunk lesions. These may arise in isolation or accompanied by deficits of other caudal cranial nerves. *Basilar impression* and *skull base tumors,* including those that arise extracranially and grow inward from the epipharynx, are among the possible causes. An *isolated unilateral deficit of CN IX and X* constitutes a separate disease entity in children and adoles-

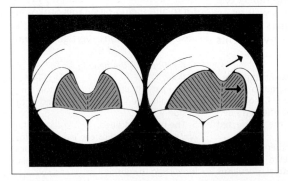

Fig. 9.**33 Curtain sign.** In right glossopharyngeal nerve palsy, elicitation of the gag reflex is followed by pulling of the palate and posterior pharyngeal wall to the unaffected left side.

cents, mainly in boys, and has been interpreted as a type of cranial mononeuropathy. The affected patients suddenly develop nasal speech and mild dysphagia, in the absence of pain or fever, and generally have normal CSF findings, without any elevation in protein concentration. The signs and symptoms regress completely in a few weeks or months in practically all cases. A *basilar skull fracture* involving the jugular foramen may produce deficits of the cranial nerves that traverse it (IX, X, XI) ("syndrome du trou déchiré postérieur," Vernet-Siebenmann syndrome). Similar findings are pro-

duced, on occasion, by herpes zoster (484), cerebral venous sinus thrombosis, or torticollis, or indeed spontaneously, with a good prognosis for recovery. A vascular mechanism presumably underlies such benign and fully reversible deficits. Tapia syndrome (p. 175), involving deficits of CN IX, X, and XII, can also be produced by an (extracranial) *carotid aneurysm,* or by carotid dissection (p. 192).

Differential Diagnosis

These cranial nerve palsies must be distinguished from the *palatal paralysis of diphtheria* and from *pseudoparalytic myasthenia gravis.*

Accessory Nerve Palsy

Anatomy

The reader is assumed to be familiar with the anatomy of the accessory nerve.

Examination Technique (Fig. 9.34).

Clinical Features

The deficit is purely motor. Lesions affecting the nerve in the lateral cervical triangle paralyze only the *superior portion of the trapezius,* producing a shoulder drop, a scapular tilt, and a weak shrug.

More proximal lesions also paralyze the *sternocleidomastoid muscle,* which turns the head to the opposite side.

The most common cause of an isolated accessory nerve palsy is *iatrogenic injury,* often incurred during *biopsy of a lymph node lying at the posterior border of the sternocleidomastoid muscle* (this complication occurs after as many as threequarters of all such procedures!). The mild motor impairment or shoulder

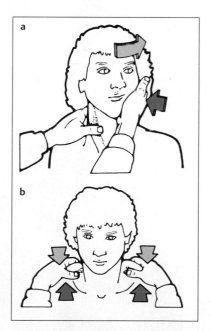

Fig. 9.**34a, b** **Testing the strength of the sternocleidomastoid (a) and trapezius (b) muscles.**

pain on movement are generally not noticed by the patient until a few weeks later, when he or she begins to use the arm again. The findings include a shoulder drop, a scapular tilt, and atrophy of the upper portion of the trapezius, without any sensory deficit and with preserved function of the sternocleidomastoid muscle (Fig. 9.**35**).

Accessory nerve palsy can also be due to anomalies of the craniocervical junction, tumors at the foramen magnum, and the jugular foramen syndrome. It is accompanied by other neurologic findings in such cases.

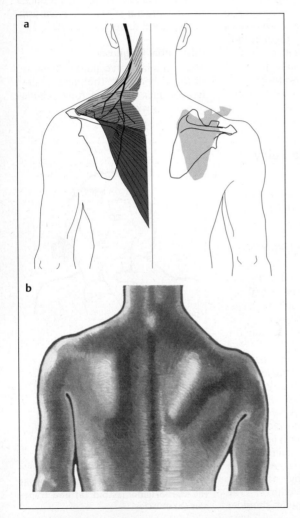

Fig. 9.**35 Right trapezius weakness due to an accessory nerve lesion in the lateral cervical triangle.**

Hypoglossal Nerve Palsy

Anatomy and Examining Technique
The reader is assumed to be familiar with the anatomy and examining technique of CN XII.

Causes of Tongue Weakness

Central tongue weakness. Central tongue weakness is seen, for example, as a component of hemiparesis in acute stroke. As the musculature of the tongue has bilateral cortical representation (176a), central tongue weakness is usually mild and is soon well compensated for by the intact contralateral innervation. *Bilateral* central tongue weakness, however, as in pseudobulbar palsy (p. 384), causes severe dysarthria and dysphagia, and thus considerable functional impairment. The tongue is not atrophic. The buccolingual apraxia and oral diplegia of Foix-Chavany-Marie syndrome were mentioned in an earlier chapter (p. 385).

Nuclear tongue weakness. Nuclear tongue weakness is most commonly a component of *true bulbar palsy* due to amyotrophic lateral sclerosis (p. 434) (cf. Fig. 3.**10**). It is also seen, together with contralateral hemiparesis, after a stroke affecting one side of the medulla (*Jackson syndrome*).

Lesions of the hypoglossal nerve (185a, 503a) (Fig. 9.**36**). These may be due to *basilar skull fractures* involving the occipital bone – e.g., condylar fractures (225b), *basilar impression,* tonsillectomy (241), brainstem or skull base tumors, or *carotid dissection* (527, 919). Reversible, isolated CN XII palsy occasionally occurs after an infection or without identifiable cause (816).

Further causes. *Pain in the tongue* may be due to local causes, such as neoplasia or infection, or to herpes zoster. Intractable *burning of the tongue* occurs in the elderly as a form of glossodynia, without any known cause (p. 826). The paroxysmal pain of *trigeminal neuralgia* may affect one-half of the tongue (which receives its sensory innervation from CN V). Paresthesiae and transient "falling asleep" of one-half of the tongue are found in the so-called *neck-tongue syndrome* (313a). *Painful trophic disturbances of the tongue* can be seen in isolation in giant cell arteritis, or accompanied by other deficits in other types of arteritis, such as Sjögren's syndrome (547a).

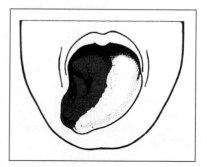

Fig. 9.**36 Unilateral atrophy and weakness of the tongue due to right hypoglossal nerve palsy.**

Multiple Cranial Nerve Palsies

Cranial Polyradiculitis

This type of radiculitis involving the spinal nerve roots and the caudal cranial nerves, particularly the facial nerve, is considered an atypical form of Guillain-Barré syndrome (p. 575). It arises after a long prodrome consisting of headache. It usually resolves without treatment, though recurrences months or years later are not uncommon. Pathologic study of such cases has revealed granulomatous inflammation of the perineural meninges. The pathophysiology of Fisher syndrome (p. 280) is presumably similar.

(Recurrent) Multiple Cranial Nerve Palsies

These have been described in sarcoidosis, Sjögren's syndrome (946a), carotid dissection (527, 919), and paraproteinemia or dysproteinemia (Bing-Neel syndrome), among other conditions. Multiple cranial nerve palsies may be the initial manifestation of vasculitis or polyarteritis nodosa (as a component of Cogan syndrome, p. 325).

Recurrent palsies of multiple cranial nerves often occur without any identifiable cause (95) and are then sometimes designated *Gougerot-Sjögren syndrome* (364). *Brown-Vialetto-Laere syndrome* involves caudal cranial nerve palsies in conjunction with bilateral hearing loss and other neurologic deficits (217).

Progressive Palsies of Multiple Cranial Nerves

These may be due to chronic meningitis, meningeal carcinomatosis, syphilis, or AIDS (963). Bilateral cranial nerve palsies have been reported as a complication of poorly controlled diabetes mellitus. Bone conditions such as Paget's disease and Albers-Schönberg marble bone disease can cause cranial nerve palsies as well. Trichlorethylene poisoning has been reported to cause a trigeminal nerve deficit, accompanied by other cranial nerve deficits (p. 612).

Garcin Syndrome

This syndrome affects the caudal cranial nerves on one side. It is usually due to a tumor of the skull base.

Rarer Causes

Progressive caudal cranial nerve deficits in conjunction with impaired autonomic regulation (the result of a combined lesion of the carotid sinus and sympathetic chain) may be due to a *thorotrastoma*, perhaps not becoming symptomatic till years after carotid angiography with Thorotrast. (This radiographic contrast medium, consisting of thorium dioxide in dextran, has not been used for many years.) Caudal cranial nerve deficits may be due to osteomyelitis of the skull base as a complication of *malignant otitis externa*. Another rare entity, the *stylokeratohyoidal syndrome*, is due to a developmental anomaly and is characterized by deficits of CN V, VII, IX, and X, along with lateral cervical pain, dysphagia, and vertigo.

10   Spinal Radicular Syndromes

Overview:

The spinal nerve roots contain both motor and sensory fibers, and spinal radicular lesions therefore produce both motor and sensory denervation of the structures they innervate. The muscles innervated by the affected root become weak and atrophic. Weakness and atrophy are most evident in muscles that receive most or all of their innervation from the affected root, less so in other muscles, including portions of the paravertebral musculature. The reflexes associated with the paretic muscles are diminished. Sensory denervation produces a dermatomal, usually band-like zone of hypesthesia, which, because of the overlap between neighboring dermatomes, is not always easy to demonstrate.

General Symptoms and Signs

Lesions of individual spinal nerve roots are clinically characterized by some, or all, of the features listed in Table 10.**1**.

- *Pain* in the distribution of the affected root (practically always present in acute lesions).

Table 10.**1**   General manifestations of spinal radicular lesions

Pain:
- Mainly in acute lesions
- Usually with dermatomal radiation

Sensory deficit:
- Not always readily demonstrable (cf. Fig. 2.**3**)
- Monoradicular; test with noxious stimulation
- Look for paravertebral sensory deficit

Paresis:
- Most severe in muscles innervated partly or wholly by affected root (cf. Table 10.**3**)
- Never total plegia

Atrophy:
- Often mild or minimal

Diminished reflexes:
- Affected reflexes are rarely entirely absent (cf. Table 10.**3**)

Fasciculations:
- Only exceptionally seen, in chronic lesions

Spinal signs and symptoms:
- When the cause is acute and spondylogenic

- *Dermatomal sensory deficit* (cf. dermatome chart, Fig. 1.**1**). This may be difficult to demonstrate in monoradicular lesions, because neighboring dermatomes overlap. It is easier to demonstrate with a noxious stimulus than with light touch.
- *Paresis* of muscles innervated by the affected root. Table 10.**2** shows the muscles innervated by each root, and Table 10.**3** shows the muscles receiving most or all of their innervation from a single root.
- *Muscular atrophy* is commonly found, but usually less pronounced than in peripheral nerve lesions, and usually does not become visible till ca. 3 weeks after the lesion arises.
- *Fasciculations* are rarely seen in radicular lesions.
- *Reflexes* subserved by the affected nerve root are diminished. Some of the relevant intrinsic muscle reflexes (proprioceptive reflexes) are listed in Table 10.**4**, some of the relevant extrinsic muscle reflexes (exteroceptive reflexes) in Table 10.**5**.
- *Spinal signs and symptoms* such as pain, abnormal posture, or blocked movement are an expression of the intra- or paraspinal location of the lesion (tumor? herniated disk?).
- *Paravertebral sensory deficits* are observed when the root lesion is located proximal to the exit of the dorsal ramus (i.e., at the intervertebral foramen or proximal to it, as in disk herniation).

Table 10.**2**   Segmental innervation of the muscles of the upper and lower limbs (adapted from R. Bing, *Kompendium der topischen Gehirn- und Rückenmarksdiagnostik*, Basle: Schwabe, 1953).

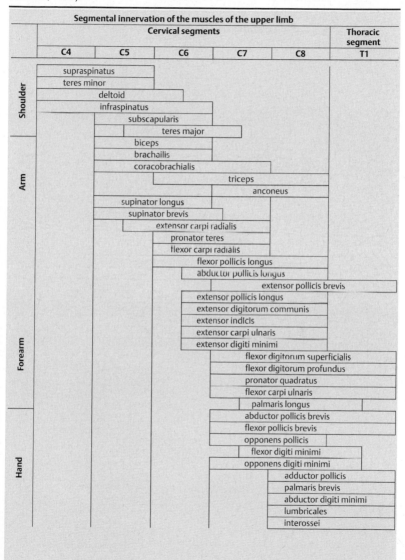

Abbreviations: add. = adductor, artic. = articularis, dig. = digitorum, f. = fasciae,
int. = internus, obt. = obturator.   *(Cont.)* →

Table 10.**2**   *(Cont.)*

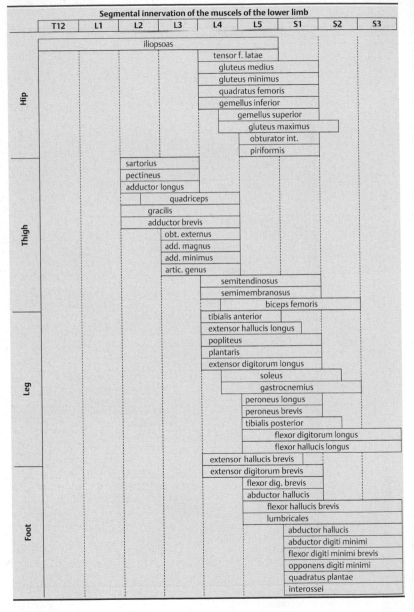

	T12	L1	L2	L3	L4	L5	S1	S2	S3
	Segmental innervation of the muscels of the lower limb								

Hip
- iliopsoas
- tensor f. latae
- gluteus medius
- gluteus minimus
- quadratus femoris
- gemellus inferior
- gemellus superior
- gluteus maximus
- obturator int.
- piriformis

Thigh
- sartorius
- pectineus
- adductor longus
- quadriceps
- gracilis
- adductor brevis
- obt. externus
- add. magnus
- add. minimus
- artic. genus
- semitendinosus
- semimembranosus
- biceps femoris

Leg
- tibialis anterior
- extensor hallucis longus
- popliteus
- plantaris
- extensor digitorum longus
- soleus
- gastrocnemius
- peroneus longus
- peroneus brevis
- tibialis posterior
- flexor digitorum longus
- flexor hallucis longus

Foot
- extensor hallucis brevis
- extensor digitorum brevis
- flexor dig. brevis
- abductor hallucis
- flexor hallucis brevis
- lumbricales
- abductor hallucis
- abductor digiti minimi
- flexor digiti minimi brevis
- opponens digiti minimi
- quadratus plantae
- interossei

Table 10.**3**   Synopsis of radicular syndromes

Seg-ment	Sensory deficit	Motor deficit	Reflex deficit	Remarks
C3/4	Pain and hypalgesia in shoulder region	Diaphragmatic paresis or plegia	None detectable	Partial diaphragmatic paresis is more ventral in C3 lesions, more dorsal in C4 lesions
C5	Pain and hypalgesia on lateral aspect of shoulder, in area covering deltoid muscle	Deltoid and biceps paresis	Diminished biceps reflex	
C6	Radial side of arm and forearm down to thumb	Biceps and brachioradialis paresis	Diminished or absent biceps reflex	
C7	Dorsolateral to C6 dermatome down to 2nd, 3rd, and 4th fingers	Triceps, pronator teres, and (occasionally) finger flexor paresis; thenar eminence often visibly atrophic	Diminished or absent triceps reflex	Triceps reflex key to differential diagnosis vs. carpal tunnel syndrome
C8	Dorsal to C7 dermatome, down to little finger	Intrinsic hand muscles visibly atrophic, particularly on hypothenar eminence	Diminished triceps reflex	Triceps reflex key to differential diagnosis vs. ulnar nerve palsy
L3	From greater trochanter crossing over the anterior aspect to the medial aspect of the thigh and knee	Quadriceps paresis	Weakness of quadriceps (knee-jerk) reflex	Differential diagnosis vs. femoral nerve palsy: sensation intact in distribution of saphenous nerve

(Cont.) →

Table 10.**3**   *(Cont.)*

Seg-ment	Sensory deficit	Motor deficit	Reflex deficit	Remarks
L4	From lateral thigh across patella to upper inner quadrant of calf and down to medial edge of foot	Quadriceps and tibialis anterior paresis	Weakness of quadriceps (knee-jerk) reflex	Differential diagnosis vs. femoral nerve palsy: involvement of tibialis anterior
L5	From lateral condyle above knee across the upper outer quadrant of the calf to the great toe	Paresis and atrophy of extensor hallucis longus, often also of extensor digitorum brevis; paresis of tibialis posterior and of hip abduction	Absent tibialis posterior reflex (of diagnostic value only when clearly elicitable on opposite, unaffected side)	Differential diagnosis vs. peroneal nerve palsy: in the latter, tibialis posterior and hip abduction are preserved
S1	From posterior thigh over posterior upper quadrant of calf and lateral malleolus to little toe	Paresis of the peronei, often also of the gastrocnemius and soleus	Absent gastrocnemius reflex (ankle-jerk or Achilles reflex)	
Combined L4, L5	Combination of L4 and L5 dermatomes	Paresis of all plantar flexors and of quadriceps	Diminished quadriceps reflex, absent tibialis posterior reflex	Differential diagnosis vs. peroneal nerve palsy: peronei spared. Note status of reflexes.
Combined L5, S1	Combination of L5 and S1 dermatomes	Paresis of toe extensors, peronei, occasionally also gastrocnemius and soleus	Absent tibialis posterior and gastrocnemius reflexes	Differential diagnosis vs. peroneal nerve palsy: tibialis anterior spared. Note status of reflexes

Table 10.4 The most important normal intrinsic muscle reflexes (proprioceptive reflexes)

Name of reflex	Stimulus	Response	Muscle(s)	Peripheral nerve	Segment(s)
Masseteric reflex (jaw jerk reflex)	Tapping on chin or an instrument laid on the lower row of teeth, with patient's mouth slightly open	Brief contraction of masseter, partially closing mouth	Masseter	Trigeminal nerve	CN V
Trapezius reflex	Tapping on lateral portion of trapezius at coracoid process	Shoulder elevation	Trapezius	Accessory nerve	CN XI, C3, C4
Scapulohumeral reflex	Tapping on medial edge of lower half of scapula	Adduction and external rotation of the dependent arm	Infraspinatus, teres major	Suprascapular and axillary nerves	C4, C5, C6
Biceps reflex	Tapping on biceps tendon with patient's elbow flexed	Elbow flexion	Biceps brachii	Musculocutaneous nerve	C5, C6
Brachioradialis reflex ("radial periosteal reflex")	Tapping on distal end of radius with patient's elbow slightly flexed and forearm pronated	Elbow flexion	Biceps brachii	Radial and musculocutaneous nerve	C5, C6
Pectoralis reflex	Tapping on scapulohumeral joint (from anterior aspect)	Ventral duction of shoulder	Pectoralis major, pectoralis minor	Medial and lateral pectoral nerves	C5–T4
Triceps reflex	Tapping on triceps tendon with patient's elbow flexed	Elbow extension	Triceps brachii	Radial nerve	C6, C7

(Cont.) →

Table 10.4   (Cont.)

Name of reflex	Stimulus	Response	Muscle(s)	Peripheral nerve	Segment(s)
Thumb reflex	Tapping on flexor pollicis longus tendon in distal third of forearm	Flexion of interphalangeal joint of thumb	Flexor pollicis longus	Median nerve	C6, C7, C8
Wrist reflex	Tapping on dorsal aspect of wrist, proximal to radiocarpal joint	Hand and finger extension (not always seen)	Hand and (long) finger extensors	Radial nerve	C6, C7, C8
Finger flexor reflex	Tapping on the examiner's finger, laid on the volar surface of the patient's hand; or tapping directly on the flexor tendons on the volar surface of the hand	Flexion of the proximal and middle phalanges of the fingers (and of the wrist)	Flexor digitorum superficialis (and wrist flexors)	Median (and ulnar) nerves	C7, C8
Trömner reflex	Patient's hand held by the middle finger; tapping on the volar surface of the distal phalanx of the middle finger	Flexion of distal phalanges (incl. thumb)	Flexor digitorum profundus	Median (ulnar) nerve	C7, C8, (T1)
Adductor reflex	Tapping medial condyle of femur	Thigh adduction	Adductors	Obturator nerve	L2, L3, L4
Quadriceps reflex (patellar reflex, knee-jerk reflex)	Tapping quadriceps tendon below patella, with knee slightly flexed	Knee extension	Quadriceps femoris	Femoral nerve	(L2), L3, L4
Tibialis posterior reflex	Tapping tibialis posterior tendon behind the medial malleolus	Supination (not always seen)	Tibialis posterior	Tibial nerve	L5

Table 10.4 (Cont.)

Name of reflex	Stimulus	Response	Muscle(s)	Peripheral nerve	Segment(s)
Peroneus reflex (plantar flexor reflex)	Foot in mild plantar flexion and supination; examiner places finger on distal portion of metatarsal bones (esp. 1st and 2nd), taps on finger	Dorsiflexion and pronation of foot	Long dorsiflexors of foot and toes, peronei	Peroneal nerve	L5, S1
Semimembranosus/ semitendinosus reflex	Tapping on tendon of medial knee flexors (patient prone, knee relaxed and in mild flexion)	Palpable muscle contraction	Semimembranosus and semitendinosus	Sciatic nerve	S1
Biceps femoris reflex	Tapping on tendon of lateral knee flexors (patient prone, knee relaxed)	Muscle contraction	Biceps femoris	Sciatic nerve	S1, S2
Gastrocnemius reflex (triceps surae reflex, ankle-jerk reflex, Achilles reflex)	Tapping on Achilles tendon (knee in mild flexion, ankle at right angle)	Plantar flexion of foot	Gastrocnemius, soleus, and other plantar flexors	Tibial nerve	S1, S2
Toe flexor reflex (Rossolimo sign)	Tapping on pads of toes	Toe flexion	Flexor digitorum longus, flexor hallucis longus	Tibial nerve	S1, S2

Table 10.5 The most important normal extrinsic muscle reflexes (exteroceptive reflexes)

Name of reflex	Stimulus	Response	Muscle(s)	Peripheral nerve	Segment(s)
Pupillary reflexes (cf. Table 9.10)	light, convergence	constriction	constrictor pupillae m.	CN II and III	diencephalon, midbrain
Corneal reflex	light touch of cornea from the side, e.g. with a strand of cotton or tissue paper, with the eye deviated nasally	lid closure (accompanied by upward movement of the globe = Bell's phenomenon)	orbicularis oculi m.	CN V and VII	pons
Bell's phenomenon (palpebrooculogyric reflex)	attempted active lid closure while the examiner keeps the upper lid open	the globes normally turn upward	superior rectus and inferior oblique mm.	CN V and III	midbra n, pons
Auriculopalpebral reflex	sudden noise, not "visible" to the patient	blink	orbicularis oculi m.	CN VIII and VII	caudal pons
Palatal and pharyngeal (gag) reflexes	stimulation of the soft palate or posterior pharyngeal wall with a tongue depressor or swab	elevation of the palatal veil and symmetric contraction of the posterior pharyngeal wall	palatal and pharyngeal muscles	CN IX and X	medulla
Mayer metacarpophalangeal joint reflex	forced passive flexion of the metacarpophalangeal joints of the 3rd and 4th fingers	adduction and opposition of the thumb	adductor pollicis and opponens pollicis mm.	ulnar and median nn.	C6–T1

Table 10.5 (Cont.)

Name of reflex	Stimulus	Response	Muscle(s)	Peripheral nerve	Segment(s)
Epigastric reflex	Rapid stroking with pin from nipple downward	Pulling of epigastrium inward	Upper fibers of transversus abdominis	Intercostal nerves	T5, T6
Abdominal reflex	Rapid stroking of abdominal skin from lateral to medial	Movement of skin and navel toward stimulated side	Abdominal muscles	Intercostal nerves, hypogastric nerve, ilioinguinal nerve	T6–T12
Cremasteric reflex	Stroking of skin at upper inner aspect of thigh (or pinching of proximal portion of adductors)	Testes drawn upward	Cremaster	Genital branch of genitofemoral nerve	L1, L2
Gluteal reflex	Stroking skin over gluteus maximus	Contraction of gluteus maximus (not always seen)	Gluteus medius, gluteus maximus	Superior and inferior gluteal nerves	L4, L5, S1
Bulbocavernosus reflex	Light pinch of glans of penis or pinprick on dorsum of penis	Bulbocavernosus contraction (palpable at root of penis, at anogenital band, or by digital rectal examination)	Bulbocavernosus	Pudendal nerve	S3, S4
Anal wink reflex	Pinprick on perianal skin or anogenital band, patient in lateral decubitus position, with hip and knee flexed	Visible anal contraction	External anal sphincter	Pudendal nerve	S3, S4, S5

Intervertebral Disk Disease as a Cause of Radicular Syndromes

Pathologic Anatomy

Each intervertebral disk is composed of a fibrous ring *(annulus fibrosus)* and the soft, cartilaginous tissue that it encloses *(nucleus pulposus)*, which is softest at the center of the disk. As the individual ages, the disk gradually dries out, changes in structure, and becomes less elastic. In response to these changes within the disk, *reactive spondylosis* occurs in the end plates of the adjacent vertebral bodies above and below. Weakened fibers of the annulus fibrosus may rupture, allowing disk material to escape. The difference between *disk protrusion* and *disk herniation* is a matter of degree (and is variably defined). The herniated disk material may consist either of fibrous tissue, or of the actual nucleus pulposus; it may protrude into the spinal canal and become separated from the parent disk as a free intraspinal fragment (sequestrum).

If there is a significant amount of disk tissue within the spinal canal, it may compress the dural sac and its contents – i.e. (depending on the level), the spinal cord, the cauda equina, or individual caudal nerve roots. On the other hand, a herniation pointing posterolaterally or laterally into the intervertebral (neural) foramen can compress a single nerve root, causing pain in a dermatomal distribution and the corresponding motor, sensory, and reflex deficits. Similar deficits can, however, be caused by reactive spondylosis as well.

General Signs and Symptoms of Disk Herniation

- *Acute onset of symptoms,* often though not always upon heavy exertion or abrupt movement.
- *Intense pain,* usually in the spine at first, limiting movement.
- Later, *radiation of pain* a shorter or longer distance into the dermatome of the affected root.
- *Exacerbation* of pain by certain movements, typically extension of the back, and by maneuvers that increase the intrathoracic pressure, such as straining, coughing, or sneezing.
- *Vertebral syndrome* with spasm affecting the corresponding segment of the spine and causing local scoliosis.
- *Pain on stretching* of the affected nerve root and the peripheral nerve trunk in which it continues (e.g., Lasègue sign in lumbar disk herniation).
- *Neurologic deficits* are not always seen in the acute phase; objectively detectable sensory, motor, or reflex abnormalities may be lacking.
- *Herniation into the spinal canal* can cause spinal cord compression if above the L1 level, or, at lower levels, compression of all or part of the cauda equina.

Cervical Disk Herniation and Spondylosis

Clinical Features

The more prominent manifestations of cervical disk herniation and spondylosis are *cervical pain, acute torticollis,* and *radicular pain* in the upper limb (brachialgia). These signs and symptoms may arise with or without an *acute precipitating event* (cervical trauma, intense physical activity, whiplash injury). Their onset may be either *acute* or, more commonly, *subacute,* increasing in severity over the course of one or two days. Spasm of the neck muscles produces a rigid, perhaps twisted neck posture (torticollis). A disk herniation, depending on its location, can compress a cervical nerve root, leading to *brachialgia* and *radicular deficits.*

The more common *spondylogenic root compression syndromes* are:

- *C6 syndrome:* the pain radiates into the entire arm, being most intense on the lateral aspect of the arm and radial aspect of the forearm down to the thumb. Hypalgesia may be present in the same distribution, especially distally. The biceps and brachioradialis muscles are weak, but not atrophic. The biceps reflex is usually markedly diminished or absent. Electromyography reveals denervation of the infraspinatus, brachioradialis, and pronator teres muscles, and occasionally also of the C7 muscles (see below).

- *C7 syndrome:* the pain radiates down the upper limb into the second, third, and fourth fingers. There is hypalgesia on both the volar and the dorsal surfaces of these fingers and in a band across the hand, which, on the dorsal surface, may continue proximally up the forearm. Marked triceps weakness is usually found, not uncommonly accompanied by weakness of the midportion of the pectoralis major and of the long finger flexors and pronator teres. The triceps reflex is diminished or absent.

- *C8 syndrome:* pain and paresthesiae are felt in the ring and little fingers, in which hypesthesia can also be demonstrated. The latter may extend in a band up the ulnar surface of the forearm. The sensory deficit is not sharply bounded by the midline of the ring finger (as it is in ulnar nerve palsy). Weakness and atrophy are found in individual interossei and in the muscles of the hypothenar eminence, but less prominently than in ulnar nerve palsy. Electromyography reveals denervation of these muscles and of the extensor indicis proprius.

The characteristics of the individual radicular syndromes are listed in Table 10.**3**. *Stretching the extended arm backward at the shoulder* may precipitate pain radiating into the arm, as may axial pressure on the head when it is slightly tilted to the affected side (*cervical compression test*). *Spinal cord compression* is rare and, when it occurs, usually chronically progressive, in the setting of cervical spondylotic myelopathy (see p. 410). In exceptional cases, however, it may arise subacutely or acutely, sometimes causing the *anterior spinal artery syndrome* (p. 420). Acute or subacute spinal cord compression is a neurosurgical emergency.

Diagnostic Evaluation

The diagnosis, once made on clinical grounds, is confirmed by imaging studies, principally *MRI,* sometimes also CT or myelographic CT. A complete series of *plain films* of the cervical spine, including oblique (foraminal) views, demonstrates the extent of spondyloarthrotic, uncovertebral, and facet joint changes.

Differential Diagnosis

A combination of spinal and radicular findings should always provoke suspicion of a *spinal tumor* (particularly metastatic). Among the rarer *tumors of the spinal nerve roots,* a "dumbbell" (or "hourglass") neurofibroma can cause radicular pain and neurologic deficits as well as widening of the intervertebral foramen, easily visible on plain radiography and CT (cf. Fig. 10.**3**). These and other tumors affecting the nerve roots, as well as *lower brachial plexus lesions,* cause radicular brachialgia without neck pain. Another cause of acute brachialgia is *neuralgic shoulder amyotrophy* (p. 765). Finally, the pain of *carpal tunnel syndrome* can sometimes ascend as high as the neck, particularly at night.

Treatment

Conservative treatment with a cervical collar, local heat application, (possibly) local anesthetic procedures, and anti-inflammatory, analgesic, and muscle relaxant medication usually suffices.
Chiropractic manipulation is contraindicated, as it may lead to massive intervertebral disk herniation, or to compression of a vertebral artery in predisposed patients, with resulting damage to the spinal cord.
Neurosurgical treatment: acute spinal cord compression due to cervical disk herniation is a neurosurgical emergency. Herniated cervical disks may also require operation if

they cause intractable and unbearable pain, or a persistent or progressive neurologic deficit. *Cervical diskectomy* is usually performed through an *anterior* approach. The intervertebral space is emptied of disk material, and any compressive disk fragments are removed. In many cases, a *fusion* (*spondylodesis*) of the vertebral bodies above and below is performed, with any of several available methods (autologous iliac crest bone graft, cadaveric bone, or metal prosthesis). Mobile cervical disk prostheses have recently been introduced as an alternative to fusion. A *posterior* (hemilaminotomy) approach is sometimes appropriate for the removal of posterolateral disk fragments.

Thoracic Radicular Syndromes

These syndromes are rare, and, when they occur, seldom spondylogenic. They are more often due to herpes zoster (shingles, p. 739), referred pain from the viscera to the corresponding zone(s) of Head, or an intraspinal tumor.

Lumbar Disk Herniation

Anatomy

The lumbar intervertebral disks are much more susceptible to symptomatic herniation than either the cervical or the thoracic disks. Lumbar disk herniation usually presents with radicular sciatica. Most lumbar disk herniations are centrolateral and therefore compress the nerve root that exits one level lower (Fig. 10.**1**). Thus, an L4–5 disk herniation usually compresses the L5 root (which exits the spinal canal between L5 and the

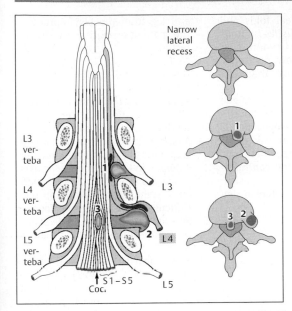

Fig. 10.**1** **Anatomic relationship of lumbar disk herniation to the exiting nerve roots.**
1 Centrolateral herniation
2 Lateral herniation
3 Central herniation

sacrum), and an L5–S1 disk herniation usually compresses the S1 root (which exits the spinal canal through the first sacral foramen). The rarer lateral herniations compress the nerve root exiting through the neural foramen at the same level. Thus, a lateral L4–5 disk herniation compresses the L4 root, a lateral L5–S1 herniation the L5 root.

Clinical History

The typical history of lumbar disk herniation is summarized in Table 10.**6**.

Physical Examination

The physical examination of the patient with a known or suspected lumbar disk herniation requires attention to the following points (Table 10.**7**):
- The configuration of the *spine* and the resulting posture, in particular,

scoliosis and flattening of the lumbar lordosis due to muscle spasm.
- Any *restriction of mobility of the spine* (forward, backward, and lateral bending).
- The *Schober index:* a point that is 10 cm above the spinous process of L5 when the patient stands upright is normally ca. 15 cm above it when the patient bends maximally forward. A diminished Schober index is abnormal.
- *The distance from the fingertips to the floor* when the patient bends maximally forward is reduced in lumbar disk herniation.
- *Reduced or painful movement* when bending forward or sideways.
- *Tenderness to palpation or tapping* on the spinous processes or paravertebral pressure points.
- *Spasm* of the erector spinae muscles.

- Position of the gluteal folds and *tone in the gluteal muscles* (gluteus maximus paresis in S1 syndrome).
- *Trophic status* of the lower extremities (calf circumference, thigh circumference).
- *Lasègue sign* (or "reverse" Lasègue sign in upper lumbar disk herniation). The "crossed" Lasègue sign is often positive in lumbar disk herniation with a large free fragment: passive elevation of the *contralat-*

Table 10.**6** Typical clinical history in lumbar disk herniation

Past medical history:
- Almost always positive for recurrent "charley-horse"
- Often earlier episodes of "sciatica"

Precipitating event:
- Lifting trauma
- Exertion in a bent or rotated posture

Initial symptoms:
- Always in the back (rather than the legs)
- Restriction of movement

Radicular radiation of pain:
- Into the leg or foot
- Constant localization
- Exacerbation on straining, coughing, sneezing

Sensory deficit:
- Often subjectively apparent ("numbness")
- Useful for localization of level

Motor deficit:
- Less often subjectively apparent
- Patient may note difficulty standing on toes or climbing stairs

Other important complaints:
- Sciatica alternating from side to side implies a large herniation
- Bladder dysfunction may indicate cauda equina compression

eral leg from the bed reproduces the patient's sciatica on the affected side.
- *Neri sign:* forward bending induces reflex flexion of the knee on the affected side.
- *Tenderness of the sciatic nerve trunk* all the way down to the Achilles tendon (Valleix pressure points).
- *Motor deficits:* look particularly for weakness of foot and great toe dorsiflexion in L5 syndrome, weakness of plantar flexion of the foot (difficulty standing or walking on toes, difficulty hopping on one foot) in S1 syndrome, quadriceps weakness (difficulty climbing onto a chair) in L4 (or L3) syndrome.
- *Reflex deficits:* diminished or absent Achilles reflex in S1 syndrome, diminished (but not absent) quadriceps reflex in L3 or L4 syndrome.
- *Sensory deficits:* dermatomal hypesthesia and hypalgesia (lateral edge of foot in S1 syndrome, dorsum of foot and great toe in L5 syndrome, see Fig. 1.**1**). For poorly understood reasons, patients with monoradicular lesions sometimes complain of mild, diffuse hypesthesia of the entire leg.

Clinical Features of the More Common Types of Lumbar Disk Herniation

S1 syndrome. This syndrome is usually produced by a herniated L5–S1 disk (the second most common level of herniation). The pain, paresthesiae, and sensory deficit are located on the lateral aspect of the foot. There is a positive Lasègue sign, and there may be tenderness at the Valleix pressure points along the course of the sciatic nerve. The Achilles reflex is diminished or absent as an early sign of S1 syndrome (734). The gluteus maximus is mildly paretic, so that the gluteal fold appears lower than normal, and tone in the gluteus maximus is diminished on the affected side during maximal contraction ("standing at attention"). Dorsiflexion of the foot is usually only mildly paretic (difficulty hopping on one foot or standing on the toes of one foot).

L5 syndrome. This syndrome is usually due to L4–5 disk herniation or far lateral L5–S1 disk herniation (in the latter case, a combined L5 and S1 syndrome is often present). L4–5 is the most common level of lumbar disk herniation. The pain radiation, paresthesiae, and sensory deficit are found on the dorsum of the foot and the lateral aspect of the calf. The Lasègue sign is positive, and there may be ten-

derness at the Valleix pressure points. The tibialis posterior reflex may be absent. (It is often difficult to elicit even in normal individuals; thus, an absent reflex on the affected side is significant only if the contralateral reflex is present; cf. Tables 10.**4** and 10.**5**.) There is practically always some degree of weakness of the extensor hallucis longus, which is innervated exclusively by L5. If the tibialis anterior is also weak, there may be a foot drop, with resulting steppage gait. In such cases, L4 may be additionally involved ("spinal pseudoperoneal palsy").

L3 and/or L4 syndrome (upper lumbar disk herniation). The much rarer herniations of the L2–3 or L3–4 intervertebral disks produce pain radiating to

Table 10.**7** Typical physical findings in lumbar disk herniation

Vertebral syndrome:
- Flattened lumbar lordosis
- Possible scoliosis
- Reduced mobility of spine (Schober less than 10–15 cm, increased finger-to-floor distance on maximal bending)
- Pain on movement (test backward and lateral bending also)
- Spinous process tenderness (when palpated or tapped)
- Often paravertebral tenderness
- Occasionally sprain-type pain

Signs of nerve irritation:
- Positive Lasègue sign
- Occasionally positive reverse Lasègue sign (with a large herniation or intraspinal fragment)
- Tenderness at Valleix pressure points
- Positive Neri sign (forward bending induces flexion of knee on affected side)

Deficits
- Motor (gluteus maximus, knee extensors, foot/toe dorsiflexors and plantar flexors)
- Muscle atrophy (measure thigh and calf circumference)
- Sensory (bandlike, radicular; anterior thigh/shin, dorsum of foot, lateral aspect of foot)
- Reflexes (quadriceps reflex weak, Achilles reflex may be absent)
- Sphincteric disturbances, particularly urinary (if cauda equina compression is suspected, check for saddle anesthesia)

the anterior portion of the thigh and the medial portion of the calf, and a sensory deficit in this distribution. The Lasègue sign is generally negative, but the femoral stretch maneuver (passive hyperextension of the hip joint, with the knee in flexion) can reproduce the patient's radicular pain ("reverse Lasègue sign"). There is tenderness over the trunk of the femoral nerve as it crosses under the inguinal ligament. The quadriceps muscle is markedly weakened (making it difficult or impossible for the patient to climb onto a chair) and the quadriceps reflex is always diminished, but never totally absent.

Lumbar spinal canal stenosis. The clinical hallmark of this condition is neurogenic intermittent claudication (see p. 846).

Ancillary Tests

Plain radiography. Plain films of the lumbar spine usually show alterations of posture due to muscle spasm, including scoliosis or straightening of the normal lordosis, as well as possible collapse of the disk space and reactive spondylotic changes. They are usually indicated for the exclusion of other processes, such as a malignant osteolytic lesion.

Radiculography (lumbar myelography). Lumbar myelography with intrathecal injection of water-soluble contrast medium is a suitable means of confirming the diagnosis of lumbar disk herniation in patients who would be candidates for surgery (Fig. 10.2), though the technique is needed much less frequently now

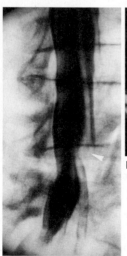

a

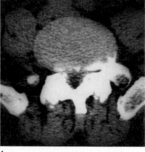

b

Fig. 10.**2a, b   Radiculography in a case of left L4–5 disk herniation** in a 41-year-old man with S1 radicular syndrome.

a The myelogram reveals broadening and shortening of the left S1 root (arrowhead), but also compression of the dural sac at this level from the right side.

b The CT reveals degenerative changes, mainly in the facet joints, and bilateral lateral recess stenosis due to spondylarthrosis.

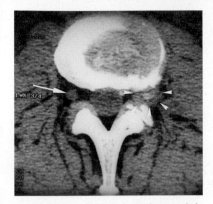

Fig. 10.**3** **CT of a left lateral L4–5 disk herniation** (arrowheads). On the right side, the normal spinal ganglion is well visualized in the intervertebral (neural) foramen (arrow).

that CT and MRI are widely available. Some 10–25% of herniated disks will be missed by myelography, and 10% of myelograms will be falsely positive for disk herniation. Far lateral ("extra-foraminal") disk herniations cannot be seen by myelography.

CT (Fig. 10.**3**) is usually the imaging study of choice when the level of the herniation can be unequivocally diagnosed on clinical grounds. CT can demonstrate far lateral herniations, which myelography cannot (262). Far lateral herniation is particularly common at upper lumbar levels.

MRI. MRI also shows disk herniation well (Fig. 10.**4**). It is primarily indi-

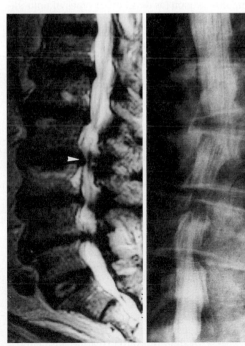

Fig. 10.**4a, b** **Lumbar disk herniation** in a 70-year-old man with neurogenic intermittent claudication due to degenerative lumbar spinal canal stenosis. The MRI and myelogram show compression of the dural sac and the nerve roots at the L2–3 (arrow) and L3–4 disk levels, as well as at L4–5 (less severe).
a MRI.
b Myelogram.

a   b

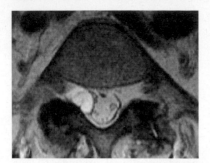 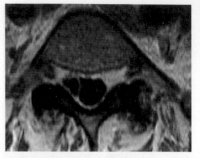

Fig. 10.**5a, b   Right L4–5 synovial cyst** in a 77-year-old man with right L5 radicular syndrome. A cystic process arising from the facet joint can be seen in the right lateral recess.
a Axial T2-weighted spin-echo image.   **b** Axial T1-weighted spin-echo image.

cated when the diagnosis of a herniated disk, or the level of the herniation, is not entirely clear on clinical grounds (e.g., in cases of neurogenic intermittent claudication). MRI can also reveal other causes of radiculopathy, such as a synovial cyst (Fig. 10.**5**).

Electromyography. EMG can contribute to the diagnosis by demonstrating a radicular pattern of denervation, perhaps involving the paravertebral and gluteal musculature as well.

Differential Diagnosis
The differential diagnosis of lumbar disk herniation consists of various pain syndromes involving the back and pelvic region (pp. 839 and 843), all other spinal lesions affecting the nerve roots (tumors, fractures), and, finally, nonradicular processes causing weakness, particularly peripheral lesions of the peroneal nerves (p. 792). Disk herniation may be difficult to distinguish on clinical grounds from other causes of weakness associated with pain, such as proximal asymmetric diabetic neuropathy in the femoral nerve distribution (p. 601), borreliosis, or retroperitoneal

hematoma (p. 787). A useful point to be remembered on physical examination is that painful plexus lesions, such as those produced by a tumor, impair sweating in the affected region (as do all other types of nonradicular peripheral nerve lesion), while lumbar radiculopathy never does (p. 449). Sciatic neuritis can be caused by a vascular process, such as an arteritis, while arteriosclerosis and other arteriopathies can also diffusely involve the lumbar plexus, causing leg weakness and atrophy.

Conservative treatment
Conservative treatment of lumbar disk herniation is usually effective. It consists of *bed rest* in a *flat position* (hard board under mattress), or else with the hips and knees flexed and the calves resting on a well-padded cushion. Cold may be applied initially and heat later; local anesthetic procedures may be useful, and anti-inflammatory, analgesic, and antispasmodic medications should be given.
A properly supervised program of *back exercises* can be initiated a short time after treatment is begun.

Operative treatment

Operative treatment of lumbar disk herniation (discectomy) is *indicated* under the following circumstances:

- Massive herniation with bilateral weakness and sphincter disturbances (absolute indication for emergency surgery).
- Major weakness of acute onset.
- Persistence of symptoms and signs for 2–4 weeks despite correct conservative management.
- Frequent recurrences with distressing symptoms and signs each time.
- Very intense pain that responds inadequately to intensive conservative treatment and that can be attributed to a nerve root lesion on the basis of objective findings.

A *relative indication* for operative treatment is present when there is clinical evidence of a large tear in the annulus fibrosus or of a large herniation – i.e., under the following circumstances:

- when sciatica alternates sides (within the present episode, or in comparison to earlier episodes); and
- when a crossed Lasègue sign is present.

Surgical technique:

The classic technique of *lumbar discectomy,* now generally performed under the operating microscope, involves *fenestration* at the involved level (i.e., partial removal of the hemilaminae above and below) to provide an extradural approach to the disk. A complete hemilaminectomy is rarely required and should be avoided, if possible, as it tends to impair spinal stability and may generate further, persistent or even lifelong pain.

Laminectomy is often necessary to treat lumbar spinal canal stenosis, but is hardly ever necessary merely for the purpose of removing a herniated disk. *Microsurgical lumbar discectomy,* when performed for correct indications, yields the best results of any currently available treatment for lumbar disk herniation (843a). *Chemonucleolysis* has not fulfilled its earlier promise as an alternative treatment. Other so-called minimally invasive techniques, such as the *percutaneous endoscopic removal of disk fragments,* are currently being tested in many clinical centers. Their results have not yet been shown to be superior to, or even as good as, those of microsurgical discectomy.

Prognosis after Surgical Treatment

The long-term outcome is very good in about two-thirds of cases, but unsatisfactory in about 10%. Poor prognostic factors include accidents on the job as the precipitating event, a preoperative course of more than 1 year, and major spondyloarthrotic changes or anomalies of the lumbosacral junction. Incomplete surgical removal of the disk, early recurrent herniation, and postoperative scarring also do their part to worsen the prognosis after surgery.

Intervertebral discitis complicates about 1% of operated cases, though the infective organism cannot always be identified. Some days or weeks after surgery, the patient develops back pain on movement. The erythrocyte sedimentation rate is elevated, CT and MRI reveal structural abnormalities of the disks, and plain radiography 3–12 weeks later shows osteolysis of the vertebral body end plates. The symptoms resolve with rest, but only after several months.

Mass Lesions in and Adjacent to the Spinal Nerve Roots

General Manifestations

These processes lead either to gradually worsening pain and neurologic deficits related to the affected nerve root or, much less commonly, to progressive but painless radiculopathy (e.g., due to nerve root neurofibroma). Tumors of the vertebrae produce local manifestations (back pain, spinal deformation, pathologic fracture, restriction of movement) and can compress the spinal cord or cauda equina if they grow into the spinal canal.

Nerve root neurofibroma.

These tumors may span the neural foramen, thus taking on an hourglass (or "dumbbell") configuration; the narrow waist of the tumor erodes the bony margins of the neural foramen, producing a widening that is easily seen on plain radiographs, and even more easily by CT (Fig. 3.**5**). The intraspinal portion of the tumor may compress the spinal cord, while its extraspinal portion may compress the nerve root itself or other structures.

Neurofibroma of the cauda equina.

This type of tumor is most commonly seen in adolescents. There may be back pain and sciatica for years before radicular weakness and sphincter disturbances appear. Plain views of the lumbar spine often reveal the characteristically widened spinal canal, thinned pedicles, and eroded dorsal surfaces of the vertebral bodies. CT and MRI confirm the diagnosis (as also in the case of lumbosacral lipoma, see below). The lumbar CSF is always abnormal; the CSF protein concentration may be markedly elevated if the tumor blocks communication of the lumbar theca with the remainder of the subarachnoid space.

Lumbosacral lipoma.

Lumbosacral lipoma can usually be recognized externally as a cushion-like protuberance on the lower back. It may extend into the spinal canal (spina bifida occulta), causing cauda equina syndrome.

Extradural lipomatosis.

Extradural lipomatosis is a rare cause of cauda equina compression.

Meningeal sarcomatosis.

This disorder always affects many nerve roots simultaneously (see discussion on p. 410).

Ankylosing spondylitis.

This rheumatologic disease (p. 839) can also cause a slowly progressive cauda equina syndrome, most often because of arachnoid cysts, which can be demonstrated by myelography (with the patient supine).

Other Radicular Syndromes

Herpes Zoster

Etiology

Herpes zoster is due to an (in principle, systemic) infection with one of the neurotropic herpes zoster viruses.

Clinical Features

The local manifestations are thus commonly, though not always, accompanied by *general manifestations* such as fatigue, myalgia, and fever. The *neurologic abnormalities* are due to *involvement of the spinal ganglia (or sensory cranial nerve ganglia)*. Unilateral, local, rather imprecisely localized pain arises first, and the typical vesicular *skin eruption* 3–5 days later. The skin eruption is in a dermatomal pattern. Once the eruption is seen, the pain takes on a sharper, more circumscribed, radicular character. It may be accompanied by a motor deficit – e.g., arm weakness in herpes zoster colli, or facial nerve palsy in herpes zoster colli or (mainly) herpes zoster oticus (p. 677); polyradiculitis; monoradicular weakness; or transverse myelitis, perhaps leading to spinal cord transection syndrome.

Cerebral manifestations may be caused by direct involvement of the brain by the virus (encephalitis). There have been multiple reports of (ipsilateral) ischemic lesions in the brain due to arteritis in the aftermath of herpes zoster ophthalmicus; it thus seems likely that the virus can attack the vascular endothelium. Analysis of the *CSF* reveals lymphocytic pleocytosis (up to 50 cells/µL) and a normal protein concentration.

▰ Late sequelae and treatment ▰

The acute syndrome is often followed, particularly in elderly patients, by a very painful *post-herpetic neuralgia* that can be very difficult to treat. *Carbamazepine* and *oxcarbazepine* are useful in some cases, as are *gabapentin* (806a), *tramadol* (350b), *oxycodone* (999d), and high doses of *tricyclic antidepressants* (75–150 mg/day).

Local *vibratory massage* and the wearing of a pressure dressing sometimes bring temporary relief. Local anesthetic ointment and irritants such as *capsaicin* (396d) are also worth trying.

Neurosurgical procedures, such as dorsal root entry zone lesions or spinal cord stimulation, may be necessary in some cases. Postherpetic pain in the face responds only to electrocoagulation of the ipsilateral descending spinal tract of the trigeminal nerve; peripheral procedures are useless in such cases.

Symptomatic Herpes Zoster

In symptomatic (i.e., secondary) herpes zoster, a pathologic process of some type in the vicinity of the spinal ganglion determines the site at which the viral infection becomes active. Tumors and granulomatous diseases are the more common causes of symptomatic herpes zoster, which predominantly strikes the elderly.

Differential Diagnosis of Radicular Syndromes

The differential diagnosis includes *lesions in the vicinity of the plexuses or peripheral nerves.* Thus, a lower brachial plexus lesion (p. 760) may clinically resemble a C8 radiculopathy, while carpal tunnel syndrome (p. 773) may clinically resemble a C6 or C7 radiculopathy. Lesions of the lumbar plexus impair sweating in the affected areas, while lumbar radicular syndromes never do (p. 457).

Certain *pain syndromes* have a pseudoradicular character (cf. p. 837 ff.)

11   Lesions of Individual Peripheral Nerves

Overview:
The brachial and lumbosacral plexuses are formed by the coming together and regrouping of nerve fibers derived from the spinal nerve roots. This chapter concerns lesions affecting the plexuses, and the peripheral nerve trunks and branches that emerge from them. The cranial nerves have been dealt with separately in an earlier chapter. Like the plexuses, almost all peripheral nerves carry both motor and sensory fibers, and autonomic (specifically, sympathetic) fibers as well. Each peripheral nerve supplies a specific muscle or muscles and innervates a well-defined area of skin. Thus, the pattern of clinical deficits usually enables a precise localization of the responsible lesion, which can then be confirmed by ancillary tests such as electromyography (EMG) and electroneurography (ENG).

General Clinical Features

The diagnostic approach to a peripheral nerve lesion is based on the following considerations, as outlined in Table 11.**1**:

- Presence of a purely *motor*, purely *sensory*, or (most often) *mixed* deficit, depending on the function of the affected nerve.
- Muscles that have been paretic for 3 weeks or more are markedly *atrophic*.
- *Fasciculations* are seen in the paretic muscles only in exceptional cases and are much more consistent with an anterior horn lesion.
- *Sweating* is deficient in the cutaneous area of the sensory deficit, because sudomotor fibers travel together with sensory fibers.
- *EMG and ENG* reveal evidence of neurogenic paresis and slowing of conduction in the affected peripheral nerve trunk.

- A topical diagnosis (localization of the lesion to a particular peripheral nerve, nerve root, or plexus) is made possible by careful consideration of the pattern of muscular involvement, and the cutaneous distribution of hypesthesia, in light of the known *anatomical organization of the PNS* (cf. Tables 10.**2**, 10.**3**).
- *Reflexes* may be impaired depending on the particular nerve or nerve root involved (cf. Tables 10.**4**, 10.**5**).
- *Sensation* is impaired in the cutaneous zone innervated by the involved nerve (cf. Fig. 1.**1**). All qualities of sensation are equally affected, and the area of the deficit is sharply demarcated.
- *Paresthesiae and pain* are not uncommon. Paresthesiae are useful for topical diagnosis, as they usually arise in the area of cutaneous hypesthesia. Pain, on the other

Table 11.**1**   Clinical features of peripheral nerve lesions

Flaccid paresis:
- Involves muscles innervated by the affected (motor or mixed) peripheral nerve
- Corresponding reflexes diminished or absent (Tables 10.**2**, 10.**3**)
- Atrophy in 3 weeks
- Fasciculations very rare

Sensory deficit:
- Present unless involved nerve is purely motor
- For all qualities of sensation
- Corresponds to autonomous area of cutaneous sensory innervation (cf. Fig. 1.1)

Pain and paresthesiae:
- At first in same area as cutaneous hypesthesia
- Later perhaps more diffuse

Diminished or absent sweating in area of cutaneous hypesthesia

Possible nerve tenderness at site of lesion, if cause is mechanical injury

Pain on stretching of affected nerve

hand, may be diffuse or even misleadingly localized. For example, a distal lesion, as in carpal tunnel syndrome, can cause pain extending proximally to involve an entire extremity (p. 773).
- Localizing clues can often be derived from the clinical history or general physical examination (trauma, fracture, chronic exogenous pressure injury, anatomic bottleneck (537, 687), mass, etc.). Practically all mononeuropathies are of mechanical origin.

Ancillary Tests

Though the correct diagnosis can be arrived at in most cases by meticulous neurological examination, ancillary tests are nonetheless often helpful for precise definition of the site and extent of the lesion, for the determination of its etiology, and for the detection of nerve regeneration.

Electromyography

EMG is the most useful ancillary test. It is performed with needle electrodes in the affected muscles, under resting and contracting conditions. The registered electrical potentials are depicted graphically on a monitor and simultaneously heard through a loudspeaker. At rest, muscle is normally electrically silent, and any spontaneous activity is pathological. When the needle is inserted into a relaxed muscle, a few positive sharp waves or fibrillations are seen transiently, but any activity after that is abnormal.

Spontaneous activity. Types of (abnormal) spontaneous activity include fibrillation potentials, positive sharp waves, fasciculations, and complex repetitive discharges.

Motor unit. *Muscle contraction* recruits a variable number of motor

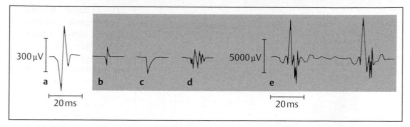

Fig. 11.**1a–e   EMG potentials of various shapes.**
a Normal motor unit potential.
b Fibrillation potential due to denervation.
c Positive sharp wave due to denervation.

d Fragmented polyphasic potential of low amplitude, as seen in reinnervation.
e Abnormally prolonged, high-amplitude potential ("giant potential") due to a chronic anterior horn process.

units, depending on its strength. A motor unit consists of all of the muscle fibers innervated by a single anterior horn cell. Individual potentials can be seen with light muscle contraction but fuse together to form an *interference pattern* with stronger or maximal contraction. The amplitude and shape of the potential derived from a single motor unit is largely a function of the position of the electrode. Normal amplitudes lie in the range of a few hundred microvolts to a few millivolts, and there are usually no more than four phases in a motor unit potential. A prolongation of the mean potential duration, higher than normal amplitude, and an increased number of polyphasic potentials are all signs of a *neurogenic process;* a shortening of the mean potential duration, lower than normal amplitude, and an increased number of polyphasic potentials indicate *muscle disease* (myopathy). Reinnervation after a peripheral nerve lesion is transiently manifested by brief, low, polyphasic potentials, which go on to renormalize.

Figure 11.**1** contains examples of spontaneous activity and abnormal motor unit potentials, while Fig. 11.**2** shows normal and abnormal EMG patterns and the corresponding interference patterns at maximal contraction. In neurogenic processes, motor units are destroyed, and the interference pattern becomes more and more sparse as axon loss progresses. In myopathic processes, on the other hand, the interference pattern remains dense, though its amplitude decreases (cf. Fig. 14.**2**) (710).

Electroneurography

ENG is a method of measuring *motor and sensory nerve conduction velocity.* What is measured is actually the conduction velocity of the most rapidly conducting fibers within the nerve. The amplitude and duration of the individual and summed nerve action potentials together provide an indication of the total number of conducting axons and the dispersion of their conduction velocities. Normal conduction velocities are 50–70 m/s in

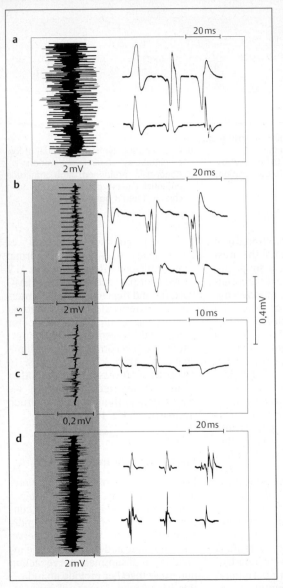

Fig. 11.**2a–d   Normal, neurogenic, and myopathic EMG tracings.**

a Normal: full interference pattern.

b Reinnervation after peripheral nerve injury: individual oscillations.

c Total denervation: fibrillation potentials and positive sharp waves.

d Myopathy: despite weakness, the interference pattern is full. The individual potentials that compose it are of low amplitude, and partially polyphasic and fragmented.

the upper limbs and 40–60 m/s in the lower limbs.

The measurement is performed through two electrodes, one for *stimulation* and the other for *recording*, which are usually placed on the cutaneous surface, though needle electrodes are also used for sensory neurography. Figure 11.3 illustrates the findings of nerve stimulation at various positions. The latency of the summed potential increases as the stimulating electrode is moved farther away from the recording electrode.

F wave. When motor nerve fibers are stimulated, action potentials are conducted not only orthodromically to the muscle, but also antidromically to the anterior horn cells. The antidromic action potentials are reflected back from the anterior horn cells in the manner of an echo and arrive at the muscle as a so-called F wave.

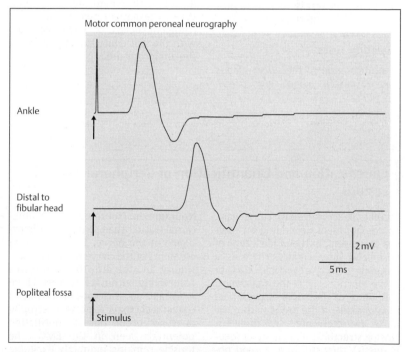

Fig. 11.**3** **ENG findings in right common peroneal pressure palsy.** As the stimulus and recording electrodes are moved farther and farther apart, the latency to the appearance of the summed potential becomes longer and longer. When the stimulus is delivered in the popliteal fossa, the summed potential is suddenly of much lower amplitude. This implies conduction block of almost all axons between the popliteal fossa and distal to the fibular head, as is typically seen in pressure palsies.

H reflex. The H reflex is the electrophysiologic correlate of the intrinsic muscle reflex. Like the F wave, it can be used to determine the conduction velocity of proximal segments of motor and sensory nerves.

Indications for EMG and ENG

The electrophysiologist who will be performing the test should be asked a precise diagnostic question, preferably one answerable with "yes" or "no." If the clinician has no such question to ask, the test is unlikely to provide any useful information.

Sweating Tests

The innervation of the sweat glands was discussed above on p. 457.

Sweating tests of the types described here can be used to provide objective evidence of deficient sweating due to a peripheral nerve lesion.

Ninhydrin test. This test enables the detection and documentation of spontaneous sweating. It is mainly useful for testing on the palms and soles.

Minor's iodine-starch test. In this test, the part of the body to be tested is painted with iodine solution, which is allowed to dry. The skin is then dusted with potato starch powder. When the patient sweats, the dark, confluent beads of sweat contrast with the still white starch powder in the anhidrotic area.

Classification and Quantification of Peripheral Nerve Lesions

Peripheral nerve lesions cause variable impairment depending on their site and extent. In the mildest type of peripheral nerve injury, there is a temporary, fully reversible loss of nerve function, while the anatomical continuity of the nerve is preserved (*neurapraxia*). If the axons within the nerve are interrupted, but their enclosing structures remain intact (*axonotmesis*), they still have a good potential for regeneration. If, however, both the axons and their enclosing structures are severed (*neurotmesis*), regeneration is impossible unless the nerve is repaired surgically.

Neurapraxia. Neurapraxia is a functional (rather than structural) disturbance of the nerve. The conducting elements of the nerve remain in continuity, and the disturbance resolves completely within a few days. There is usually no sensory deficit, though dysesthesia may be present. Atrophy does not occur, nor are fibrillation potentials seen in the EMG. The muscle remains indirectly excitable by conventional electric stimulation – i.e., galvanic stimulation through the nerve. Sleep pressure palsies, for example, are a variety of neurapraxia.

Axonotmesis. In axonotmesis, the axons themselves are interrupted, but their enclosing structures are intact. The fully developed picture of a peripheral nerve palsy results, with weakness, atrophy, and a sensory deficit. The anatomic situation is, however, conducive to axon regeneration, so that full recovery usually follows, unless prolonged, chronic compression has already led to irreversible fibrosis of the perineural structures. Axonotmesis occurs, for example, in carpal tunnel syndrome (p. 773).

Neurotmesis. When both the axons and their enclosing structures are interrupted, the axons find no scaffold upon which to regenerate, and regeneration in random directions produces a neuroma (see below). This type of lesion is seen in plexus avulsion as well as in sharp transections or avulsions of peripheral nerves. Surgical nerve repair is indicated.

Grading scales for motor and sensory deficits due to peripheral nerve (or other) lesions are presented in Table 11.2.

Table 11.2 Grading of motor and sensory deficits: the M and S scales

Motor deficit	
M0	No visible muscle activity
M1	Visible contraction, but no movement
M2	Movement, but cannot overcome gravity
M3	Strength sufficient to overcome gravity
M4	Strength sufficient to overcome moderate resistance
M4–5	Intermediate strength between M4 and M5
M5	Normal strength
Sensory deficit	
S0	No sensation whatever
S1	Sensation only to pain or deep pressure in the autonomous zone
S2	Slight, superficial cutaneous sensation to noxious and tactile stimuli, only in autonomous zone
S3	Superficial cutaneous sensation to noxious and tactile stimuli in entire autonomous zone; no hypersensitivity
S3+	Like S3, but also with a certain degree of two-point discrimination in the autonomous zone
S4	Normal sensation

Peripheral Nerve Regeneration

Axons can regrow from the site of injury to the periphery as long as the continuity of the nerve has not been disrupted by the injury, or has been restored by surgical repair. Nerves regenerate at a speed of approximately 1 mm per day, or about one inch per month. The course of regeneration can be followed by clinical examination, by EMG, and by testing of the Tinel sign (sometimes called the Hoffmann-Tinel sign): lightly tapping on the nerve at precisely the point that has been reached by the regenerating axons evokes paresthesia in its peripheral distribution.

A positive Tinel sign is a good, though not infallible, predictor of nerve regeneration. The typical electrophysiologic features of denervation and reinnervation are shown in Fig. 11.**4**.

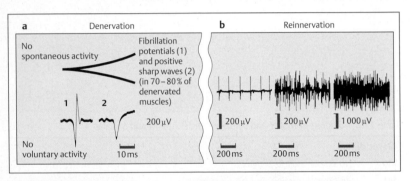

Fig. 11.**4a, b   EMG findings in denervation and reinnervation**
a Denervated muscle.

b Reinnervated muscle. Observe the increasing density of the interference pattern.

Pain Syndromes due to Peripheral Nerve Lesions

Painful Neuroma

This is the most common pain syndrome after transection of a nerve. A neuroma is formed by axons sprouting in all directions from the proximal stump of the severed nerve. The pain is mostly limited to the site of the neuroma and is evoked by pressure or a blow. Small, post-traumatic neuromas of peripheral nerve branches – e.g., digital branches of the median nerve – can cause not only intense local pain, but also intense pain radiating proximally ("algie diffusante"), with tenderness of the entire nerve trunk to pressure.

A *pseudoneuroma* is a swelling (often painless) of a nerve trunk due to proliferation of endoneural connective tissue at a site of chronic pressure (e.g., in the ulnar groove). Most pseudoneuromas need no treatment.

Phantom Limb Pain

Phantom limb pain is pain felt in an amputated limb. It may be spontaneous or evoked by external stimuli. If the pain is due to a neuroma at the stump, it can sometimes be successfully treated by resection of the neuroma. In other cases, peripheral nerve stimulation, either transcutaneous or through implanted electrodes, can bring relief.

Causalgia

This syndrome of extremely severe pain is characterized by burning dysesthesiae of waxing and waning intensity, induced by external stimuli. Tactile stimuli are needed at first; in the later course of the condition, even an acoustic or visual stimulus can provoke a painful attack. A cool and moist cloth draped over the affected body part can lessen the pain. Severe autonomic and trophic disturbances complete the picture of this disorder. The very distressing symptoms often affect the patient's personality and behavior.

Causalgia is usually the result of a direct (partial) peripheral nerve injury and may develop immediately after the injury or within a few hours of it. Wartime injuries to the median and tibial nerves are typical causes. All peripheral surgical procedures are ineffective, but sympathetic blockade or sympathectomy often brings relief.

▌ Brachial Plexus Palsies

Anatomy

The anatomy of the brachial plexus is shown in Fig. 11.**5**.

As it descends from the cervical spine to the proximal end of the arm, the brachial plexus occupies an hourglass-shaped space whose narrowest point lies at the passage between the clavicle and the first rib. The ventral rami of the cervical nerves, which join together to form the brachial plexus, lie at first between the small anterior and posterior intertransverse muscles, then dorsal to the vertebral artery, vein, and nerve, and finally arrive at the scalene hiatus, which is delimited by the anterior and middle scalene muscles and the first rib. The ventral branch of T1 reaches the scalene hiatus along the posterior surface of the dome of the pleura, which is reinforced by the costopleural ligament. The subclavian artery occupies the most ventral position in the scalene hiatus, directly superior to the first rib. The scalene hiatus is also the site of certain typical anatomical variations. A cervical rib is present in only about 0.5–1 % of persons. Short cervical ribs merely touch the ventral ramus of C7, but a long cervical rib can narrow the scalene hiatus from below. The subclavian artery and the brachial plexus always cross over a cervical rib. A fibrous band may be present as a continuation of a short cervical rib or rib stump and compress the costoclavicular space from below.

Brachial Plexus Lesions
The brachial plexus is particularly susceptible to injury because of its proximity to the highly mobile structures of the shoulder girdle. In our experience, the topical localization of brachial plexus lesions is not always an easy matter, because of the complicated anatomy of the plexus. As the plexus is constructed out of the coalescing and regrouping fibers of the C5 through T1 nerve roots (some-

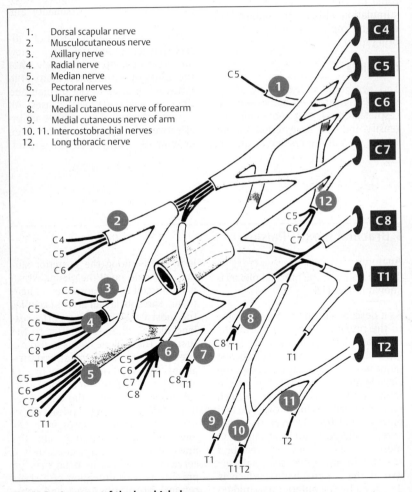

1.   Dorsal scapular nerve
2.   Musculocutaneous nerve
3.   Axillary nerve
4.   Radial nerve
5.   Median nerve
6.   Pectoral nerves
7.   Ulnar nerve
8.   Medial cutaneous nerve of forearm
9.   Medial cutaneous nerve of arm
10. 11. Intercostobrachial nerves
12.   Long thoracic nerve

Fig. 11.**5   Anatomy of the brachial plexus.**
Schematic diagram showing the distribution of the axons of the individual nerve roots to the peripheral nerves.

times with contributions from C4 and/or T2), plexus lesions affect the multisegmentally innervated muscles of the shoulder girdle and upper limb more or less severely depending on the precise location of the lesion.

The important clinical aspects of lesions of the brachial plexus and the peripheral nerves of the upper limb are summarized in Table 11.**3**. Figure 11.**6** is intended as an aid to the clinical localization of brachial plexus lesions based on the pattern of upper limb muscles involved.

Traumatic Brachial Plexus Palsies

Trauma is the most common cause of brachial plexus palsy.

Mechanism

Direct trauma to the shoulder, causing a sudden, intense pull on the brachial plexus, is the usual mechanism. Motorcycle drivers are at elevated risk for this sort of injury, as are snowboarders and devotees of various other sports. The shoulder need not be dislocated for a brachial plexus injury to occur; a strong pull on the arm suffices in some cases. The subclavian artery can be injured simultaneously, even in non-penetrating trauma. Birth injury is a further cause (see below).

Upper Brachial Plexus Lesions

Upper brachial plexus palsy (*Erb's* or *Erb-Duchenne palsy*) reflects loss of

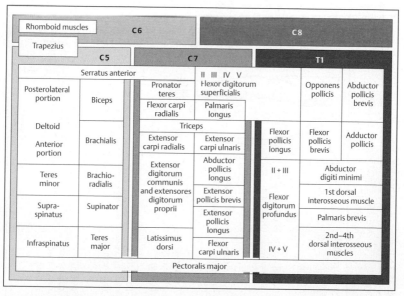

Fig. 11.**6** **Localization of brachial plexus lesions from the pattern of muscle weakness.**

Table 11.3   Lesions of the brachial plexus and the nerves of the upper limb (778)

Nerve	Muscle involved	Sensory deficit	Function	Special tests	Etiology	Remarks	Differential diagnosis
Upper brachial plexus:							
• C5–C6							
• Dorsal scapular nerve, C4–C5	Rhomboids (major and minor)		Adduction of scapula toward spine	Standing, hand on hip, elbow backwards			
• Suprascapular nerve C5–C6	Supraspinatus, infraspinatus		Abduction and external rotation of the shoulder	First 15° of shoulder abduction			
• Axillary nerve (see below)							
• Long thoracic nerve (see below)				Trauma (with or without shoulder dislocation)	Motorcycle riders at risk		
• Musculocutaneous nerve (see below)			Most commonly disturbed in upper brachial plexus palsies:		Backpack palsy, pressure on shoulder from carrying heavy loads	Long thoracic nerve often involved	Root lesions (spondylosis, disk herniation), familial proximal neurogenic muscle atrophy

Table 11.3 (Cont.)

Nerve	Motor	Sensory area	Function	Causes		
• Radial nerve (see below)			Shoulder abduction, elbow flexion, supination, occasionally shoulder external rotation	Neuralgic shoulder amyotrophy, serogenic neuritis, tumor infiltration	Bilateral in 25% of cases	Arm vein thrombosis, amyotrophic lateral sclerosis
Lower brachial plexus:						
• C8–T1						
• Medial brachial cutaneous nerve C8–T1	None	Medial brachial cutaneous nerve	Finger adduction and abduction, flexion of finger joints (and wrist)	Trauma, birth trauma, scalene syndrome (with or without cervical rib), costoclavicular syndrome, Pancoast tumor of lung apex, lymphomatous infiltration	Occasionally with Horner's syndrome; sometimes additional symptoms from subclavian artery, early pain and Horner syndrome	Root lesions, peripheral ulnar nerve palsy, amyotrophic lateral sclerosis, myopathies with distal muscle atrophy (e.g., myotonic dystrophy), syringomyelia
• Medial antebrachial cutaneous nerve C8–T1	None	Medial antebrachial cutaneous nerve				
• Median nerve (see below)						
• Ulnar nerve (see below)						

(Cont.) →

Table 11.3 (Cont.)

Nerve	Muscle involved	Sensory deficit	Function	Special tests	Etiology	Remarks	Differential diagnosis
Long thoracic nerve C5–C7	Serratus anterior		Pulls scapula ventrolaterally, rotates angle of scapula	Pressing palms of extended arms against a wall (reveals winging of scapula)	Surgical procedures in the axilla, heavy lifting, pressure palsies (backpack), "inflammatory-allergic"	A component of neuralgic shoulder amyotrophy	Winged scapula in shoulder girdle form of progressive muscular dystrophy
Axillary nerve C5–C6	Deltoid		Shoulder abduction	Lateral raising of the arm past 15°	Trauma (often with shoulder dislocation)		Muscular dystrophy, rotator cuff tear
	Teres minor		Shoulder external rotation				
Musculocutaneous nerve C5–C7	Coracobrachialis		Stabilizes shoulder (flexion and adduction of the arm at the shoulder)				

Table 11.3 (Cont.)

	Biceps brachii	Arm and forearm flexion, supination	Elbow flexion with supinated forearm	Traumatic; rarely isolated without trauma	Tear of long biceps tendon
	Brachialis (partly supplied by radial nerve)	Arm flexion			
Radial nerve C5–C7 (T1)	Triceps brachii and anconeus	Elbow extension			
	Brachioradialis	Elbow flexion	In intermediate position between pronation and supination		
	Brachialis (also supplied by musculocutaneous nerve)	Elbow flexion			
	Extensor carpi radialis brevis et longus	Wrist extension (and radial abduction)	With flexed finger joints	Humeral fracture	Triceps spared
	Supinator	Supination	With extended elbow	Pressure palsy at humerus	Spontaneous recovery

1 Axillary nerve
2 Lateral antebrachial cutaneous nerve (branch of musculocutaneous nerve)
3 Superficial branch of radial nerve

(Cont.) →

Table 11.3 (Cont.)

Nerve	Muscle involved	Sensory deficit	Function	Special tests	Etiology	Remarks	Differential diagnosis
	Extensor digitorum communis		Extension at metacarpophalangeal joints	Fingers flexed at interphalangeal joints	"Lead neuritis"	Often purely motor	
	Extensor carpi ulnaris		Wrist extension (and ulnar abduction)	Fingers flexed			
	Extensor digiti minimi		Extension of the little finger		Isolated palsy of the deep branch at the level of the supinator		Pressure lesions of the terminal sensory branch to the thumb (cheiralgia paresthetica)
	Abductor pollicis longus		Thumb abduction (at metacarpophalangeal joint)				
	Extensor pollicis longus		Extension of thumb at interphalangeal joint	Distal phalanx flexed			Tear of extensor tendon
	Extensor pollicis brevis		Extension of thumb at metacarpophalangeal joint				
	Extensor indicis		Extension of index	Other fingers flexed			

(Cont.) →

Table 11.3 (Cont.)

Median nerve C5–T1	Median nerve			
Pronator teres et quadratus		Pronation		
Flexor carpi radialis		Radial volar flexion of wrist	Traumatic – e.g., supracondylar fracture of humerus	"Preacher's hand" with proximal lesion
Palmaris longus		Pure volar flexion of wrist		
Flexor digitorum superficialis		Finger flexion at proximal interphalangeal joint	Pressure palsy at humerus	Good prognosis
				Volkmann contracture
Flexor digitorum profundus (II–III)		Flexion of 2nd and 3rd fingers at distal interphalangeal joint	At the supracondylar process of the humerus	(Lower) brachial plexus lesions
Flexor pollicis longus		Flexion of thumb at interphalangeal joint	Cut injury at wrist	
Flexor pollicis brevis (superficial head)		Flexion of thumb at metacarpophalangeal joint	Carpal tunnel syndrome	Symptoms of brachialgia paresthetica nocturna
Abductor pollicis brevis		Abduction of 1st metacarpal	(Occupational) pressure palsy at the root of the hand	Often purely motor
		Thumb abduction while grasping an object ("bottle sign")		Amyotrophic lateral sclerosis

(Cont.) →

Table 11.3 (Cont.)

Nerve	Muscle involved	Sensory deficit	Function	Special tests	Etiology	Remarks	Differential diagnosis
	Lumbricals I–III		Rotation of thumb, flexion at MP joints, extension at IP joints of 2nd and 3rd fingers	Touching the base of the little finger with the volar pad of the thumb			
Ulnar nerve C8–T1	Flexor carpi ulnaris	**Ulnar nerve**	Volar and ulnar wrist flexion	Abduction of little finger (tendon prominent)			
	Flexor digitorum profundus (IV–V)		Flexion at distal interphalangeal joint of 4th and 5th fingers		Pressure lesion at elbow	Occupational injury; bedridden patients	C8 root lesion lower brachial plexus palsy
	Palmaris brevis		"Skin muscle" at hypothenar eminence	Dimpling of hypothenar skin when the little finger is abducted	Dislocation of ulnar nerve at elbow	With or without additional trauma, can be bilateral!	
	Abductor digiti minimi		Abduction of little finger				

(Cont.) →

Table 11.3 *(Cont.)*

Opponens digiti minimi Flexor digiti minimi brevis	Opposition of little finger Flexion of metacarpophalangeal joint of little finger			Medial epicondylitis Muscular dystrophy with distal atrophy
		Traumatic, in elbow fractures Late paresis after old elbow fracture	Esp. medial epicondyle Esp. lateral portion (radial condyle)	
Lumbricals III–IV	Flexion of MP and extension of IP joints of 3rd and 4th fingers	Sometimes bilateral		(Dupuytren's contracture) amyotrophic lateral sclerosis
		Paresis in arthroses and chondromatoses of the elbow joint		
Interossei	Ad- and abduction of the fingers	Pressure palsy at the root of the hand	Usually purely motor	
		Lateral movement of the middle finger		
Adductor pollicis	Thumb adduction	Abnormally frequent flexion and extension of the elbow	E.g., in die cutting, or work on drilling machines	
		Froment sign (cf. p. 777)		
Flexor pollicis brevis (deep head)	Flexion of metacarpophalangeal joint of thumb			

nerve fibers derived from the C5 and C6 roots. The commonest form of brachial plexus palsy, it is characterized by weakness of shoulder abductors and external rotators, elbow flexors, and the supinator, and variable, partial weakness of the elbow extensors, wrist extensors, and some of the muscles around the scapula. There may be a sensory deficit over the shoulder, the lateral aspect of the arm, and the radial aspect of the forearm, but there may also be no sensory deficit at all (Fig. 11.**7**).

Lower Brachial Plexus Lesions

Lower brachial plexus palsy (*Klumpke's* or *Dejerine-Klumpke palsy*) reflects loss of nerve fibers derived from the T1 nerve root, and sometimes also C8. It is rarer than Erb's palsy. All of the small muscles of the hand are paretic, as are some-times the long flexors of the fingers, and, rarely, the wrist flexors. The triceps is usually spared. There may also be a deficit of the cervical sympathetic, producing Horner's syndrome (ptosis, miosis, enophthalmos, and, occasionally, conjunctival injection); this implies injury to the T1 root proximal to the exit of its white ramus communicans to the sympathetic chain (p. 458). The sensory deficit usually covers the ulnar portion of the hand and the ulnar aspect of the forearm (Fig. 11.**8**).

C7 Palsy

Lesions affecting the C7 portion of the brachial plexus, rather than the C7 root, are rare. The corresponding deficit is usually found in the distribution of the radial nerve. The brachioradialis is spared, as it is innervated by C5 and C6 as well as C7.

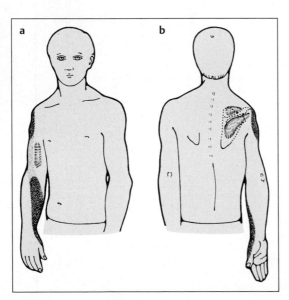

Fig. 11.**7a, b**   **Upper limb posture and sensory deficit in right upper brachial plexus palsy.**

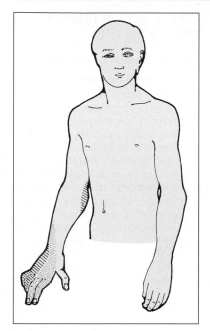

Fig. 11.8 **Upper limb posture and sensory deficit in right lower brachial plexus palsy.**

at first but is later confined to its upper or, more commonly, lower portion.

Nerve Root Avulsion and Tandem Lesions

Trauma often leads to nerve root avulsion or a combination of peripheral brachial plexus injury with nerve root avulsion (tandem lesion). Bloody CSF and spinal cord signs commonly accompany nerve root avulsion. Horner's syndrome does not necessarily imply nerve root avulsion, as it only indicates some degree of injury to the C8 and T1 roots proximal to the exit of their white rami communicantes to the sympathetic chain. Nerve root avulsion and other nerve root injuries, hematoma, and tandem lesions of the plexus (if present) are best seen by MRI; CT sometimes provides useful additional information.

Birth Injuries to the Brachial Plexus

The brachial plexus may be injured even in spontaneous vaginal delivery with a normal presentation if the infant's shoulders are disproportionately wide in relation to the pelvis. Injury is more common, however, in forceps deliveries, caused by direct pressure from the forceps on the plexus. Upper brachial plexus palsy (Erb's palsy) is the most common type.

Prognosis of Traumatic Brachial Plexus Injuries

Upper brachial plexus injuries generally have a better prognosis than lower ones; more than half of pa-

Fascicular Palsies

Three types of *fascicular palsy* affect the brachial plexus:
- a dorsal type, with combined axillary and radial nerve deficits,
- a lateral type, affecting the musculocutaneous nerve and the lateral fibers contributing to the median nerve, and
- a medial type, affecting the ulnar nerve and the medial fibers contributing to the median nerve.

Total Brachial Plexus Palsy

Paralysis after a traumatic injury often affects the entire brachial plexus

tients with upper brachial plexus injuries recover completely. Pain is an unfavorable prognostic indicator in nerve root avulsion. The electrophysiologic correlate of nerve root avulsion is intact peripheral sensory nerve conduction on ENG, despite analgesia in the cutaneous distribution of the root. This finding demonstrates continuity between the cell bodies (in the dorsal root ganglion) and the peripheral nerve fibers, so that the interruption in the nerve pathway must lie proximal to the ganglion – i.e., at the root.

Treatment of traumatic brachial plexus injuries

Initial management consists of *prevention of stiffening of the shoulder joint* (proper positioning, perhaps an abduction sling, passive motion exercises). *Active motion exercises* are begun later.

Primary operative treatment by *nerve suture* is indicated in sharp cutting injuries. A surgical approach is now increasingly used in other cases where the expected recovery fails to occur, and in documented nerve root avulsion (see above). *Autogenous nerve transplantation* (autograft) is performed. Reinnervation generally cannot restore function to totally denervated muscle after an interval of 12–18 months from the injury. In such cases, *orthopedic procedures* may help restore some degree of arm function.

Other Causes of Brachial Plexus Palsy

Chronic Exogenous Pressure

Backpack palsy, caused by carrying an excessively heavy pack on the shoulders, is sometimes seen in fresh military recruits. It is essentially an upper brachial plexus palsy, though it often also involves the long thoracic nerve. A similar syndrome results from carrying other types of load on one or both shoulders. Likewise, women may suffer an iatrogenic brachial plexus palsy, due to shoulder pressure, in gynecologic procedures requiring elevation of the pelvis, in which shoulder rests are used to secure the patient to the operating table. These pressure palsies all share a good prognosis, though several months may be needed for recovery.

Compression Syndromes at Anatomical Bottlenecks

The *thoracic outlet* is a natural anatomical bottleneck at which the brachial plexus may be subject to chronic compression in the presence or absence of other contributing factors. The lower portion of the plexus is particularly vulnerable. The precise mechanism of compression is not always clear; thus, the general term *thoracic outlet syndrome* is often used to describe such cases.

■ Scalene Syndrome and Cervical Rib Syndrome

The brachial plexus, and sometimes the subclavian artery as well, can be compressed as these two structures pass through the hiatus delimited by the anterior and middle scalene muscles. Compression is much more likely when there is an anatomical variant at this site; the most common type is a *cervical rib*. The rudimentary analogue of a cervical rib is a *fibrous band*, which may be, but need not be, attached to a cervical rib stump. Fibrous bands are not seen in plain radiograms but are sometimes seen on MRI or CT. It should be borne in mind, however, that cervical ribs are seldom symptomatic when present. Surgical excision of a cervical rib is indicated only in exceptional cases.

■ Costoclavicular Syndrome

The brachial plexus can be compressed if the space between the clavicle and the first rib (the costoclavicular space) is unusually narrow, as in asthenic individuals with sloping shoulders. This syndrome, and other brachial plexus compression syndromes at bottleneck sites, are much rarer than commonly supposed, and not every brachialgia of unclear cause can be ascribed to such a syndrome. The diagnosis must be based on objective evidence of a lesion of the plexus, usually affecting its lower portion, perhaps with accompanying compression of the subclavian artery. In such cases, the symptoms often first become evident after the patient carries a heavy load. Certain movements, such as bending the head backward and simultaneously turning it to the affected side (the Adson maneuver), may bring out the symptoms or cause the radial pulse to disappear. It should be noted, however, that pulling downward on the shoulders causes the radial pulse to disappear in nearly half of all normal persons.

■ Hyperabduction Syndrome

Symptomatic compression of the neurovascular bundle between the coracoid process and the pectoralis minor on hyperelevation of the arm is a rare phenomenon. It presents with paralysis and insensibility of the entire upper limb that may begin while the patient sleeps.

> ### Treatment of compression syndromes
>
> Most cases without an objectively detectable motor or sensory deficit can be treated adequately with *posture exercises* to strengthen the shoulder girdle muscles, and avoidance of precipitating factors.
> *Surgical division of the anterior scalene muscle,* followed by removal of a cervical rib, or of part of the first rib in costoclavicular compression, is indicated only if a neurologic deficit can be documented. These procedures can be performed through either an axillary or a supraclavicular approach. The latter, though more difficult, is nevertheless preferred, as it provides better exposure of the anatomical relationships at the thoracic outlet. In the larger surgical series that have been reported to date, anomalies of the thoracic outlet were nearly always found on the preoperative imaging studies, and were seen at surgery in every case without exception.

Pancoast Tumor of the Apex of the Lung

Clinical Features

Small-cell bronchial carcinoma in its early stage is an easily overlooked cause of pain in the upper limb and of lower brachial plexus palsy. Tumors of other histologic types (sarcoma, Hodgkin's lymphoma) present less commonly in this manner. Patients initially complain of severe pain in the C8 and T1 distribution, radiating to the ulnar side of the hand, and then go on to develop a lower brachial plexus palsy. In three-quarters of patients, the first objective sign is ipsilateral Horner's syndrome and loss of sweating in the corresponding quadrant of the body, due to involvement of the cervical sympathetic pathway. The tumor occasionally grows into the spinal canal and compresses the spinal cord.

Diagnostic Evaluation

Chest radiography and CT point to the diagnosis.

> ### Treatment
> Treatment of Pancoast tumors generally fails to provide a good outcome, but *radiotherapy* can often eliminate the pain, at least temporarily.

Radiation Injury to the Brachial Plexus

Pathogenesis

Animal experiments have shown that radiation can injure the brachial plexus not only by a direct mechanism, but also through compression from the adjacent indurated and scarred connective tissue.

Clinical Features

Radiotherapy can cause progressive brachial plexus palsy after a latency of one or more years. Pain is a promi-

nent symptom in ca. 15% of patients, and frequently the initial symptom. The palsy may affect the upper or lower portion of the plexus, or, rarely, the entire plexus. The prognosis for recovery is poor, as strength never returns to the affected muscles, and the pain rarely improves.

It is often hard to tell whether brachial plexus palsy has been caused by radiation therapy or by regrowth of the original tumor. A few criteria for making this distinction can be derived from a clinical study that compared 78 patients with tumor-related brachial plexus palsy, of whom 34 had also undergone radiation therapy, with 22 patients with radiation-induced brachial plexus palsy. Very severe pain was present in 80% of tumor-related palsies, but only 20% of radiation-induced palsies; the lower portion of the plexus was involved in 75% of tumor-related palsies, the upper portion in 75% of radiation-induced palsies; Horner's syndrome was more common in tumor-related palsies, while lymphedema was more common in radiation-induced palsies. Palsies that arose within 1 year of radiation therapy were always due to tumor infiltration, unless the radiation dose had exceeded 60 Gy (538a).

> ### Treatment
> *Early operative neurolysis* has been performed for this condition, with disappointing results.

Asymmetric, purely motor paresis of both upper or lower limbs. This rare complication of radiotherapy in the midline was recently described in a group of six patients – in the upper limbs in one, in the lower limbs in five (549c). It arises many years after treatment (mean latency, 15 years). Electrophysiologic study suggests that it reflects radiation injury to the nerve roots, rather than to the spinal cord.

Neuralgic Shoulder Amyotrophy ("Brachial Plexus Neuritis," Parsonage-Turner syndrome)

Pathogenesis

This is an inflammatory allergic affection of the brachial plexus that sometimes arises 4–12 days after an immunization (see p. 613), but is more often spontaneous.

Clinical Features

Most patients are young adults, probably more often male than female. The onset is acute, usually of unknown cause, and only rarely in the setting of an atypical infection or cold exposure. Patients are afebrile and do not feel generally unwell.

The initial symptom is *very severe pain in the shoulder*, often of a tearing quality, often beginning at night. It may radiate into the arm, rarely as far down as the forearm. *Weakness* of one or more of the proximal muscles of the shoulder and arm usually ensues within a few hours, but sometimes only after several days. The pain may be so intense as to restrict arm movement, so that weakness may not be detected until some time after it arises.

The pain usually abates within a few days, leaving the weakness behind. In rare cases, however, mild pain may persist for weeks or even months, or reappear whenever the arm is put back in full use.

Physical Examination

Weakness is found in multiple muscles of the shoulder girdle and upper arm (all of which are usually innervated by the upper portion of the brachial plexus). Distal weakness is seen only in rare cases, perhaps creating a clinical picture resembling radial nerve palsy. The syndrome occurs more commonly on the right side. Sensory disturbances are present in only one-quarter of cases, usually on the lateral aspect of the shoulder and arm.

Diaphragmatic paresis is also found in some cases. The question thus arises whether cases of isolated diaphragmatic paresis might be due to a variant form of this syndrome if no other process affecting the C3 and C4 roots, and the fibers derived from them, can be found. The CSF is always normal.

Prognosis

The prognosis is good. The severe pain resolves within a week in half of cases, within 3 months in nearly all the rest, though milder residual pain may persist for months afterward. Weakness, too, usually resolves, though it may not begin to improve till 9–12 months after onset, and maximal recovery may take 2 years. Permanent residual weakness is uncommon. The manifestations recur in a rare familial form of this condition and in rare sporadic cases.

Treatment

Anti-inflammatory agents and cortisone in the acute phase, later local application of heat and physical therapy.

Differential Diagnosis of Brachial Plexus Palsies

The differential diagnosis includes palsies of individual nerves or nerve roots of the upper limb, as well as certain CNS processes that tend to cause distal weakness. Certain pain syndromes of the upper limb must also be considered (p. 834).

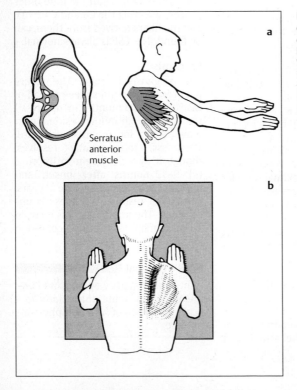

Serratus anterior muscle

Fig. 11.**9a, b   Winging of the scapula (right) due to a lesion of the long thoracic nerve.** Winging of the scapula is easiest to see when the patient stretches out his arms and presses his hands against a wall (**b**).

Long Thoracic Nerve

Anatomy
The long thoracic nerve, a purely motor nerve, draws its fibers from the C5 through C7 nerve roots. It innervates the serratus anterior.

Clinical Features
A lesion of the long thoracic nerve produces weakness of the serratus anterior, clinically evident as a displacement of the medial edge of the scapula away from the chest, so-called winging of the scapula (Fig. 11.**9**). This is most evident when the patient stretches his arms forward and presses his hands against a wall.

Causes
Many cases are due to *mechanical injury,* to which this nerve, with its long course, is particularly vulnerable. The nerve may be injured in isolation – e.g., in transport workers or persons wearing backpacks. It may also be affected in *neuralgic shoulder amyotrophy* and after *infectious illnesses.*

Axillary Nerve

Anatomy
The axillary nerve, deriving its fibers from the C5 and C6 roots, innervates the deltoid and teres minor muscles. Its sensory innervation is to a small area, the size of the palm of a hand, on the lateral surface of the upper arm.

Clinical Features
Lesions of the axillary nerve impair forward elevation and abduction of the arm (functions of the deltoid) as well as external rotation of the shoulder joint (the function of the teres minor). The lateral portion of the deltoid is often markedly atrophic.

Causes
The most common cause of axillary nerve palsy is (anteroinferior) dislocation of the shoulder. The diagnosis may be missed at first because movement of the shoulder is limited by pain. Sensation should be tested before the dislocation is reduced.

Prognosis
The prognosis is usually good.

Differential Diagnosis
The differential diagnosis includes arthrogenic deltoid atrophy, painful scapulohumeral periarthritis, rotator cuff tear, and muscular dystrophy (which is bilateral).

Suprascapular Nerve

Anatomy
This nerve, composed of fibers from the C4 through C6 roots, passes through the scapular groove to innervate the supraspinatus and infraspinatus muscles.

Clinical Features
Paralysis of the muscles supplied by the suprascapular nerve causes a mild impairment of the initial component of shoulder abduction and a moderate impairment of external rotation of the arm. There is no sensory deficit, but chronic irritation of the nerve may be painful.

Causes
The causes include trauma (shoulder dislocation) and compression of the nerve in the scapular groove – e.g., by a ganglion. In the latter case, neurolysis is indicated.

Musculocutaneous Nerve

Anatomy
This nerve, derived from the C5 through C7 roots, supplies the biceps brachii, the coracobrachialis, and a portion of the brachialis. Its terminal branch is the lateral cutaneous nerve of the forearm, a purely sensory nerve.

Clinical Features
An isolated palsy of the musculocutaneous nerve (which is rare) causes weakness of elbow flexion and supination. The sensory deficit, which is often mild, is on the radial edge of the forearm.

Causes
Trauma is the most common cause of an isolated musculocutaneous nerve palsy, though one may arise spontaneously for no clear reason. Dysfunction of this nerve is usually a component of an upper brachial plexus palsy affecting multiple nerves.

Differential Diagnosis
Palsy must be distinguished from rupture of the long biceps tendon.

Radial Nerve

Anatomy
The radial nerve derives its fibers from the C5 through C8 nerve roots. Early in its course, it gives off a motor branch to the triceps, as well as one or more sensory branches, a posterior brachial cutaneous branch, and sometimes a cutaneous branch to the forearm. It then passes around the shaft of the humerus in the radial groove. At the level of the elbow, it gives off motor branches to the brachioradialis, the extensor carpi radialis longus, and the lateral portion of the brachialis. It then divides, ventral to the lateral humeral condyle, into a sensory superficial branch and a purely motor deep branch to the

extensors of the hand and fingers. The sensory branch innervates on the radial side of the dorsum of the hand, with an autonomous zone over the first interosseous space. The deep motor branch is vulnerable to chronic damage at the point where it passes through the supinator, which it supplies (see below).

Clinical Features

The pattern of sensory and motor deficits depends on the site of the lesion. Lesions of the radial nerve characteristically produce a *hand drop,* reflecting inability to extend the wrist and the metacarpophalangeal joints (Fig. 11.**10**). A pad of edematous tissue is often found on the back of the hand (Gubler's swelling). Very proximal lesions of the nerve paralyze the triceps muscle as well, impairing elbow extension, but the nerve is usually affected lower than this, in its course along the humerus. Sensation is impaired only in a small area on the back of the hand over the first interosseous space.

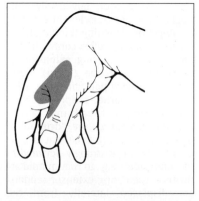

Fig. 11.**10   Typical hand drop in radial nerve palsy.**

Causes of Radial Nerve Palsy

■ Traumatic Palsy

Radial nerve palsy is often a component of *traumatic brachial plexus palsy.* Radial nerve palsy due to a *fracture of the humeral shaft* is by far the most common peripheral nerve injury due to a long bone fracture. This type of injury produces hand drop, brachioradialis weakness, and a sensory deficit on the back of the hand. If paresis or paralysis appears at the moment of injury, only the further course can reveal whether the nerve or its fascicles remain in continuity. Contusion of the nerve is far more common than transection and is generally followed by good spontaneous recovery.

If weakness is present from the moment of injury and fails to improve, operative intervention may be indicated. EMG can be of considerable use in the often difficult decision whether and when to operate. Surgical exploration is clearly indicated if there is no evidence of reinnervation in the brachioradialis or extensor carpi radialis longus 5–6 months after the injury. Earlier exploration may be indicated in individual cases, depending on the severity of the injury, the degree of initial displacement of the bone fragments, etc. Complete rupture of the nerve is rare.

If a radial nerve palsy is not present at first, but then develops 3 or 4 weeks after the fracture, or if an initially incomplete palsy worsens over this interval, it must be assumed that the nerve has become embedded in scar tissue, or even in bony callus. Surgical exploration and neurolysis are indicated and confer a good prognosis.

■ Pressure Palsies

Pressure in the axilla. Chronic pressure on the nerve in the axilla (arm pit) – e.g., crutch palsy – causes hand drop and triceps weakness.

Pressure at mid-humeral level. Radial nerve palsy is most often due to pressure at mid-humeral level, where the nerve winds around the humeral shaft in close apposition to the bone and is thus unusually vulnerable to a pressure injury. Such injuries usually arise during sleep or a drunken stupor. The patient awakens with a wrist drop and, at least initially, a sensory deficit over the first interosseous space on the back of the hand. This condition has been nicknamed "parkbench paralysis," "Saturday night palsy," and rather bluntly, in French, *"la paralysie des ivrognes"* (drunkards' palsy). The prognosis is excellent: spontaneous recovery may begin within a few days and be complete within a few weeks.

Handcuff palsy, cheiralgia paresthetica. *Handcuff palsy* is an isolated sensory deficit on the back of the hand due to pressure around the wrist (from handcuffs, or simply a tight bracelet or wristband). *Cheiralgia paresthetica* is an isolated sensory deficit on the lateral aspect of the distal phalanx of the thumb due to a lesion of the sensory (and usually lateral) superficial branch of the radial nerve, which is a terminal branch. The most common cause is pressure – e.g., from prolonged use of scissors, a painter's palette, etc. The condition is harmless and resolves spontaneously.

■ Compression Syndromes

The radial nerve has little freedom of movement *as it passes through the supinator muscle* and is vulnerable to mechanical injury at this point. The deep branch (dorsal interosseous branch) of the nerve is affected, resulting in a purely motor palsy that slowly worsens over weeks or months, affecting the ulnar finger extensors first and then gradually producing a partial hand drop. The brachioradialis and extensor carpi radialis longus are usually spared. This condition, the *supinator syndrome,* can be caused by a lipoma or neurofibroma but is usually merely the result of chronic mechanical injury in the absence of any other pathology. Surgical exploration is indicated.

■ Differential Diagnosis of Radial Nerve Palsy

Central (cerebral) distal paralysis of the upper limb must first be excluded. In such cases, weakness of the extensor muscles is always accompanied by other motor deficits and by exaggerated reflexes. When a patient with central hand drop powerfully contracts the flexor muscles (in grasping an object or clenching the fist), there is accompanying reflex contraction of the extensors, causing extension of the hand (Wartenberg sign). Hand drop due to *lead poisoning* was mentioned in an earlier chapter (p. 610). Extension of the thumb may be impaired by *tendon rupture* ("drummer's palsy," which is not a palsy at all).
If the fingers are strongly deviated to the ulnar side – e.g., in rheumatoid arthritis – their long extensor tendons are displaced laterally from the digital axis. Thus, when the fingers are flexed, these tendons may slide

around the fingers and come to lie under, rather than over, the finger joints. Contraction of the extensor muscles in this situation only pro-

duces additional flexion. The inability to extend the fingers may falsely suggest a radial nerve palsy.

Median Nerve

Anatomy

The median nerve (C5–T1) arises from the medial and lateral cords of the brachial plexus. At the level of the elbow, it gives off branches that innervate flexor muscles of the forearm (the pronator teres, flexor carpi radialis, palmaris longus, and flexor digitorum superficialis muscles). It then passes through the pronator teres and gives off further branches to the flexor pollicis longus, flexor digitorum profundus (radial portion), and pronator quadratus muscles. At the

wrist, it passes under the flexor retinaculum (= transverse carpal ligament), together with the tendons of the long flexors of the fingers, to reach the palm of the hand. Here, it gives off motor branches to the abductor pollicis brevis and opponens pollicis muscles and to the superficial head of the flexor pollicis brevis. A terminal branch provides sensory innervation to the radial half of the palm, the volar surface of the radial $3^1/2$ fingers, and the dorsal surface of the middle and distal phalanges of the second and third finger and the radial side of the fourth finger (cf. Fig. 1.1 and Table 11.3).

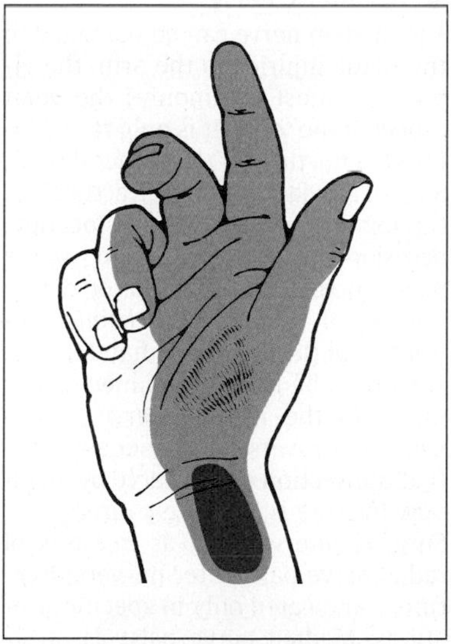

Clinical Features

A high lesion of the median nerve prevents the patient from making a fist, as he can flex only the fingers supplied by the ulnar nerve. The resulting deformity is the so-called "preacher's hand" (Fig. 11.11). This is not seen, however, if the lesion lies distal to the mid-forearm, in which case it only affects the intrinsic muscles of the hand that are supplied by the nerve. Weakness of thumb abduction can be demonstrated by having the patient try to grasp a large tumbler or bottle in his hand; a gap appears between the object and the web between the thumb and index finger ("bottle sign," Fig. 11.12). When the patient tries to approximate the thumb to the little finger, the thumb

Fig. 11.**11** **"Preacher's hand" in median nerve palsy, with thenar atrophy.**

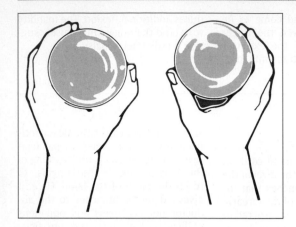

Fig. 11.**12 Bottle sign in right median nerve palsy.**
Inadequate abduction of the right thumb makes the patient unable to grip a round object (= positive bottle sign). The thumb is insufficiently rotated.

is insufficiently pronated, so that its side, rather than its tip, contacts the tip of the little finger or the palm of the hand. The examiner sees the patient's thumbnail tangentially, rather than head-on (Fig. 11.**13**). Atrophy of

Fig. 11.**13 Poor approximation of the thumb and little finger in right median nerve palsy.**
Because the thumb is insufficiently rotated, the fingernail is seen tangentially rather than head-on.

the lateral portion of the thenar eminence is also typical.

Causes of Median Nerve Palsy

■ Traumatic Palsy

The median nerve can be damaged in traumatic injuries to the arm, the elbow, or (most commonly) the volar aspect of the wrist. It is only rarely injured in *fractures of the humeral shaft.* Supracondylar humeral fractures of the extension type, with dislocation, occasionally cause median nerve palsy. In such cases, the later development of *Volkmann's ischemic contracture* of the finger and hand flexors is more to be feared than mechanical injury to the median nerve, which usually recovers spontaneously. Actual transection of the nerve by an elbow fracture is extremely rare.

Surgical intervention, as in cases of radial nerve palsy after humeral fracture, is indicated only in specific situations. Median nerve palsy is rarely due to distal forearm fractures. Any cutting injury to the wrist, however superficial it may appear, should prompt careful examination for signs of median (and ulnar) nerve injury. Sensory deficits are often easier to detect than weakness in the acute setting, because a painful injury may considerably limit movement.

■ Pressure Palsies

The median nerve may be compressed by the weight of the head of the patient's bedmate ("*la paralysie des amoureux,*" lovers' palsy) or iatrogenically by a tourniquet (Esmarch bandage). Both of these types of palsy have a good prognosis. A chronic, occupational pressure injury to the median nerve at the wrist may produce a purely motor deficit with thenar atrophy. A similar picture arises after prolonged bicycle riding (cyclist's palsy, p. 778).

■ Carpal Tunnel Syndrome

Anatomy

The median nerve can be compressed in the carpal tunnel – i.e., as it passes under the flexor retinaculum (transverse carpal ligament) into the hand, accompanied by the tendons of the long finger flexors and their sheaths.

Pathogenesis

Chronic compression of the nerve at this anatomical bottleneck is the decisive factor. In some cases, an old, healed wrist fracture or arthrosis involving the carpal bones may contribute to the generation of the syndrome. Hypothyroidism, amyloidosis, gout, and diabetes mellitus, and the presence of an artificial arteriovenous fistula for nephrodialysis are further predisposing conditions. Most of the time, however, the syndrome arises without any other underlying pathology.

Clinical Features

Women are much more commonly affected than men, often at the menopause, and sometimes during or immediately after pregnancy. Rare cases arise after rapid, marked weight gain. The disturbances are purely *subjective* at first, and many patients may not develop objective signs till years later, if ever. The classic clinical picture is that of a more or less pure, nocturnal *brachialgia paresthetica,* which is by no means pathognomonic of carpal tunnel syndrome, but is caused by it in the vast majority of cases.

The patient is awakened from sleep by the feeling that one hand (sometimes both) is numb and swollen. Finger movements are difficult and clumsy, and pain may affect the entire upper limb, sometimes ascending even into the shoulder and neck. Shaking or massaging the hands brings temporary relief, enabling the patient to go back to sleep for a short time, until she is reawakened by the same symptoms. In the morning, the first activities of the day are often made difficult by stiffness and clumsiness of the fingers. Painful episodes may occur during the day as well, less frequently and in milder form than the nocturnal episodes. On specific questioning, some but not all patients clearly describe involvement of the thumb and middle three fingers. Strenuous physical activity, such as washing clothes or housework, or certain postures, such as gripping the steering wheel during prolonged driving, can also bring on the symptoms.

The brachialgia and the objective deficits usually begin in the dominant hand, but tend to appear sooner or later in the other hand as well.

Physical Examination

There are usually no objective findings in the early stage of the condition, though pain may be elicited by pressure on the median nerve trunk in the carpal tunnel. Weakness and atrophy of the thenar muscles, with or without a sensory deficit, may not be seen until nerve compression has been present for several years. Occasionally there is isolated sensory loss without weakness, but weakness of thumb adduction and a positive bottle sign (see Fig. 11.**12**) are usually readily demonstrable.

The typical symptoms of carpal tunnel syndrome can be brought on during the examination by *provocative testing* with forced extension or flexion of the wrist for about 1 minute (Phalen test). Tapping of the volar surface of the wrist over the carpal tunnel may evoke electrical paresthesia in the thumb or index finger (Tinel test).

Ancillary Tests

Electroneurography reveals a prolonged distal motor latency in the median nerve, as well as slowing of the distal motor and orthodromic or antidromic sensory conduction velocities.

> ### Treatment
>
> In the stage of nocturnal brachialgia paresthetica with mild or minimal objective deficits, the condition is often satisfactorily treated by resting the wrist at night with a well-padded volar splint. If this is ineffective, or if a distressing deficit is present, *surgical division of the* flexor retinaculum (carpal tunnel release) is the treatment of choice. Marked thenar atrophy, if present, is often irreversible, but the sensory disturbances respond well to surgical treatment. In particular, the nocturnal pains usually disappear at once.
>
> Milder cases can be treated by injection of 1 mL of corticosteroid into the carpal tunnel. Relief ensues in two-thirds of patients, but persists for a year or more in only one-quarter.

Other Median Nerve Compression Syndromes

■ Supracondylar Process of the Humerus

The median nerve trunk is closely apposed to this bony spur, present in about 1% of persons, that projects from the humeral shaft about a hand's breadth above the medial epicondyle. The ligament of Strutter runs from this process, over the nerve, to the ulnar epicondyle. Symptomatic nerve compression occasionally results.

■ Pronator Teres Syndrome

The median nerve is susceptible to chronic mechanical injury at the site in the forearm where the median nerve passes under this muscle, particularly if the patient engages in certain types of activity involving prolonged extension of the upper limb. The syndrome is characterized by paresthesiae of the radial fingers as well as tenderness to pressure over the pronator teres muscle.

■ Anterior Interosseous Nerve Syndrome (Kiloh-Nevin Syndrome)

Anatomy

This purely motor branch of the median nerve in the forearm innervates the flexor pollicis longus, the flexor digitorum profundus (second and third fingers), and the pronator teres.

Pathogenesis

The anterior interosseous nerve can be injured by a forearm fracture, but the syndrome is more often due to other local causes; almost half of all cases are spontaneous, among them those due to compression by a fibrous band.

Clinical Features

There is weakness of flexion of the interphalangeal joint of the thumb and the distal interphalangeal joint of the index finger, so that the patient cannot form a ring with these two fingers.

Treatment

Surgical exploration is advisable in post-traumatic or rapidly progressive cases. Other cases usually resolve spontaneously.

■ Rarer Causes of Median Nerve Palsy

An artificial arteriovenous fistula created to facilitate nephrodialysis may cause ischemic neuropathy distal to it, mainly in the median nerve.

■ Differential Diagnosis

Median nerve palsy must be distinguished from lower brachial plexus palsy and C8 or T1 nerve root processes, as these conditions, too, can produce thenar atrophy. The different patterns of sensory loss usually point to the correct diagnosis. Central astereognosis, due to a lesion in the cerebral cortex or cervical spinal cord, can also mimic a peripheral sensory deficit involving the thumb, index, and middle finger.

Ulnar Nerve

Anatomy

The ulnar nerve emerges from the lower brachial plexus, deriving its fibers from the C8 and T1 nerve roots. Its first muscular branches arise below the elbow to supply the flexor carpi ulnaris and the ulnar portion of the flexor digitorum profundus. It gives off only one, dorsal branch in the forearm, which provides sensory innervation to the ulnar side of the back of the hand. It divides terminally at the wrist, giving off a deep motor and a superficial sensory branch. The former innervates all of the interossei and lumbricals on the ulnar side, which are the most important muscles for fine movements of the fingers. The latter provides sensory innervation to the ulnar side of the palm and ulnar $1^{1}/_{2}$ fingers, as well as motor innervation to a single, minor muscle, the palmaris brevis (cf. Fig. 1.**1a**).

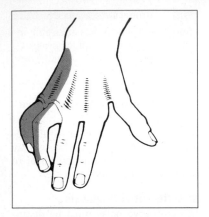

Fig. 11.**14 Typical claw hand in ulnar nerve palsy.** Atrophy of the interossei; hyperextension of the metacarpophalangeal joints and flexion of the interphalangeal joints, particularly in the fourth and fifth fingers; hyperextension of the metacarpophalangeal joint of the thumb ("signe de Jeanne").

The function of the flexor carpi ulnaris can be tested by observing and palpating its tendon during flexion and extension of the wrist. The ulnar portion of the flexor digitorum profundus is the only muscle that flexes the distal interphalangeal joint of the little finger. The palmaris brevis causes dimpling of the skin on the proximal portion of the hypothenar eminence when the little finger is abducted.

Clinical Features

Paralysis of the interossei dominates the clinical picture, producing hyperextension of the fourth and fifth fingers at the metacarpophalangeal joints, and mild flexion of the interphalangeal joints *("claw hand,"* Fig. 11.**14**). The fourth and fifth fingers are abducted. Incomplete finger abduction and adduction are still possible through the respective actions of the long extensor and long flexor muscles. *Froment's sign* indicates weakness of the adductor pollicis muscle: a flat object can be firmly grasped between the thumb and index finger only with the aid of the flexor pollicis longus muscle (median nerve), which flexes the thumb at its interphalangeal joint (Fig. 11.**15**). The area of sensory loss is always sharply bounded by the midline of the 4th finger. Muscle atrophy is most obvious on the dorsal aspect of the hand between the thumb and index finger.

Causes of Ulnar Nerve Palsy

Ulnar nerve palsy is the most common peripheral nerve palsy, both as a result of trauma and as a nontraumatic event. The lesion is usually at the elbow, less commonly at the wrist.

■ Traumatic Palsy

Direct trauma – e.g., from a blow, knife wound, or glass fragments – presents no diagnostic problem. The wrist is the most common site. Primary ulnar nerve palsy rarely occurs in *elbow fractures* (usually of the medial condyle).

■ Delayed Palsy

Ulnar nerve palsy may develop insidiously, becoming evident only months, years, or even decades after an elbow injury (fracture, dislocation, other). Most of the affected patients are adults, and most will recall the original elbow injury when asked specifically about it. Often, but not always, the cause is a healed lateral condylar fracture, and examination of the elbow reveals a vagus deformity.

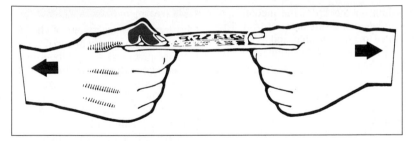

Fig. 11.**15   Froment sign in right ulnar nerve palsy.** On the right side, the patient can only grip the paper by contracting the flexor pollicis longus (innervated by the median nerve), because the adductor pollicis is paralyzed.

Palpation in the ulnar groove behind the medial epicondyle may yield the typical finding of an abnormally immobile, thickened, and sometimes painful nerve; it may, however, be embedded in connective tissue so that it cannot be readily felt. The forearm muscles are far less severely affected than the hand muscles; the first interosseous muscle is usually markedly atrophic. The sensory deficit is often very mild.

■ Chronic Pressure Injury at the Ulnar Groove

Chronic pressure injuries of the ulnar nerve are often misdiagnosed. Some 80% occur at the ulnar groove on the medial aspect of the elbow, where the nerve lies exposed and closely apposed to the underlying bone. *Pressure palsy* at this site, caused by prolonged resting of the elbow on a hard surface, is common. The patient may not, at first, realize what specific activity brought on the problem; this may be discoverable only by thorough, direct questioning. Most injuries are occupational (telephone operators, precision grinders) or due to

habitual postures. In *bedridden patients,* even the light pressure of the elbows on the bedclothes can cause ulnar nerve palsy, which may appear suddenly, and not necessarily only in cachectic or gravely ill persons. The neurologic deficit may be wrongly attributed to a surgical or other therapeutic procedure. It is more commonly found on the side nearer the patient's bedside table.

Prognosis

The prognosis of pure pressure palsies is good.

■ Treatment

Treatment consists solely in preventing further nerve damage. Anterior transposition of the ulnar nerve is seldom indicated.

Anomalies at the Ulnar Groove

■ Ulnar Nerve Dislocation

This congenital anomaly is found in 5% of persons, nearly always on both sides. When the elbow is flexed, the nerve slides out of the ulnar groove, riding on the tip of the medial epi-condyle or passing anterior to it. The nerve may be visible and is always palpable on careful examination. The examiner sits opposite the patient and palpates the right ulnar groove with his right index and middle fingers while the elbow joint is flexed and extended. The continually repeated dislocation of the nerve as the patient flexes and extends the elbow in the course of everyday activities suffices to cause permanent injury.

■ **Excessive Elbow Movement**

Even in the absence of ulnar nerve dislocation, excessive movement about the elbow joint can cause cumulative, chronic trauma to the nerve as it passes between the bones, ligaments, and medial head of the triceps. Pain, paresthesiae, and weakness can result – e.g., in drilling and die-cutting workers.

> **Treatment**
>
> Recovery can be promoted by the prevention of excessive movement, including perhaps a change of occupation, and deliberate avoidance of elbow flexion, combined with local measures such as soft padding of the medial side of the elbow. Surgery is hardly ever indicated.

■ **Degenerative Processes at the Elbow**

Arthrosis can chronically damage the ulnar nerve, producing the clinical picture described above for delayed palsies. The same is true of *chondromatosis* and *ganglion cysts* of the elbow joint.

> **Treatment**
>
> Surgery is the treatment of choice for ulnar nerve palsy due to degenerative processes at the elbow, and should be performed at the earliest opportunity to prevent progression. The ulnar nerve should be transposed to the anterior surface of the joint beneath the origin of the ulnar flexor group. Timely surgery confers a good prognosis.

Chronic Pressure Injury at the Wrist

Clinical Features

Chronic pressure injury to the ulnar nerve at the wrist often does not involve its superficial palmar (sensory) branch. The associated, purely motor weakness may also spare the hypothenar muscles, leading to difficulties in differential diagnosis, as a purely motor deficit with atrophy of the intrinsic muscles of the hand immediately raises the suspicion of spinal muscular atrophy. The diagnostic importance of the preservation of palmaris brevis function has already been pointed out. If the hypothenar muscles are spared, the little finger is held in an abducted position. In advanced cases, the contrast between the severely atrophic first dorsal interosseous muscle (between the thumb and the index finger) and the virtually normal hypothenar muscles is the most important clue to the correct diagnosis.

Causes

This condition is an occupational hazard of workers using *tools* such as knives, woodworking tools, sledgehammers, pneumatic drills, etc. *Cy-*

clist's palsy is also due to pressure on the ulnar nerve at the wrist (a median nerve injury may be present as well). Ulnar palsy is occasionally a late complication of *scarring* after traumatic injury to the hypothenar soft tissues or an infection (phlegmon) involving the palmar aponeurosis. Other causes are a *wrist ganglion* or a gouty tophus. In rare cases, chronic mechanical injury to the ulnar nerve may occur in the absence of any external factors as it passes through the narrow space between the pisiform bone and the hook of the hamate bone, the so-called *loge de Guyon*.

Differential Diagnosis

Ulnar palsy must be carefully distinguished from lower brachial plexus palsy and lesions affecting the medial cord of the plexus or the C8 and T1 roots. A distal, purely motor deficit caused by isolated involvement of the deep branch may be misdiagnosed as spinal muscular atrophy. In Dupuytren's contracture, flexion of the 4th and 5th fingers is always accompanied by the characteristic skin changes and thickening of the palmar aponeurosis; the metacarpophalangeal joints are not hyperextended, as they always are when the interossei are paralyzed. Nonetheless, Dupuytren's contracture is often seen in association with ulnar nerve dislocation at the ulnar groove, and there may be a causal connection between these two conditions. The same is true of camptodactyly and clinodactyly, two rare deformities of the little finger.

The appearance of paralysis is sometimes created by locking of the fingers in a specific position for purely mechanical reasons. For example, the cause may be an abnormality of the lateral attachment of the extensor tendon on the posterior surface of the metacarpophalangeal or interphalangeal joint, as in rheumatoid arthritis (discussed above under the differential diagnosis of radial nerve palsy). Conditions causing abnormal laxity of connective tissue can create a similar problem.

Treatment

The treatment of such conditions depends on their etiology. In all cases, *further pressure damage is to be prevented* by eliminating the responsible mechanism. If, for some reason, the causative activity cannot be discontinued, the volar surface of the wrist should be heavily padded. *Surgical exploration* is indicated in exceptional cases – e.g., for neurolysis or excision of a ganglion.

Lumbosacral Plexus

Anatomy
The lumbosacral plexus is formed by the L1–S3 nerve roots. It lies in the retroperitoneal space, well protected from exogenous injury. It gives rise to the following:

- the superior gluteal nerve, which emerges through the suprapiriform foramen;
- the inferior gluteal nerve and the sciatic nerve, both of which emerge through the infrapiriform foramen;
- the obturator nerve, which exits the pelvis through the obturator foramen; and
- the femoral nerve, which exits the pelvis between muscle heads under the inguinal ligament.

Clinical Features
Lesions of the lumbosacral plexus cause highly varied patterns of paralysis, depending on the portion of the plexus that is affected. Clinical features of plexus lesions and of peripheral nerve lesions in the lower limb are presented in Table 11.4.

Causes of Lumbosacral Plexus Palsies
The lumbosacral plexus is most commonly affected by a *retroperitoneal mass* (metastatic tumor, lymphoma, endometriosis, or local malignancy, particularly of the rectum, urogenital tract, or female reproductive tract). It can also be affected by a hematoma (see below) or aneurysm, or by *radiotherapy* or intra-arterial chemotherapy. *Chronic progressive lumbosacral plexopathy* is a disorder of the lumbosacral plexus that is analogous to neuralgic shoulder amyotrophy affecting the brachial plexus (977). It is characterized by the acute onset of usually unilateral pain and neurologic deficits that tend to improve spontaneously within several months but may require treatment with cortisone or intravenous immunoglobulins. For intermittent claudication of the lumbosacral plexus, see p. 847.

Diagnostic Evaluation
Ultrasonography, CT, MRI, and electrophysiologic studies are very helpful.

Genitofemoral and Ilioinguinal Nerves

Anatomy
These two mainly sensory nerves arise from the L1 and L2 segments. Their cutaneous distributions in the inguinal and genital areas are shown in Fig. 1.1.

Clinical Features
Lesions of these nerves produce a *sensory deficit* in their cutaneous distribution in the groin, the upper medial aspect of the thigh, and the scrotum or labium majus. The cremasteric reflex is absent. A partial paralysis of the abdominal muscles is present but may not be clinically detectable. These nerves can also be the site of origin of very painful syndromes, such as *genitofemoral neuralgia*. Ilioinguinal nerve lesions cause severe

Table 11.**4** Lesions of the lumbosacral plexus and the nerves of the lower limb

Nerve	Muscle involved	Sensory deficit	Function	Special tests	Etiology	Remarks	Differential diagnosis
Lumbar plexus L1–L4	Hip flexors and rotators, thigh adductors, knee extensors	1 Iliohypogastric nerve 2 Posterior femoral cutaneous nerve 3 Lateral femoral cutaneous nerve 4 Obturator nerve 5 Ilioinguinal nerve	See individual muscles		Trauma, retroperitoneal processes (tumor, hematoma), squatting position, diabetes mellitus		
Sacral plexus L5–S3	Glutei, hamstrings, dorsiflexors and plantar flexors of foot and toes		See individual muscles		Pelvic tumors, pregnancy, childbirth, surgery		Multiple root lesions, cauda equina syndrome, pelvic arterial occlusion

(Cont.) →

Table 11.4 (Cont.)

Nerve	Muscle involved	Sensory deficit	Function	Special tests	Etiology	Remarks	Differential diagnosis
Femoral nerve L2–L4	Iliacus Pectineus		Hip flexion and internal rotation	Test with patient seated and legs dangling	Surgery, trauma, hyperextension of hip, hemophilia		High lumbar disk herniation, progressive muscular dystrophy (isolated involvement of thigh), muscle atrophy due to knee joint disease, femoral form of diabetic neuropathy
	Sartorius	**6 Saphenous nerve** **7 anterior cutaneous branch of femoral nerve**	Hip flexion, adduction, and external rotation				
	Quadriceps femoris		Knee extension (and hip flexion)				
Obturator nerve L2–L4	Obturator externus Pectineus Adductor brevis		Thigh adduction and external rotation				

(Cont.) →

Table **11.4** (Cont.)

Nerve	Muscle involved	Sensory deficit	Function	Special tests	Etiology	Remarks	Differential diagnosis
	Adductor longus Adductor magnus		Thigh adduction				
	Gracilis		Thigh adduction and internal rotation, knee flexion				
Lateral femoral cutaneous nerve L2–L3	None		Purely sensory	Tenderness just medial to anterior superior iliac spine, pain on hyperextension of the hip	Chronic mechanical injury at point of emergence from inguinal ligament	Meralgia paresthetica	High lumbar disk herniation
Ilioinguinal nerve L1(–L2)	None		Mainly sensory	Hyperextension of the hip	Chronic mechanical injury at point of emergence from abdominal wall musculature		Hip disease

(Cont.) →

Table 11.4   (Cont.)

Nerve	Muscle involved	Sensory deficit	Function	Special tests	Etiology	Remarks	Differential diagnosis
Superior gluteal nerve L4–S1	Gluteus medius, gluteus minimus		Internal rotation of the slightly flexed hip; hip abduction	Leg abduction in the lateral decubitus position, pelvic tilt downward to opposite side on walking (Trendelenburg sign)	Trauma, esp. iatrogenic due to incorrectly placed intramuscular injection		Pelvic girdle form of progressive muscular dystrophy
	Tensor fasciae latae		Hip abduction				
Inferior gluteal nerve L5–S2	Gluteus maximus	8 Sural nerve 9 Tibial nerve 10 Lateral plantar nerve 11 Medial plantar nerve	Hip extension	Lifting thigh from examining table in prone position with knee flexed to 90°			Muscular dystrophy
Tibial nerve L4–S3	Gastrocnemius, soleus, plantaris		Plantar flexion (and knee flexion)	First 15° of knee flexion	Trauma in popliteal fossa, trauma to sciatic nerve (may present with tibial nerve findings only)		L5–S1 disk herniation

(Cont.) →

Table 11.4 (Cont.)

Nerve	Muscle involved	Sensory deficit	Function	Special tests	Etiology	Remarks	Differential diagnosis
	Popliteus		Knee flexion	Knee flexed to 90°			
	Tibialis posterior		Supination and plantar flexion of the foot	Toes should not be flexed			
	Flexor digitorum longus		Flexion at distal interphalangeal joints				
	Flexor hallucis longus						
	Flexor digitorum brevis		Flexion at proximal interphalangeal joints				
	Flexor hallucis brevis						
	Abductor digiti minimi						
	Adductor hallucis						
	Quadratus plantaris						
	Lumbricals						
	Interossei						

(Cont.) →

Table 11.4   (Cont.)

Nerve	Muscle involved	Sensory deficit	Function	Special tests	Etiology	Remarks	Differential diagnosis
Common peroneal nerve L4–S2	Tibialis anterior	12 Common peroneal nerve / 13 Superficial peroneal nerve / 14 Sural nerve / 15 Deep peroneal nerve	Dorsiflexion of foot				
	Extensor digitorum longus Extensor hallucis longus		Extension at distal interphalangeal joints, dorsiflexion of foot	Heel walk	Direct trauma, fibular fracture		
Deep peroneal nerve	Peroneus tertius extensor digitorum brevis		Extension at metacarpophalangeal joints	Steppage gait	Pressure palsy	Good prognosis	L4/L5 disk herniation, other root lesions, polyneuropathy, peroneal muscular atrophy, distal muscular atrophy in myopathy (Steinert), tibialis anterior syndrome
	Extensor hallucis brevis		Eversion and plantar flexion of foot				
Superficial peroneal nerve	Peroneus longus						
	Peroneus brevis						

pain in the groin when the patient is erect and thus force the patient into an antalgic position, with slight flexion and rotation of the hip, whether the patient is standing or lying down *(ilioinguinal syndrome).*

Causes

These syndromes are usually caused by surgical injury to the nerves, either through direct trauma or through postoperative scarring (e.g., after inguinal hernia repair, nephrectomy, or

retrocecal appendectomy). The ilioinguinal nerve can also be chronically compressed where it passes through the abdominal wall musculature, even without additional trauma.

Treatment

These conditions are treated by neurolysis or resection of the nerve proximal to the site of compression.

Femoral Nerve

Anatomy

This nerve derives its fibers from the L2 through L4 roots. As it arises from the lumbar plexus, it passes between the iliacus (which it innervates) and the psoas, and then leaves the pelvis with the latter muscle as it passes under the inguinal ligament. It innervates the quadriceps femoris muscle and provides sensory innervation to the anterior aspect of the thigh and the ventromedial aspect of the calf (saphenous nerve).

Clinical Features

Femoral nerve lesions cause paralysis of all knee extensors, making it impossible for the patient to climb stairs, and diminishing or abolishing the knee-jerk reflex. Hip flexion, too, is weak, because part of the quadriceps also serves to flex the hip, and it is even weaker if the lesion lies within the pelvis, compromising the innervation of the iliacus as well. A sensory deficit is found on the anterior aspect of the thigh and the ventromedial aspect of the calf (saphenous nerve distribution).

Causes

The femoral nerve can be damaged in its intra-abdominal course under the inguinal ligament by a *psoas hematoma* or by *surgical trauma* (appendectomy, hernia repair, hysterectomy). Sudden hyperextension of the hip is a rare cause of injury to the femoral nerve; the prognosis for recovery in such cases is poor. Femoral nerve palsy is common in persons who suffer from a bleeding tendency. Isolated damage to the *saphenous nerve* from chronic compression at the site of its *passage through the crural fascia* causes pain and a sensory deficit on the anteromedial aspect of the calf. Neuropathia patellae is discussed on p. 844. Involvement of a peripheral sensory terminal branch in a bodybuilder is a rare event (736a).

Differential Diagnosis

Quadriceps weakness, the most prominent sign of femoral nerve palsy, may also be due to L3 or L4 *radiculopathy,* which is usually the consequence of a centrolateral L2-3 or L3-4 disk herniation, or, less commonly, a lateral

L3–4 or L4–5 disk herniation. Clues to the diagnosis of disk herniation include the accompanying back pain (usually present), radicular pattern of weakness affecting other muscles beside those supplied by the femoral nerve, dermatomal pattern of sensory loss, and corresponding anatomical findings on plain radiographs, CT, and MRI. Monoradicular quadriceps weakness never completely abolishes the knee-jerk reflex. An isolated (bilateral) atrophy and purely motor weakness of the thigh extensors is, in rare cases, due to *myopathy of old age. Proximal diabetic neuropathy* can cause (unilateral) femoral nerve palsy. Inactivity and knee lesions can lead to "arthritic muscle atrophy" in the thigh.

Visible wasting of the anterior aspect of the thigh is not always due to muscle atrophy; the pathological change may rather lie in the subcutaneous fat. *Lipoid atrophy* develops in diabetics who inject themselves with insulin. Horizontal bands of atrophy of the subcutaneous fat *(lipoatrophia semicircularis)* were once commonly seen in washerwomen and are nowadays found in persons, still mainly women, who habitually lean the upper thigh against the edge of a table or similar object.

Lateral Femoral Cutaneous Nerve (Meralgia Paresthetica)

Anatomy

The lateral femoral cutaneous nerve (L2–L3) is purely sensory. It exits the pelvis just medial to the anterior superior iliac spine between the fibers of the inguinal ligament – i.e., between the fibers of the thickened lower end of the external oblique aponeurosis. It is tightly enclosed by these fibers at this point, where it also makes a 90° turn from a horizontal course within the pelvis to a vertical course down the thigh. In phylogenetic terms, the turn is necessitated by the upright human stance.

Clinical Features

An acute lesion of this purely sensory nerve causes a sensory deficit on the anterolateral aspect of the thigh. Chronic lesions, however, are more common and lead to the syndrome of *meralgia paresthetica,* which consists of paresthesiae and aching, sometimes burning pain in the cutaneous distribution of the nerve. The symptoms are almost always exacerbated by hip extension, which stretches the nerve ("reverse Lasègue sign"), and alleviated by flexion – e.g., when the foot is elevated. The syndrome affects men roughly three times more commonly than women and is bilateral in ca. 10 % of cases.

The paresthetic phase is often followed by permanent hypesthesia or anesthesia and analgesia in the distribution of the nerve (Fig. 1.1). Cases with an intermittent course are not uncommon. The site where the nerve penetrates the inguinal ligament, two finger-breadths medial to the anterior superior iliac spine, is tender in three-quarters of cases. Spontaneous remission occurs in only about one-quarter of cases.

Causes

The nerve can be *directly injured* where it traverses the inguinal ligament, sometimes iatrogenically during hip surgery or harvesting of a bone graft from the pelvis. Chronic mechanical injury, due to compression at this site, is much more common. The anatomical relationships described above play a major role in pathogenesis, but other factors often contribute as well. The leading ones are tight clothing or belts, abnormal fat distribution (paunch), habitual vigorous contraction of the abdominal muscles attaching to the inguinal ligament (internal and external oblique and transversus abdominis muscles; pregnancy, military marching, heavy exertion, gait abnormalities due to musculoskeletal disease, etc.), and unusually long maintenance of the hip joint in hyperextension (positioning of an immobilized patient, sleeping on the floor, etc.). Chronic injury of the nerve causes meralgia paresthetica.

Differential Diagnosis

A *high lumbar disk herniation* is the leading element in the differential diagnosis but usually causes a clearly distinct clinical syndrome, including back pain, a differently distributed sensory deficit, and perhaps a detectable motor deficit as well. In meralgia paresthetica, but not in lumbar radiculopathy, the sensory deficit is entirely lateral to the midline of the thigh.

Treatment

The symptoms of meralgia paresthetica are usually only mildly distressing, and only rarely severe enough to require intervention. The contributing factors listed above should be eliminated. *Hydrocortisone injections,* or a *neurolysis* at the point where the nerve penetrates the inguinal ligament, can be performed but is rarely necessary.

Obturator Nerve

Anatomy

This nerve, which derives its fibers from the L2–L4 roots, exits the pelvis through the obturator foramen. It innervates the adductor muscles of the thigh and provides cutaneous sensory innervation to the distal portion of the medial aspect of the thigh.

Clinical Features

Obturator nerve palsy produces weakness of thigh adduction, impairment of the adductor reflex, and a sensory deficit in the area described above. Chronic irritation of the nerve can produce a painful syndrome at the medial aspect of the knee (Howship-Romberg phenomenon). EMG is required to distinguish the latter from primary pathology of the knee itself.

Causes

Pelvic fracture, tumor, and obturator hernia are the common causes of obturator nerve palsy.

Gluteal Nerves

Anatomy

The *superior gluteal nerve* is derived from the L4–S1 roots and supplies the hip abductors (gluteus medius and minimus) and the tensor fasciae latae. It exits from the pelvis through the suprapiriform portion of the sciatic foramen (also called the suprapiriform foramen). The *inferior gluteal nerve* (L5–S2) innervates the gluteus maximus, the most important exten-

sor of the hip. It exits from the pelvis through the infrapiriform portion of the sciatic foramen.

Clinical Features

Weakness of the hip abductors causes the pelvis to tilt downward on the affected side when the patient walks (*Trendelenburg sign*). If the weakness is only partial, the pelvic tilt can be compensated for by lateral bending of the trunk away from the affected side

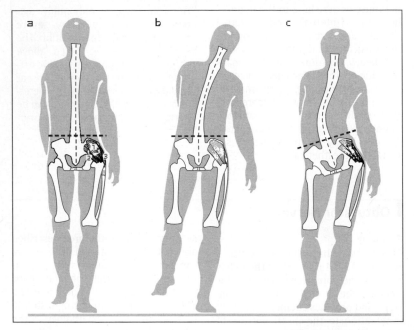

Fig. 11.**16a–c   Degrees of gait impairment due to weakness of right hip abductors.**

a Normal configuration.
1 Gluteus medius
2 Gluteus minimus
3 Tensor fasciae latae

b In *mild* abductor weakness, the trunk is bent to the side of weakness to displace its center of gravity and thus prevent tilting of the pelvis toward the normal side (Duchenne sign).

c In *severe* abductor weakness, trunk bending is insufficient to overcome the pelvic tilt toward the normal side, which is now evident (Trendelenburg sign).

(*Duchenne phenomenon*) (Fig. 11.**16**). Loss of function of the gluteus maximus impairs hip extension, so that the patient has difficulty ascending a staircase or climbing onto a chair.

Causes

Gluteal nerve palsy may result from direct trauma to the nerve(s), an injury during delivery, or a misplaced intragluteal injection (injection palsies, see below).

Differential Diagnosis

A *radicular lesion* (e.g., a lumbar disk herniation causing S1 syndrome) can produce partial weakness of the glutei (in this case, the gluteus maximus). Furthermore, involvement of the pelvic girdle should prompt suspicion of *progressive muscular dystrophy,* as well as of (congenital) *hip dislocation* with its characteristic waddling gait.

Sciatic Nerve

Anatomy

The sciatic nerve (L4–S3) is the longest and thickest peripheral nerve in the body. It is composed of fibers from all portions of the lumbosacral plexus and leaves the pelvis through the infrapiriform portion of the sciatic foramen. The motor branches to the knee flexors and the posterior femoral cutaneous nerve (a sensory nerve) branch off the nerve trunk in the proximal portion of the thigh. At a level that varies between individuals, but no lower than the point where it enters the popliteal fossa, the sciatic nerve divides into its terminal branches, the tibial and common peroneal nerves. The nerve fibers belonging to these two branches are, however, entirely separate from each other within the sciatic nerve at a much higher level, and a clear morphologic differentiation between them is often already visible where the nerve comes out of the sciatic foramen. In the thigh, the *tibial portion* gives off branches to the semitendinosus and semimembranosus, the long head of the biceps femoris, and a portion of the adductor magnus,

while the *common peroneal portion* gives off muscular branches to the short head of the biceps and articular branches to the knee joint.

Thus, the sciatic nerve provides *motor* innervation to the ischiocrural musculature as well as all muscles of the calf and foot, and cutaneous *sensory* innervation to a large portion of the lateral and dorsal surfaces of the calf and all of the foot, with the exception of the medial malleolar region and a small strip on the medial edge of the foot, which are innervated by the saphenous nerve.

Clinical Features

Sciatic nerve lesions causes varying combinations of the manifestations of tibial and common peroneal nerve palsies (see below). High (proximal) injuries of the nerve can also cause weakness of the knee flexors and impair the reflexes they mediate (cf. Tables 10.**4**, 10.**5**, and 11.**4**).

Causes

The more common causes of injury to the sciatic nerve are *penetrating trauma* (stab or gunshot wound), *pel-*

vic fractures (especially fracture-dislocations with acetabular separation), and *dislocation of the hip*. We have seen *pressure palsies* in extremely thin individuals and in persons who were unconscious for long periods. *Ischemic injury* of the sciatic nerve may be caused by atherosclerosis, abdominal aortic occlusion (Leriche syndrome), or arteritis. Iatrogenic injury by intragluteal injection will be described below (injection palsy, p. 793).

Common Peroneal Nerve

Anatomy

This nerve, which derives its fibers from L4 through S2, emerges from the popliteal fossa and winds laterally just distal to the head of the fibula. It lies directly apposed to the bone at this point and divides here into the *superficial* and *deep peroneal nerves*. The former provides motor innervation to the peroneus muscles, weakness of which impairs elevation of the lateral edge of the foot, and cutaneous sensory innervation to the lateral edge and most of the dorsum of the foot. The latter provides motor innervation to the muscles of the anterior compartment of the leg – i.e., the tibialis anterior, extensor digitorum longus, and extensor hallucis longus – and, through its terminal branch on the dorsum of the foot, to the extensor digitorum brevis and extensor hallucis brevis. Its only autonomous sensory area is a small zone on the dorsum of the foot over the first interosseous space.

Clinical Features

Common peroneal nerve palsy is one of the more frequent peripheral nerve palsies. The characteristic clinical feature of a common (or deep) peroneal nerve palsy is *steppage gait:* unable to dorsiflex the foot and toes, the patient has a foot drop and must there-fore raise the affected foot high in the air with each step so that the tips of the toes clear the ground. If the superficial peroneal nerve is involved as well, the lateral edge of the foot sinks down with each step also; this is easily observed from behind.

Causes

■ Traumatic Palsy

Fracture of the fibular head is not uncommonly accompanied by a peroneal nerve palsy. *Knee dislocation* can injure the nerve, often severely. A *false step* that sprains the ankle joint can suddenly stretch the peroneal nerve as well, causing acute weakness.

■ Pressure Palsy

The most common type of pressure palsy occurs at the *fibular head*. The legs-crossed posture, improper positioning of an unconscious, immobile, or anesthetized patient, pressure from a cast, and certain types of activity in the kneeling position can cause a pressure palsy at this site. Thin individuals are at higher risk. The prognosis for recovery is good.

A *ganglion* of the tibiofibular joint can chronically damage the common peroneal nerve. We have seen several cases of pressure palsies of cutaneous branches on the *dorsum of the foot* caused by excessively tight shoes (usually mountain hiking or ski boots), with resulting dysesthesia and hypesthesia. Hypesthesia of the *medial portion of the distal phalanx of the great toe* results from the pressure of a rigid shoe in the presence of either hallux valgus or an osteophytic change of the unguicular process. A painful syndrome of the sciatic nerve, the piriformis syndrome, will be described below (p. 843).

■ Injection Palsies

Pathologic Anatomy

Injections improperly placed into or in the vicinity of a nerve cause an intense foreign body reaction around the nerve, leading to dense fibrosis which may penetrate between the nerve fascicles.

Clinical Features

Weakness develops immediately after injection in about two-thirds of patients, while only one-sixth have immediate pain. In about 10% of cases, the weakness develops only after an interval of hours or even days. The weakness is at its worst 24–48 hours after its onset. A causalgia-like pain syndrome may develop and dominate the clinical picture.

Causes

Injection palsies are most often due to injections into or near the sciatic nerve (less commonly, the gluteal nerves). They usually cause paresis in the muscles supplied by the common peroneal nerve (lateral half of the sciatic trunk) and are therefore discussed in this section.

The occurrence of an injection palsy is largely determined by the site of injection rather than by the substance injected, as many different substances can produce harm in this way. In general, intramuscular injections should be avoided unless absolutely necessary.

Differential Diagnosis

An injection into a gluteal artery can cause *Nicolau syndrome,* in which part of the gluteal musculature becomes discolored (blue) and may become necrotic.

Prophylactic Measures: Proper Injection Technique

Intragluteal injections should be carried out exclusively in the upper outer quadrant of the buttock, and with the needle perpendicular to the body surface, rather than pointing dorsomedially or caudally. If, on insertion of the needle or on injection, the patient complains of shooting, shock-like pain, or even of pain that radiates only to the periphery, the needle should be immediately withdrawn and the injection performed correctly on the other side.

Treatment

If an injection palsy occurs, prompt *surgical exploration* is indicated to remove all pockets of injection fluid from the nerve trunk and its vicinity, and for lysis of any adhesions that may be present.

General Differential Diagnosis of Peroneal Nerve Lesions

Syndromes resembling peroneal nerve palsy have many causes. First among these is *L4–5 intervertebral disk herniation with L5 root compression,* which leads to marked weakness of dorsiflexion of the great toe, and often to sensory loss on the dorsum of the foot (mimicking a peroneal nerve palsy). The sensory loss usually extends far up the limb in the L5 dermatome; this, together with back pain, points to the correct diagnosis.

L5 radiculopathy differs from peroneal nerve palsy on motor examination in that the former may impair hip abduction and foot inversion (= supination), while the latter does not.

Many polyneuropathies begin distally in the lower limb and can produce a steppage gait resembling that of peroneal nerve palsy. This can be unilateral, at least initially, in *(vascular) mononeuropathy multiplex* (p. 607). In *advanced HMSN* (p. 588), weakness resembling that of peroneal nerve palsy is accompanied by calf muscle weakness and atrophy, loss of the Achilles reflexes, and, rarely, distal sensory deficits. This familial disease also usually causes pes cavus. The muscle weakness and atrophy (without sensory deficit) of *Steinert's myotonic dystrophy* are usually accompanied by other signs of this autosomal dominant inherited disease.

Tibialis Anterior Syndrome (Tibial Compartment Syndrome)

This syndrome, caused by ischemia of the dorsiflexor muscles of the foot and toes in the anterior compartment of the leg, is often confused with a peripheral peroneal nerve palsy.

Pathogenesis

The condition is due to ischemic necrosis of the muscles of the anterior compartment of the leg (tibialis ante-rior, extensor hallucis longus, and extensor digitorum longus). This compartment is sealed on all sides by walls of bone and connective tissue, so that edematous tissue within it has no room to expand. If ischemia should arise because of thrombosis, embolism, or occlusion of a proximal artery, a vicious circle of edema and vascular compression ensues. The same may occur in association with a tibial fracture or a traumatic or postoperative hematoma within the compartment, or with overuse of the leg muscles (military marching, football, etc.).

Clinical Features

There is intense pain, redness, and swelling in the pretibial region. At the same time, dorsiflexion of the foot and toes becomes painful, and complete paralysis may develop within hours. Concomitant ischemic damage to the deep peroneal nerve, which traverses the compartment, may cause paralysis of the extensor digitorum brevis and extensor hallucis brevis muscles on the dorsal surface of the foot, as well as sensory loss in the first dorsal interosseous space. The superficial peroneal nerve becomes ischemic in some cases as well, as it is sometimes supplied by a branch of the anterior tibial artery. In such cases, there is additional paralysis of the peroneal muscles, with a corresponding sensory deficit. Thus, in its early stage, the pattern of weakness in tibial compartment syndrome closely resembles that of common peroneal nerve palsy. A correct differential diagnosis is possible only on the basis of a careful history, the presence of pain in the tibial compartment, and the frequent but not invariable absence of a pulse in the dorsalis pedis artery. EMG reveals no activity in the necrotic muscles ("silent EMG"), but there is still electrical activity in the neurogenically paretic extensor digitorum brevis and peroneal muscles.

Prognosis

Usually only the neurogenic component of the paralysis can recover spontaneously as the muscles of the anterior compartment of the leg undergo fibrosis, retraction, and perhaps calcification. In the later stages,

they are as hard as wood, the ankle cannot be plantar flexed beyond 90°, and there is a hammer-toe deformity due to shortening of the extensor hallucis longus muscle.

Treatment

Early diagnosis is essential, as fasciotomy (splitting of the anterior crural fascia) must be performed within the first 24 hours to preserve the muscles from infarction. The same holds for compartment syndromes at other sites as well.

Tibial Nerve

Anatomy

The tibial nerve arises from the L4–S3 roots, its fibers lying on the medial side of the sciatic trunk. It supplies the plantar flexors of the foot and toes, and all of the small muscles of the foot except the extensor digitorum brevis and extensor hallucis brevis. It provides cutaneous sensory innervation to the heel and sole of the foot. It also carries many autonomic fibers.

Clinical Features

A lesion of the posterior tibial nerve causes paralysis of the plantar flexors of the foot and toe. Even an incomplete paralysis impairs toe-walking and diminishes the Achilles reflex. In complete paralysis, there is a valgus posture of the foot, because the peronei, innervated by the superficial peroneal nerve, prevail over the paralyzed invertors. The toes can no longer be spread or maximally flexed. Sensation on the sole of the foot is impaired.

Causes

The tibial nerve is well protected in the popliteal fossa and is thus rarely injured – e.g., by a gunshot wound. A supracondylar femoral fracture may damage the sciatic trunk or either of its main divisions. Dislocation of the knee injures the tibial nerve much less frequently than the common peroneal nerve. A dorsally angulated or dislocated fracture of the proximal portion of the tibial shaft can damage the trunk of the tibial nerve, and primary surgical exploration is justified in such cases. In other cases, sensory changes on the sole of the foot and weakness may only appear in the course of fracture healing; as this is likely due to perineural scarring, surgical exploration for neurolysis is indicated. The same applies to fractures of the distal third of the tibia. Persons in certain occupations requiring continuous pedaling movements (e.g., potters) are at risk of chronic mechanical injury to both the tibial and the common peroneal nerves, because of the anatomical relationship of these nerves to the muscles around the knee joint.

Tarsal Tunnel Syndrome

Pathogenesis and Clinical Features

The tibial nerve and its two branches, the lateral and medial plantar nerves, can be chronically compressed under the flexor retinaculum in the region of the medial malleolus. This can occur in the aftermath of an ankle or heel fracture, or merely an ankle sprain, or for no apparent reason. The resulting *tarsal tunnel syndrome* is characterized by painful paresthesiae of the sole of the foot that are aggravated by walking. Physical examination reveals a sensory deficit in the distribution of the plantar nerves, diminished or absent sweating on the sole of the foot, and weakness of the small muscles of the sole. The toes cannot be maximally spread. There is often tenderness to palpation over the course of the tibial nerve.

There are also cases with painful paresthesiae of the sole, aggravated by walking, in which there is no motor deficit. The symptoms can be immediately relieved by *tibial nerve block* with injection of local anesthetic behind the medial malleolus, but this is not a specific test.

Diagnostic Evaluation

The diagnosis can be confirmed by electromyography.

> **Treatment**
> *Tarsal tunnel release* by division of the flexor retinaculum is justified if the symptoms are distressing and the diagnosis clear. A pannus-like

> tissue reaction is found, sometimes accompanied by pseudoneuroma formation in the nerve trunk.

Metatarsalgia (Morton's Toe)

Pathogenesis

This condition is caused by a fusiform pseudoneuroma of a digital nerve just proximal to its division, usually in the third or fourth interdigital space. Chronic pressure from the metatarsal head on the nerve is the cause.

Clinical Features

Patients complain of neuralgic, often burning pain in the sole of the foot, usually in the region of the third and fourth metatarsal heads and the corresponding two toes. The pain first appears when the patient walks but later becomes continuous and may radiate proximally. The pains are often incorrectly attributed to a splayfoot (valgus) deformity. On physical examination, intense pain can be provoked by pressure on the sole of the foot, or by pressing the metatarsal heads on either side of the lesion against each other. The diagnosis is confirmed by the cessation of pain on infiltration of local anesthetic at the site of division of the plantar nerve in the third or fourth interdigital space. The approach is from the dorsum of the foot.

> **Treatment**
> Adequate relief can be obtained in mild cases with special shoes, or foot supports within the shoes, that hold up the arch of the foot just behind the metatarsal heads. If the pain persists, the lesion can be excised.

12   Headache and Facial Pain

Overview:
Headache and facial pain are due to the irritation of sensitive structures in these regions, among them the major vessels of the base of the brain, portions of the basal dura and pia mater, the cerebral venous sinuses, and the cranial nerves that have a sensory component, as well as all extracranial structures. The brain itself is not sensitive to noxious stimuli. Headache and facial pain are sometimes due to a specific disease involving the cranial structures, but are more often the expression of idiopathic disturbances of vasomotor or neural regulation, in which case no anatomical abnormality of these structures can be found.

Table 12.**1**   Headache history

Family history of headache?	**Treatment/ medication(s) used:**
	• Frequency
How long have headaches been present?	• Dose
	• Efficacy
Nature of headache:	
• Site?	**Neurologic abnormalities between headache episodes**
• Continuous or episodic?	• Memory?
• Timing of onset?	• Neurologic/neuropsychological deficits?
• Speed of development?	
• Nature of pain?	• Epileptic seizures?
• Precipitating factors?	• General symptoms (fatigue, weight gain, circulatory problems, etc.)?
• Duration of episodes?	
• Accompanying signs?	**Personality**
	• Character?
Frequency?	• Occupation?
	• Private life?
Headache-free intervals?	• Conflicts?
	• Alcohol, tobacco, caffeine, drugs of abuse?
Intensity?	
• Impairment of activities at home and at work?	• Medications?

General Aspects

History-Taking from Patients with Headache

A thorough and precise headache history often suffices to lead the clinician to the correct etiologic diagnosis. The aspects of headache that should be asked about specifically are listed in Table 12.**1**. It is also important to assess the degree to which the headache impairs the patient's functioning in everyday life – e.g., with the Migraine Disability Assessment Scale (MIDAS; Table 12.**2**) (590a, 910a).

Classification of Headache and Facial Pain

A sample etiologic classification is shown in Table 12.**3**. The very extensive table of the International Headache Society is reproduced in abbreviated form in Table 12.**4**; the original also contains specific criteria for each diagnosis, and is mainly of use in clinical research. Table 12.**9**, at the end of this chapter, contains a list of the various headache and facial pain syndromes according to their clinical features and localization, as an aid to differential diagnosis.

Table 12.**2**   Migraine Disability Assessment Scale (MIDAS) questions (590a)

Question	Days (n)
1 On how many days in the last 3 months did you miss work or school because of your headaches?	
2 How many days in the last 3 months was your productivity at work or school reduced by half or more because of your headaches? *(Do not include days you counted in question 1 where you missed work or school)*	
3 On how many days in the last 3 months did you not do household work because of your headaches?	
4 How many days in the last 3 months was your productivity in household work reduced by half or more because of your headaches? *(Do not include days you counted in question 3 where you did no household work)*	
5 On how many days in the last 3 months did you miss family, social or leisure activities because of your headaches?	

Total days (n)	Disability:
• 0–5	None or mild
• 6–10	Mild
• 11–20	Moderate
• > 21	Severe

Table 12.**3**   Classification of the major headache and facial pain syndromes by etiology

Primary headache:
- Tension headache
- True migraine
  - Ophthalmic migraine
  - Migraine accompagnée
  - Ophthalmoplegic migraine
  - Abdominal migraine
  - Basilar migraine
  - Dysphrenic migraine
- Cluster headache (erythroprosopalgia, Horton's neuralgia)
- Rarer forms:
  - "Ice-cream headache"
  - Acute postcoital headache
  - Carotidynia
  - Cough headache
  - Hemicrania continua
  - Hypnic headache

Headache in organic vascular disease:
- Ischemic stroke
- Hemorrhagic stroke
- Subarachnoid hemorrhage
- Cranial (temporal) arteritis
- Carotid or vertebral artery dissection

Headache due to an intracranial mass:
- Brain tumor
- Subdural hematoma
- Brain abscess

Headache due to impaired CSF circulation:
- Obstruction to CSF flow
- CSF malresorption
- Intracranial hypotension

Spondylogenic headache:
- Cervical spondylosis
- Cervical migraine
- Whiplash injury

Tension headache
("psychogenic" headache)

Other "non-neurological" causes of headache:
- Arterial hypertension
- Intracranial inflammatory/infectious processes
- Toxic and iatrogenic headache
- ENT diseases
- Eye diseases
- Dental diseases

Facial neuralgia and atypical facial pain:
- True neuralgia
- Trigeminal neuralgia
- Glossopharyngeal neuralgia
- Auriculotemporal neuralgia
- Sluder's neuralgia
- Temporomandibular joint "neuralgia" (Costen syndrome)
- Atypical facial pain

Table 12.**4**   Abbreviated etiologic classification of the more important causes of headache and facial pain, following the proposal of the Headache Classification Committee of the International Headache Society (Cephalagia 1988; 8 [Suppl. 7]: 1–96).

1.	**Migraine**
1.1	Migraine without aura
1.2.1	Migraine with typical aura
1.2.2	Migraine with prolonged aura
1.2.3	Familial hemiplegic migraine
1.2.4	Basilar migraine
1.2.5	Migraine aura without headache
1.3	Ophthalmoplegic migraine
1.4	Retinal migraine

(Cont.) →

Table 12.**4**   *(Cont.)*

1.5	Childhood periodic syndromes that may be precursors to or associated with migraine
1.5.1	Benign paroxysmal vertigo of childhood
1.5.2	Alternating hemiplegia of childhood
1.6	Complications of migraine
1.7	Migrainous disorder not fulfilling above criteria
2.	**Tension-type headache**
2.1	Episodic tension-type headache
2.2	Chronic tension-type headache
2.3	Headache of the tension type not fulfilling above criteria
3.	**Cluster headache and chronic paroxysmal hemicrania**
3.1	Cluster headache
3.1.1	Cluster headache periodicity undetermined
3.1.2	Episodic cluster headache
3.1.2	Chronic cluster headache
3.2	Chronic paroxysmal hemicrania
3.3	Cluster headache-like disorder not fulfilling above criteria
4.	**Miscellaneous headaches unassociated with structural lesion**
4.1	Idiopathic stabbing headache
4.2	External compression headache
4.3	Cold stimulus headache
4.4	Benign cough headache
4.5	Benign exertional headache
4.6	Headache associated with sexual activity
5.	**Headache associated with head trauma**
5.1	Acute post-traumatic headache
5.2	Chronic post-traumatic headache
6.	**Headache associated with vascular disorders**
6.1	Acute ischemic cerebrovascular disease
6.2	Intracranial hematoma
6.3	Subarachnoid hemorrhage
6.4	Unruptured vascular malformation
6.5	Arteritis
6.6	Carotid or vertebral artery pain
6.6.1	Carotid or vertebral dissection
6.6.2	Carotidynia (idiopathic)
6.6.3	Post endarterectomy headache
6.7	Venous thrombosis
6.8	Arterial hypertension
6.9	Headache associated with other vascular disorder
7.	**Headache associated with non-vascular intracranial disorder**
7.1	High cerebrospinal fluid pressure
7.1.1	Benign intracranial hypertension
7.1.2	High pressure hydrocephalus
7.2	Low cerebrospinal fluid pressure
7.3	Intracranial infection
7.4	Intracranial sarcoidosis and other noninfectious inflammatory diseases

(Cont.) →

Table 12.**4**   *(Cont.)*

7.5	Headache related to intrathecal injections
7.6	Intracranial neoplasm
7.7	Headache associated with other intracranial disorder
8.	**Headache associated with substances or their withdrawal**
8.1	Headache induced by acute substance use or exposure
8.2	Headache induced by chronic substance use or exposure
8.3	Headache from substance withdrawal (acute use)
8.4	Headache from substance withdrawal (chronic use)
8.5	Headache associated with substances but with uncertain mechanism
9.	**Headache associated with non-cephalic infection**
10.	**Headache associated with metabolic disorder**
10.1	Hypoxia
10.2	Hypercapnia
10.3	Mixed hypoxia and hypercapnia
10.4	Hypoglycemia
10.5	Dialysis
10.6	Headache related to other metabolic abnormality
11.	**Headache or facial pain associated with disorder of cranium, neck, eyes, ears, nose, sinuses, teeth, mouth or other facial or cranial structures**
11.1	Cranial bone
11.2	Neck
11.3	Eyes
11.4	Ears
11.5	Nose and sinuses
11.6	Teeth, jaws and related structures
11.7	Temporomandibular joint disease
12.	**Cranial neuralgias, nerve trunk pain and deafferentation pain**
12.1	Persistent (in contrast to tic-like) pain of cranial nerve origin
12.1.1	Compression or distortion of cranial nerves and second or third cervical roots
12.1.2	Demyelination of cranial nerves
12.1.3	Infarction of cranial nerves
12.1.4	Inflammation of cranial nerves
12.1.5	Tolosa-Hunt syndrome
12.1.6	Neck-tongue syndrome
12.1.7	Other causes of persistent pain of cranial nerve origin
12.2	Trigeminal neuralgia
12.2.1	Idiopathic trigeminal neuralgia
12.2.2	Symptomatic trigeminal neuralgia
12.3	Glossopharyngeal neuralgia
12.4	Nervus intermedius neuralgia
12.5	Superior laryngeal neuralgia
12.6	Occipital neuralgia
12.7	Central causes of head and facial pain other than tic douloureux
12.7.1	Anaesthesia dolorosa
12.7.2	Thalamic pain
12.8	Facial Pain not fulfilling criteria in groups 11 or 12
13.	**Headache not classifiable**

Examination of Patients with Headache

Patients with headache should be examined thoroughly and meticulously, though the findings will be normal in almost all cases. Aspects requiring special consideration are listed in Table 12.**5**.

Pathogenesis of (Primary) Headache

Tension headache and migraine are thought to be due to the interplay of three main types of causative factor.

Vascular and Humoral Factors

It has long been presumed that, in the *first phase* of migraine, *vasoconstriction* produces focal cortical ischemia (accounting for the neurologic deficits seen in migraine accompagnée). Recent measurements of intracranial blood flow, however, have cast some doubt on this hypothesis. In the *second phase, vasodilatation* occurs. Dilatation of the large extracranial vessels causes typically unilateral, often pulsating pain. The patient appears pale, because the facial capillaries are constricted; only in cluster headache are they dilated, producing a red face. The *third phase,* characterized by *edema of the periarterial tissue,* manifests itself in a dull, continuous pain. These vascular changes are partly due to, and accompanied by, *humoral processes* of various kinds; *serotonin* seems to be the most important transmitter substance involved. For unexplained reasons (perhaps because of exogenous factors), serotonin is released at the onset of a migraine attack from stored reserves in the intestinal wall, the brain, and, most of all, the blood platelets and mast cells. Serotonin at high concentration in the bloodstream then induces, not only the initial intracranial vasoconstriction, but also (in concert with histamine released from mast cells) an increase in capillary perme-

Table 12.**5** Examination of patients with headache

General considerations:	**Neurological examination, with particular attention to:**
• Blood pressure	• Meningismus
• Circulatory function	• Evidence of intracranial hypertension
• Renal function	• Focal neurologic signs
• Evidence of infection	• Cranial nerve deficits
• Evidence of meningitis	
• Evidence of malignancy	**Mental status, with particular attention to:**
• ENT diseases	• Psycho-organic syndrome
• Eye diseases	• Neuropsychological deficit
• Dental diseases, jaw diseases	• Impairment of consciousness
	• Psychological conflicts
	• Depression
	• Neurotic personality traits

ability. This, in turn, promotes transudation of a type of plasma kinin called neurokinin, which acts to lower the pain threshold. The concentration of serotonin in the blood then declines, which induces the vasodilatation and pain of the second phase. Serotonin is degraded through the enzymatic action of monoamine oxidases and excreted in the urine as 5-hydroxyindoleacetic acid.

CNS Factors

These factors have recently drawn increased attention. Impulses arising in the diencephalon are thought to be responsible for the episodic character, accompanying vegetative signs, epileptiform EEG changes, and unilaterality of migraine headache. A decisive role is played by excitatory processes mediated by fibers of the trigeminal nerve.

The Major Primary Headache Syndromes

Tension-Type Headache

Terminology

Tension-type headache, earlier known as "cephalea vasomotorea," is also somewhat confusingly called "common migraine." *The International Headache Society's definition* recognizes two types of tension-type headache, episodic and chronic, which are distinguished according to the following criteria.

Episodic Tension-Type Headache:
- **A**: At least 10 earlier episodes fulfilling criteria B–D, occurring fewer than 180 days per year.
- **B**: Headache episodes last 30 minutes to 7 days.
- **C**: At least two of the following pain characteristics are present:
  - pressing, not pulsatile,
  - mild to moderate intensity, not impairing everyday activities,
  - bilateral,
  - not exacerbated by exertion, walking, or climbing stairs.

- **D**: Both of the following characteristics:
  - no nausea or vomiting,
  - no or very rare photophobia or phonophobia.
- **E**: At least one of the following is true:
  - The history and physical findings are not consistent with another known type of headache; or
  - other types of headache can be excluded with ancillary tests; or
  - another type of headache, if present, is different from and not correlated with the tension-type headache.

Chronic Tension-Type Headache:
- **A**: Moderately frequent headaches (15 or more days/month) for at least 6 months, fulfilling criteria B through D.
- **B**: The pain has at least two of the following characteristics:
  - pressing, not pulsatile,
  - mild to moderate intensity, without impairment of daily activities,

- bilateral,
- not exacerbated by exertion, walking, or climbing stairs.
- **C**: Both of the following characteristics:
  - no vomiting,
  - no nausea, photophobia, phonophobia (or at most one of these phenomena).
- **D**: At least one of the following is true:
  - The history and physical are not consistent with another known type of headache; or
  - other types of headache can be excluded with ancillary tests; or
  - another type of headache, if present, is different from and not correlated with the tension-type headache.

Clinical Features

Tension-type headache is the most common type of chronic headache. The pain is usually diffuse, generally most severe over the forehead, temples, or vertex, and often of dull, perhaps throbbing character. It increases when the patient bends over or strains. It appears at unpredictable times over the course of the day, but most often in the morning on awakening or just after arising. There are usually no accompanying signs or symptoms, but there are transitional forms between this condition and migraine (see below). Tension-type headache most commonly affects young and middle-aged adults, both sexes about equally frequently, though the symptoms are, as a whole, more severe in women. Weather changes, lack of sleep, alcohol abuse ("hangover") an mental tension are common precipitating causes.

A diagnostic distinction is drawn between the *episodic type,* in which the attacks are rare, and the *chronic type,* in which they occur at least 15 days in each month for at least 6 months.

Neurologic Examination

There are no abnormal findings in the neurological examination of patients with tension-type headache, though there is often evidence of abnormal autonomic tone (constipation, possibly a tetaniform tongue).

Treatment

Tension-type headaches are treated by appropriate adjustments in *life-style,* the *elimination of internal and externals sources of tension,* and *medication* including ergot alkaloids, β-blockers, sedatives, and antidepressants. Among the last-named class of agents, the *nonselective* serotonin reuptake inhibitors are preferred (e.g., amitriptyline) (84a). All of these medications must be taken continuously for months. An effect of acupuncture has often been claimed, but was not confirmed in a randomized study (658a).

Post-Traumatic Headache

Post-concussive headaches after head trauma have the same subjective character as tension-type headaches. Their exacerbation by bending forward, shaking, noise, alcohol, and sunlight is particularly evident. Other forms of headache can, however, be seen after head trauma (see below). The organic nature of these complaints is a subject of ongoing controversy in the literature, as it is affirmed by some authors and disputed by others. We do not doubt that posttraumatic headache is a genuine phenomenon, but the resulting impairment in some cases depends on factors beyond the pain itself. The intensity of post-traumatic headache (287b, 504a, 999c) seems to be inversely proportional to the severity of the precipitating trauma (777c).

Migraine (298a, 723c)

Pathogenesis
This has been discussed above (see p. 802).

Epidemiology
Some 5% of school-age children are said to suffer from migraine; among older children, it affects girls more than boys. Epidemiologic studies in adults have yielded the surprisingly high prevalence estimates of 25% in women and 17% in men. Most migraineurs (as migraine patients are traditionally called) have a family history of headache, though not necessarily of migraine. Women are more commonly affected than men, or at least seek medical assistance more often. Persons suffering from narcolepsy have an increased prevalence of migraine (200c; cf. p. 565).

Classification of Migraine

Migraine is characterized, on the one hand, by the typical headache attacks (and by these alone in *simple migraine*), and, on the other hand, by highly diverse accompanying phenomena, which are sometimes more prominent than the headache itself. A classification scheme for migraine is suggested in Table 12.**6**.

Table 12.**6** Classification of migraine

Simple (classic) migraine

Complicated migraine
- Ophthalmic migraine
- Migraine accompagnée with:
  - Sensory symptoms
  - Motor symptoms
  - Aphasia
- Migraine with Jacksonian seizure
- Migraine with vertigo ("vestibular migraine")
- Migraine with ataxia ("cerebellar migraine")
- Ophthalmoplegic migraine
- Basilar migraine
- Dysphrenic migraine
- Abdominal migraine
- Cardiac migraine
- Meningeal migraine

Cluster headache

■ Simple Migraine
Clinical Features
This form of migraine headache is not associated with an aura and is characterized by headache alone. About half of all patients with migraine suffer from simple migraine. The International Headache Society (IHS) has promulgated the following defining criteria for simple migraine (migraine without aura):

- **A**: At least five episodes fulfilling criteria B through D, below.
- **B**: The headache episodes last 4–72 hours (or, in children under 15 years of age, 2–48 hours), either when untreated or when treated unsuccessfully.
- **C**: The headache has at least two of the following features:
  - unilateral localization,
  - pulsating character,

- moderate or marked intensity (makes everyday activities difficult or impossible),
- exacerbation by climbing stairs or other habitual physical activities.

- **D**: At least one of the following symptoms is present during the headache:
  - nausea and/or vomiting,
  - abnormal sensitivity to light and noise.

One often finds that the patient with migraine already suffered from atypical episodic headaches as a child. A past history of episodic abdominal pain and vomiting (sometimes called "cyclic vomiting syndrome") is also present in many cases; in French, these episodes have been termed *crises ombilicales* (umbilical crises). The headache is truly hemicranial in only about 65% of adult patients. (The word "migraine" is derived from Latin *hemicrania*.) It usually begins in the frontotemporal area and then spreads to the entire half of the head. It is often throbbing, aching, and deep-seated, and is exacerbated by external stimuli such as light and noise. The patient appears pale, and the temporal artery is tender. The pain rises to a maximum within a few hours and is accompanied by nausea and vomiting in 60% of cases. Because of the photo- and phonophobia, the patient withdraws into a quiet, dark room. Smells, too, may be intolerable. Allodynia has been described in 70% of patients during the headache episode, i.e., the perception of pain on mere touching of certain areas of the skin (153c). The side of the headache is almost always the same for most patients, but absolute constancy of side without exception should prompt the suspicion of symptomatic rather than migraine headache.

If the pain is not hemicranial, then it is mostly diffuse, particularly in children, many of whom go on to develop typical, hemicranial migraine headaches. Localization of the pain in the neck or elsewhere, instead of the head, has been described (224a). Among the not uncommon vegetative (autonomic) manifestations of migraine episodes are sweating, abdominal colic, diarrhea, tachycardia, dryness of the mouth, oliguria, and (after the episode) polyuria. The episodes usually last one or a few hours and may occur at any frequency from a few times a year to practically every day.

Precipitating Factors:

- *Atmospheric changes* can precipitate migraine headache, as can *photic stimuli,* the *menses, relaxation,* and *prolonged bed rest* (Sunday migraine, vacation migraine), and especially *mental stress* (responsibility, worries, inability to cope with demands, other conflicts).
- Migraine bears a complex relationship to the *menses* (696b). Episodes strictly limited to the menstrual period are seen only in very rare patients. Most female patients have no episodes during pregnancy, and migraine headache often resolves at the menopause. In some patients, oral contraceptive drugs can precipitate migraine-like headaches with certain atypical electroencephalographic features. The headaches persist in these patients even after the medication is stopped, implying a predisposition of some type. If a woman first develops migraine while taking oral

contraceptives, and particularly when migraine accompagnée appears in this situation, there is a danger that permanent neurologic deficits may ensue. The danger is even higher in patients who smoke. At least in patients who continue to smoke, the medication must be discontinued and replaced by another form of contraception.

- The pressor substance *tyramine*, which is present in some varieties of cheese and which can cause hypertensive crises in patients taking monoamine oxidase inhibitors, can rarely precipitate migraine headache (diet-related migraine).
- The role of *allergies*, however, is generally overstated.
- Traumatic migraine ("footballer's migraine") is occasionally seen, particularly in younger patients (692c). It clinically resembles basilar migraine (p. 812).

Physical Examination

The *neurologic examination* is normal in patients with simple migraine. The EEG, however, is truly normal in only half of all cases. In the rest, there are nonspecific dysrhythmic changes and focal disturbances (usually seen in patients with paralytic manifestations during episodes); about 16% have paroxysmal hypersynchronia with θ-waves and scattered sharp waves, as seen in clinical epilepsy. Migraine with these electroencephalographic features is termed hypersynchronous headache.

Migraine bears a complex relationship to epilepsy. In our own experience, the two conditions tend to occur in the same patient more frequently than chance would predict; this is especially true of temporal lobe epilepsy. The literature, too, supports the hypothesis of true comorbidity (733). Thus, it is sometimes necessary to treat both conditions at once (617).

Treatment

The treatment of simple migraine consists of two components: treatment of acute episodes as they occur, and interval treatment for prophylaxis of further episodes.

Treatment of acute episodes:
These therapeutic guidelines are equally valid for complicated migraine (to be described in the following sections). Treatment of the acute episodes alone, without interval treatment, is justifiable if the patient suffers no more than 3 episodes per month, or if the episodes, though more frequent than this, are generally mild and do not all require treatment. The principles of the treatment of acute episodes are summarized in Table 12.7.

The choice of agent depends on the severity of the episode. If the patient's headaches are usually mild, a new episode can be treated with acetylsalicylic acid, other analgesics, and nonsteroidal anti-inflammatory agents, perhaps combined with an antiemetic. If the patient's headaches are usually severe, one should not hesitate to prescribe a triptan ("stratified care": cf. Ref. 590a).

Prophylactic (interval) treatment:
More frequent headaches necessitate prophylactic (interval) treatment. This is justified, generally speaking, when the patient suffers from more than one episode weekly, or when rarer episodes are

unusually intense, prolonged, and disabling. The goal of prophylactic treatment is to make the episodes less frequent, less intense, and shorter. Some of the medications given for this purpose are listed in Table 12.**8**.

Side effects:
The use of ergotamine derivatives, perhaps in combination with other drugs, can rarely cause ergotism, while the use of agents that alter serotonergic transmission, such as lithium, imipramine, amitryptiline, and the triptans, can produce the serotonin syndrome (623a). Manifestations of the latter include agitation or confusion, tremor, myoclonus, ataxia, dysarthria, fever, and diarrhea. Chronic intake of analgesics can lead to drug-induced headache (see below).

We shall merely mention the following curious observation: persons with a patent foramen ovale sometimes undergo surgical or endovascular procedures to close the foramen so that they can go diving at lesser risk. When this was done in patients who also suffered from migraine, the frequency of migraine episodes declined (1028d).

■ **Complicated Forms of Migraine**

By this term, we refer to all forms of migraine in which the episodes are accompanied, some or all of the time, by manifestations other than those described above. On occasion, there may be striking neurologic deficits. These forms of migraine are apparently due to vasoconstriction, the pathogenesis of which was de-

scribed above. It has also been hypothesized that there may be an underlying, primary functional disturbance of a specific area of the brain, of which the local circulatory abnormalities are merely an epiphenomenon. The accompanying manifestations sometimes occur in the absence of headache *("migraine sans migraine")*. Complicated migraine can be precipitated by the same factors as simple migraine. If complicated migraine first appears or worsens in women using oral contraception, a switch to another contraceptive method is recommended.

Treatment

The treatment follows the same lines as that of simple migraine (q.v.)

■ **Ophthalmic Migraine**

This most common form of complicated migraine is characterized by visual manifestations preceding the headache, and is thus equivalently termed *migraine with (visual) aura.* About one-third of patients with migraine have this form of migraine. (A note on terminology: English-speaking clinicians differ from the rest of the world in referring to ophthalmic migraine as "classic migraine," a term elsewhere used synonymously with "simple migraine." We avoid "classic migraine" in this book in order not to confuse our international readers.)

A typical type of visual aura is the *scintillating scotoma,* in which the patient first sees a bright, colored, lightning-like figure with a zigzag border proceeding from the center to the periphery of the homonymous visual field (*fortification specter*). The

Table 12.**7**   Treatment of acute migraine episodes. (This form of treatment can be used alone, without interval treatment, if the episodes occur less than once a week and are not unusually intense or prolonged.)

Drug	Dose	Remarks
Drugs for self-administration		
Acetylsalicylic acid	500–1000 mg	May cause stomach upset
Acetaminophen (paracetamol)	500–1000 mg	P.o. or p.r.
Antiemetics, e.g.:		
• Domperidone	10 mg	P.o. or p.r.
• Metoclopramide	20 mg	
Codeine combinations		
Nonsteroidal anti-inflammatory drugs, e.g.:		
• Naproxen	500 mg	
Prostaglandin inhibitors, e.g.:		
• Flufenaminic acid	250 mg	Repeat q2h, maximum 750 mg
Ergotamine tartrate with caffeine	1 mg / 100 mg	2 doses, further tablet or suppository 30 min later (maximum 6 per episode)
Sumatriptan		
P.o.	50–100 mg	May repeat in 2 h
S.c.	6 mg	Not if concurrently taking an ergotamine preparation
P.r.	25 mg	
nasal spray	10 – 20 mg	
Naratriptan p.o.	2.5 mg	Takes effect more slowly, lasts longer
Zolmitriptan p.o.	2.5 mg	Can be taken without fluids
Rizatriptan		
P.o.	5–10 mg	
Sublingual	5–10 mg	Can be taken without fluids
Eletriptan	40–80 mg	
Drugs to be administered by a physician		
Noramidopyrine (metamizole sodium)	0.5–1.0 mg slowly i.v. or i.m.	In addition to metoclopramide
Metoclopramide	10–20 mg i.m. or (slowly) i.v.	
Ergotamine	0.5 mg s.c. or i.m.	
Dihydroergotamine	1.0 mg s.c. or i.m.	Or very slowly i.v.
Sumatriptan	6 mg s.c.	

Table 12.**8** Prophylactic (interval) treatment of migraine. This form of treatment should be used if the episodes occur more frequently than once per week or are particularly intense, prolonged, or refractory to treatment. Treatment must be continued for several months.

Drug	Daily dose	Remarks
β-blockers:		
• Propranolol	40–160 mg	May increase to full β-blockade
• Nadolol	30–60 mg	(160–240 mg)
• Metoprolol	100–200 mg	
Calcium antagonists:		
• Flunarizine	5–10 mg h.s.	Weight gain, depression; very
• Verapamil	240–400 mg	effective in cluster headache
• Cyclandelate	1200–1600 mg	
Dihydroergotamine	2.5 mg t.i.d.	Not to be combined with triptan therapy for acute episodes
Serotonin antagonists:		
• Pizotifen	1.5 mg h.s.	
• Methysergide	3–6 mg	Risk of retroperitoneal fibrosis with long-term use
Antidepressants:		
• Tricyclics, e.g. amitryptiline	10 – 150 mg	
• SSRI	20 mg	
• MAO-A inhibitors	150–300 mg	
Anticonvulsants:		
• Gabapentin	1200–2800 mg	Gradually increasing dose; sedating
• Valproic acid	500–1500 mg	Baseline liver function tests; not to be used in pregnant women
Other substances:		
• Magnesium	24 mmol	
• Dibenzepin	240 mg, a.m.	

figure reaches the periphery in 5–15 minutes and leaves a transient visual field defect behind. *Horizontal visual field defects* due to retinal ischemia are less common, and transient monocular blindness *(amaurosis fugax)* as a manifestation of retinal migraine is quite rare.

Scintillating scotomata of this type are followed by a *headache episode* of the type described above, usually on the side opposite the homonymous visual field defect. In rare cases, the scintillating scotoma remains the only manifestation of migraine, and the headache or other manifestations never develop. A permanent visual field defect may be present in such cases.

A small number of patients with ophthalmic migraine who, for various reasons, underwent surgical repair of a right-left intracardiac shunt went on to have attacks at lower frequency, or no attacks at all. It thus seems that this type of anomaly may rarely be of pathogenetic importance.

■ Ophthalmoplegic Migraine

This form of migraine is characterized by the appearance of an extraocular muscle paresis, usually an oculomotor nerve palsy, on the side of the headache. The paresis may take months to resolve. Probably most cases with this clinical picture are due to an underlying structural abnormality, such as an aneurysm of the posterior communicating artery (p. 216) or a process involving the cavernous sinus, rather than migraine. Other manifestations of ophthalmoplegic migraine include unilateral, but alternating, pupillary dilatation (or constriction).

■ Migraine Accompagnée

We use this term somewhat restrictively to refer to cases of migraine with an aura consisting of neurologic deficits other than the visual and oculomotor disturbances just described. Most, but not all, patients experience the aura in association with a migraine headache. Paresthesiae are present in some cases, usually in the upper limbs, but sometimes in the face. These may alternate sides during an episode, or affect both sides simultaneously. There are also cases with mono- and hemiparesis ("hemiplegic migraine"), aphasia, homonymous hemianopsia, and sensory disturbances, as well as Jacksonian seizures.

The headache usually follows the aura, thereby providing the clue to the diagnosis, but it can also precede the aura in not a few cases. In rare cases, the headache is entirely absent, so that one may speak of "*migraine accompagnée sans migraine.*" This condition tends to appear in childhood and is the initial manifestation of migraine in nearly half of all persons suffering from it.

A few cases of this type are due to a genetic disorder called *familial hemiplegic migraine,* which may result from a mutation at any of several different loci: just over half of the time, the mutation is on the short arm of chromosome 19 (930e), just as it is in CADASIL, another condition associated with migraine (p. 196). In about 10% of CADASIL cases, however, the mutation is on chromosome 1q or elsewhere (250a). Among the cases due to a mutation on chromosome 19, there is a subgroup of patients who additionally suffer from progressive cerebellar atrophy.

The neurologic deficits in migraine accompagnée generally resolve within 1 hour but occasionally last longer or even become permanent. There seems to be a somewhat higher risk of a permanent deficit in patients with ophthalmic migraine who have previously suffered a prolonged deficit in the wake of a migraine episode (112, 809).

The putative connection between migraine and stroke has not, however, been conclusively demonstrated, and expert views on this issue are highly divergent. At any rate, the danger that migraine accompagnée will produce a permanent deficit is low. In one study, a group of young women who had suffered a stroke contained more migraine patients than a control group without stroke (166d, 660b) (p. 196).

The EEG recorded just after an episode of migraine accompagnée reveals a massive focal abnormality that takes days to regress. Episodes are not uncommonly accompanied by CSF pleocytosis (802). *Familial fatal migraine* has also been described, a condition in which mild head trauma can precipitate cerebral edema, migraine with aura, and MRI signal abnormalities.

■ Basilar Migraine

Migraine in the territory of the basilar artery is characterized by occipital headache and is presumably due to vasoconstriction in the posterior circulation. Many cases of ophthalmic migraine, and cases involving bilateral visual loss, can be classified as basilar migraine, as can cases with vertigo, gait ataxia, dysarthria, or tinnitus. Bilateral paresthesiae of the hands, the head, and the tongue may also be manifestations of basilar migraine. Basilar migraine mainly affects women and almost always begins in adolescence. The migraine episodes are often accompanied by unconsciousness, and the EEG may reveal typical epileptic discharges.

Treatment

Basilar migraine responds to treatment with antiepileptic drugs.

■ Alternating Hemiplegia of Childhood

This condition may be a special form of basilar migraine. It usually begins in the first year of life and is associated with progressive psychomotor retardation. It is characterized by hemiplegic attacks on alternating sides that last from 15 minutes to several days. The attacks are accompanied by dystonia, choreoathetosis, tonic crises, nystagmus, and irritability.

Treatment

Naloxone and the calcium antagonist *flunarizine* are effective.

Special Forms of Complicated Migraine

Abdominal crises (p. 806) are not uncommon, particularly in children. Complicated migraine may also present with abnormal fluctuations of mood (anxiety, depression), cognitive disturbances, confusion, or agitation, perhaps severe enough to represent an actual "migraine psychosis" (*dysphrenic migraine*). Recurrent attacks of vertigo (*vestibular migraine*) (234c) and episodic ataxia (*cerebellar migraine*) have been described. *Cardiac migraine* is characterized by episodes of retrosternal pain in migraine patients, either simultaneously or nonsimultaneously with migraine headache, accompanied by nonspecific T-wave changes on ECG. The pain and the ECG changes respond to β-blockers (575a). Migraine patients are more susceptible than other persons to *acute amnestic episodes* (p. 387), reportedly also to *coital amnesia* (551a).

Cluster Headache
(547, 551, 607)

Synonyms
Alternative names for cluster headache include "erythroprosopalgia," "Horton's neuralgia," "Bing-Horton neuralgia," and *céphalée en grappes* (i.e., headache in clusters).

Pathogenesis
This hemicranial type of vasomotor headache has many similarities to migraine, as well as a number of distinctive characteristics. It is about one-tenth as common as migraine, occurs much more frequently in men than in women (especially smokers), and tends to begin in middle or old age. The attacks seem to have their origin in a functional disturbance of the hypothalamus (646c, 913b).

In 20% of patients, there is a family history of episodic headache. In 7%, there is a family history of cluster headache itself; an autosomal dominant inheritance pattern with incomplete penetrance, but greater penetrance in men, has been postulated (814b). A number of authors have reported individual cases of apparently traumatically induced cluster headache, but this finding was not corroborated in a larger case series (735a).

Characteristics of Headache Episodes
Cluster headache is diagnosed from the typical clinical features of the attacks. The headache attains maximum intensity within 20 minutes of onset, then subsides again in 1–2 hours. It consists of extremely intense, stabbing, locally circumscribed pain in the orbital and supraorbital region, always on the same side of the head, sometimes accompanied by nausea and photophobia. About one-third of patients are awakened by the headache at specific times of night, and most experience one to three attacks within 24 hours.

Unlike patients with migraine, those with cluster headache do not seek a dark, quiet room to lie down, but rather sit down, or pace restlessly back and forth. Periods of one or more weeks with very frequent episodes (clusters) alternate with months, or even years, in which episodes do not occur.

Objective Findings during an Attack
Attacks are typically accompanied by conjunctival injection, lacrimation, and a running or congested nose, often also by erythema of the face. All of these phenomena appear on the same side as the pain.

Transitional Forms between Cluster Headache and Migraine
Transitional forms are not uncommon. Some patients have headaches of both types, at different times; in others, each headache episode has some of the characteristics of each of the two types of headache.

Chronic Cluster Headache
This rather paradoxical term refers to the same type of headache occurring without episode-free intervals (i.e., without clusters).

Differential Diagnosis
Cluster headache is to be distinguished from various forms of neuralgia occurring in the face, i.e., *trigeminal*, (p. 822) *nasociliary*, (p. 823) and *Sluder's neuralgia* (p. 824), and from *SUNCT syndrome* (p. 815) and *hypnic headache* (p. 814).

Nor should it be forgotten that the clinical picture of cluster headache is

occasionally *symptomatic* of an intracranial mass or inflammatory process, or of multiple sclerosis.

████ **Treatment** ████

Acute attacks can be treated with
sumatriptan, 6 mg s.c., or with the
inhalation of 100% oxygen (6 L/
min). *Verapamil* can be given to
lessen the frequency of attacks, at
an initial daily dose of 80–160 mg,
gradually   increasing   to
360–480 mg. *Indomethacin* 75 mg/
day and *thymoleptic agents* can also
be used. *Prednisone* can be given
for 2–3 weeks during a cluster,
starting at 1 mg/kg per day. To treat
chronic cluster headache, lithium
can be given in a gradually increasing dose till a serum concentration
of 0.6–0.8 mmol/L is reached. See
also Tables 12.**7** and 12.**8**.

Rarer Primary Headache Syndromes

Carotidynia. This type of headache is
similar to cluster headache in some
respects. It affects women almost exclusively. The headache is always on
the same side, either on the side of
the neck or (occasionally) in the maxillary or periorbital area. There is a
continuous, dull ache on which acute
attacks are superimposed, which last
minutes or hours and may occur several times a day. During attacks, the
carotid artery pulsates strongly and is
painful, and the area around the artery appears swollen.
Pain in the side of the neck due to
acute carotid artery dissection should
not be called carotidynia.

████ **Treatment** ████

This type of headache responds to
the same medications as migraine.
Indomethacin is particularly effective, sometimes in combination
with a *tricyclic antidepressant.*

Hemicrania Continua

This is a continuous unilateral headache.

████ **Treatment** ████

Hemicrania continua responds to
indomethacin and sometimes to
acetylsalicylic acid.

Paroxysmal (episodic) hemicrania.
This condition is characterized by recurrent, brief unilateral headaches.

████ **Treatment** ████

This type of headache also responds to *indomethacin.*

Hypnic headache. This condition is
often difficult to distinguish from
paroxysmal (episodic) hemicrania
and chronic cluster headache. It is
characterized by uni- or bilateral attacks of intense headache that
awaken the patient from sleep
("alarm-clock headache syndrome")
(238a). It affects patients aged 65 or
older. The attacks last 15–60 minutes,
rarely hours. The condition is benign.

Exploding head syndrome (814d).
This term refers to a sudden, extremely intense headache. The headache resembles that of subarachnoid
hemorrhage, but is not accompanied
by meningismus, and resolves much
more rapidly.

SUNCT syndrome. The name is an acronym for "short-lasting unilateral neuralgiform headache with conjunctival injection and tearing." The headaches of SUNCT syndrome are less intense than those of cluster headache in the temporal and periorbital areas, but the accompanying autonomic manifestations are very prominent.

"Ice-Cream Headache"

Ice-cream headache is a special type of primary headache. A cold stimulus on the palate is followed in 20–30 seconds by headache, usually in the temporal area and sometimes very intense. The headache resolves again in a further 20 seconds.

Cough Headache

This form of headache is provoked by coughing, and in some cases also by straining or bending over. Each epi-sode lasts no more than a few seconds. Cough headache is harmless in most cases, but it is occasionally symptomatic of a mass or other process (e.g., arachnoiditis) in the posterior fossa (743a). The headache of elevated intracranial pressure is exacerbated by coughing.

Coital Headache

This type of headache occurs suddenly during coitus or other activities that acutely raise the intracranial pressure. Intense headache begins suddenly and lasts for minutes or hours. There is no meningismus. The clinical picture often prompts suspicion of subarachnoid hemorrhage, which is then ruled out by a normal emergency CT scan and bloodless CSF on lumbar puncture. It has been hypothesized that coital headache is a type of migraine (meningeal migraine).

Headache in Organic Vascular Disease

Cranial Arterial Occlusion

Intracranial arterial occlusion only rarely causes headache. Carotid occlusion can cause headache in the orbital area, basilar occlusion diffusely or in a ring encircling the head. Spontaneous dissection of the internal carotid artery causes very intense pain on one side of the face (p. 192). Dissection of the vertebral artery causes pain on one side of the neck and occiput (920) (p. 193).

Aneurysmal Subarachnoid Hemorrhage

Ninety percent of patients with an acute subarachnoid hemorrhage have headache; 45% experience the sudden onset of an extremely intense headache ("the worst headache of my life"), which then persists. In almost half of all cases, the headache begins in the occipital or nuchal region and then rapidly spreads to the whole head (1012) (p. 215). There can also be persistent headache in the months and years after subarachnoid hemorrhage (298c). Secondary normal pressure hydrocephalus should be ruled out (p. 41).

Arterial Hypertension

It is not known for certain whether hypertensive persons suffer from headache more than normotensives other than during hypertensive crises. If they do have headaches, these generally resemble tension-type headaches in their clinical pattern. They tend to appear in the morning and to persist diffusely and in moderate intensity for the rest of the day. The clinical evaluation includes measurement of blood pressure as well as a general medical and neurologic examination. If a patient with severe hypertension and headache is found to have papilledema, the differential diagnosis is between hypertensive headache and raised intracranial pressure from a mass (brain tumor). Patients sustaining a spontaneous intracranial hemorrhage due to hypertension present with acute headache combined with a unilateral neurologic deficit (p. 210).

Pheochromocytoma

In this condition, headache episodes begin suddenly and last a few minutes to an hour, accompanied by pallor, sweating, and palpitations. They are not uncommonly triggered by bending over, turning, exertion, or excitement.

Temporal Arteritis

Synonyms

This condition is alternatively known as cranial arteritis, Horton's syndrome, and giant-cell arteritis.

Pathogenesis

Temporal arteritis is a local manifestation of an autoimmune giant-cell arteritis affecting the tunica media and internal elastic layer of larger and medium-sized arteries. It mainly affects the branches of the external carotid artery but may also affect other major arteries of the body. The internal carotid artery is involved only in very exceptional cases (see also vasculitis, pp. 197 and 324).

Clinical Features

Almost all patients are over 50 years old. Headache is often the first symptom. It is very severe, usually in the temple or forehead, and often bilateral. It may be a throbbing and continuous ache, or a pain in the jaw during chewing ("intermittent claudication of the jaw"). The temporal artery is often thick, tortuous, and tender to palpation, though it may seem normal in some cases. Headache may also be outside the temporal region. As giant-cell arteritis is a systemic disease, there are also cases without headache, but with other manifestations such as ischemic optic neuropathy, retinal artery occlusion, ophthalmoplegia, polyneuropathy, etc.

The involvement of other major arteries in the body may produce highly varied manifestations such as Takayasu's aortic arch syndrome, an aortic aneurysm, or coronary ischemia. Granulomatous giant cell arteritis of the CNS can involve the temporal arteries.

General manifestations such as fatigue, anorexia, weight loss, night sweats, and low-grade fever are common. They are also seen in the other major form of giant-cell arteritis, namely *polymyalgia rheumatica*, which causes pain in the larger joints, particularly in the proximal segments of the limbs. The most serious complication of giant-cell arteritis is sudden *blindness* caused by the occlusion of the posterior long ciliary arteries.

Ancillary Tests

The *erythrocyte sedimentation rate* (ESR) is markedly elevated in practically every case, with values of more than 50 mm in the first hour. The *C-reactive protein* is also usually elevated.

Color-duplex sonography reveals the thickened, inflamed wall of the superficial temporal artery in cross-section as a dark halo (844b) (p. 145).

Temporal artery biopsy confirms the diagnosis and is indicated even when the artery appears normal to examination if there are other grounds for suspecting the diagnosis. Histologic sections at multiple levels of the artery are required.

Differential Diagnosis

The differential diagnosis includes, on the one hand, other unusual causes of headache in the elderly, and, on the other hand, occlusion of the internal carotid artery, which may cause the superficial temporal artery to become enlarged and pulsate more vigorously if it serves to provide collateral circulation around the occlusion (847). Lastly, in rare instances, young patients may present with painful swelling of the temporal artery combined with marked eosinophilia. This process can involve other organs and is called "juvenile arteritis of the temporal artery with eosinophilia" (149).

Treatment

Corticosteroids – e.g., prednisone at a dosage of 1–2 mg/kg/day – must be given until the ESR has returned to normal and must be continued in a smaller dose for many months or, in many cases, years. Recurrent elevation of the ESR after the cessation of corticosteroids represents a recrudescence of the process, which usually takes several years to "burn out."

Treatment should be begun as soon as the diagnosis is suspected, without waiting for the result of the biopsy, because of the risk of sudden blindness.

Spondylogenic Headache and Cervical Migraine

Pathogenesis

Pathologic changes in the upper cervical spine can produce pain radiating into the head. As cervical spondylosis is a very common radiologic finding in older persons, spondylogenic headache is probably too frequently diagnosed (14b, 575e, 746a, 746b, 765d, 885a). Yet it is certainly true that degenerative or post-traumatic changes of the upper three cervical segments sometimes cause transient occipital pain; they can also reactivate a pre-existing headache tendency (746a, 746b). Spondylogenic headache should be diagnosed only if the following conditions are met:

- other local, radicular, or vegetative signs of cervical spondylosis are present (p. 729), or
- there has been documented injury to the cervical spine, e.g., a whiplash injury in an automobile accident (p. 402); and
- the headache has the characteristic features of spondylogenic headache (see below).

Clinical Features

Spondylogenic headache tends to occur in older patients. It is typically, though not always, unilateral. It may be confined to the neck or radiate from the occipital to the frontal region (headache of the latter type is often mimed by the patient with a helmet-removing gesture). The pain may also be felt in the face. Headache is not uncommonly triggered by certain positions or movements of the head – e.g., during prolonged reading, or at night if the patient sleeps in an unfavorable position.

There is often a history of acute torticollis. On physical examination, there is tenderness of the cervical spine and paravertebral muscles and restricted mobility of the neck and head. Imaging studies reveal spondylosis, spondylarthrosis, and deformation of the uncovertebral joints.

Treatment

This condition is difficult to treat. *Extension treatment* can be tried in acute cases, particularly in those accompanied by torticollis. If a brief manual extension is effective, this also implies that the diagnosis of spondylogenic headache was probably correct. In chronic cases, or in acute cases after extension has been performed, appropriate treatment includes partial immobilization of the cervical spine for a few days in a *soft or hard collar*, attention to proper *positioning of the head in bed, local heat application followed by active exercise, muscle relaxants,* and *anti-inflammatory drugs.*

Neck-Tongue Syndrome

In this rare condition, sudden turning of the head induces an attack of occipital headache and, simultaneously, paresthesia of one half of the tongue (313a). The problem is presumably caused by mechanical irritation of the C2 nerve root by the inferior articular process of the atlantoaxial joint when the head is turned (105a). In rare cases, another lesion at the same location may be responsible – e.g., a tuberculoma (16a).

Other Symptomatic Forms of Headache

Headache Due to an Intracranial Mass

Headache is an early or late symptom in about half of all patients with brain tumors and in more than half of those with posterior fossa tumors. It can be the sole manifestation of a cerebellar tumor in a child long before other symptoms or signs develop. Headache due to a supratentorial tumor is usually, but not always, on the side of the tumor. The etiologic diagnosis is generally made on the basis of the history, physical examination, and imaging studies.

Headache Due to Intermittent Obstruction of CSF Flow (pp. 72 and 38)

The pain usually arises suddenly at maximal intensity, accompanied by nausea, vomiting, and sometimes a brief loss of consciousness or opisthotonus. Attacks last seconds or minutes, rarely longer, and usually subside somewhat less rapidly than they began.

This type of headache can be caused by any process intermittently obstructing the flow of CSF, but is particularly characteristic of *colloid cyst of the third ventricle* and other intraventricular tumors. These may also cause sudden, brief episodes of leg weakness with falling ("drop attacks") in the absence of headache or loss of consciousness.

Syndrome of Low Cerebrospinal Fluid Volume (Hypoliquorrhea)

Pathogenesis and Clinical Features

This syndrome can arise after head trauma or loss of CSF by lumbar puncture (981a), in association with a subdural hematoma or hygroma (in rare cases), or without any apparent cause (81, 445a, 671b). Idiopathic cases are more common in women. Its clinical hallmark is a very severe headache that develops when the patient stands up and subsides when the patient lies down. The headache can also be abolished by compression of the jugular veins. Drowsiness and vomiting are not uncommon accompanying signs. The neurologic examination is generally normal, though meningismus (sometimes severe), abducens palsy, tinnitus, and hearing loss may be found in some cases.

In the recent past, this syndrome was variously known as hypoliquorrhea, aliquorrhea, orthostatic headache, acute pseudomeningitis, and the syndrome of intracranial hypotension. Accumulating evidence now seems to suggest that the most important pathogenetic factor is not low intracranial pressure, but rather low intracranial cerebrospinal fluid volume (indeed, the measured ICP is sometimes normal).

Note on terminology: The term "CSF hypovolemia" was introduced into the literature in 1999 and has been perpetuated in a number of subsequent papers. This is a regrettable misnomer, as "hypovolemia" means low blood volume ("-emia" is from Greek *haima*, blood; cf. "heme"). We recommend calling this condition "the syndrome of low cerebrospinal fluid volume."

Diagnostic Evaluation

When a lumbar puncture is performed with the patient in the lateral decubitus position, the CSF pressure is usually found to be below 5 cm H_2O; it may be so low that the fluid does not drip out of the needle spontaneously and a sample must be gently aspirated. The CSF may be xanthochromic, the protein concentration may be increased up to 1 g/dL, and the cell count is often elevated. MRI reveals diffuse pachymeningeal contrast enhancement in some, but not all cases. This radiologic sign is distinct from the pachymeningeal and leptomeningeal enhancement seen in chronic meningitis (671b) (cf. Fig. 2.**15**).

> **Treatment**
>
> Bed rest, copious hydration, and slow infusion of half-normal saline solution.

Pseudotumor Cerebri

Clinical Features

This syndrome of spontaneous intracranial *hypertension* is in some respects the opposite of the one just described (above). Its major symptom is daily, diffuse headache; most patients are young, markedly obese women. The neurologic examination is usually normal, though there may be papilledema, which, if long untreated, can cause permanent visual impairment.

Diagnostic Evaluation

The *CSF pressure* is found to be markedly elevated on lumbar puncture. Imaging studies of the brain reveal *narrowing of the ventricles*.

> **Treatment**
>
> The treatment generally consists of *fluid restriction* and possibly *diuretics, repeated lumbar punctures,* and, above all, *weight loss.* Neurosurgical *CSF shunting* is sometimes indicated in intractable cases. Patients whose vision is threatened can be treated with *optic nerve fenestration* (an invasive neuroophthalmologic procedure).

Headache Due to Ocular Disorders

Disorders of the eye that cause headache include refractive anomalies and, most of all, heterophorias in childhood. The headache tends to increase over the course of the day. Appropriate treatment of the ocular problem leads to resolution of the headache. In an attack of acute glaucoma, the intense, usually frontal headache is accompanied by vomiting, bradycardia, and visual disturbances.

Headache Due to Disorders of the Ear, Nose, and Throat

Sinusitis can cause intractable, often focal headache. The same is true of chronic otitis and masses in the ear, nose, or throat. Supraorbital neuralgia, a cause of focal headache, is due either to frontal sinusitis or to mechanical irritation of the supraorbital nerve. A special form of this disorder is caused by the wearing of swimming goggles that are too tight ("goggle headache").

Headache Due to Systemic Disease

Certain *infectious diseases,* such as Q fever, tend to cause very severe headache that may persist long after resolution of the acute illness. *Chronic iron deficiency* – e.g., in hemorrhagic anemia – can cause intractable headache. Headache due to *hypothyroidism* has been described (674b). *Morgagni-Morel syndrome,* a disorder of unknown and probably heterogeneous cause affecting elderly women, consists of frontal internal hyperosto-

Facial Pain **821**

sis, obesity, hirsutism, abnormal carbohydrate metabolism including diabetes mellitus, sleep disturbances, dysequilibrium, and headache.

Psychogenic Headache

Not all headaches affecting persons under stress or in conflict situations are psychogenic headaches. The diagnosis is made too often. Psychogenic factors are said to play an important role in so-called *tension headache.* This not entirely unproblematic term refers to a variety of forms of headache, mostly in the occipital region, that are said to be due to shorter- or longer-lasting spasmodic contraction of the nuchal musculature, particularly at times of mental stress. Tension headache is not the same thing as tension-type headache (p. 803). It is not always easily differentiated from *occipital neuralgia* (another overdiagnosed condition; resection of the greater occipital nerve only rarely brings improvement) (508). Head-

ache may also herald an incipient *psychosis.*

Drug-Induced Headache

Prolonged, regular intake of analgesics can produce persistent, diffuse headache (66a, 287d, 371a). Drug-induced headache often results when multiple analgesics are used daily, or nearly so, for 6 months or longer. It is seen in patients who take analgesics to treat a pre-existing headache, never in patients who take them for other chronic pains in the absence of headache.

Treatment

This condition is difficult to treat (371a). A close working relationship must be established with the patient so that the analgesic consumption can be effectively reduced (behavior-therapeutic treatment). Antidepressants may be indicated.

Facial Pain

Neuralgias

Neuralgia is pain in the distribution of a particular peripheral nerve, generally of a wrenching or boring kind. Various types of neuralgia in the face are characterized by brief and lightning-like or, less commonly, prolonged and intense bouts of pain. Often, the pain can be brought on by touching a particular point or points on the face (trigger points), or through specific activities such as

speaking, swallowing, or chewing. Neuralgia in the face is usually idiopathic, but a minority of cases are symptomatic of an underlying pathologic process (tumor, infection/inflammation, adhesion, etc.) in the vicinity of a sensory nerve. Objective neurologic signs are present only in symptomatic cases, and not in all such cases. A very precise clinical history is essential to the diagnosis.

Trigeminal Neuralgia (Tic Douloureux)

Epidemiology

The prevalence of this condition is estimated at 100–400 cases per million individuals. Its incidence is just under five cases per million per year in men, a bit more than seven cases per million per year in women. The average age of onset for idiopathic trigeminal neuralgia is 50 years.

Pathophysiology

This condition is generally thought to be due to aberrant ("ephaptic") transmission of nerve impulses from somatosensory to nociceptive fibers within the trigeminal nerve at a site of local damage to myelin sheaths. The myelin lesion is, in turn, attributed to mechanical factors relating to old age, or to the compressive effect of a pulsating vascular loop making contact with the trigeminal nerve near the brainstem at its root entry zone. Other mechanical factors account for the development of symptomatic trigeminal neuralgia from pathologic processes in the vicinity of the nerve.

Clinical Features

Idiopathic (essential) trigeminal neuralgia. This condition only affects persons at least 50 years of age. The pain is usually in the distribution of the second and third trigeminal divisions – i.e., in the maxillary and mandibular regions. Thus, the first specialist the patient consults is often a dentist. The pain is always unilateral and always in the same place (at least at first). It is lightning-like (lancinating), usually lasts no more than a few seconds, and is unbearably intense. Attacks may occur as often as every few minutes – i.e., hundreds of times a day – driving the patient to despair, perhaps even to the brink of suicide. When the condition first arises, the patient is entirely asymptomatic between attacks of pain, but over time a dull background pain establish itself between attacks, and the attacks themselves can become longer. The attacks can be provoked by chewing or speaking, or by touching a particular point or points on the face or in the mouth (trigger points). Thus, some patients hardly venture to open their mouths even to eat or speak. In idiopathic trigeminal neuralgia, the neurologic examination is entirely normal. In the natural, untreated course of the disease, periods of more frequent attacks may alternate with months or years of freedom from pain. If the pain disappears and then returns, it is not necessarily in the same trigeminal division as before. Bilateral trigeminal neuralgia (usually staggered in time, rather than simultaneous) is seen in ca. 3% of cases.

Symptomatic trigeminal neuralgia. The common causes of symptomatic trigeminal neuralgia are multiple sclerosis (p. 469), pontine ischemia (49a), and mass lesions in the vicinity of the trigeminal nerve. Symptomatic cases are distinct from idiopathic cases in several respects: the patients are generally younger, bilaterality is more common, and there is more likely to be continuous background pain and/or an objective neurologic deficit. Yet occasional cases of symptomatic trigeminal neuralgia may be clinically indistinguishable from the idiopathic variety. In cases where a vascular loop makes contact with the trigeminal root, the loop can often be seen on MRI.

Treatment of trigeminal neuralgia (298d)

Symptomatic trigeminal neuralgia is treated by treatment of its cause. The more common idiopathic condition is initially treated pharmacologically, usually with anticonvulsants such as *carbamazepine* in a gradually increasing dose, up to three to five tablets of 200 mg daily. If the patient cannot tolerate carbamazepine, another anticonvulsant is substituted: *gabapentin* 400–600 mg t.i.d., *oxcarbazepine* 200–600 mg t.i.d., *clonazepam* 2 mg q.i.d. (maximum), *phenytoin* 100 mg b.i.d. or t.i.d. *Levo-baclofen* is occasionally useful instead of, or in addition to, carbamazepine. Levo-baclofen is not the same as the more commonly used racemic form of the drug (Lioresal).

If conservative treatment fails, a *neurosurgical procedure* is indicated. In the past, the more commonly performed procedures were infiltration of the Gasserian (semilunar) ganglion, electrocoagulation of the ganglion by the Kirschner technique, and open retroganglionic neurotomy (the Spiller-Frazier operation). At present, the best available methods are *differential thermocoagulation* of the Gasserian ganglion and *glycerol injection* into the cistern of the Gasserian ganglion.

In view of the pathogenetic role of a vascular loop making contact with the nerve trunk in its intracranial course, particularly at the root entry zone, *neurosurgical exploration of the posterior fossa* is recommended, just as in hemifacial spasm (589). The procedure has a high success rate: 70% of patients are permanently free of symptoms. Nonetheless, initial success can be followed by a recurrence of pain, particularly in the first 2 years after operation (59a, 140a). About 1% of patients undergoing this operation lose hearing in the ipsilateral ear as an operative complication (59a).

Symptomatic trigeminal neuralgia in multiple sclerosis responds to cortisone infusions, anticonvulsants, or a prostaglandin E analogue (782).

Auriculotemporal Neuralgia

In this rare condition, the pain is in front of the ear and in the temple. It usually arises after a disease affecting the parotid glands, at a latency of days to months, but may also come about spontaneously. It is assumed that faulty regeneration of the auriculotemporal nerve after damage to in its intraparotid portion leads to ingrowth of parasympathetic fibers into the sensory cutaneous branches and sweat glands. Chewing and gustatory stimuli, especially from sour or hot foods, induce burning pain, skin erythema, and marked sweating in the distribution of the nerve, i.e., mainly in front of the ear (gustatory sweating). Worsening of pain as the patient chews may lead to misdiagnosis of this condition as trigeminal neuralgia of the third (mandibular) division (see above), or as temporomandibular joint syndrome (p. 825).

Nasociliary Neuralgia

This condition, which is also rare, is due to a functional disturbance of the ciliary ganglion. It is characterized by episodic or continuous pain in the region of the nose, at the inner canthus, and in the globe, accompanied by erythema of the forehead, swelling of the nasal mucosa and, sometimes, conjunctival injection and lacrimation. The pain may be provoked by chewing or by touching a trigger zone (e.g., at the inner canthus), in which case it is commonly misdiagnosed as trigeminal neuralgia. This syndrome can also appear symptomatically as the result of a carotid aneurysm or dissection.

▰▰▰▰Treatment▰▰▰▰

Local application of *5% cocaine solution* to the nasal mucosa instantly abolishes the pain in some cases, establishing the diagnosis. As local infection and inflammation may be the cause, a trial course of *antibiotics and cortisone* is indicated.

Sluder's Neuralgia

This condition closely resembles nasociliary neuralgia but is due to a functional abnormality of the pterygopalatine ganglion. Sneezing attacks are a characteristic but not invariable feature. An underlying inflammatory process is sometimes found in the sphenoid, ethmoid, or maxillary sinus.

Glossopharyngeal Neuralgia

This type of neuralgia is also rare. It most commonly affects the elderly but can occur at any age. It is characterized by sudden, intense attacks, or, more rarely, by continuous pain. The pain is strictly unilateral and located in the base of the tongue, the tonsillar area, and the hypopharynx. It may radiate to the ear, mimicking the pain of auriculotemporal neuralgia. Swallowing, especially of cold liquids, provokes intense pain, as does speaking or sticking out the tongue. There are trigger points in the tonsillar area and in the throat.

Glossopharyngeal neuralgia is bilateral on occasion, and, in 10% of cases, it is combined with trigeminal neuralgia. It is rarely accompanied by syncope. Spontaneous regression is not uncommon.

▰▰▰▰Treatment▰▰▰▰

Pharmacotherapy as for trigeminal neuralgia. *Neurosurgical treatment* by division of the glossopharyngeal nerve and the upper rootlets of the vagus nerve is almost always effective.

Neuralgia of the Geniculate Ganglion

This type of neuralgia was originally described as a sequela of herpes virus infection of the geniculate ganglion, manifested by a vesicular eruption in the area of the tragus and mastoid process and peripheral facial palsy *(Ramsay Hunt syndrome)*. It can, however, arise just as well in the absence of either vesicles or facial palsy. The pain is in front of the ear and in the external auditory canal, and also deep in the roof of the palate, the maxilla, and the mastoid process. It is of lancinating quality, comes in attacks, and may be accompanied by abnormal gustatory sensations localized to the anterior half of the tongue, as well as copious salivation.

Treatment

If pharmacotherapy (as for trigeminal neuralgia, see above) is unsuccessful, neurosurgical treatment should not be delayed, as it has been found to be effective in three-fourths of cases (813). Depending on the localization of the pain, the neurosurgeon divides the nervus intermedius, the geniculate ganglion, the glossopharyngeal nerve, or the vagus nerve.

Other Neuralgias of the Face

Neuralgia of the superior laryngeal nerve. This rare condition is characterized by attacks of pain over the thyrohyoid membrane on one side.

Neuralgia of the auricular branch of the vagus nerve. This type of neuralgia is characterized by pain in the suboccipital region and shoulder, and by acute, retroauricular pain that can be evoked by local pressure.

Occipital neuralgia. This disorder causes occipital and nuchal pain. It is diagnosed too often.

Other Types of Facial Pain

Temporomandibular Joint Syndrome

Pathogenesis

This pain syndrome is of neuralgiform character and is due to a functional disturbance of the temporomandibular joint. There is sometimes an underlying disease of the joint or its associated muscles, but, in most cases, the primary problem is one of *malocclusion*. Premature contact of the teeth leads to a reflexive, compensatory adaptation of the pattern of muscle contraction, resulting in abnormal jaw posture and mechanics.

Nomenclature

Temporomandibular joint syndrome is also called myofascial syndrome and Costen syndrome.

Clinical Features

Most patients are young or middle-aged women. The initial symptom is preauricular pain aggravated by chewing. About half of all patients also complain of facial pain and headache, worst in the preauricular area but radiating to the forehead, the mandible, or the occiput. This pain is usually unilateral and is occasionally evoked or aggravated by chewing. Less common symptoms include vertigo, tinnitus, hearing loss, oscillopsia, buccofacial dystonia, toothache, and dysphagia.

Diagnostic Evaluation

The major findings on physical examination are tenderness of the jaw joint, possible restriction of jaw opening and closing, and malocclusion of the bite. Plain radiographs and CT scanning of the temporomandibular joint, with visualization of the disk in various functional positions, may be helpful. MRI often reveals an abnormality of the joint meniscus.

In our experience, this condition is overdiagnosed. The search for temporomandibular joint syndrome also leads to the performance of an excessive number of MRI scans of no therapeutic consequence.

Treatment

The only etiologic treatment is the correction of malocclusion, if present, by a dentist. Symptomatic relief can be obtained from local anesthetic procedures and injection of hydrocortisone into the joint.

Atypical Facial Pain

Pathogenesis and Clinical Features

This term refers to diffusely localized facial pain of a burning and distressing nature. The pain may arise spontaneously or in the aftermath of comparatively minor and uncomplicated dental procedures. It is unilateral, always on the same side, and continually present, albeit in fluctuating intensity. There are generally no objective physical findings. The affected patients are typically middle-aged women. The distressing nature of the pain leads them to seek help repeatedly. The unfortunate result is often a succession of dental and maxillofacial procedures of escalating invasiveness.

Atypical facial pain is rarely accompanied by facial erythema, Horner's syndrome, and tenderness of the carotid artery; the term "sympathalgia" is applied to such cases, which were once designated as carotidynia.

Treatment

The treatment of atypical facial pain usually brings disappointing results. *Ergotamine tartrate, serotonin reuptake inhibitors, indomethacin,* and *tricyclic antidepressants* can be tried.

■ Tolosa-Hunt Syndrome

This syndrome is characterized by intense periorbital pain accompanied by a palsy of one or more of the nerves supplying the extraocular muscles.

Treatment

The pain responds very rapidly to corticosteroids. The differential diagnosis includes a number of steroid-resistant conditions (311a); nonresponse thus implies the need to reconsider the diagnosis.

■ Glossodynia

Glossodynia (381) consists of a more or less continuous, dull, burning pain of the tongue, sometimes accompanied by paresthesiae. It is a complex of symptoms rather than a clearly defined disease entity. It mainly affects elderly women. The pain tends to become increasingly severe toward evening and is often unbearable, leading the patient to seek medical help urgently. The objective examination is usually normal; many patients have the expected dental problems of old age, but these are hardly ever relevant to the pathogenesis of glossodynia. Systemic conditions of possible pathogenetic importance (such as iron deficiency) are only very rarely present. Psychological factors seem to play an important role, especially latent depression.

Other Types of Facial Pain

Mass lesions and infectious processes in the face, a wide variety of disorders of the ear, nose, and throat, ocular disorders, and dental disorders can all cause chronic facial pain, or, less commonly, episodic facial pain. Habitual bruxism (grinding of the teeth) can also lead to muscle pain in the face. A selection of such conditions is listed in Table 12.**9**.

General Differential Diagnosis of Headache and Facial Pain

A precise clinical history is essential for the correct diagnosis of pain syndromes in the head and face. The nature, temporal characteristics, and localization of the pain, any precipitating factors, and any accompanying phenomena should be inquired about and documented. A thorough physical examination is equally important. A classification of headache and facial pain for use in differential diagnosis is given in Table 12.**9**.

Table 12.9 Differential diagnosis of headache and facial pain

Clinical features	Syndrome	Site of pain	Duration	Time of onset, precipitating factors	Accompanying phenomena	Objective findings	Remarks
Recurrent episodes of (acute) headache	Migraine	Often unilateral, head and temple, switches sides	Hours to days	Weather, tension, menses	Vomiting, scintillating scotoma, occas. focal signs	Neurologic exam normal, EEG occas. abnormal	May increase with oral contraceptives
	Cluster headache	Temple and eye, always unilateral and on the same side	30 min to several hours	Often "on schedule," often at night	Facial reddening, lacrimation, vomiting	Normal; conjunctival injection during attack	Differential diagnosis: nasociliary neuralgia
	Hypertensive crises	Diffuse	Minutes to hours	Irregular	Sometimes vomiting or confusion	Hypertension, changes in fundus, stroke	Rule out pheochromocytoma
Recurrent episodes of intense facial pain	Trigeminal neuralgia	2nd and 3rd divisions of CN V, always on same side	Seconds	Trigger points (touch, eating, speaking)	Grimace	Normal	
	Auriculotemporal neuralgia	Preauricular	Minutes	Chewing	Local sweating, cutaneous erythema	Normal	Often follows parotid disease
	Nasociliary neuralgia	Inner canthus	Minutes to hours	Local pressure, chewing	Conjunctivitis, lacrimation	Normal	May be continuous. Differential diagnosis: Sluder's neuralgia, cluster headache

Table 12.**9** (Cont.)

	Sluder's neuralgia	Inner canthus	Minutes		Sneezing	Occas. sinusitis	Differential diagnosis: nasociliary neuralgia
	Glossopharyngeal neuralgia	Base of tongue, tonsillar fossa	Seconds	Swallowing, trigger zone		Normal	
	Geniculate ganglion neuralgia	Auditory canal, roof of palate	Seconds	Often after herpes zoster oticus	Gustatory sensations, salivation	Normal	
More or less continuous facial pain	Atypical facial pain	One side of face, diffuse	Virtually continuous		Sometimes erythema and sweating	Normal	Often burning pain, often intractable
Sudden headache	Subarachnoid hemorrhage	Diffuse (rarely occipital or unilateral)	Days	Straining	Occas. loss of consciousness, vomiting, seizures	Meningismus, focal signs, Terson's syndrome	CT
	Intracerebral hemorrhage	Unilateral	Days		Sometimes vomiting	Focal signs	CT
	Intermittent obstruction of CSF flow	Diffuse (may be unilateral)	Minutes to hours	Sometimes sudden on change of position	Vomiting, confusion, somnolence	Occas. meningismus	May disappear on change of position
	Cough headache	Diffuse		Coughing, straining		Rarely due to posterior fossa lesion	Sometimes posttraumatic

(Cont.) →

Table 12.**9**   (Cont.)

Clinical features	Syndrome	Site of pain	Duration	Time of onset, precipitating factors	Accompanying phenomena	Objective findings	Remarks
Chronic headache, usually diffuse	Tension-type headache	Diffuse	Hours to days	Stress, alcohol			Sometimes post-traumatic
	Headache due to hypertension	Diffuse	Hours to days	Worst in the morning	Occas. intermittent neurologic deficit	Hypertension	
	Headache due to intracranial mass	Diffuse, rarely localized	Continuous		Occas. vomiting, signs of intracranial hypertension	Occas. focal signs, papilledema	
	Post-traumatic headache	Diffuse	Days	Worse with alcohol, sunlight, shaking		Usually normal	Trauma history
	Headache due to systemic illness; toxic/iatrogenic headache; psychogenic or depressive headache	Diffuse	Virtually continuous		Depending on etiology		Carbon monoxide, lead, bromine, oral contraceptives, analgesics
Subacute headache, usually persistent and diffuse	Meningitis, encephalitis	Diffuse	Virtually continuous		Depending on underlying illness	Meningismus, occas. focal signs	

Table 12.9 (Cont.)

	Localization	Duration	Provoking factors	Associated symptoms	Findings	Remarks
Cerebrovascular disorders	Diffuse	Hours to days		Occas. vomiting, impairment of consciousness	Occas. focal signs	
Post-infectious headache	Diffuse	Days to months				Note prior disease
Intracranial hypotension	Diffuse	Hours	Sitting or standing	Occas. vomiting	LP to measure pressure, analyze CSF. Elevated CSF protein concentration	Better on lying down and with pressure on jugular veins
Chronic localized headache Spondylogenic headache	Occipital, may be unilateral, radiating anteriorly	Hours to days	Prolonged unchanging head posture (e.g., reading, bed rest)	Neck pain, occas. arm pain	Occipital trigger points, occas. cervical radiculopathy	Usually older patients, sometimes after cervical whiplash injury; overdiagnosed
Cranial (temporal) arteritis	Often temporal	Continuous			Tender temporal arteries, elevated sedimentation rate	Usually older patients
Eye diseases	Frontotemporal	Hours to days	After reading, particularly in the evening	Depending on etiology		
ENT diseases	Depending on etiology	Often in the morning				
Dental diseases	Face, temple	Virtually continuous	Chewing; warmth or cold			E.g., temporomandibular joint disease

13 Pain Syndromes of the Limbs and Trunk

Overview:

As pain is often neurogenic, the neurologist is often asked to examine patients with painful conditions of no immediately evident cause. The differential diagnosis in such cases will include both neurogenic and non-neurogenic pain syndromes. A number of such syndromes of both types form the topic of this chapter. Some have already been discussed in detail elsewhere in this book and are only briefly mentioned here with respect to differential diagnosis.

The first important step in the evaluation of a painful condition is to obtain a detailed history of the character of the pain itself. As for *psychogenic factors* that may generate or maintain pain, the following can be said: Pain is likely to be organic if it is precisely localized, if it is regularly brought on by specific physical activities, positions, or other precipitating factors, and if it is regularly alleviated by a different set of factors. Conversely, pain is likely to be psychogenic if it is diffusely or variably localized, and if there is no clear pattern of factors by which it can be brought on or alleviated. Among patients with chronic pain, a larger number than would be predicted by chance have had to deal extensively with chronically ill persons over the course of their lives, or were themselves the victims, or at least witnesses, of physical abuse.

Some important aspects of the *pain history* are summarized in Table 13.1.

Table 13.1 Pain history

Where is the pain?
- Precisely localized or diffuse?
- Constant or varying localization?
- Radiating?

How long has it been present?
- For what length of time?
- Since what precipitating event, if any?

Continuous or intermittent?
- If continuous: constant or variable intensity?
- If intermittent: how long and how frequent are the episodes of pain?

Quality?
- Hammering?
- Throbbing?
- Stabbing?
- Dull?

Intensity?
- On a scale of 0 (no pain) to 10 (intolerable pain)

Precipitating and/or aggravating factors?
- None?
- Constant or variable factors – which, if any?
- Dependence on posture?

Alleviating factors?
- None?
- Constant or variable factors – which, if any?
- Medications – which ones, with what effect, lasting how long?

How severely is the patient impaired by the pain?
- At work?
- In the personal sphere?

To what does the patient attribute the pain?

Current complaints other than pain?

Other medical history?

Living conditions?

Pain in the Shoulder and Arm (Cervicobrachialgia) (692)

Cervical Disk Herniation and Cervical Spondylosis

Typical clinical features of cervico-brachialgia caused by these two common conditions include torticollis, neck pain, worsening of pain on coughing, and possibly weakness, sensory deficit, and/or paresthesiae in a radicular distribution.

Lesions at the Thoracic Outlet

Scalene syndrome, with or without a cervical rib (p. 762), is characterized by lower brachial plexus palsy and compression of the subclavian artery. Apical lung tumors (Pancoast tumors, p. 763) cause very severe pain that is soon accompanied by a progressive lower brachial plexus palsy and Horner's syndrome due to involvement of the cervical sympathetic chain.

Neuralgic Shoulder Amyotrophy

This condition (p. 765) is characterized by shoulder pain that arises acutely overnight and is soon followed by weakness of the shoulder muscles.

Brachialgia Paresthetica Nocturna

This is the most common type of arm pain encountered in neurological practice. In its typical form, it is almost always due to carpal tunnel syndrome (p. 773). Pain and paresthesiae awaken the patient at night; the hand feels swollen and stiff. The entire arm is painful, up to the shoulder and beyond to the nuchal area. Objective signs of median nerve palsy are often not detectable till years after the onset of pain.

Causalgia

This syndrome of burning pain most commonly results from a median nerve injury (p. 749).

Intramedullary Lesions of the Spinal Cord

Cervical syringomyelia, in particular, can cause severe pain in the upper limb.

Scapulohumeral Periarthritis

This is the most common cause of shoulder pain. It is characterized by "tendinitis" and degenerative changes of the rotator cuff tendons, particularly that of the supraspinatus muscle. Calcific deposits may irritate the subdeltoid bursa, causing chronic bursitis. Radiographic studies reveal calcification in just over half of all cases.

This condition affects middle-aged or older patients. It occasionally begins just after a powerful pull on the arm or a local injury to the shoulder. It seems to occur more commonly than chance would predict in association with coronary artery disease, which may have similar symptoms; shoulder pain can arise acutely in either condition. The pain of scapulohumeral periarthritis can be brought on by active abduction, which brings the affected tendon into contact with the coracoacromial roof of the shoulder joint. It can be alleviated by passive raising of the arm with the shoulder muscles relaxed, a maneuver that lowers the head of the humerus. Patients typically complain of pain on abduction and external rotation of the arm – e.g., while putting on a jacket. The diseased tendon and joint capsule are often tender.

Shoulder-Hand Syndrome (Frozen Shoulder)

Causes

This condition may be a sequela of scapulohumeral periarthritis, shoulder trauma, or myocardial infarction. It often arises after a period of immobilization of the shoulder, for whatever reason. Bilateral shoulder-hand syndrome is a rare complication of phenobarbital use.

Clinical Features

In this syndrome, gradually worsening pain is accompanied by progressive limitation of shoulder movement over a long period of time. Severe arthrosis of the shoulder joint and tenosynovitis of the long bicipital tendon are found. The syndrome affects patients aged 40–60, and particularly women with cardiovascular disease. The pain eventually recedes, but the limitation of movement continues to worsen. There are often trophic changes as well.

Complex Regional Pain Syndrome (CRPS)

Pathogenesis

This term refers to the group of conditions previously known as reflex sympathetic dystrophy, algodystrophy, and Sudeck's dystrophy (99a). CRPS is divided into types I and II, depending on whether it is or is not as-

sociated with a peripheral nerve lesion (751b).

The sympathetic nervous system plays a role in the pathogenesis of CRPS; in particular, abnormal sympathetic activity seems to cause the characteristic swelling of the affected limb. A further role is played by altered information processing in the posterior horn of the spinal cord.

Clinical Features

CRPS is most often seen in the hand, often as an accompaniment to shoulder-hand syndrome. It may develop gradually after a traumatic injury of greater or lesser severity, with or without fracture. It is clinically characterized by edema of the soft tissues; smooth, cold, often cyanotic skin; restricted movement in the finger joints; patchy osteoporosis; and intense, often burning pain.

▌Treatment

Treatment with *guanethidine sulfate* in a dose of 20–30 mg/day is often beneficial. Other medications that may help include *nonsteroidal anti-inflammatory drugs, calcitonin,* corticosteroids, and β-blockers.

Lateral Humeral Epicondylitis ("Tennis Elbow")

This condition is characterized by pain at the origin of the long extensor muscles of the wrist and fingers on the lateral side of the elbow. Local tenderness is aggravated by extension of the wrist and fingers. The condition is caused by overuse of these muscles at work or in sporting activities. A similar mechanism underlies *radial styloiditis*.

Medial Humeral Epicondylitis ("Golfer's Elbow")

This is an analogous condition affecting the origin of the ulnar elbow flexors at the medial epicondyle. The pain can be produced by forced flexion of the hand and fingers.

Gout Attacks

These can cause very severe, localized pain in the hand, often but not always in the first metacarpophalangeal joint (*cheiragra* or *cheiralgia*).

Snapping Scapula

This abnormality in the region of the shoulder blade produces pain and an unsettling noise ("snap") accompanying movement of the shoulder.

Overuse Brachialgias

Terminology

This anatomical term refers to pain syndromes in the upper limb in which the action of certain muscles is restricted because of pain. Alternative terms for it include "muscular rheumatism" and "tenomyalgia."

Pathogenesis

These conditions are mainly encountered after long-standing overuse of a certain muscle or muscles, or as a consequence of pain in a joint (of whatever cause). The tone and functional characteristics of the muscles moving the joint are changed, sometimes markedly so. Assessment of these conditions must take the complex interplay of the nervous and musculoskeletal systems into account (145a, 145b).

Clinical Features

The pain is induced by movement. The condition most often affects the (upper) arm, but can also be found anywhere else in the musculoskeletal system (223). Dull, boring, wrenching pain in the muscle is by no means the only manifestation; a wide variety of reactive changes can usually be noted in the affected muscles, sometimes referred to as "tenomyosis." These include rapid fatigability of the muscles, painful contractures, and sometimes even fasciculations or an increase in muscle tone (rigidity). The pain may radiate from proximal to distal along the limb, in a so-called *pseudoradicular* pattern.

Treatment

The treatment consists of the *elimination of contributing factors* – e.g., the correction of improper posture or excessive mechanical stress at work, or the alleviation of joint pain with procaine or hydrocortisone injections. Manual triggerpoint therapy is also used (223).

Scapulocostal Syndrome

This is probably no more than a proximal variety of overuse syndrome, caused by an abnormal functional relationship between the scapula and the rib cage. The abnormality may be due to a lesion in the shoulder region (secondary type), paralysis or amputation of the upper limb (static type), or improper posture or unilateral overuse of certain muscles of the shoulder girdle (primary type). The primary type is the most common.

Treatment

Local anesthetic injections are recommended. Shoulder girdle exercises may also help. A change of occupation is sometimes necessary.

Arteriopathies

Occlusion of the subclavian artery, due to aortic arch syndrome or a cervical rib, can cause exercise-induced arm pain, a true *intermittent claudication* of the arm. In the subclavian steal syndrome, the arm pain may be accompanied by lightheadedness (see p. 191).

Vasomotor Disturbances

Raynaud's syndrome is characterized by blanching of individual fingers *(doigts morts),* particularly on exposure to cold, with subsequent reddening and cyanosis, occasionally leading to ulceration of the fingertips. It may be accompanied by paresthesiae, stiffness, and aching pain in the fingers. Most patients are young women. The syndrome may occur without apparent cause (the idiopathic form, or *Raynaud's disease*), or as a manifestation of another underlying disease. In men with Raynaud's syndrome, a collagen disease – e.g., scleroderma – should be suspected.

Venous Thrombosis

Causes

Paget-Schrötter syndrome (effort syndrome) consists of compression or postcompressive thrombotic occlusion of the axillary or subclavian vein. It often arises immediately after very intensive use of the arm, but may also occur without any apparent cause. Bi-lateral *sternoclavicular hyperostosis,* in which the sternum and clavicle are affected by spongiosclerosis, is a rare cause of venous thrombosis. In such cases, local pain and swelling of the clavicle are found.

Clinical Features

Men are much more commonly affected than women, usually on the right side. Most patients are between the ages of 20 and 30. The pain usually begins suddenly or over no more than a few hours, then progresses over the next few days. The shoulder pain and tension in the arm are usually accompanied by arm swelling or discoloration. The veins are often prominently distended. Paresthesiae and weakness are present in some cases, and the tender, thrombosed vein can occasionally be palpated in the axilla.

Diagnostic Evaluation

Doppler ultrasonography and/or *venography* are essential for confirmation of the diagnosis.

Treatment

Treatment is not always needed, as the acute manifestations usually regress spontaneously over a few days or, at most, weeks. Nonetheless, *anticoagulation* should be given whenever thrombosis is discovered in the acute phase. *Surgical treatment* is only rarely necessary.

Glomus Tumors

Pathogenesis

These small, almost always benign growths are derived from the glomus organs of the skin, which are arteriovenous anastomoses tightly linked to autonomic nerve fibers. They are most numerous in the fingers and toes. Glomus tumors can appear at these or other sites – e.g., on the forearms or the lower limbs, and can also be multiple.

Clinical Features

Typically, there is at first no more than local tenderness at the site of the tumor, often on a finger. The tumor appears blue if it is located under a fingernail, as is sometimes the case. The pain on palpation becomes very intense and radiates into the entire limb. There is also pain in the limb at rest, particularly when it is dependent, which develops into a more or less continuous, dull dysesthesia. Local autonomic disturbances may be seen in connection with these tu-

mors. For glomus jugulare tumors, cf. p. 687.

Diagnostic Evaluation

The diagnosis can be confirmed by CT.

> **Treatment**
>
> Glomus tumors are treated by surgical excision.

Referred Pain

Pain arising from the internal organs can be referred into the shoulder and upper limb. Chest pain radiating into the arm in *angina pectoris* may not be immediately recognized as such if it is present at rest, as in Prinzmetal's angina. The pain of *gallbladder disease* is referred to the right shoulder.

Pain Syndromes of the Trunk and Back

Pain in the Trunk

Pain in the trunk is often due to diseases of the internal organs that will not be discussed here (appendicitis, etc.). There are, however, a number of conditions (rheumatologic, orthopedic, other) of which pain can be the initial or only manifestation. These will be discussed here.

Bandlike Pain

Bandlike pain always suggests the possibility of intraspinal disease, such as a tumor, or of a disease of the spine causing uni- or bilateral radicular irritation. The pain often radiates from back to front and is characteristically demonstrated by the patient with a

movement of both hands from the spine around the flanks to the chest or abdomen. If herpes zoster is the cause, it generally declares itself with a vesicular eruption soon after the onset of pain. The chronic, often intractable pain of postherpetic neuralgia is described above on p. 739.

Abnormally Mobile 9th (or 10th) Rib

Rib fractures can produce an intractable pain syndrome of the costal arch. This occurs more often in women than in men, usually on the right side. Pain is evoked whenever the patient executes certain movements, such as bending forward or lifting. Less commonly, there is a dull, sometimes burning, continuous pain. Complete relief on local anesthetic block of the intercostal nerve establishes the diagnosis. Resection of the free end of the broken rib cures the pain.

Abdominal Wall Pain

Pain in the abdominal wall may arise acutely through *hemorrhage into the rectus abdominis muscle* – e.g., in certain gymnastic exercises (abdominal roller). A *compression syndrome of the ventral rami* of the caudal thoracic segmental nerves produces strictly localized, motion-induced pain, sometimes accompanied by a half-dollar-sized area of sensory deficit. The pain disappears upon infiltration of the corresponding nerves with local anesthetic. Pain in the inferolateral portion of the abdominal wall may be due to a *Spigelian hernia*. Such hernias are often difficult to diagnose when covered by the intact external oblique aponeurosis. In women, the pain of *endometriosis* can be referred to a localized, superficial area on the trunk.

Back Pain

Back pain is among the more common complaints for which patients seek medical attention. It is often difficult to determine which of the many possible causes has produced it (200b).

Ankylosing Spondylitis (Marie-Strümpell disease, Bekhterev's Disease)

This is an autosomal dominant genetic disease of incomplete penetrance that mainly affects young men. The sacroiliac, intervertebral, and costovertebral joints are usually affected first, causing progressively severe back pain, worst at night, often accompanied by sciatica. Rarer symptoms include pain in the chest, the heels, or the proximal joints of the limbs. The diagnosis is supported by the findings of iritis, an elevated erythrocyte sedimentation rate, and the characteristic radiographic appearance of the sacroiliac joints and, later, the spine. (For cauda equina syndrome in ankylosing spondylitis, cf. p. 739).

Spondylolisthesis

Pathogenesis

This condition comes about when the partes interarticulares (interarticular portions) on both sides of the posterior arch of a lumbar vertebra are either abnormally elongated or actually disrupted (*spondylolysis*). The vertebra is no longer held securely over the vertebra below by the intervertebral joints and thus slides forward on it, leaving its posterior arch and inferior articular facets behind. Spondylolisthesis affects the L5 vertebra in 80% of cases, less commonly the L4 or L3 vertebra. Its prevalence in the general population is about 5%. If the anterior displacement is very large, equaling the anteroposterior dimension of the underlying vertebra, the term *spondyloptosis* is used.

Clinical Features

At least 90% of cases of spondylolisthesis are asymptomatic (i.e., an incidental radiologic finding). Spondylolisthesis is found with roughly equal prevalence in the two sexes, though it is twice as likely to be symptomatic in men. One may infer from this that the nature and intensity of the patient's physical activity determine whether spondylolisthesis will cause pain.

The symptoms usually arise after the patient has attained full adult stature and are, at first, nonspecific, usually involving only a vague discomfort and feeling of weakness in the low back, particularly after prolonged sitting or carrying of heavy loads.

Physical examination usually reveals full mobility of the lumbar spine. In very thin patients, the anterior displacement of a spinous process over the one below can be directly seen and palpated on the back. The pelvis is tilted backward to compensate for the slip, returning the patient's center of gravity to a position above the feet (necessary for a stable upright stance). Radicular manifestations may be present; true sciatica is rare.

Treatment

Depending on the severity of symptoms, a *three-point brace* may be required, or even operative *spinal fusion* (spondylodesis). The latter is usually performed through an anterior approach.

Baastrup's Sign (Osteoarthritis Interspinalis, Kissing Spine)

These terms refer to a radiologic finding in which the spinous processes of two adjacent lumbar vertebrae touch each other. Baastrup's sign is a consequence of degenerative processes of the spine, rather than a disease in its own right. Resection of a spinous process to treat this condition is excessively performed and rarely, if ever, justified. A case can be made for this form of treatment only if pain is consistently induced by backward bend-

ing, the interspinous space is tender to palpation, the radiologic findings are consistent with the diagnosis, local anesthetic infiltration abolishes the pain, and other, more common causes of pain have been ruled out.

Sacroiliac Joint Syndrome (Sacroiliac Strain)

The pain of this condition is located at the sacroiliac joint, in the low back, and radiating down the posterior aspect of the leg. The condition is sometimes brought on by a forceful twisting movement; pain is consistently produced by lifting, and by standing erect from a stooped position. Physical examination reveals local tenderness at the sacroiliac joint and reproduction of symptoms by extension of the joint – e.g., by the Mennell maneuver, in which the patient lies in the lateral decubitus position and holds one knee to the chest while the examiner pulls the other leg strongly backward. Standing on one leg on the affected side also reproduces the pain. The diagnosis is supported if the pain is relieved by the wearing of a trochanter belt.

Coccygodynia

Coccygodynia is an aching, often burning pain in the region of the coccyx. It can be caused by a sprain, fracture, or surgically induced lesion of the coccyx, by root sleeve or arachnoid cysts (especially Tarlov cysts), or, most commonly, by chronic, repetitive microtrauma, such as prolonged sitting on a hard surface ("television bottom"). There is usually no neurologic deficit. The pain is reproduced on rectal examination when the coccyx is palpated and moved from within by the tip of the examiner's finger. Infectious and neoplastic processes of the anogenital region must be ruled out.

Spinal Nerve Root Compression Syndromes

Low back pain is sometimes due to irritation of the dorsal rami of the spinal nerves where they directly contact the facet joint capsules. Examination reveals tenderness of the articular facets and of the iliac crest. The dorsal rami innervate the paravertebral muscles and then penetrate the muscular fascia to innervate the deep fascia of the back (thoracolumbar fascia). Intractable local pain can be caused not only by facet joint disease, but also by posture-dependent mechanical strain on dorsal rami where they penetrate the muscular fascia, or by the pressure of small herniations of fatty tissue on the dorsal rami at these points.

Notalgia paresthetica is localized thoracic paravertebral pain due to compression of the terminal sensory branch of a dorsal ramus at the point where it penetrates the fascia. Local trauma may induce this condition. Examination reveals an area of sensory deficit the size of a quarter.

Other Types of Back Pain

Although the cause of back pain is at least partly understood in the syndromes just described, *nonspecific, chronic back pain of unclear etiology* is by far the most common syndrome. Only a minority of cases can be convincingly attributed to intervertebral disk degeneration (317a) or an arachnoid cyst (814a). Back pain of this type, for which there is no ready ex-

planation, is a major cause of human suffering and a major medical and socio-economic problem. In most cases, the pain is local and intractable; it may be present either continuously or intermittently, in relation to exertion. Nonorganic factors (psychological and social) certainly play a role in the development and maintenance of this type of pain (1034b).

Treatment

This type of pain often prompts physicians to search for one or more degenerated intervertebral disks. The search generally succeeds, as practically every adult has some degree of radiologically demonstrable disk degeneration. The inference that disk degeneration is the cause of pain is, however, not justified. Treatments based on this notion – e.g., *extension therapy* – fail to bring relief (96a). Many cases respond to *manual trigger point therapy* (223a). *Lumbar fusion* (of the appropriate segment!) is effective in a small number of cases, perhaps with the recently developed technique of *intersomatic composite cage implantation*.

Pelvic Pain and Pain in the Lower Limb

Pelvic Pain

Pelvic pain is more common in women and may be due to varicosities of the pelvic veins (as revealed by transvaginal ultrasonography or transuterine venography) or a gynecologic condition, usually endometriosis.

Pain in the Groin

Ilioinguinal nerve syndrome, which causes pain in the groin and an antalgic, flexed and internally rotated posture of the hip joint, is discussed above on p. 780. A *snapping iliopsoas tendon* produces an audible noise, but rarely any more than minimal pain. Slow extension of the hip from a flexed position with simultaneous contraction of the iliopsoas muscle causes the tendon to slide audibly over the iliopectineal eminence. Pain in the groin should always prompt a search for an *inguinal hernia.*

Pain in the Buttock

Piriformis syndrome is characterized by severe pain in the gluteal region, arising shortly after a mechanical trauma. The pain may radiate toward the sacrum or the hip joint, or down the leg, and is exacerbated by bending and lifting. Examination reveals focal tenderness at the greater sciatic foramen, as well as pain in the same area on forced flexion and internal rotation of the hip.

Ischial bursitis is another cause of pain in the buttock. The ischial bursa is located between the gluteus maximus muscle and the ischial tuberosity. It can become inflamed after prolonged sitting – e.g., in certain occupations ("tailor's bottom"). *Myofascial trigger points* in the gluteus medius muscle can produce intractable local pain as well as radiating lumbosacral pain and sciatica. They can be identified by palpation and successfully treated by local anesthetic injection or suitable manual techniques (223).

■ Pain in the Hip

In osteoarthrosis of the hip joint (coxarthrosis), the pain typically occurs when the patient starts to walk. It may be pseudoradicular, radiating down the side of the leg ("general staff stripe"). The patient walks with his hip held stiff, and rotational movements are particularly restricted (tested with the patient seated on the edge of the bed).

Three of the numerous *bursae around the hip joint* can become chronically irritated and painful through overuse of the neighboring tendons and joints:

- the *trochanteric bursa* between the greater trochanter and the tendinous attachment of the gluteus maximus,
- the *iliopectineal bursa* between the iliopsoas muscle and the iliopectineal eminence, and
- the *ischial bursa* (see above).

Periarthropathy of the hip is a disorder of the elderly. It causes local tenderness of the hip and intense pain on movement, while hip mobility remains full and plain radiographs are normal, though they may later show periarticular calcification.

Algodystrophy of the hip ("disappearing hip") mainly affects middle-aged men. Exertional pain in the hip progresses over a few days or weeks, producing a limp, while hip mobility remains full. Plain radiographs 1–2 months later reveal osteopenia of the femoral head with preservation of the articular surface. The symptoms resolve, and the radiographic appearance renormalizes, within a few months. The cause of this condition usually remains obscure. It is only rarely preceded by a local process of some type. Cases have been reported after surgery on the aortic bifurcation.

Pain in the Knee

Apart from the common local causes of an orthopedic and rheumatologic nature, there are rare neurologic causes, such as *patellar neuropathy.* This condition is due to compression of the infrapatellar branch of the saphenous nerve as it penetrates the fascia. Pain is felt under the patella. In the *Howship-Romberg syndrome* (p. 789), irritation of the obturator nerve at the level of the obturator foramen produces pain on the medial aspect of the knee.

Pain in the Leg

The intense pain in the shin encountered in *anterior tibial compartment syndrome,* in which there is ischemic necrosis and paralysis of the foot and toe extensors, was described above on p. 794. *Nocturnal cramps of the calf muscles,* though harmless, are a painful nuisance. The patient is awakened by attacks of intense calf pain, as a rule on one side, usually in the early morning hours. The foot is held in plantar flexion by rigid involuntary contraction of the calf muscles and cannot be actively dorsiflexed. Passive extension of the calf muscles by standing or walking on the affected foot brings immediate relief. The attacks are more frequent in cool surroundings; they may arise at any age. Their cause is unknown. They can sometimes be prevented by covering the legs with a warm blanket or by resting the knees on a cushion. *Symptomatic calf cramps* with fasciculations are found in amyotrophic lateral sclerosis (p. 434) and after myelitis.

Treatment

Calf cramps usually respond well to *quinine* 200–400 mg/day, *chloroquine phosphate* 250 mg/day, *tocopherol* 100 U t.i.d. (also effective in restless legs syndrome), or *diphenhydramine* 25–75 mg/day.

Pain in the Foot

A *calcaneal spur,* which causes local pain in the heel on walking, will be visible in a plain radiograph. *Plantar fasciitis* is characterized by tenderness of the heel and plantar fascia and is occasionally misdiagnosed as *tarsal tunnel syndrome.* The latter syndrome often arises after a twisting injury of the foot and is due to chronic compression of the tibial nerve under the flexor retinaculum behind the medial malleolus. It causes pain in the foot on walking. The diagnosis is confirmed by the typical sensory deficit on the sole of the foot, and weakness of spreading of the toes (p. 796). The pain of *Morton's metatarsalgia* is also induced by walking (p. 796).

Burning Pain in the Leg or Foot

The autonomic nervous system seems to play a role in the pathogenesis of these conditions.

Erythromelalgia (erythermalgia) affects middle-aged men and women. Patients complain of burning and often painful sensations in the feet and hands, especially while walking, but also in bed under the bedclothes. Warmth aggravates the symptoms. The painful limbs are often red or cyanotic, and the skin is warm. Local cooling and elevation often brings relief. The tricyclic antidepressant clomipramine is also effective. Most cases are idiopathic, but there are also symptomatic cases due to heavy metal poisoning, hypertension, or polycythemia vera.

A very similar condition, *burning feet syndrome*, is encountered in various types of polyneuropathy, particularly in hereditary sensory neuropathy. There is also a *syndrome of myalgia and fasciculations* due to mild axonal degeneration in peripheral nerves. It is characterized by aching myalgia, cramps, burning sensations, and (less commonly) paresthesiae of the legs, sometimes also of the limb girdles and the arms. The symptoms are aggravated by physical activity and relieved by rest. Benign fasciculations are always present, usually in the calves. The Achilles reflex is occasionally diminished. The clinical picture remains stable for years.

Restless Legs and Toes

Restless legs. The most common disorder of this group is *restless legs syndrome* ("anxietas tibiarum"), whose *prevalence* is usually estimated at ca. 5% of the general population. Most patients are women. Most cases are *idiopathic*, but about one-third are found in familial clusters, with an autosomal dominant inheritance pattern. *Symptomatic cases* are rare; the underlying etiology may be iron deficiency, end-stage renal failure (949a), polyneuropathy, pregnancy, or a spinal cord lesion (392b). The pathogenesis of this disorder is unclear, though structures in the brain appear to play a role (150a, 957a).

The major symptom is a poorly defined, unpleasant sensation, neither a pain nor a paresthesia, localized in both lower limbs from about mid-thigh to mid-calf level. It usually arises toward evening and in the night, particularly when the patient is recumbent or sitting on an upholstered chair (recliner, theater seat, first-class seat on a train or airplane). The ambient temperature has no consistent effect. Typically, the patient has an irresistible urge to exercise the legs, becomes restless, and paces up and down. This symptom is occasionally accompanied by myoclonic twitching of the legs as the patient falls asleep. Physical examination reveals no objective neurologic or circulatory abnormalities. Periods of severe symptoms alternate with symptom-free intervals.

Treatment

The medications of first choice are *dopaminergic agonists* such as *pergolide* (1017a), *pramipexole* (672a), or *cabergoline* (910b). *Levodopa* preparations at a daily dose of 100–200 mg, taken in the evening, has also been used with success (949a). Other effective treatments include *clonidine, benzodiazepines, a combination of vasodilators with phenobarbital*, and *tramadol*.

Restless toes. This is a separate syndrome consisting of pain in the legs and a continuous, no more than temporarily resistible urge to move the toes. Cases have been described as the result of trauma or polyneuropathy. This condition is probably due to a lesion causing spontaneous discharges in the afferent fibers of the posterior roots and, in turn, reflex movement of the corresponding muscles. Sleep disturbances are a frequent accompaniment.

Treatment

Local anesthetic block of the lumbar sympathetic chain brings no more than transient relief; *lumbar sympathectomy* unfortunately also brings no more than transient relief.

Intermittent Claudication

The Latin word *claudicatio* means "limping" (from *claudus*, "lame"). In medical usage, "intermittent claudication" refers specifically to pain in the lower limbs that is brought on by walking and forces the patient to stand still. The coincidental resemblance of the word "claudication" to "occlusion," as of a blood vessel, routinely causes confusion. Intermittent claudication may be either vasogenic or neurogenic.

Vasogenic intermittent claudication. Insufficiency of either arterial or venous blood flow to the lower limbs can cause intermittent claudication. *Arterial insufficiency* causes exercise-dependent pain in the area of ischemia, which may be limited to the calf muscles or involve the hip and thigh muscles as well, depending on the

site of arterial stenosis or occlusion. The pain may even be felt in an amputation stump. It forces the patient to stop walking ("window-shopping disease"), then resolves after a brief period of standing at rest, so that the patient can start walking again. The diagnosis is made on the basis of these characteristic symptoms, along with correlated angiologic findings (palpation, auscultation, Ratschow's test – i.e., reproduction of pain by moving the foot while the leg is elevated, oscillometry, Doppler ultrasonography). Muscle atrophy is occasionally present. The causative lesion is usually arteriosclerosis. Occlusive peripheral vascular disease is often amenable to surgical or interventional radiologic treatment (arterial grafting, transluminal angioplasty, stenting). In younger persons, intermittent claudication of the calf may be due to an aberrant course of the popliteal artery medial to the medial head of the gastrocnemius in the popliteal fossa; this anomaly can be corrected surgically.

Inadequate return of venous blood from the lower limbs can also cause intermittent claudication. Stenosis or occlusion of the pelvic veins causes diffuse pain, a feeling of overdistension, and leg cramps on walking. The pain recedes slowly when the patient stops walking (102a), in distinction to the pain caused by arterial insufficiency. Elevation of the lower limbs brings relief.

Neurogenic intermittent claudication. Chronic compression of the cauda equina in lumbar spinal stenosis causes bilateral sciatica that is induced by walking and accompanied by a transient loss of lower limb reflexes. The pain is often more severe on descending a staircase (because of the accompanying accentuation of the lumbar lordosis), rather than on ascending, as in vasogenic intermittent claudication. Simply standing still is not enough to relieve the pain; rather, the patient must alter the configuration of the lumbar spine by sitting or crouching. This phenomenon can be exploited in a diagnostic "stoop test": the pain is provoked by standing in hyperlordosis and disappears on sitting with pronounced kyphosis of the lumbar spine (255). MRI is the best and least invasive method of demonstrating lumbar spinal stenosis (Fig. 10.**4**), which can also be seen by myelography and myelographic CT. Neurogenic claudication need not affect the entire cauda equina; it may be manifest in symptoms relating to a single root only (*root claudication*).

Cauda equina compression by distended veins. In rare cases, the symptoms of intermittent claudication may arise because the cauda equina is compressed within the spinal canal by intermittently distended veins (102a). When the pelvic veins are occluded, muscular activity in the lower limbs may induce distension of the intraspinal veins, which serve as a collateral pathway for venous return.

Ischemia of the lumbosacral plexus (1031b). Occlusive disease of the pelvic arteries with ischemia of the lumbosacral plexus is a further rare cause of intermittent claudication. The pain begins in the pelvic girdle, then radiates into the lower limb, perhaps accompanied by paresthesiae, hyporeflexia, and (rarely) muscle paresis. It may be on one side or both. Treatment by endovascular dilatation of the stenotic arteries is usually successful.

Intermittent claudication of the spinal cord. Transient spinal cord ischemia on walking is a rare condition (cf. p. 420) whose main symptom is usually weakness of the lower limbs, rather than pain. The cause is usually spondylogenic myelopathy, which can be diagnosed by MRI (Fig. 13.**1**).

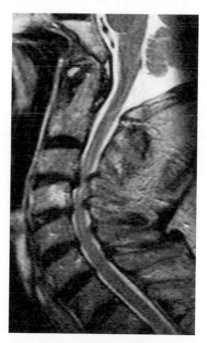

Fig. 13.**1 Cervical myelopathy.** Cervical myelopathy due to degenerative spinal canal stenosis and secondary spinal cord ischemia. The most pronounced narrowing is seen at the C3–4 level.

Other Regional and Generalized Pain Syndromes

Complex regional pain syndrome (CRPS). See p. 836.

Fibromyalgia syndrome. This intractable condition consists of diffuse pain in many different areas of the body, with tenderness in at least 11 of 18 defined "tender points," most of which correspond to sites of tendinous insertion. The diagnosis is based entirely on clinical criteria (765e), but affected patients are more likely than the general population to have a particular form of the polymorphic 5AT2c receptor gene, a low serum serotonin concentration, and an elevated concentration of substance P in both CSF and muscle tissue. The cause of fibromyalgia is unknown. Muscle biopsy reveals only nonspecific changes (765f).

Other chronic pain syndromes. It is often difficult to distinguish fibromyalgia from other chronic conditions, such as *myofascial pain syndrome.* Psychological factors often play a major role in chronic pain conditions, and sometimes even the most important role. The term *somatoform pain disorder* is applied to such cases (1034b).

The major distinguishing features of neurogenic and somatoform pain are listed in Table 13.**2**.

Table 13.**2**   Differentiating features of organic and somatoform pain

| Category | Differentiating features | |
	Organic pain	Psychogenic pain
Quality of pain	Burning Stabbing Shock-like Wrenching	Deep Dull Throbbing Pulsating Cramping
Localization of pain	Constant localization	Variable localization Ubiquitous
Patient's description of pain	Matter-of-fact Appropriate affect	Dramatic Vague Diffuse Perhaps inappropriate affect (la belle indifférence)
Other aspects	Objective abnormal findings Constant precipitating factors Specific alleviating factors	Excessive preoccupation with pain Variable precipitating factors Prolonged, fruitless search for organic cause Agrees readily to invasive procedures, including surgery Excessive use of analgesics History of having been physically abused as a child
Differential diagnosis		Still unidentified organic cause Depression Hypochondriasis Coenesthetic schizophrenia Malingering
Synonyms		Psychogenic pain Somatoform pain disorder Chronic idiopathic pain

14 Myopathies (276, 361, 465, 996)

Overview:
Myopathies are primary diseases of muscle. Their clinical manifestations include muscle weakness, atrophy, pseudohypertrophy, diminished reflexes, and hypotonia, and sometimes contractures, muscle spasms or myotonic reactions. The most important diagnostic tests in myopathy are measurement of serum muscle enzyme concentrations, electromyography, electroneurography, muscle biopsy, and genomic analysis. The etiology of myopathy may be dystrophic, infectious, inflammatory, metabolic, or myotonic. Abnormalities of muscle can also be produced by systemic diseases, as well as by medications, exogenous substances, and neoplastic processes elsewhere in the body. Disorders of neuromuscular transmission, of which myasthenia gravis is the most common, are also considered to be types of myopathy. Depending on its cause, myopathy may be treatable. Persons suffering from hereditary myopathies can prevent the appearance of disease in their descendants by undergoing genetic counseling and following the recommendations.

General Aspects

Myopathies are primary diseases of muscle. Although some myopathies have additional manifestations in other organ systems, muscular involvement is their most prominent feature.

Clinical Manifestations and Physical Findings

Muscle weakness. The weakness of myopathy is usually symmetric, affects proximal more than distal muscles, and may also involve the muscles of the face, neck, and throat. Occasionally, certain muscle groups are affected asymmetrically or distally. The weakness may cause gait abnormalities (Duchenne sign, Trendelenburg sign, steppage gait) and make it difficult for the patient to climb stairs, climb onto a chair, stand up from a sitting or lying position, hold an object, keep the arms extended, or comb the hair. Severe weakness renders the patient dependent on such aids as splints and crutches, or on assistance from other persons. Abnormalities of posture and movement resulting from myopathic weakness are depicted in Fig. 14.1. Weakness of individual muscles or muscle groups can be graded on the scale of the Medical Research Council (U.K.)

(Table 11.2, p. 747). In most types of myopathy, the muscle weakness is present at all times; in some, however, it is episodic (as in the dyskalemic paralyses), exercise-induced (as in metabolic myopathies and myasthenia), or progressively severe over the course of the day in connection with activity (myasthenia). The age of onset is an important datum for the differential diagnosis of myopathy. The speed of progression is another.

Muscle atrophy. Muscle atrophy is usually present, but sometimes absent – e.g., in myasthenia or when the muscle fibers have been replaced by fat and connective tissue.

Pseudohypertrophy. In the muscular dystrophies, replacement of muscle by fat and connective tissue can lead to pseudohypertrophy, particularly in the calves and in the deltoid muscle.

True hypertrophy of muscle. True hypertrophy is seen in Thomsen's myotonia congenita and, rarely, in other types of myopathy in which there is continuous spontaneous activity of muscle fibers (632).

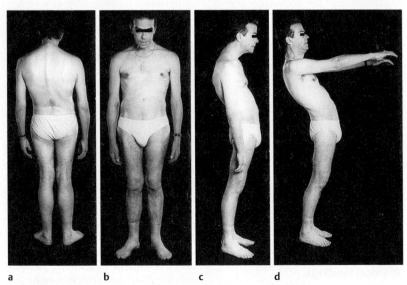

a   b   c   d

Fig. 14.**1e–h**
A 52-year-old man with polymyositis and predominantly proximal quadriparesis.

a–c The body posture is sunken rather than upright, with the head bent forward, the shoulders hanging, the back kyphoscoliotic, and the hips hyperextended. Atrophy mainly of the thigh muscles.

d When the patient stretches his arms forward, the compensatory backward displacement of the trunk is greater than normal.

Muscle tone. The muscle tone is normal or diminished.

Reflexes. The reflexes are *diminished or absent,* roughly in parallel to the extent of weakness. Preserved reflexes despite marked weakness are seen only in myasthenia.

Pain. Only a few types of myopathy are painful. Most infectious myopathies (myositides) produce continuous pain, as does ischemic necrosis of muscle. Metabolic myopathy can cause exercise-induced myalgia.

Myotonic reaction. A myotonic reaction is clinically observable in most forms of myotonia. It consists of the inability of skeletal muscle to relax rapidly immediately after a contraction.

Contracture. Contracture (shortening of a muscle), like pathologic processes in and around the joints, limits passive movement. Contracted muscles show no electromyographic activity.

Muscle spasms. These are painful contractions of one or more muscles that occur either spontaneously (as in the myotonias) or on voluntary innervation (as in the metabolic myopathies). Electromyography reveals high-frequency discharges in many muscle fibers. Muscle spasms are not specific to myopathy.

Paresthesia, dysesthesia, hypesthesia. These sensory abnormalities are always due to peripheral or central nervous system dysfunction and are thus not found in myopathy.

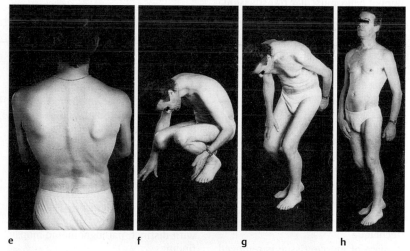

e   f   g   h

Fig. 14.**1e–h**

e The same maneuver induces bilateral winging of the scapula.

f–h To stand up from a squatting position, the patient pushes with his hand against his own thigh (part of the Gowers maneuver).

Fasciculations. Fasciculations reflect the activation of individual motor units. They are a characteristic finding of anterior horn processes, and can also be seen in radiculopathy and neuropathy, but not in myopathy (pp. 427 and 435).

Ancillary Tests in Myopathy

Myopathy can be demonstrated and differentiated from a neurogenic process with the aid of the following ancillary tests:

- ■ **Electromyography and Electroneurography** (pp. 742 and 743)

These procedures are a noninvasive or minimally invasive means of demonstrating primary diseases of muscle. They are also indispensable for the diagnosis of myotonias and disorders of neuromuscular transmission.

- ■ **Muscle Biopsy** (465)

Muscle biopsy is helpful in differentiating myogenic and neurogenic processes from each other and in establishing a specific diagnosis within one or the other category.

Indications

Muscle biopsy is indicated when there is suspicion of a disorder affecting peripheral motor neurons, a primary myopathy, a metabolic disorder of muscle, or a systemic illness affecting muscle.

Technique

A piece of muscle tissue is removed, under sterile technique and local anesthesia, from a muscle that is known to be affected on clinical grounds but is not maximally paretic or atrophic.

Muscle biopsy should not be performed at a site of previous needle puncture for EMG or intramuscular injection. Tissue is usually obtained for light and electron microscopy and histochemical and biochemical study. In our experience, the best results are obtained when the surgeon is well versed in biopsy technique and hands the tissue specimens to a laboratory technician for further processing as soon as they are obtained (i.e., during the operation). Punch biopsies with a hollow needle can also be performed, but these produce smaller specimens and have a lower diagnostic yield.

Histopathology

The histological picture allows differentiation between neurogenic muscular atrophy and primary myopathy. As shown in Figs. 14.**2** and 14.**3**, the atrophic muscle fibers in neurogenic atrophy lie next to each other in small groups. They are usually of elongated polygonal shape, and they are structurally intact. Their nuclei are peripheral, and otherwise appear normal. In primary myopathy, on the other hand, the affected fibers appear randomly distributed in the muscle, and are atrophic to varying degrees. They are usually still round, and they display various structural changes, often without atrophy. Their nuclei are often multiple and centrally located. There may be abnormal proliferation of fat and connective tissue, and inflammatory infiltrates may be found (not only in polymyositis). Certain types of myopathy are associated with distinct, pathognomonic biopsy findings.

Histochemical Studies

Histochemical studies enable a distinction between slow (oxidative)

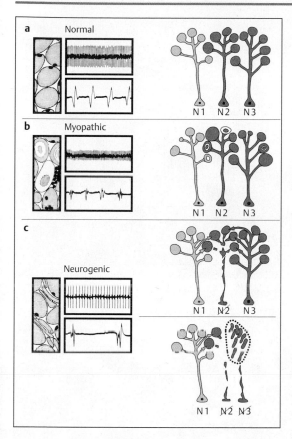

Fig. 14.**2a–c
Motor unit.**

a Normally, the muscle fibers are all of the same caliber. Three motor units are shown. EMG: full interference pattern, normally configured individual motor unit potentials.

b Myopathy. The fibers of different motor units are involved to individually varying degrees. EMG: a full interference pattern is still present, but the amplitude is reduced, and the motor unit potentials are smaller and misshapen.

c Neurogenic lesion affecting a motor ganglion cell or peripheral nerve axon. The muscle fibers belonging to the involved motor unit are denervated; some have been reinnervated by neighboring motor units. If a neighboring motor unit is also lost, a pattern of equally severely atrophic muscle fibers results. EMG: sparse interference pattern on maximal voluntary innervation, and widened, misshapen motor unit potentials.

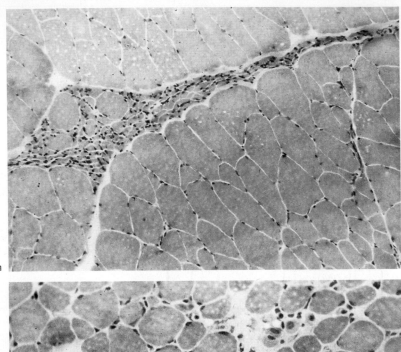

Fig. 14.**3a, b   Muscle biopsy.**
a Spinal muscular atrophy. The muscle fibers are all atrophic to the same degree.
b Progressive muscular dystrophy. The muscle fibers are of varying caliber, some atrophic, some hypertrophic. Central nuclei and regenerating fibers are seen. Mild proliferation of connective tissue.

and fast (glycolytic) muscle fibers (= *type I and type II fibers,* respectively). Systemic illness or inactivity causes loss of type II fibers. Certain enzyme defects can be detected histochemically – e.g., phosphorylase deficiency (McArdle's disease). Lipid stains are useful in the diagnosis of myopathies with abnormal lipid metabolism (carnitine deficiency, carnitine palmitoyltransferase deficiency). Additional *biochemical studies* are often needed for the diagnosis of metabolic myopathies.

■ Serum Muscle Enzymes

Many myopathies elevate the serum concentration of creatine kinase (CK) and other muscle enzymes (aspartate aminotransferase, alanine aminotransferase, lactate dehydrogenase, aldolase). The CK may be only mildly elevated, or not at all, if there is severe muscle atrophy or in the setting of corticosteroid use, collagen diseases, alcoholism, or hyperthyroidism. On the other hand, it may be mildly elevated in the absence of myopathy when a denervating process has led to loss of muscle fibers – e.g., in anterior horn disorders, or after athletic activity.

■ Serum Immunologic Studies

These are mainly helpful in the etiologic diagnosis of the inflammatory myositides.

■ Demonstration of Circulating Antibodies

The demonstration of circulating antibodies – e.g., against the acetylcholine receptor, is important for the diagnosis of myasthenia.

■ Serum Electrolytes

Measurement of serum electrolytes is essential for the diagnosis of episodic paralyses. Abnormal values may also be a sign of an endocrine or metabolic disorder, or of malignancy (e.g., hypercalcemia).

■ Testing with Acetylcholinesterase Inhibitors

This is an easy way of testing for myasthenia.

■ CSF Studies

The CSF is normal in most types of myopathy, with rare exceptions (e.g., elevated CSF protein concentration in hypothyroid myopathy).

■ CT and MRI

CT and MRI of muscle can reveal atrophy, elevated water content, or replacement of muscle tissue by fat.

■ General Medical Examination and Specific Laboratory Tests

These are needed for the detection of systemic conditions affecting muscle (pp. 285 and 299 ff.).

■ Genetic Analysis (98)

Genetic analysis plays an important role in the diagnosis of hereditary myopathies, the identification of carriers, prenatal diagnosis, and prevention. Hereditary myopathy may be of autosomal dominant, autosomal recessive, X-linked, or mitochondrial inheritance, and the underlying genetic defect may be a substitution, deletion, insertion, or duplication of DNA base pairs in the genome.
DNA expansions within a gene are of both diagnostic and prognostic significance. In myotonic dystrophy (p. 874) and in Huntington's disease

(p. 256), the length of the abnormal trinucleotide repeat is correlated with the age of onset of disease, and with its severity. Because the number of repeats increases with each successive generation, the disease tends to appear at younger and younger ages. This clinically observed phenomenon is called *anticipation*.

Classification of Myopathies

The systematic classification of myopathies outlined in Table 14.**1**, based on a combination of clinical, pathophysiological, and genetic considerations, will serve as an organizing framework for the remainder of this chapter.

Table 14.**1**   Classification of myopathies

Group of diseases	Individual diseases	Mode of inheritance
Muscular dystrophies	Progressive muscular dystrophy: Duchenne type Becker type Emery-Dreifuss type Dilated cardiomyopathy	X-linked
	Scapuloperoneal form Steinert's myotonic dystrophy Myotonic dystrophy, proximal form (PROMM) Facioscapulohumeral dystrophy Scapuloperoneal dystrophy Limb girdle forms Distal myopathies (hereditary late-onset distal myopathies of Welander and Markesbery-Griggs) Oculopharyngeal dystrophies	Autosomal dominant
	Limb girdle forms Distal myopathies (Nonaka type, Miyoshi type) Quadriceps myopathy Congenital dystrophies	Autosomal recessive
Spinal muscular atrophy and other motor neuron diseases	See p. 430	

(Cont.) →

Table 14.**1**   *(Cont.)*

Group of diseases	Individual diseases	Mode of inheritance
Myotonias and periodic paralyses ("channelopathies")	Myotonia congenita (Thomsen) Paramyotonia congenita (Eulenburg) Other congenital myotonias Hypokalemic periodic paralysis Hyperkalemic periodic paralysis	Autosomal dominant
Metabolic myopathies	Disorders of carbohydrate metabolism Lipid storage myopathies Disorders of the purine nucleotide cycle	Autosomal recessive
Mitochondrial myopathies and encephalomyopathies	Progressive external ophthalmoplegia and ragged red fibers Kearns-Sayre syndrome MERFF syndrome MELAS syndrome NARP syndrome (and others)	Maternal
Congenital myopathies	Central core myopathy Nemaline (rod) myopathy Centronuclear myopathy (and others	Autosomal dominant, X-linked
Inflammatory myopathies	Polymyositis Dermatomyositis Juvenile dermatomyositis Poly- and dermatomyositis in malignancy Polymyositis in collagen disease Sarcoidosis Eosinophilia-myalgia syndrome Infectious myositis	Not hereditary
Myopathy in endocrine disorders	Hypothyroidism Hyperthyroidism Cushing's disease Steroid myopathy Acromegaly Hypoparathyroidism Hyperparathyroidism	Not hereditary

(Cont.) →

Table 14.**1** *(Cont.)*

Group of diseases	Individual diseases	Mode of inheritance
Toxic and drug-induced myopathies	Muscle injury due to alcohol abuse (rhabdomyolysis, acute alcoholic myopathy, subacute and chronic alcoholic myopathy), cocaine, heroin, "self-crush" in drug-induced coma, vacuolar myopathy due to colchicine, chloroquine, or vincristine, hypokalemic myopathy due to diuretics, laxatives, licorice or alcohol Emetine, ipecac Gasoline fumes, toluene Cholesterol-lowering drugs Inflammatory myopathy due to penicillamine or cimetidine Nutritional deficiency, vitamin E deficiency	Not hereditary
Disorders of neuromuscular transmission	Myasthenia gravis pseudoparalytica Congenital myasthenia gravis Lambert-Eaton myasthenic syndrome Botulism Bungarotoxins Familial infantile myasthenia Slow channel syndrome	Not hereditary Autosomal recessive or dominant
Tumors		
Trauma		
Ischemia		

Muscular Dystrophies

Overview:
The muscular dystrophies are a group of hereditary diseases caused by abnormalities of the dystrophin-associated membrane complex. The clinical features of most types of muscular dystrophy were described many decades ago, but the underlying genetic defects and the associated abnormal or deficient gene products have only begun to be identified in recent years as a result of major progress in molecular biology. In muscular dystrophy of the Duchenne or Becker type, for example, a genetic defect leads to deficient or absent expression of the structural protein dystrophin; these diseases are thus referred to as *dystrophinopathies*. On the other hand, the *sarcoglycanopathies* are caused by deficient sarcoglycan expression and clinically characterized by limb girdle dystrophy. Another disease, *myotonic dystrophy*, is due to a trinucleotide repeat mutation in the DM gene; its clinical manifestations are more or less severe depending on the number of trinucleotide copies present. Molecular genetic advances have made it much easier to assign a specific diagnosis in cases of muscular dystrophy, and genetic counseling has come to play a major role in patients' family planning decisions. It is hoped that further advances will point the way to effective therapies in the near future.

The proteins of the dystrophin-associated membrane complex, which have been discovered only in the last few years, play a vital role in maintaining the normal structure and function of muscle cells. The complex includes the extracellular protein laminin-2 (= merosin), the intra- or juxtamembranous dystro- and sarcoglycans, and the intracellular syntrophins and dystrophins (Fig. 14.**4**). The absence or deficient expression of one of these proteins is clinically expressed as a muscular dystrophy, which, depending on the protein involved, may first become symptomatic in childhood or adulthood. The particular protein involved also determines whether the disease will affect all muscles or will preferentially affect the oculopharyngeal muscles, the limb girdles, or the distal limb muscles. The functions of the individual proteins are not known in detail; they are thought to play mechanical and structural roles and to regulate the permeability of the muscle cell membrane – e.g., to calcium. These functions are essential prerequisites for normal muscle contraction. The major types of muscular dystrophy, to be discussed in the following sections, are listed in Table 14.**2**.

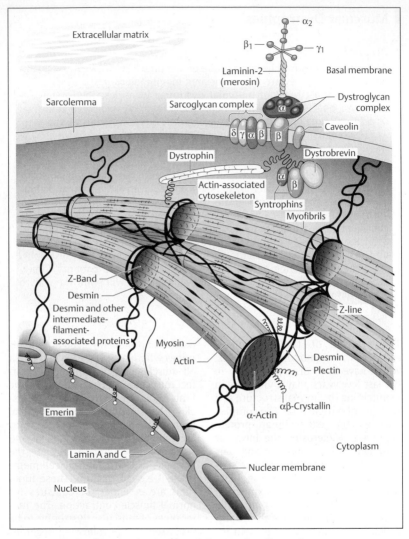

Fig. 14.**4 Dystrophin protein complex of the muscle cell membrane**
(adapted from Dalakas et al., 2000).

Table 14.2 The muscular dystrophies

Type	Inheritance pattern	Chromosomal or genomic defect	Missing or abnormal gene product	Incidence (i.e., frequency with respect to live births)	Age of onset	Clinical features	Prognosis
Duchenne	X-linked, 30% sporadic	Xp21.2	Dystrophin absent	20–30/100,000 boys	2nd–3rd year	Onset in pelvic girdle, pseudohypertrophy of calves	Rapidly progressive, most patients die by age 25
Becker	X-linked	Xp21.2	Dystrophin abnormal	3/100,000 boys	1st(–4th) decade	Same as in Duchenne muscular dystrophy, but milder; sometimes cardiomyopathy	Ambulatory till age 15 or later, death in 4th or 5th decade or later
Emery-Dreifuss	X-linked, rarely autosomal-dominant	Xp28	Emerin	1/100,000	Childhood, adolescence	Scapuloperoneal dystrophy, contractures, and cardiopathy may be prominent	Ambulatory till 3rd decade or for entire life; cardiac arrhythmia a frequent cause of death
Facioscapulohumeral dystrophy (Duchenne-Landouzy-Dejerine)	Autosomal-dominant	4q35	Homeobox gene	5/100,000	Childhood to young adulthood	Weakness of facial, shoulder girdle, and calf muscles	Practically normal life expectancy

(Cont.) →

Table 14.2 The muscular dystrophies

Type	Inheritance pattern	Chromosomal or genomic defect	Missing or abnormal gene product	Incidence (i.e., frequency with respect to live births)	Age of onset	Clinical features	Prognosis
Scapuloperoneal dystrophy	Autosomal dominant, autosomal recessive, or sporadic	Unknown	Unknown	Rare	Childhood to adulthood	Weakness of shoulder girdle and dorsiflexors of the feet and toes	Usually normal life expectancy
Limb girdle dystrophy in adults and severe autosomal-recessive muscular dystrophy in children	Autosomal recessive, autosomal dominant (only the caveolin-3 type), or sporadic	17q12-q21.33 4q12 13q12 5q33-q34 15q15.1-q21.1 3q25	α-sarcoglycan β-sarcoglycan γ-sarcoglycan δ-sarcoglycan calpain-3 caveolin-3	3–4/100,000	Childhood to adulthood	Mainly proximal weakness of pelvic or shoulder girdle	Depending on type, premature death or only minor disability into old age
Distal myopathies (Welander and Markesbery-Grigg types, Finnish variant)	Autosomal dominant	2p13 (Welander type) 2q31 (Markesbery-Griggs type)	Unknown	Rare	Middle age	Mainly distal atrophy and weakness	Only minor disability into old age
Distal myopathies (Nonaka and Miyoshi types)	Autosomal recessive	Miyoshi: 2p12-14 Nonaka: unknown	Unknown	Rare	Adolescence to young adulthood	Mainly distal weakness	Progression to inability to walk

(Cont.) →

Table 14.2 The muscular dystrophies

Oculopharyngeal dystrophies	Autosomal dominant	14q11.2-q13	Poly-(A-) binding protein 2	Rare	Middle age	Oculofaciobulbar paresis	Often premature death due to dysphagia and aspiration pneumonia
Congenital dystrophies (for variants, see text)	Autosomal recessive	6q2	Merosin	Rare	At birth	Depending on type: involvement of muscles, eyes, and brain; contractures, arthrogryposis multiplex	Ranging from mild disability to severe mental retardation
Steinert's myotonic dystrophy	Autosomal dominant	19q13.3	Myotonin protein kinase	13.5/100,000, prevalence 5/100,000	Young adulthood, rarely congenital, earlier age of onset in each successive generation ("anticipation")	Mainly distal weakness, faciobulbar paresis, myotonia, cataracts	Age of significant disability depends on age of onset, usually middle age; premature death
Proximal myotonic myopathy (PROMM)	Autosomal dominant	Unknown	Unknown	0.5/100,000	3rd and 4th decades, sometimes earlier	Mainly proximal weakness, myotonia, and cataracts	Disability in old age

Progressive Muscular Dystrophy of Duchenne Type (142)

Epidemiology and Pathogenesis

This disorder is due to a lack of expression of the structural protein dystrophin, leading to progressive destruction of muscle fibers (626, 736). Dystrophin is located within the cell and is a part of the muscle cell membrane (sarcolemma). It probably plays a role in the interaction of the con- tractile and stationary elements of the muscle fiber. It is inherited in X-linked recessive fashion. The responsible gene is found on the short arm of the X chromosome at the site Xp21.2. It is present in 20–30 per 100,000 boys at birth, and its prevalence in the male population is three per 100,000. As many as 30 % of cases are sporadic (the result of new mutations).

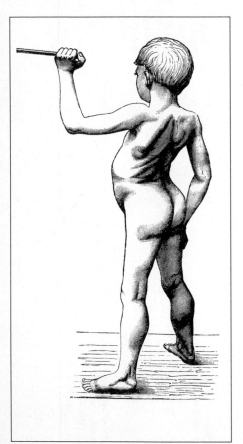

Fig. 14.**5 Progressive muscular dystrophy.**
Drawing of a child with muscular dystrophy, from the original publication by Erb (W. Erb, Dystrophia muscularis progressiva. Klinische und pathologisch-anatomische Studien. Dtsch Z Nervenheilkd 1891; 1: 13–94, 173–261).

Involvement of Muscle

Delivery and early childhood development are normal. Development usually slows before age 3, as the child learns to stand and walk. The child's movements become clumsy, coarse, and uncoordinated, with particular worsening of walking, jumping, and climbing stairs. The proximal muscles of the pelvic girdle are prominently involved at first, less so the shoulder girdle and the neck flexors. The muscle involvement is roughly symmetric.

Loss of muscle fibers leads to clinically evident muscle atrophy. In some muscles, however, the replacement of muscle fibers by fat and connective tissue can compensate for the lost muscle volume or even produce pseudohypertrophy (Fig. 14.5), particularly in the calves and buttocks, but also in the deltoids, the muscles of mastication, and the tongue. Some muscles may have atrophic portions intermingled with zones of preserved contractility ("boules musculaires").

The weakness of the hip muscles leads to a bilateral *Duchenne gait abnormality,* and later to a bilateral *Trendelenburg gait abnormality,* with a characteristic waddling appearance. To stand up from a lying position, the affected boys turn themselves prone, spread the legs or pull them together, raise the buttocks, and then climb with their arms and hands up their own thighs till they are upright *(Gowers sign).* Furthermore, the hip weakness, in combination with weakness of the abdominal and paraspinal musculature, causes severe *spinal lordosis when the patient stands or walks,* which is accompanied by a backward thrust of the shoulders that gives the patient a characteristic posture. The scapulae are projected forward in wing-like fashion. If the examiner tries to pick up the patient by holding him under the axillae, he tends to slip out of the examiner's hold *("loose shoulder sign").* When the patient is supine, he cannot raise his head from the pillow. *The tongue is pseudohypertrophic,* and, in advanced stages of the disease, a mildly *myopathic facies* is not uncommon.

The *intrinsic muscle reflexes* are diminished, with the exception of the Achilles reflexes, which long remain normal. Contractures arise as the disease progresses, producing a tiptoe gait.

Course

Duchenne muscular dystrophy progresses rapidly. It affects first the pelvic girdle, then the shoulder girdle. Most patients become unable to walk at some time between the ages of 8 and 15. Most die between the ages of 18 and 25.

Involvement of Other Organs

Dystrophin is expressed, not only in skeletal muscle, but also in smooth muscle and in the brain. Patients with Duchenne muscular dystrophy almost always have demonstrable involvement of the myocardium and intracardiac conducting system, but heart failure and arrhythmia are seen only in advanced disease. Smooth muscle involvement may cause acute gastric distension and intestinal pseudo-obstruction. CNS involvement accounts for the occasional finding of mild mental retardation in a Duchenne child.

Ancillary Tests (586b)

The *serum creatine kinase concentration* is already markedly elevated in the preclinical stage. It reaches a maximum in the third year of life (50–100 times normal), then declines thereafter by about 20% per year. A merely mild elevation of the creatine kinase concentration is inconsistent with the diagnosis of Duchenne muscular dystrophy, except in a very late stage.

The *EMG* reveals a myopathic pattern with as many as 50% low polyphasic potentials and spontaneous activity in the form of fibrillation potentials, positive sharp waves, and complex repetitive discharges (= pseudomyotonic discharges). The nerve conduction velocities are normal.

Muscle biopsy reveals a pathological variation of muscle fiber caliber, isolated or small focal groups of necrotic fibers with macrophages, regenerating fibers, and hypertrophic fibers, often with central nuclei. Moreover, round-cell infiltrates may be present, and intramuscular fat and connective tissue become more and more prominent as the disease progresses. The diagnosis is definitively established by immunohistochemical staining for the absent dystrophin molecule (Fig. 14.**6**).

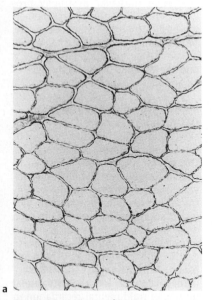
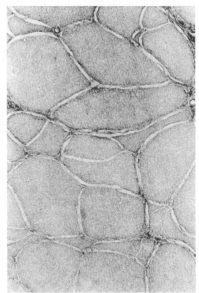

Fig. 14.**6a–c Dystrophin stain.**
a Normal skeletal muscle. Regular, homogeneous distribution of dystrophin on inner surface of sarcolemma.

b Duchenne dystrophy. Dystrophin is absent.

DNA analysis (e.g., of leukocyte DNA) reveals deletions, duplications, or point mutations of the dystrophin gene. These findings are important for prenatal diagnosis and for the detection of female carriers.

Differential Diagnosis

Important entities in the differential diagnosis are *congenital muscular dystrophies, spinal muscular atrophy,* and *acid maltase deficiency.*

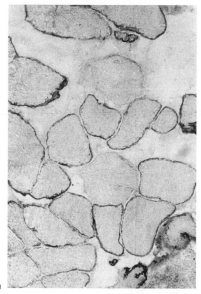

a

c Becker dystrophy. Dystrophin is expressed to a varying extent on the individual muscle fibers, in diminished quantity and abnormal distribution.

Treatment

The first important therapeutic step after establishment of the diagnosis is *psychological counseling* of the parents. The child, too, will require counseling as he grows older.

Somatic therapy consists of *physical therapy* and *orthopedic aids.* Important measures to be taken in early childhood to prevent contractures include regular exercise, swimming, and passive stretching of the limbs by the patient's parents and physiotherapists. Night splints may also be useful.

In the late stage of the disease, *assisted respiration* – e.g., continuous positive airway pressure (CPAP) at night – may considerably improve the patient's quality of life in the daytime. *Prednisone* (0.75 mg/kg/ day) improves muscular strength at the cost of side effects such as weight gain and slowing of vertical growth (362). Cyclosporine, too, improves strength (865). The utility of these medications in the long term remains an open question. The same can be said for *myoblast transfer* and *gene therapy.*

Benign Muscular Dystrophy of Becker Type (78, 154)

Becker muscular dystrophy is one-tenth as common as the Duchenne type. It resembles the latter in all respects except that its progression is much slower and relatively benign. The genetic defect is at the same site. Dystrophin is expressed, but in abnormal fashion. The initial manifestations of the disease are evident in the first decade of life in about half of all patients. They consist of mainly proximal weakness and atrophy, with pseudohypertrophy of the calves. On average, patients become unable to walk in their thirties. Most die in the fifth decade of life.

Nonetheless, the phenotype is highly variable. The *milder forms* of Becker muscular dystrophy produce only myalgia and muscle cramps, exercise intolerance, and myoglobinuria, or mild truncal girdle atrophy, or benign quadriceps myopathy (984). The life expectancy in such cases is practically normal. The *more severe forms* of the disease begin in early childhood and are clinically indistinguishable from Duchenne muscular dystrophy. The serum creatine kinase concentration is elevated 20–100-fold. The findings of EMG and muscle biopsy resemble those in Duchenne muscular dystrophy. Dystrophin is present in diminished quantity and/or abnormal distribution (cf. Fig. 14.**6c**).

X-Chromosomal Dilated Cardiomyopathy (947)

This disorder, another X-linked dystrophinopathy, is characterized by dilated cardiomyopathy with progressive heart failure, leading to end-stage heart failure in the second or third decade of life.

Progressive Muscular Dystrophy of Emery-Dreifuss Type (274)

Genetics

This type of muscular dystrophy is X-linked or, rarely, autosomal dominant. The responsible genetic defect lies on the long arm of the X chromosome, in the Xq28 band. The gene product, emerin, is a protein of the nuclear membrane. In this condition, emerin is absent not only in muscle cells, but also in cells of other types (blood, skin).

Clinical Features

Prominent contractures appear early, particularly in the elbow flexors and calf muscles. These result in an inability to straighten the upper limb, and in pes equinus. At first, the muscle atrophy affects mainly the biceps, triceps, tibialis anterior, and peroneus muscles, but it later comes to involve the upper and lower limb girdles as well. Frequently, the heart, too, is involved, with bradycardia and conduction abnormalities that usually necessitate pacemaker placement. The onset of disease is in childhood or adolescence. Most patients remain able to walk into their third decade, some of them for life.

Prevention of Muscular Dystrophy of the Duchenne, Becker, and Emery-Dreifuss Types

The mothers of patients with muscular dystrophy of these three types are carriers of the disease (unless a new mutation is responsible). So, too, are all daughters of patients, and 50% of their sisters. Occasionally, female carriers show signs of a mild form of myopathy, with mild atrophy or calf pseudohypertrophy, myalgia, cramps, elevation of the creatine kinase concentration, and ECG and EMG changes.

Female carriers can be identified with certainty only through DNA analysis. If a specific DNA mutation can be identified in an affected patient, the same mutation can be easily sought in female relatives by PCR testing. If no such mutation is found, linkage analysis of the patient's family can be helpful. The information derived from these tests serves as a basis for genetic counseling. A female carrier who becomes pregnant can be offered prenatal DNA analysis, the results of which will weigh in the decision whether to terminate the pregnancy, if this is in accordance with her ethical and religious views.

Facioscapulohumeral Muscular Dystrophy (Duchenne-Landouzy-Dejerine) (143, 308a)

Genetics

Facioscapulohumeral muscular dystrophy is inherited in autosomal dominant fashion. There are also occasional sporadic cases. Linkage analysis has shown the underlying genetic defect to be a deletion in the 4q35 region of chromosome 4. The incidence of this disorder is relatively high: four per 100,000 births.

Clinical Features

The disease initially affects the face and the shoulder girdle. Eye closure may be incomplete, or the patient may be unable to whistle, drink through a straw, or lift an object above shoulder height. The objective findings include a myopathic facies without ptosis and weakness and atrophy of the shoulder girdle muscles, with winging of the scapula. The strength and bulk of the deltoids are preserved to the greatest degree and for the longest time. At first, the pattern of muscular involvement is often markedly asymmetric. Sensorineural deafness is also common. The disease first appears in the second and third decades of life and progresses very slowly thereafter. Over the course of time there may develop peroneal atrophy, foot drop, and, later, weakness of the pelvic girdle and of the distal muscles of the upper limb. The life expectancy is minimally shortened, if at all.

Ancillary Tests

The serum creatine kinase concentration is normal to mildly elevated. EMG and muscle biopsy reveal myopathic changes. The appearance of inflammatory infiltrates in a biopsy specimen may make it difficult to differentiate this condition from polymyositis.

Treatment

The treatment consists of symptomatic measures, such as orthopedic aids. Surgical fixation of the scapula to the chest wall occasionally improves function.

Scapuloperoneal Muscular Dystrophy

The weakness in this condition (unlike the one last discussed above) mainly affects the shoulder muscles and the dorsiflexors of the feet and toes. The differentiation of this condition from spinal muscular atrophy with a similar distribution can sometimes be made only with the aid of ancillary tests. The serum creatine kinase concentration is normal to mildly elevated. The progression is slow, and the life expectancy mostly normal.

Autosomal Recessive and Autosomal Dominant Limb Girdle Dystrophies (871)

The limb girdle dystrophies, sometimes also called truncal girdle dystrophies, make up a heterogeneous spectrum of mainly autosomal recessive and, less commonly, autosomal dominant inherited disorders. The underlying genetic defects and the corresponding deficient or absent gene products are listed in Table 14.**2** (586a).

The clinical manifestations are highly variable. They range from childhood onset and rapid progression to onset in late adulthood and barely discernible myopathy. Muscular involvement in these dystrophies usually begins in the pelvic girdle and later ascends to the shoulder girdle, though the reverse pattern is also found. The oculopharyngeal and distal limb muscles are also affected.

An autosomal dominant variant, *Bethlem myopathy* (named after its describer), usually begins at an early age and progresses slowly. Many adult patients become disabled by contractures (465a).

Some of the limb girdle dystrophies are associated with cardiomyopathy, which may even be their most prominent manifestation. The differential diagnosis encompasses most neuro- and myogenic processes causing mainly proximal weakness.

Distal Myopathies (711b)

A number of myopathies primarily affect the distal musculature. The following forms can be distinguished on clinical grounds:

Hereditary tardive distal myopathy of Welander type. This condition, the first distal myopathy to be described, is most common among persons of Scandinavian descent and is due to a genetic defect on chromosome 2p13 (1013). It begins in middle age and affects first the hand muscles and, later, the distal muscles of the lower limb. The serum creatine kinase concentration is normal to mildly elevated, and the progression is slow.

Distal myopathies beginning in adolescence or adulthood. *Distal myopathy of Markesbery-Griggs type* is an autosomal dominant disease of late onset that begins with weakness and atrophy in the feet and later involves the hands and arms as well. This disease differs from myopathy of Welander type in that it frequently causes severe cardiomyopathy. A *Finnish variant* of distal myopathy is restricted to the lower limbs (961). The genetic defect in both Markesbery-Griggs myopathy and the Finnish variant is on chromosome 2q31 (385b). Splints to support the extensor muscles can be of therapeutic benefit, improving both hand function and mobility. Early-onset distal myopathies – i.e., those beginning in adolescence or young adulthood – have an autosomal recessive inheritance pattern. The *Nonaka type* initially involves the anterior muscular compartment of the leg, while the *Miyoshi type* initially involves the calf muscles. These disorders often progress to inability to walk. They are caused by genetic defects on chromosomes 9p1-q1 and 2p13, respectively.

Distal myopathies beginning in infancy or childhood. It is not clear at present whether the forms beginning

---

in infancy and childhood (the latter referred to as hereditary juvenile distal myopathy of Biemond) are a single disease or different diseases. Ancillary tests must be performed to distinguish these types of myopathy from Steinert's myotonic dystrophy, neuropathies (particularly Charcot-Marie-Tooth disease), and the distal form of spinal muscular atrophy.

Myofibrillar myopathies. Diseases in this group can also present with mainly distal weakness. One member of the group, *desmin myopathy,* is caused by a missense mutation in the desmin gene. The disease first becomes evident in young adulthood with mainly distal myopathy, accompanied by a cardiomyopathy that can cause conduction abnormalities and heart failure (205b).

Oculopharyngeal Dystrophy

Genetics
This type of muscular dystrophy is of autosomal dominant inheritance. The underlying genetic defect is on chromosome 14q11.2-q13, and the defective gene product is the Poly-(A-) binding protein.

Clinical Features
Oculopharyngeal dystrophy begins in middle age with mild weakness of the extraocular muscles and mild ptosis. These findings gradually progress until total ophthalmoplegia is present. By this time, the facial and bulbar musculature is also weak, and the shoulder and hip muscles may be as well. When dysphagia becomes severe, cachexia and recurrent aspiration pneumonia ensue.

Diagnostic Evaluation
The *serum creatine kinase concentration, EMG,* and *histology* all point to a myopathy. Rimmed vacuoles and typical tubular filaments are seen on muscle biopsy.

Differential Diagnosis
The most important element in the differential diagnosis is *myasthenia gravis* (p. 911). *Myotonic dystrophy* (see below), *Kearns-Sayre syndrome* (p. 897), and *inclusion body myositis* can present similarly. Ocular muscular dystrophies almost always involve other muscles beside those of the eyes.

Congenital Muscular Dystrophies

These are muscular dystrophies that are clinically evident at birth, producing a number of different clinical syndromes. Currently, five kinds of congenital muscular dystrophy are recognized:
- A relatively *nonprogressive congenital muscular dystrophy* with or without *arthrogryposis multiplex.* The latter term refers to congenital joint contractures with often grotesquely deformed postures and severely impaired mobility of the affected joints. A number of different neuromuscular processes may be the cause.
- *Congenital muscular dystrophy of Fukuyama type,* which is always combined with a developmental disturbance of the brain.
- *Congenital muscular dystrophy of Walker-Warburg type,* involving the muscles, eyes, and brain.
- *Congenital muscular dystrophy of Santavuori type,* also involving the muscles, eyes, and brain.

- *Rigid spine syndrome,* in which contractures of the paraspinous musculature restrict mobility of the spine and mainly proximal limb weakness may be present. In the patient's later years, this syndrome resembles Becker muscular dystrophy.

Steinert's Myotonic Dystrophy (389)

Epidemiology and Genetics

This disease, described by Steinert in 1909, is the most common type of myopathy in adults. It is found in 13.5 of 100,000 live births and has a prevalence of 5 per 100,000. The responsible genetic defect is on chromosome 19q13.3, a site encoding myotonin protein kinase. The mutation consists of an unstable expansion of CTG trinucleotide sequences within the gene, in which the usual length of 5–30 trinucleotide repeats is exceeded.

The disease is inherited in autosomal-dominant fashion. In each successive generation, the trinucleotide repeat expansion is longer and the disease becomes evident at an earlier age (anticipation, cf. p. 858). This is particularly true when the patient inherits the disease from his or her mother; if the inheritance is paternal, the expansion may become shorter. The expansion is very long (more than 750 CTG repeats) in congenital myotonic dystrophy (see below). These facts explain why almost all mothers of children with congenital myotonic dystrophy have clinically evident disease themselves, and why affected fathers can have children who are only mildly affected (39, 720).

Clinical Features of Muscular Involvement

The disease usually becomes clinically evident in young adulthood but may do so either earlier or later. *Myotonia* is often the most prominent manifestation of the disease in its initial stage. Later on, *dystrophy* becomes increasingly marked, making myotonia difficult or impossible to elicit. Myotonia is elicited by quick percussion or powerful voluntary contraction of a muscle, producing a visible dent or visibly slowed relaxation. The muscles of the thumb and of the tongue are good ones to test for myotonia. Another sign of myotonia is the inability to extend the fingers quickly after the fist is clenched.

The dystrophy, and with it the *weakness* and *atrophy,* affect the facial and distal limb muscles first, the proximal limb muscles later. Involvement of the face and forehead produces a characteristic facial appearance: sunken temples, atrophic masseters, flaccid periocular and perioral muscles, and, later, bilateral ptosis.

Ptosis in this disease is hardly ever severe enough to impair sight (in distinction to mitochondrial myopathies and myasthenia gravis). The atrophic sternocleidomastoid muscles contrast with the preserved neck extensors. Weakness and atrophy in the extremities are mainly distal and affect extensors more than flexors. The muscles of the shoulder and pelvic girdles are affected only in a late stage of the disease, if at all, so that a Trendelenburg gait abnormality hardly ever appears and the patient usually remains able to walk till shortly before death.

Involvement of Other Organs

The protein kinase abnormality has consequences for many organ systems other than muscle. Sometimes, involvement of another organ system can become a greater problem for the patient than the muscular dystrophy itself:

- In the eyes, cataracts and involvement of the ciliary body with low intraocular pressure are present as a rule. Voluntary eye movements, including saccades, may be restricted or slowed.
- Smooth muscle involvement in the esophagus and stomach can lead to dysphagia. Smooth muscle involvement in the colon and anal sphincter can lead to dysfunctional defecation with megacolon and stool retention.
- Cardiac involvement is usually seen in the advanced stage of the disease, mostly in the form of intracardiac conduction abnormalities. Dilated cardiomyopathy is also encountered. Sudden cardiac death is not uncommon.
- In the advanced stage of the disease, there are repeated attacks of aspiration pneumonia, and chronic hypoventilation can manifest itself in abnormal fatigue and daytime somnolence.
- Peripheral nerve involvement may cause a mild sensory deficit.
- Patients with the congenital form of the disease are severely mentally retarded. In adult-onset disease, involvement of the brain may produce a mild cognitive deficit.
- Endocrine disturbances are common.
- Affected men usually have testicular atrophy, and affected women often have irregular menstrual cycles.
- Cranial hyperostosis is the most prominent skeletal abnormality.

Ancillary Tests

The *serum creatine kinase concentration* is normal or mildly elevated. The *EMG* reveals signs of myopathy combined with myotonic discharges, mainly in the distal muscles, less so in the proximal muscles (Fig. 14.**7**). *Electroneurography* may reveal mildly slowed nerve conduction velocities. *Muscle biopsy* reveals signs of dystrophy. The prominent (though nonspecific) findings include a large number of central nuclei, which are arranged in rows on longitudinal section; ring fibers; and sarcoplasmic masses. The diagnosis is definitively established by *DNA analysis*. DNA can be obtained from leukocytes or from chorionic or amniotic cells for prenatal diagnosis. Some 50–75 CTG trinucleotide repeats are found in patients with milder forms of the disease, and as many as several hundred in patients with more severe forms. The normal number is below 30.

Prognosis

Among patients who develop symptoms in young adulthood, more than half will become disabled from work at a young age. Most die between the ages of 45 and 50. The course of the disease, however, is highly variable. Persons with mild forms may attain old age with no more serious problem than a cataract. Patients and their relatives should undergo genetic counseling, whenever possible, before they marry and have children.

Treatment

Only symptomatic treatment can be provided. Whatever symptomatic improvement can be achieved for the patient's *dysphagia and respiratory difficulties* will substantially improve his or her quality of life. *Cardiac arrhythmias* may necessitate pacemaker placement. *Orthopedic procedures* to correct abnormal postures should be resorted to sparingly, as they generally do not improve function.

The *myotonia* itself can be very disturbing in the early stage of the disease. It can often be ameliorated with *antiepileptic and antiarrhythmic drugs* such as *phenytoin* 100 mg t.i.d.,. *quinidine sulfate* 1–1.5 g/day, or *procainamide* 0.5–1.0 g q.i.d.

Caveat: These medications can be dangerous, as they may worsen an intracardiac conduction abnormality, if present.

Congenital Myotonic Dystrophy

Genetics

Congenital myotonic dystrophy is generally transferred to the child from a mother who herself has a long trinucleotide expansion. The disease affects both boys and girls.

Clinical Features

From birth onward, the patient suffers from dysphagia for solids and liquids. The face appears weak, flaccid, and mask-like. The upper lip forms an inverted V. A high palate is invariably found. Muscle tone is diminished, motor development is slowed, and the patient is mentally retarded. The sternocleidomastoid and temporalis muscles are atrophic. Myotonia is evident on EMG tracings and sometimes clinically as well. Deformities of the foot, scoliosis, and micrognathia are common.

Cause

This disorder is caused by a very long CTG trinucleotide repeat expansion (more than 2000 copies in some cases).

Proximal Myotonic Myopathy (PROMM) (787, 939)

Genetics

This disorder is genetically heterogeneous, and the underlying genetic defects have not yet been identified. A further form of dystrophic myotonia is linked to a lesion of chromosome 3q21 (221a).

Clinical Features

PROMM resembles myotonic dystrophy in one of its milder forms: its manifestations are myotonia, myopathy, and cataract, and cardiac arrhythmias and testicular atrophy may also be present. It is distinguished from myotonic dystrophy by the mainly proximal myopathy, the only mild muscular atrophy, and the absence of anticipation.

Course

The course is benign. The patient's gait is not impaired till old age.

▌Myotonias and Periodic Paralyses (442)

Overview:
The primary function of skeletal muscle is to contract and perform mechanical work. Necessary preconditions for this are: normal depolarization of the nerve terminals, secretion of acetylcholine into the synaptic cleft, depolarization of the postsynaptic membrane and spread of the action potential through the transverse tubular system, entry of calcium into the sarcoplasm, and, finally, the interaction of actin and myosin. If one of these processes is inoperative, the contractile mechanism cannot function. The myotonias and periodic paralyses are genetic diseases that impair the functioning of the chloride and sodium channels of the muscle cell membrane and thereby prevent normal muscle contraction and relaxation.

Though most of the diseases in this group have been well-defined clinical entities for many years, their underlying genetic defects have only been discovered recently, and with them the common underlying pathogenetic mechanism – i.e., a disturbance of one of several different voltage-dependent, ligand-controlled transmembrane ion channels. These diseases have thus come to be known as "ion channel diseases" or, more informally, "channelopathies." They include the following:
- the periodic paralyses,
- the myotonias,
- cardiac arrhythmias,
- types of hereditary epilepsy, such as nocturnal frontal lobe epilepsy (p. ■) (an autosomal dominant disease),
- types of migraine (776a).

Major features of the more common ion channel diseases – i.e., the myotonias and the periodic paralyses – are summarized in Table 14.**3**.

The Myotonias (775)

Myotonia is a prolonged relaxation phase after a voluntary muscle contraction. It can be detected either mechanically, as a dent in a percussed muscle or an abnormally slow reopening of the eye or fist after forced closure, or electrically, as repetitive discharges in the EMG. It is usually more pronounced in low ambient temperatures and tends to improve on repeated muscle contraction (warm-up phenomenon). *Paramyotonia* is different, in that it is markedly worsened by cold, but also by repeated muscle contraction.

Mild myotonic reactions are sometimes seen in diseases other than the hereditary myotonias – e.g., in polymyositis, progressive muscular dystrophy, glycogen storage diseases (particularly acid maltase deficiency), centronuclear myopathy, small-cell lung cancer, and hypothyroidism.

Table 14.3 Myotonias and periodic paralyses ("channelopathies")

Type	Inheritance pattern	Chromo-somal or genomic defect	Missing or ab-normal gene product	Incidence (i.e., frequency with respect to live births)	Age of onset	Clinical features	Prognosis
Myotonia congenita, Thomsen type	Autosomal dominant	7q35	Abnormal chloride channels	1/23,000	Early childhood	Generalized myotonia	Stable, nonpro-gressive
Myotonia congenita, Becker type	Autosomal recessive	7q35	Abnormal chloride channels	1/23,000 – 1/50,000	End of 1st decade	Generalized myotonia	Stable, nonpro-gressive
Myotonia fluctuans, myotonia permanens, acetazolamide-sensitive myotonia	Autosomal dominant	17q23-25	Abnormal sodium channels	Very rare	Childhood; myotonia fluctuans in adolescence	Generalized, myotonia fluctuans only episodic, other types severe, potassium loading worsens myotonia, acetazolamide-sensitive myotonia is painful	Nonprogressive
Paramyotonia congenita of Eulenburg	Autosomal dominant	17q23-25	Abnormal sodium channels	Very rare	Childhood	Generalized myotonia induced by cold and worsened by exertion, occasionally combined with paramyotonic and hyperkalemic paralyses	Persistent, tends to improve over time

(Cont.) →

Table 14.3 (Cont.)

Hyperkalemic periodic paralysis	Autosomal dominant	17q23-25	Abnormal sodium channels	Very rare	Childhood	Paralysis occurring on fasting, or rest after physical activity	Persistent, often improves over time. Permanent myopathy and weakness are less severe than in hypokalemic paralysis.
Hypokalemic periodic paralysis	Autosomal dominant	1q31-32	Calcium channels	Very rare	age 5–30, usually in 2nd decade	Paralysis occurring after carbohydrate consumption or physical activity	Persistent, often slowly developing permanent myopathy and weakness

Myotonia Congenita (Thomsen and Becker Types)

Genetics

The inheritance pattern of myotonia congenita is either autosomal dominant (Thomsen type) or autosomal recessive (Becker type). The underlying genetic defect in either case is on chromosome 7q35 at the chloride channel locus. The resulting abnormality of chloride channels lowers the chloride conductance, the net effect of which is to increase the electrical excitability of muscle fibers.

Clinical Features

Myotonia congenita becomes manifest at a very early age, sometimes "in the cradle." Its characteristic feature is the myotonic reaction that is common to all striated muscles, proximal as well as distal. The muscles display delayed relaxation after voluntary or electrically induced contraction, or even after stretching by percussion. A tightly gripped object cannot be let go at once, the clenched fist cannot be rapidly opened, and tapping of the tongue with the edge of a tongue depressor leaves a dent that remains apparent for some time.

At first, the patient cannot carry out any rapid movement, but this becomes possible after repeated attempts (warm-up phenomenon). Sudden, forceful movements may be impossible because of *transient myotonic paralysis*, rather than myotonic rigidity per se. When a patient with myotonia lifts a heavy suitcase, the handle may simply slide out of the patient's hand rather than remain tightly gripped. In some patients, myotonia of the lid muscles manifests itself as blepharospasm after forced lid closure.

The severity of myotonia may fluctuate, but it is not affected by cold, stress, sporting activities or diet. The muscles are of normal strength and bulk. In many cases, indeed, they are more prominent than normal, so that patients may actually have an athletic habitus. The hypertrophic masseter muscles lend a characteristic appearance to the face. Myotonia tends to become less severe over time, and patients are generally fully able to work. The life expectancy is normal.

Ancillary Tests

The *EMG appearance* is characteristic. Low-amplitude, high-frequency potentials continue to be seen for several seconds after the end of voluntary contraction and are heard in the audio channel as a characteristic "motorcycle" or "dive-bomber" sound (Fig. 14.7). The same occurs when the EMG needle is mechanically displaced. When a nerve is electrically stimulated, even at low intensity, what results is not a motor unit contraction, but tetany.

Muscle biopsy reveals nothing on conventional staining, but the absence of type IIb fibers can be demonstrated with *histochemical* stains.

Differences between the Thomsen and Becker Types of Myotonia Congenita

Clinical and electromyographic study of near relatives never reveals myotonia in anyone but the patient if he or she suffers from the Becker type of myotonia congenita (autosomal recessive), but always does so if he or she suffers from the Thomsen type (autosomal dominant). The onset of myotonia is somewhat later in the Becker type, sometimes not until age 14 or 15, but the myotonia is more pronounced than in the Thomsen type, and may be accompanied by a mild, mainly distal dystrophy, with mild elevation of the serum creatine kinase concentration. Myotonic paralysis, too, is more severe in the Becker type.

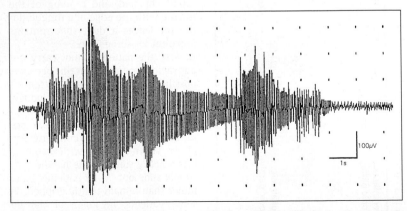

Fig. 14.**7** **Myotonic discharges in the EMG of a patient with Steinert's myotonic dystrophy.**

Other Nondystrophic Myotonias
(442, 776)

Myotonia fluctuans, myotonia permanens, and *acetazolamide-sensitive myotonia* are further nondystrophic types of myotonia. They are all due to a genetic defect on chromosome 17q23-25 (allelic for paramyotonias and dyskalemic paralyses) which leads to dysfunction of sodium channels. A potassium load alters the manifestations of myotonia. Myotonia fluctuans first appears in adolescence, while the other two diseases appear in the first decade of life. In myotonia fluctuans, myotonia is only episodically present ("fluctuating"). In the other two diseases, myotonia is permanent and severe, and in acetazolamide-sensitive myotonia it is also painful.

▌Treatment▐

Myotonic rigidity and myotonic paralysis can be ameliorated by various types of medications that lower membrane excitability, among them *local anesthetics, antiarrhythmics,* and *anticonvulsants* such as *procainamide, mexiletine, quinidine,* and *phenytoin.* Of these, mexiletine is the most effective (549a). Many patients, however, decline to take medication around the clock, either going without medication entirely or taking it only before planned physical activities. The side effects of such medications may be significant, particularly in the elderly, in whom they may induce disturbances of intracardiac conduction. *Acetazolamide* has a palliative effect in the Thomsen form of myotonia congenita as well as in acetazolamide-sensitive myotonia.

Paramyotonia Congenita of Eulenburg (775)

Genetics

This autosomal dominant inherited disease is caused, like a number of other congenital myotonias, by an abnormality of the sodium channel. The genetic defect is at the same locus, namely chromosome 17q23-25.

Clinical Features

From birth onward, patients with this disease suffer from myotonia that can be induced by cold, as well as attacks of flaccid weakness mainly affecting the proximal muscles that can appear in warm surroundings too and last for minutes to hours. So-called paradoxical myotonia may be present – i.e., rigidity that worsens as a muscle is repeatedly contracted. Some families with this disease also suffer from paralytic attacks resembling those of hyperkalemic periodic paralysis. In between paralytic attacks, physical examination reveals nothing abnormal except myotonia. The manifestations tend to regress somewhat over the years.

Ancillary Tests

The *EMG* always shows myotonic discharges, even at room temperature. The serum creatine kinase concentration is often mildly elevated.

▌Treatment▐

The treatment is similar to that of the congenital myotonias. *Acetazolamide* can ameliorate paradoxical myotonia, but it simultaneously worsens the cold-induced weakness. *Hydrochlorothiazide* is used prophylactically in patients who concomitantly suffer from hyperkalemic periodic paralysis.

Differential Diagnosis of Congenital Myotonias vs. Myotonic Dystrophy

The distinction between these two entities can be difficult to draw in the early stages, when the dystrophic features of myotonic dystrophy are still only mild. Myotonia is mainly distal in myotonic dystrophy, but present proximally as well in the congenital myotonias. DNA analysis can help in the differential diagnosis.

Paramyotonia congenita is made worse by cold or exercise (see above). Certain other syndromes involving continuous muscle fiber activity enter into the differential diagnosis of the myotonias, among them Schwartz-Jampel syndrome, neuromyotonia, and stiff man syndrome (see below).

Heterogeneous Syndromes Involving Excessive Muscle Fiber Activity

Aside from the myotonias, there are a number of other diseases that are characterized by clinically or electromyographically demonstrable overactivity of muscle fibers, and which can also be associated with skeletal deformities.

Schwartz-Jampel Syndrome (Myotonia Chondrodystrophica) (896)

This disease becomes manifest in the first few years of life and is characterized by muscle stiffness at rest that worsens on exertion, short stature, multiple skeletal deformities such as Perthes-type dysplasia of the femoral head, and myopia. The autosomal-recessive form is caused by a genetic defect on chromosome 1p34-p36.1 (143a). The EMG reveals continuous muscle fiber activity and pseudomyotonic discharges. The pathogenesis is not understood.

Neuromyotonia (Syndrome of Continuous Muscle Fiber Activity; Isaacs Syndrome) (453, 604, 705, 966)

Definition:
This disease, first described by Isaacs, is characterized by muscle rigidity, spontaneous fine wave-like contractions in muscle (myokymia), and continuous spontaneous muscle fiber activity on EMG.

Pathogenesis

Cases of neuromyotonia are usually sporadic and only rarely familial. It is thought to be secondary to a mild, possibly autoimmune polyneuropathy.

Clinical Features

There are spontaneous, fine, wave-like muscle contractions (myokymia) and permanent spasms of all skeletal muscles, with resulting postural abnormalities. The muscles are hard to the touch, and all movements are viscous, as they must be carried out against the resistance of the antagonist muscles. Contractures may appear in the late stage of the disease.

A further typical feature is pseudomyotonia, which clinically resembles true myotonia but can be distinguished from it by EMG.

Course

The disease can appear relatively suddenly at any age. It may progress in spurts thereafter, and perhaps later disappear (453).

Electromyography

The typical finding is of continuous spontaneous activity despite optimal relaxation, consisting of partly increased and partly diminished motor unit potentials, as well as repetitive discharges of shorter potentials (doublets, triplets, etc.). These findings persist during sleep and after peripheral nerve block with local anesthetic, but disappear when the muscle is curarized. Myotonia, in contrast, is not affected by curare.

Differential Diagnosis

This disorder must be differentiated from tetanus, the myotonic syndromes, and stiff man syndrome (see below) (966). In the syndrome of fasciculations and myalgia (p. 845), which is presumably also due to a polyneuropathy, pain is more prominent and the EMG does not reveal continuous muscle fiber activity (441).

Treatment

Antiepileptics such as *phenytoin* and *carbamazepine* have a prompt beneficial effect. Plasmapheresis is also helpful in rare cases.

Stiff Man Syndrome (Stiff Person Syndrome, Moersch-Woltman Syndrome) (59c, 596)

Clinical Features

Stiff man syndrome is characterized by a mainly axial and proximal appendicular rigidity with painful muscle spasms resembling those of chronic tetanus. It thus differs from neuromyotonia, in which the rigidity is mainly distal. The facial and pharyngeal muscles can be affected as well, but trismus does not occur. The painful muscle spasms are exacerbated by external stimuli, movement, or strong emotion but improve during sleep and under general anesthesia. Passive stretching of a muscle induces a reflex contraction that lasts for several seconds. The spasms may lead to deformities of the joints and spine, and may even be intense enough to cause muscle ruptures or bony fractures. Motor and sensory function is otherwise intact.

Pathogenesis and Course

Stiff man syndrome progresses over months or years, then becomes stable. It affects men and women at equal frequency (despite its name). Familial cases are rare. In most patients, the presence of anti-GAD antibodies (GAD = glutamic acid decarboxylase) supports the hypothesis of an autoimmune mechanism (205a). Paraneoplastic cases are also said to occur. Though the muscular rigidity is presumed to be due to a central lesion of some kind, no histopathologic or neuroradiologic abnormality has been found to date in the brain or spinal cord that might account for it. The long-term prognosis of stiff man syndrome is not known with any certainty.

Electromyography

Continuous activity of motor units is seen, with intervening silent periods (these are absent in tetanus and are thus useful in differential diagnosis). Local anesthetic nerve block, sleep, and general anesthesia abolish the continuous muscle activity.

Differential Diagnosis

Stiff man syndrome can usually be distinguished with some confidence from the myotonias, neuromyotonia, and tetanus on clinical grounds alone, and with certainty by EMG.

Treatment

The treatment of choice is *diazepam*. A favorable symptomatic effect can also be obtained with phenytoin, baclofen, or tizanidine. Long-term remissions after the intravenous administration of immunoglobulins have been reported (514a).

Periodic Paralyses

Familial Periodic Paralyses (442)

The familial, or primary, periodic paralyses are associated with an abnormality of the serum potassium concentration and with inexcitability of muscle during the paralytic episodes. The underlying molecular abnormality is at the muscle cell membrane. These diseases are to be distinguished from secondary periodic paralyses, which are due to abnormalities of potassium metabolism that may arise from a wide variety of causes.

The following features are common to all of the familial periodic paralyses:

- Attacks of paralysis lasting from a few hours to a few days, which may be either focal or generalized, and usually spare the muscles of respiration and facial expression (though not always).
- During the attacks, the intrinsic muscle reflexes are diminished or unelicitable, and muscle fibers are electrically unexcitable.
- In later stages of the disease, permanent weakness and irreversible changes in muscle may develop.

Cardiac arrhythmia is a rare concomitant finding in all types of periodic paralysis but is not a component of the typical clinical syndrome.

Hypokalemic Periodic Paralysis

Genetics

This autosomal dominant inherited disease is caused by an abnormality of the dihydropyridine-sensitive calcium channels in the transverse tubular system of muscle cells, which is in turn due to a genetic defect on chromosome 1q31-32.

Pathogenesis

The pathogenetic mechanism remains poorly understood. The disorder is less penetrant in women, and thus more prevalent in men.

Clinical Features

The first attacks occur some time between the ages of 5 and 30, usually in the second decade of life. They may occur only once or twice per year, or more frequently, even daily. They sometimes last only 1 hour or several hours, but usually up to 1 day. The usually involve the muscles of the upper and lower limbs, sparing the respiratory, facial, and pharyngeal muscles, though deaths due to respiratory failure or cardiac arrhythmia have been described. A myotonic reaction is absent, or present only in the eyelids.

Thyrotoxic Periodic Paralysis

A thyrotoxic crisis may present as hypokalemic paralysis without any other obvious signs of thyrotoxicosis, particularly in persons of East Asian ancestry. This etiology should be suspected if a patient presents with new hypokalemic paralysis without any relevant family history.

Diagnostic Evaluation

The typical paralytic attacks, hypokalemia, and positive family history point to the correct diagnosis. The serum creatine kinase concentration is normal to mildly elevated. The EMG reveals few or no motor unit potentials on attempted voluntary contraction. The summed motor potential is abnormally small or absent. The ECG shows flat T and U waves.

The diagnostic evaluation in the interval between attacks is discussed in further detail below.

Treatment and prevention of paralytic episodes

The paralysis of each attack generally recedes in the reverse order to that in which it arose. *Oral administration of potassium* (2–10 g in 10–25% aqueous solution) or *intravenous KCl* (0.05–0.1 mEq/kg as a bolus), in addition to *mild exercise*, can speed recovery from an attack. A *low-carbohydrate, low-salt diet*, possibly combined with *oral potassium administration* and *acetazolamide* (125–500 mg/day), can lessen the frequency and intensity of attacks.

A randomized study revealed a significant reduction of the frequency of attacks with *dichlorphenamide*, a carbonic anhydrase inhibitor previously used to treat glaucoma (1034a). If this fails, *triamterene* or *spironolactone* can be tried.

Thyrotoxic hypokalemic paralysis is managed by *treatment of the underlying thyrotoxicosis*.

Hyperkalemic (= Potassium-Sensitive) Periodic Paralysis (Adynamia Episodica Hereditaria of Gamstorp)

Genetics and Pathogenesis

The genetic defect responsible for this autosomal dominant disorder has been localized to chromosome 17q23-25. This locus encodes the sodium channels of the muscle fiber membrane. The disorder is highly penetrant. Sporadic cases due to new mutations are also seen.

Clinical Features

Potassium-sensitive periodic paralysis appears at an earlier age than hypokalemic periodic paralysis, namely, almost always before age 10. The attacks are shorter and milder, lasting from a quarter of an hour to an hour, rarely as long as 4 hours. They can be provoked by fasting or by rest after physical activity. They mainly affect the proximal muscles of the upper and lower limbs but can also be predominantly distal and asymmetric, depending on which muscles are voluntarily activated.

Paresthesiae and a Chvostek sign are sometimes present, but there is no objectively detectable sensory deficit. Many, though not all, patients have myotonia or paramyotonia during and between the attacks. The progressive muscle weakness between attacks is less pronounced than in hypokalemic periodic paralysis, and many patients experience spontaneous improvement as the years go by.

In hyperkalemic periodic paralysis, low ambient temperatures induce no more than mild weakness, which rapidly improves as soon as the patient returns to a warm area. Patients who simultaneously suffer from paramyotonia, however, may develop severe weakness on exposure to cold. This implies that the pathogenetic mechanisms underlying this disease differ in patients with and without paramyotonia.

Diagnostic Evaluation

The characteristic paralytic episodes and hyperkalemia point to the diagnosis, which is supported by the presence of concomitant myotonia or paramyotonia, if any. The EMG at the beginning of an attack reveals strongly increasing fibrillations, as well as myotonic or paramyotonic discharges in patients who have myotonia or paramyotonia. Attempted voluntary contraction yields only a few or no motor unit potentials. The ECG reveals sharp T waves of greater than normal amplitude.

Treatment and prophylaxis

A *high-carbohydrate diet* and *copious hydration* have a beneficial effect, as do *thiazide diuretics* or *acetazolamide* at the beginning of an attack, or β-adrenergic agonists such as *salbutamol*. As in hypokalemic periodic paralysis, the carbonic anhydrase inhibitor *dichlorphenamide* reduces the frequency and intensity of attacks (1034a). *Mild exercise* also speeds recovery from an attack.

Intravenous potassium-lowering therapy, with glucose and insulin, calcium gluconate, or sodium bicarbonate, is rarely necessary.

Prophylaxis of attacks is important for the long-term prevention of permanent weakness. This is accomplished by the consumption of *frequent high-carbohydrate meals low in potassium*, and by the *avoidance of fasting, rigorous exercise, and exposure to cold*. If these measures are not sufficient, *thiazide diuretics* (e.g., chlorothiazide 250–1000 mg/day) are given, or *acetazolamide* (125–1000 mg/day) as a second choice.

Normokalemic Periodic Paralysis

Rare patients have a normal serum potassium level during their attacks. Most of these patients have potassium-sensitive periodic paralysis. The underlying genetic defect and pathogenesis are presumed to be the same as those of hyperkalemic periodic paralysis.

Diagnostic Evaluation of the Periodic Paralyses in between Attacks

Other conditions such as thyroid and adrenal disease should be excluded. The EMG may show myotonia and thereby suggest the diagnosis of a hyperkalemic periodic paralysis, or it may show myopathic changes, implying that a muscle biopsy is indicated. Biopsy reveals large, centrally located vacuoles within muscle fibers in hypokalemic periodic paralysis, but fewer such vacuoles in hyperkalemic periodic paralysis.

Serial determinations of the serum potassium concentration may also provide clues to the diagnosis. In hyperkalemic periodic paralysis, the potassium level is often elevated in between attacks, while, in hypokalemic periodic paralysis, it is normal. Low or high values in the interval between attacks suggest the possibility of a secondary periodic paralysis and prompt a search for the cause; possible causes are listed in Tables 14.**4** and 14.**5**.

DNA analysis may also aid in the diagnosis.

Table 14.**4** Differential diagnosis of hypokalemia

Gastrointestinal	Inadequate intake Abnormal losses (diarrhea, ureterosigmoidostomy, etc.)
Renal	Metabolic alkalosis Diuretics Mineralocorticoid excess (Conn syndrome, Cushing syndrome, secondary hyperaldosteronism, licorice consumption) Renal tubular disease
Shift into cells (no absolute deficiency)	Hypokalemic periodic paralysis Alkalosis Insulin β-adrenergic agents

Table 14.**5** Differential diagnosis of hyperkalemia

Inadequate excretion	Renal diseases (acute and chronic renal failure, tubular diseases) Hypoaldosteronism Extracellular volume deficiency Potassium-sparing diuretics
Abnormal potassium shift	Tissue injury (e.g., rhabdomyolysis) Acidosis Insulin deficiency Medications (e.g., β-blockers) Hyperkalemic periodic paralysis
Excessive intake	Dietary Improper electrolyte therapy
Artefactual hyperkalemia	Faulty venipuncture technique Hemolysis

Insufficient clinical characterization of periodic paralysis usually results in suboptimal treatment. Thus, it is advisable to perform *provocative tests* while monitoring the patient's strength, serum potassium concentration, and ECG (361). Hypokalemic paralysis can be induced by glucose and insulin, while hyperkalemic paralysis can be induced by oral potassium administration or by exposure to cold (e.g., the immersion of one arm in cold water).

Metabolic Myopathies (361)

Overview:

The main sources of energy for muscle are glycogen for brief anaerobic activity and long-chain fatty acids for longer aerobic activity. Disturbances of energy metabolism generally lead to dynamic manifestations such as exercise-induced weakness, myalgias, and contractures. Less common are disease states involving permanent and progressive weakness, with clinical signs resembling those of a muscular dystrophy or myositis.

General Aspects of Energy Metabolism in Muscle

Normal muscle contraction requires energy in the form of ATP molecules. This energy is made available through glycogenolysis, lipid catabolism, phosphocreatine, and the purine nucleotide cycle.

The sequential steps that constitute the glycolytic pathway break down glycogen to pyruvate, which is then decarboxylated to acetyl-CoA so that it can enter the Krebs cycle. Glycogenolysis takes place outside the mitochondrion, the Krebs cycle within it. *Long-chain fatty acids* in the cytoplasm are bound to carnitine and, with the aid of carnitine palmitoyltransferase I and II, transported across the mitochondrial membrane and incorporated in fatty acyl CoA, which, in turn, is β-oxidized within the mitochondrion. Electrons liberated in this process are transported by the hydrogen carriers NADH+H$^+$ and FADH$_2$ to the respiratory chain on the inner mitochondrial membrane, in which ATP is synthesized. Alternatively, energy can be stored in muscle in the form of *phosphocreatine*. ATP and phosphocreatine are in equilibrium with each other. ATP can also be produced in muscle from *adenosine monophosphate* (AMP). The deamination of AMP to inosine monophosphate (IMP), a reaction catalyzed by the enzyme myoadenylate deaminase, is an important step in the physiologic regulation of the ATP concentration in muscle. This reaction liberates ammonia as a "waste product."

Glycolysis makes energy available for brief, intense muscle activity, which requires more energy than can be derived from oxygen in the short time available. Under these anaerobic conditions, pyruvate is converted to lactate rather than to acetyl CoA. Brief and very intense muscle activity also derives energy from *phosphocreatine* and from the *purine nucleotide cycle.* Under aerobic conditions, in which the energy consumption does not outstrip the amount of energy delivered in the form of oxygen, pyruvate can directly enter the Krebs cycle and respiratory chain. This pathway is used for activities lasting up to ca. 45 minutes. For longer-lasting activities, or when the individual is at rest, energy is derived mainly from fat.

The above sketch of energy metabolism in muscle facilitates understanding of the clinical syndromes of the metabolic myopathies and the techniques used to diagnose them. The signs and symptoms also depend on whether the enzyme deficiency is restricted to muscle or also affects other organs, particularly the central nervous system. Table 14.**6** provides an overview of the metabolic myopathies.

Clinical Presentation and Diagnostic Evaluation of the Metabolic Myopathies

Clinical Features

Metabolic myopathies have both dynamic and static clinical manifestations in muscle.

Table 14.**6** Metabolic myopathies with exercise-induced manifestations

Group of diseases	Enzyme defect or deficiency	Clinical manifestations	Diagnostic evaluation
Glycogen metabolism	Phosphorylase Phosphorylase b kinase Phosphofructokinase Phosphoglycerate kinase	Exercise-induced weakness, myalgias, contractures, and sometimes myoglobinuria, even after brief exertion	Lactate ischemia test Electromyography Muscle biopsy with histochemistry, biochemical study of muscle, DNA analysis
Lipid metabolism	Carnitine Carnitine palmitoyltransferase	Exercise-induced weakness, myalgias, and sometimes myoglobinuria, with prolonged muscle activity	Muscle biopsy with histochemistry and perhaps biochemical analysis; in systemic carnitine deficiency, the serum carnitine concentration is low
Mitochondrial myopathies	See p. 895 and Table 14.**8**	Muscle involvement almost always includes progressive external ophthalmoplegia; the brain is usually involved as well; see p. 897 ff.	Serum lactate concentration, muscle biopsy with electron microscopy and biochemical analysis DNA analysis
Purine nucleotide cycle	Myoadenylate deaminase	Rarely clinically relevant, exercise intolerance	Absence of rise in ammonia concentration with exercise

Dynamic manifestations. These include exercise-induced weakness, myalgia, and contractures. If not enough energy can be made available to meet the metabolic demand of muscle, structural injury results – i.e., rhabdomyolysis with release of myoglobin. This, in turn, produces myoglobinuria, which lends the urine a dark color.

Static manifestations. These generally consist of muscle weakness and atrophy resulting from the abnormal deposition of glycogen and fat in muscle, mostly within lysosomes. Metabolic myopathies with static manifestations have a clinical appearance closely resembling that of muscular dystrophy.

Diagnostic Evaluation

Ancillary tests. The *serum creatine kinase concentration* may be elevated, especially in the glycogenoses, carnitine deficiency, and malignant hyperthermia. The *lactate concentration* may be elevated in mitochondrial diseases.

EMG. The EMG reveals myopathic changes in some types of metabolic myopathy, but a normal EMG does not rule out metabolic myopathy.

Ischemia test (forearm ischemia test). This provocative test is easy to carry out (465). An intravenous catheter is placed in a cubital vein for blood drawing, and a sphygmomanometer cuff is placed around the ipsilateral arm and inflated to above the systolic blood pressure to produce ischemia. The patient then repeatedly squeezes a second, partially inflated blood pressure cuff with his or her hand up to a pressure of 200 mmHg. Blood

samples are drawn at 1, 3, 5, and 10 minutes from the start of this ischemic muscle activity for the measurement of serum lactate and ammonia levels. In the normal individual, both of these levels increase approximately fourfold over the course of the test. The lactate level fails to rise in disorders of glycogenolysis and glycolysis, while the ammonia level fails to rise in myoadenylate deaminase deficiency. A lower than normal rise of both levels simultaneously indicates insufficient effort on the subject's part, rather than a disease state. A lactate level that is already elevated at rest, or rises disproportionately high with minimal exertion, indicates a mitochondrial disorder.

SATET test. The sub-anaerobic threshold exercise test can be used to screen for mitochondrial disorders.

Muscle biopsy. Light microscopy may reveal storage of glycogen or fat, or mitochondrial changes with ragged red fibers. Histochemical stains may reveal deficiencies of phosphorylase, phosphofructokinase, or myoadenylate deaminase, which can then be quantified with biochemical techniques. Other enzyme defects, including some cases of carnitine and carnitine palmitoyltransferase deficiency, cannot be detected by muscle biopsy and must be sought biochemically.

Magnetic resonance spectroscopy. This technique can be used to study muscle metabolism but is not routinely available at present.

Specific Metabolic Myopathies (276, 361, 465, 633)

The glycogen storage diseases are summarized in Table 2.**72**. Metabolic myopathy can be the most prominent manifestation of a number of them. The known enzymatic defects of glycogenolysis and glycolysis are listed in Table 14.**6**.

Phosphorylase Deficiency (McArdle Syndrome, Muscle Phosphorylase Deficiency, Myophosphorylase Deficiency, Glycogenosis Type V) (236)

Genetics

This is a hereditary disorder of either autosomal recessive or autosomal dominant inheritance, for which the causative genetic defect lies on chromosome 11q13-qter and produces a deficiency of the enzyme phosphorylase in muscle.

Clinical Features

The onset of illness is generally in childhood or adolescence, rarely in early adulthood. The manifestations include exercise-induced myalgia, weakness, muscle stiffness, and contractures that are usually rapidly reversible. Many patients must rest even after minimal exertion. About half of all patients report experiencing a "second wind" phenomenon – i.e., they are able to engage in prolonged activity relatively well by carefully dosing the degree of exertion. This phenomenon is presumably explained by the mobilization of energy sources other than glucose. Greater exertion can lead to rhabdomyolysis and myoglobinuria, and thereby to renal failure, loss of consciousness, and grand mal seizures.

Mainly proximal muscle atrophy is sometimes seen in older patients, while, in younger patients, the neurological examination is entirely normal.

Ancillary Tests

The *serum creatine kinase concentration* is usually mildly elevated. In the *ischemia test,* the lactate level does not rise, or rises less than normal. The *EMG* at rest often reveals mild myopathic changes. When contractures are present, no action potentials can be recorded. *Muscle biopsy with PAS staining* often reveals an increased number of glycogen-containing vacuoles. *Histochemical study* reveals the lack of phosphorylase.

> **Treatment**
>
> No etiologic treatment is available. As a symptomatic treatment, *oral creatine* can raise the patient's exercise tolerance (987a). Some patients benefit from *exercise programs* emphasizing aerobic activities.

Phosphofructokinase Deficiency (236)

Phosphofructokinase is the limiting enzyme in glycolysis. A deficiency of this enzyme is much rarer than phosphorylase deficiency. Its clinical presentation is likewise characterized by exercise-induced manifestations. There is also a mild hemolytic anemia.

Acid Maltase Deficiency
(236, 280)

Pathogenesis and Genetics

Unlike the enzyme deficiencies just discussed, acid maltase deficiency causes static rather than dynamic changes and thus more closely resembles muscular dystrophy in its clinical presentation.

The enzyme deficiency is inherited in an autosomal recessive pattern. The genetic defect is located on chromosome 17q21-23. The deficiency causes accumulation of glycogen in muscle lysosomes.

Clinical Features

In cases of acid maltase deficiency that become manifest in infancy, patients present as "floppy infants" with progressive weakness, enlargement of the heart, liver, and tongue, respiratory insufficiency, and dysphagia. They die before reaching the age of 2 years. In the *juvenile* and rarer *adult* forms of the disease, the principal manifestation is progressive, mainly proximal muscle weakness. Subsequent involvement of the respiratory musculature leads to premature death. The clinical picture resembles that of limb girdle or scapuloperoneal muscular dystrophy.

Ancillary Tests

The *serum creatine kinase concentration* is mildly elevated. The *EMG* reveals myotonic discharges and abbreviated, low-amplitude, and often polyphasic motor unit potentials, fibrillations, positive sharp waves, and complex repetitive discharges. The lactate level rises normally in the *ischemia test*. *Muscle biopsy* reveals many glycogen-laden vacuoles and lysosomes. The enzyme deficiency can be demonstrated in cultivated fibroblasts, in lymphocytes, or in the urine.

Treatment
There is no known treatment.

Muscle Carnitine Deficiency
(234)

Pathogenesis and Genetics

Carnitine deficiency causes fat storage in muscle, mainly in type I fibers. Its inheritance pattern is autosomal recessive. It may present as a *systemic disease* or as a *myopathic form* restricted to muscle.

Clinical Features

The *myopathic form* of the disease begins in childhood or early adolescence with progressive, mainly proximal weakness and atrophy. Exercise intolerance, myoglobinuria, cardiomyopathy, and heart failure are further manifestations. Cardiomyopathy is usually the most prominent manifestation of *systemic carnitine deficiency*.

Ancillary Tests

The *serum creatine kinase concentration* is usually mildly elevated. The *EMG* shows mild myopathic changes. *Muscle biopsy* with Oil-red-O staining may reveal fatty droplets in muscle, in which case the diagnosis can be definitively established by *biochemical testing*. The *serum carnitine concentration* is low only in the systemic form of the disease.

Treatment
The treatment consists of a *low-fat diet* and *oral L-carnitine supplementation* (2–4 g/day).

Carnitine Palmitoyltransferase Deficiency (1048)

Pathogenesis and Genetics
This genetic disease, due to a defect on chromosome 1, is the most common cause of recurrent myoglobinuria. Its inheritance pattern is autosomal recessive.

Clinical Features
Prolonged physical exertion leads to myalgia, muscle stiffness, and myoglobinuria. These symptoms can also be induced by fasting, infections, cold, or low-carbohydrate, high-fat meals.

Ancillary Tests
The *serum creatine kinase concentration, EMG, ischemia test,* and *muscle biopsy* are all normal except for the *histochemical and biochemical studies* that reveal the enzyme defect.

Treatment
The treatment consists of frequent meals rich in carbohydrates, and the avoidance of prolonged exertion.

Myoadenylate Deaminase Deficiency

Genetics
This enzyme deficiency, due to a lesion on chromosome 1, is transmitted in an autosomal recessive inheritance pattern.

Clinical Features
This enzyme deficiency has often been reported to cause either ordinary muscle cramps or exercise-induced myalgia and weakness – e.g., after jumping (in children). It occasionally causes myoglobinuria.

Ancillary Tests
The *serum creatine kinase concentration* may be mildly elevated. The *EMG* is normal. In the *ischemia test,* the ammonia level rises too little, or not at all.

Treatment
There is no known effective treatment. This clinical entity remains controversial at present, as myoadenylate deaminase deficiency has also been found in many clinically healthy persons.

Myoglobinuria

Myoglobinuria is visible as a dark, beer-brown discoloration of the urine. It is the result of rhabdomyolysis (breakdown of striated muscle), which, in turn, has many different causes, both genetic and exogenous (Table 14.7). Myoglobinuria can lead to renal tubular necrosis and acute renal failure. This can usually be prevented with forced diuresis, brought about by the administration of sodium bicarbonate, copious intravenous fluids, and furosemide.

Malignant Hyperthermia (880)

Pathogenesis and Genetics
Malignant hyperthermia is an autosomal dominant inherited disorder of which myopathy is sometimes a

Table 14.**7**   Causes of myoglobinuria

Excessive physical stress
Metabolic myopathies (cf. Table 14.**6**)
Myotonias
Myositis
Infection (viral, bacterial)
Muscular dystrophy
Ischemic necrosis of muscle
Mechanical trauma, crushing injury, burn, status epilepticus
Medications and toxic substances (alcohol, gasoline vapors, anesthetic gases, succinylcholine, illicit drugs, hypnotics, neuroleptics, clofibrate, statins, snake venom, insecticides, etc.)
Malignant hyperthermia (see above)
Malignant neuroleptic syndrome
Electrolyte disturbances (hypokalemia, hypophosphatemia [785])

component. The responsible genetic defects are located on chromosomes 19q13.1 and 17q11.2-24. The defect at the former locus causes faulty expression of the ryanodine receptor of the calcium channels of the sarcoplasmic reticulum. A defect at the same locus is the genetic basis of central core myopathy, a disorder that predisposes to malignant hyperthermia. This explains why patients with certain kinds of myopathy are at elevated risk of malignant hyperthermia.

Clinical Features

Most patients are asymptomatic until they undergo general anesthesia and, while anesthetized, develop an unexpected and potentially lethal hyper-

metabolic disorder of muscle. Halogenated inhalational anesthetics, such as halothane, and depolarizing muscle relaxants, such as succinylcholine, are among the more common precipitating agents.

The hallmarks of this syndrome are difficult intubation, tachycardia, arrhythmia, possible cardiac arrest, hyperventilation, muscle rigidity, and, above all, extreme hyperthermia. The syndrome is similar in some respects to malignant neuroleptic syndrome (p. 307).

Identification of Persons at Risk

The best indicator of risk is a positive personal or family history of similar events. Uncomplicated general anesthesia in the past unfortunately does not mean that malignant hyperthermia cannot occur during a subsequent operation under general anesthesia. As mentioned above, certain types of myopathy, including the dystrophinopathies (p. 866) and central core myopathy (p. 899), are associated with an elevated risk of malignant hyperthermia. In persons at risk, the serum creatine kinase concentration is often mildly elevated.

Treatment

In the acute stage, dantrolene (2.5 mg/kg) is rapidly infused. If there is no improvement in 45 minutes, an additional dose of 7.5 mg/kg is given.

Mitochondrial Encephalomyopathies
(235, 467, 575b, 575c, 676, 807)

Overview:
The diseases in this clinically heterogeneous group are all due to structural, biochemical, or genetic abnormalities of the mitochondria. Mitochondrial diseases affect all organ systems of the body. We discuss them here in the chapter on myopathy because myopathy and encephalopathy are often among their more prominent manifestations.

Mitochondria are intracellular organelles. Carbohydrates, fat, and protein are broken down in the liver and other organs into pyruvate, fatty acids, and amino acids that can be

Table 14.8 Biochemical classification of the mitochondrial myopathies and encephalomyopathies

Transport disorders:
- Carnitine deficiency
- Carnitine palmitoyltransferase deficiency

Substrate utilization defects:
- Pyruvate dehydrogenase deficiency
- Pyruvate carboxylase deficiency
- β-oxidation defects

Defects of the Krebs cycle:
- Fumarase deficiency
- Aconitase deficiency

Defects in which oxidative phosphorylation is uncoupled:
- Luft syndrome

Defects of the respiratory chain:
- Complex I deficiency*
- Complex II deficiency
- Complex III deficiency*
- Complex IV deficiency*
- Complex V deficiency*
- Combined defects of complexes I–V*

* Encoded by mtRNA.

transported into the mitochondria, where they are used to generate ATP. Like the metabolic myopathies, the mitochondrial myopathies, too, can be classified according to their underlying biochemical defects (Table 14.8). Some of the defects listed here have been documented in no more than a few case reports but share genetic and clinical features with the other, more common ones.

Genetics
In addition to the DNA contained in the nucleus of each cell (nuclear DNA, nDNA), each mitochondrion contains multiple copies of its own mitochondrial DNA (mtDNA). Mitochondrial DNA encodes 22 transfer RNA molecules, two ribosomal RNA molecules, and most of the enzymes of the respiratory chain. Nuclear DNA is inherited autosomally according to the familiar mendelian rules. Mitochondrial DNA, in contrast, is transmitted independently of the nuclear genome, directly in the mitochondria of the sperm cell and oocyte that join to form the zygote. The oocyte contains far more mitochondria than the sperm cell, as it is much larger, and thus contributes the overwhelming majority of mitochondria to the zygote. It follows that the inheritance

Table 14.**9**   Clinical manifestations of mitochondrial diseases

Organ	Manifestation
Muscle	Myopathy with ragged red fibers
	Progressive external ophthalmoplegia
	Exercise intolerance
Nervous system	Myoclonus and generalized seizures
	Stroke in younger individuals
	Ataxia
	Dementia
	Polyneuropathy
	Deafness
	Optic neuropathy
	Migraine
	Basal ganglionic calcification (Fahr syndrome)
	Dystonia
	Elevated CSF protein
Eye	Retinitis pigmentosa
	Cataract
Heart	Cardiomyopathy
	Conduction abnormalities
Gastrointestinal system	Intestinal pseudo-obstruction
	Diarrhea
Endocrine system	Short stature
	Diabetes
	Goiter
	Hypogonadism
Skin	Multiple lipomas
	Ichthyosis

pattern of mitochondrial diseases is nearly exclusively maternal.

Further characteristics of mitochondrial DNA include a high incidence of mutation, and *heteroplasmia* – i.e., the coexistence, within a single cell, of both normal and mutated mtDNA. In the normal case, of course, there is homoplasmia, as the cell contains nothing but normal (unmutated) mtDNA. When mutated mtDNA is present, the relative proportions of normal and mutated mtDNA determine the clinical phenotype. Disease is clinically evident only when the percentage of mutated mtDNA exceeds a certain *threshold*. In persons harboring mutated mtDNA, the proportions of normal and mutated mtDNA typically vary from organ to organ, and also change over the course of the individual's life and with every cell division. It follows that the mitochondrial genotype changes over the years, and there may not be any overt disease until the threshold value for mutated mtDNA is crossed (if it is ever crossed).

Mitochondrial diseases due to mtDNA mutations are much more common than those due to nDNA mutations.

Clinical Features (236a)

Mitochondrial disorders may display a predilection for a particular organ. Generally, however, multiple organs are affected to differing degrees. The manifestations of mitochondrial disorders in different organ systems are listed in Table 14.**9**.

Mitochondrial Disease Syndromes

Carnitine deficiency and carnitine palmitoyltransferase deficiency are two types of mitochondrial disorder that are autosomally inherited – i.e., based on a defect in nuclear DNA. The disorders of the pyruvate dehydrogenase complex and of the Krebs cycle are also of this type.

Disorders of the pyruvate dehydrogenase complex. These disorders cause lactic acidosis and progressive cerebral dysfunction. In the more severe forms, the abnormality is already apparent immediately after birth. Forms of intermediate severity are characterized by episodic lactic acidosis and progressive encephalopathy, or by Leigh syndrome (p. 296). The mild phenotype manifests itself in *episodic ataxia* in childhood and adolescence.

Disorders of the Krebs cycle. These include fumarase deficiency, which manifests itself in early childhood with progressive encephalopathy, and aconitase deficiency, which causes exercise intolerance and myoglobinuria.

Disorders of the respiratory chain. These disorders all display a mitochondrial inheritance pattern (with one exception). Most of them cause myopathy with ragged red fibers, though not always as the most prominent manifestation. The individual disorders are briefly discussed in the following paragraphs.

Progressive external ophthalmoplegia with ragged red fibers (235, 467, 724). This syndrome consists of a combination of bilateral ptosis, limitation of ocular motility, a usually mild, generalized myopathy, and ragged red fibers on muscle biopsy. The latter are created by the accumulation of mitochondria in muscle fibers, which are stained red by the Gomori stain. The disorder progresses inexorably over the years. Further clinical and laboratory evidence of a mitochondrial disorder may be present. Progressive external ophthalmoplegia is found as a familial syndrome with a maternal or autosomal dominant inheritance pattern, and as a component of Kearns-Sayre syndrome.

Kearns-Sayre syndrome (KSS). KSS is caused by a single deletion mutation in mtDNA in patients with a negative family history. Its cardinal manifestations are progressive external ophthalmoplegia, mitochondrial myopathy with ragged red fibers, retinal pigment degeneration (retinitis pigmentosa), and intracardiac conduction disturbances. Further clinical manifestations (Table 14.**9**) may also be present in varying combinations. The disease appears before age 20 and confers a risk of sudden cardiac death.

MELAS syndrome (mitochondrial myopathy, encephalopathy, lactic acidosis, and stroke-like episodes) (746). This syndrome usually makes its appearance in childhood with TIAs, cerebral infarction, and episodic vomiting. Lactic acidosis is present. In the full-fledged syndrome, patients become demented and die before the age of 20. Myoclonic and generalized epileptic seizures occur as well. In such cases, only DNA analysis can establish the differential diagnosis between MELAS and MERRF syndrome.

MERRF syndrome (myoclonus epilepsy with ragged red fibers) (993). Phenomenologically, this syndrome consists of myoclonic and generalized epileptic seizures, myopathy and weakness of the limb muscles, mental retardation or dementia, ataxia, and hearing loss, and usually lactic acidosis. Ophthalmoplegia is not part of the syndrome. There may, however, be cerebral calcifications, short stature, neuropathy, and other mitochondrial manifestations. The clinical course is highly variable; some patients die before reaching adulthood, while others live a full normal life span with no more than mild myopathy.

NARP syndrome (neuropathy, ataxia, and retinitis pigmentosa) (427). A point mutation of mtDNA causes NARP syndrome, which is characterized by proximal muscle weakness, sensory neuropathy, developmental disturbances, ataxia, epileptic seizures, dementia, and retinitis pigmentosa. Some patients suffering from Leigh syndrome (p. 296) have the same mutation.

COX (cytochrome c oxidase) deficiency. This disorder is clinically manifested by fatal infantile myopathy, benign infantile myopathy, or Leigh syndrome. Aside from myopathy, it can also cause encephalopathy and renal tubular defects of a type designated separately as Debré-de Toni-Fanconi syndrome.

MNGIE syndrome (myoneurogastrointestinal encephalopathy) (940). This syndrome consists of myopathy, neuropathy, encephalopathy, and gastrointestinal manifestations (intestinal pseudo-obstruction, chronic diarrhea). Ophthalmoplegia with ptosis is usually also present, along with further mitochondrial manifestations.

LHON syndrome (Leber's hereditary optic neuropathy) (p. 630) (466). Patients with this syndrome suffer from loss of visual acuity and optic nerve atrophy, which usually arises acutely or subacutely and then progresses, first in one eye and then in the other as well. Further manifestations may include ataxia, polyneuropathy, intracardiac conduction abnormalities, or ragged red fibers on muscle biopsy.

DAD syndrome (deafness and diabetes syndrome). Deafness in the early years of life, diabetes mellitus, and often also migraine-like headaches characterize this syndrome.

Luft syndrome (mitochondrial hypermetabolism). This disorder consists of euthyroid hypermetabolism with progressive muscle weakness, hypotonia, and heat intolerance.

Succinate dehydrogenase deficiency. This is the only respiratory chain disorder that is purely nDNA dependent and inherited in an autosomal recessive pattern. It becomes evident in childhood and is characterized by exercise intolerance with dyspnea, palpitations, and rhabdomyolysis.

Diagnostic Evaluation and Ancillary Tests

If there is clinical suspicion of a mitochondrial myopathy, this can be followed up with the following tests: in the *serum*, the concentrations of pyruvate, lactate, and alanine are often elevated, and the *creatine kinase* concentration is normal or mildly elevated. In the *ischemia test* (p. 890), the lactate concentration may rise disproportionately. In the *CSF*, the protein concentration may be elevated. The *EMG* is normal or displays myopathic changes. The sensory and motor *nerve conduction velocities* may be mildly slowed. Intracardiac conduction abnormalities are found mainly in Kearns-Sayre syndrome. *CT* may reveal calcifications in the basal

ganglia and cerebellar nuclei, while *MRI* shows nonspecific signal abnormalities in the basal ganglia, cerebellum, and cerebral white matter (cf. Fahr syndrome, p. 299).

The keys to diagnosis are *muscle biopsy* and *DNA analysis*. Muscle biopsy may be pathognomonic if a modified trichromatic stain reveals the presence of ragged red fibers. Mitochondrial abnormalities are visible by electron microscopy. DNA analysis may reveal (for example) deletions or point mutations in mitochondrial DNA.

> **Treatment**
>
> There is no etiological treatment for any of the mitochondrial disorders. They progress inexorably as the patient ages. The possibilities for treatment are limited to *symptomatic measures*, such as eyelid surgery for ptosis.

Congenital Myopathies

> **Overview:**
>
> By definition, congenital myopathies are present at birth, progress little or not at all, and are characterized by specific morphological abnormalities visible on muscle biopsy. They are thus distinct from progressive neuromuscular diseases such as dystrophies, spinal muscular atrophies, and others. They are presumed to be due to specific genetic defects, though the underlying defect has only been identified in a few of them to date.

In their description of central core myopathy, Shy and Magee defined a congenital myopathy as one that is present at birth and does not progress (874). In this particular disorder, there was also a well-defined morphologic abnormality (i.e., the central

cores). Today, the term "congenital myopathy" refers to any of an etiologically heterogeneous group of myopathies that are present at birth, may or may not be hereditary, are histologically well-defined, and progress little or not at all (Table 14.**10**).

Table 14.**10** Congenital myopathies

Well-recognized forms	Central core myopathy Nemaline (rod) myopathy Centronuclear myopathy Multicore myopathy Fingerprint body myopathy Sarcotubular myopathy Hyaline body myopathy (= myopathy with disintegration of myofibrils in type I fibers)
Inadequately character-ized or questionable congenital forms	Myopathy with congenital fiber type disproportion Congenital hypotonia with type I fiber predominance X-linked myotubular myopathy Fingerprint body myopathy Reducing body myopathy Cytoplasmic body myopathy Myopathy with tubular aggregates Zebra body myopathy Trilaminar fiber myopathy Spheroid body myopathy

Genetics

Most congenital myopathies are of autosomal dominant or X-linked recessive inheritance (myotubular myopathy, centronuclear myopathy). Sporadic cases are also found, and, for some of these disorders, the pattern of inheritance is not yet clearly defined. In central core myopathy, the gene defect lies on chromosome 19q13.1, while in X-linked hereditary centronuclear myopathy it is on chromosome Xq28 (524).

Clinical Features

In *infancy*, patients manifest "myotonia congenita" (floppy infant, Oppenheim disease). Motor development and learning to walk are almost always delayed. In *childhood and adulthood,* there is mainly proximal weakness affecting the lower and, to a lesser extent, the upper limbs. These children often use the Gowers maneuver to stand up – i.e., they climb up their own legs with their arms and hands. Occasionally, the extraocular and facial muscles are also involved. The face and head are usually narrow and high (dolichocephaly) and the palatal vault is high (Gothic palate). Deformities such as pectus excavatum, scoliosis, hip dysplasia, pes cavus, pes planus, and clubfoot are common. The intrinsic muscle reflexes can be either normal or diminished.

The disease progresses little, if at all; progression and premature death from myopathy occur only in exceptional cases. Cardiomyopathy is a rare component of the syndrome. Some types of congenital myopathy are associated with mental retardation (e.g., fingerprint body myopathy).

Ancillary Tests

The *serum creatine kinase concentration* is usually normal or only mildly elevated. The *EMG* generally shows myopathic changes. *Muscle biopsy* reveals specific structural abnormali-

Table 14.**11** Differential diagnosis of congenital myopathy

| Spinal muscular atrophy |
| Congenital muscular dystrophy |
| Congenital myotonic dystrophy and other congenital myotonias |
| Congenital myasthenic syndromes |
| Glycogenoses, particularly types II, III, and IV (cf. Table 2.72) |
| Carnitine deficiency |
| Mitochondrial myopathies |
| Congenital polyneuropathies |

ties in the muscle fibers, establishing the diagnosis. Examples are the central cores of central core disease, the rods of nemaline myopathy, and rows of central nuclei in centronuclear myopathy.

Differential Diagnosis

The differential diagnosis may be difficult, particularly in infants. The important entities to be considered are listed in Table 14.**11**.

Treatment

No etiologic treatment is available to date for the congenital myopathies. Their treatment is thus limited to *symptomatic measures* such as physical therapy and corrective orthopedic procedures. Precise diagnosis of these syndromes is nonetheless justified and important, as they must be clinically differentiated from entities such as muscular dystrophies, spinal muscular atrophies, neuropathies and others that may be at least partly treatable. The diagnosis of a congenital myopathy also provides the basis for prognostication and genetic counseling.

Myositis (203, 401)

Overview:

The term "myositis" refers to an inflammation of muscle of any cause (sterile or infectious). A classification of the myositides based on their historical, clinical, histologic, electromyographic, and serologic features, such as that found in Table 14.**12**, is useful for clinical purposes. *Autoimmune* and *infectious* myositides are the two main categories. Inflammation of muscle can also result from any type of muscle damage – e.g., muscular dystrophies; inflammation of this type should not be confused with primary myositis.

Table 14.**12** Inflammatory myopathies (myositides)

Autoimmune inflammatory disorders mainly affecting muscle	Dermatomyositis and polymyositis in adults Dermatomyositis and polymyositis in children Dermatomyositis and polymyositis accompanying malignancy Inclusion body myositis
Autoimmune inflammatory disorders affecting muscle as well as other organ systems	Scleroderma (progressive systemic sclerosis) Sjögren syndrome Systemic lupus erythematosus Rheumatoid arthritis (=primary chronic polyarthritis) Mixed collagenosis (mixed connective tissue disease, Sharp syndrome) Polyarteritis nodosa Behçet's disease
Other noninfectious myositides	Giant-cell myositis Diffuse fasciitis with eosinophilia Eosinophilic polymyositis Polymyalgia rheumatica Sarcoidosis Myositis in Crohn's disease Myositis ossificans Myosclerosis
Infectious myositides	Viral Bacterial Borrelial Fungal Protozoal Helminthic

Polymyositis and Dermatomyositis (117, 203, 401)

Overview:
These are generalized, usually symmetric, more or less rapidly progressive inflammatory diseases of muscle. Inflammation of the skin is additionally present in dermatomyositis.

Epidemiology

Poly- and dermatomyositis are rare diseases with an incidence of 5–10 cases per million persons per year. The age-specific incidence of dermatomyositis has two peaks, one before puberty and another around age 40. Polymyositis appears almost exclusively after age 35 and affects more women than men. In both disorders, the family history is usually negative.

Pathogenesis

These disorders are presumed to have an autoimmune basis. Dermatomyositis seems to be produced mainly by humoral and polymyositis mainly by cell-mediated immune mechanisms. Thus, the two disorders differ in both their pathophysiology and their clinical manifestations. The following *subgroups* are, to some extent, independent of one another:

- polymyositis without known concomitant illness,
- dermatomyositis in adults,
- dermatomyositis in children,
- polymyositis or dermatomyositis accompanying malignancy,
- polymyositis in collagenoses.

Clinical Features

In dermatomyositis, manifestations appear in both skin and muscle, usually simultaneously. The skin manifestations may proceed those in muscle by some weeks, but the reverse is hardly ever seen. The manifestations of polymyositis, on the other hand, are purely those of a myopathy.

A *general feeling of illness,* arthralgias, myalgias, and sometimes even fever are common initial symptoms. The involved *muscles* are tender to pressure. The progressively developing, symmetric weakness involves proximal more than distal muscles and makes it difficult for the patient to raise the arms above shoulder level, lift objects, take objects down from a shelf, arise from a low chair, climb stairs, or even walk straight ahead. It may be weeks, or in rare cases months, before the weakness has progressed to maximum severity.

In at least one-third of all patients there is a disturbance of pharyngeal and esophageal motility causing *dys-phagia.* Dysarthria is unusual. In dermatomyositis, muscle involvement is accompanied by *livid patches* on the skin. These may appear on the face in a butterfly shape over the ridge of the nose, on the cheeks, or on the eyelids, but also on the back of the hands, in the nail folds, or on the chest. Subcutaneous calcifications (calcinosis) resembling those of scleroderma are not uncommon.

Other manifestations of poly- and dermatomyositis involve the heart and lungs, causing heart failure, atrial and ventricular arrhythmias, or pulmonary fibrosis. Marked dysphagia may lead to aspiration pneumonia. Joint involvement usually causes no visible changes, but sometimes produces joint effusions and contractures. Raynaud's syndrome also occurs at increased frequency in patients with myositis.

About 10% of cases of polymyositis and dermatomyositis appear in patients with malignant disease. (N.b., this statement does not apply to dermatomyositis in children.) The malignancy is usually a carcinoma of the lung, breast, ovary, or stomach. Polymyositis in such cases is usually one manifestation of a disease process affecting multiple organ systems. No disease other than scleroderma is associated with dermatomyositis. Patients with both are said to suffer from "sclerodermatomyositis."

Ancillary Tests

The *serum creatine kinase concentration* is markedly elevated (10-fold or more above normal). It becomes normal again only in long-standing, "burnt-out" myositis. The erythrocyte sedimentation rate and C-reactive protein concentration are usually elevated as well, and protein electrophoresis usually shows an acute inflammatory pattern.

EMG reveals a myopathic pattern with low-amplitude, often polyphasic motor unit potentials and spontaneous activity, mostly in the form of fibrillations and positive sharp waves.

Muscle biopsy reveals diffusely distributed necrosis of muscle fibers. The endo- and perimysial connective tissue and perivascular spaces are infiltrated by lymphocytes, histiocytes, and plasma cells. In dermatomyositis, the infiltrate consists mainly of B and CD4 lymphocytes, while, in polymyositis, it consists mainly of CD8 lymphocytes.

Diagnostic Evaluation and Differential Diagnosis

The diagnosis is based on the finding of rapidly progressive, symmetric, mainly proximal muscle weakness, the results of the ancillary tests just discussed, and the exclusion of other diseases. In dermatomyositis, the typical constellation of skin and muscle changes points to the diagnosis. Collagenoses often affect the kidneys, blood vessels, eyes, lungs, heart, skin, skeleton, and peripheral nerves and are associated with specific antibodies for each type of collagenosis; the demonstration of such antibodies rules out primary myositis. Inclusion body myositis typically causes mainly distal weakness. Drug-induced toxic myopathy is most easily diagnosed by careful history-taking, sarcoidosis by muscle biopsy, endocrine myopathy by hormone analysis, and limb girdle dystrophy by family history and muscle biopsy.

Course and Prognosis

About one-quarter of all patients die within 10 years of disease onset, but about half of those for whom optimal treatment can be provided are cured or markedly improved. In about one-quarter of patients, the disease continues to progress despite treatment or recurs as soon as immunosuppressive therapy is stopped. The duration of treatment is usually 1–2 years or more.

Treatment (203b, 530a, 623a)

Children with dermatomyositis almost always respond to *corticosteroids*, which can be slowly tapered to off once remission occurs.

Adults often require *immunosuppressive therapy* in addition to steroids, particularly in order to avoid the complications of long-term steroid use. *Prednisone* is recommended at a dose of 1–1.5 mg/kg daily. Once the disease has stabilized, as judged from the lack of further progression of weakness and decline of the sedimentation rate and creatine kinase concentration, the daily prednisone dose can be reduced by 10 mg every month down to a dose of 30–40 mg/day, then by 5 mg every month down to a dose of 15–20 mg/day, and thereafter by 2.5 mg each month, always with careful monitoring of the patient's clinical status, sedimentation rate, and creatine kinase concentration. Patients should be informed of the potential side effects of corticosteroid therapy, which should be actively looked for at each follow-up examination. These include electrolyte disturbances, osteoporosis, peptic ulcer, skin changes, endocrine disturbances, sleep disturbances, cataracts, glaucoma, reactivation of old tuberculosis, and other problems.

Likewise, women at risk for osteoporosis who are being treated with corticosteroids should be given *vitamin D supplements* and *calcium* as *prophylaxis*, as well as *alternating corticosteroid treatment* (every second day). The immunosuppressive agent of first choice is *azathioprine*, 2–3 mg/kg daily. The treatment must be continued at least 1 year after remission. *Cyclophosphamide* and *methotrexate* are alternative medications.

Intravenous immunoglobulin therapy is also useful in the acute stage of the disease. Steroids should not be given concomitantly. *Plasmapheresis* is ineffective against polymyositis and variably effective against dermatomyositis.

Inclusion Body Myositis
(97, 568, 723b)

Clinical Features

This disorder usually appears after age 50 and is more common in men. It clinically resembles polymyositis but affects both proximal and distal muscles. In the forearms, the flexors are more severely affected than the extensors. Dysphagia is common. Inclusion body myositis is not associated with malignant disease but may appear in combination with other autoimmune processes. Its etiology is unknown.

Diagnostic Evaluation

The *erythrocyte sedimentation rate* is usually normal. The *serum creatine kinase concentration* is mildly elevated (up to fivefold the normal value). *EMG* reveals a myopathic pattern, but also prolonged potentials resembling those seen in neuropathy. On *muscle biopsy*, there are vacuoles with basophilic borders (rimmed vacuoles) in multiple muscle fibers, and electron microscopy shows filamentous inclusions in cell nuclei and cytoplasm, as well as mitochondrial changes.

Course

Inclusion body myositis usually progresses inexorably.

> **Treatment**
> Immunosuppressive therapy usually fails to halt the progression of the disease. Intravenous immunoglobulin therapy may be effective.

Other Noninfectious Myositides

■ Diffuse Fasciitis with Eosinophilia (Shulman Syndrome)

This disorder consists of fasciitis with scleroderma-like skin changes, an elevated erythrocyte sedimentation rate, eosinophilia, and mild fever (680). The inflammatory infiltrates of the fasciae are sometimes accompanied by myositis.

> **Treatment**
> Steroids bring prompt improvement.

■ Eosinophilic Polymyositis

This disorder of unknown cause is frequently associated with cerebral infarction, diffuse encephalopathies, and neuropathies.

Treatment
Eosinophilic polymyositis is treated by aggressive immunosuppressive therapy, which, however, often fails to improve its unfavorable course.

■ **Eosinophilia-Myalgia Syndromes**
Syndromes of this type may be induced by the consumption of chemically contaminated tryptophan and denatured cooking oil ("Spanish toxic oil syndrome," p. 611).

■ **Polymyalgia Rheumatica**
This syndrome is a manifestation of giant cell arteritis (p. 816). Its main symptom is myalgia, usually in the early morning, without any significant weakness. The erythrocyte sedimentation rate is markedly elevated, while the serum creatine kinase concentration is only mildly elevated, if at all, and the EMG and muscle biopsy reveal normal findings or nonspecific changes.

Treatment
Steroids rapidly relieve the pain.

■ **Sarcoidosis**
Sarcoidosis often affects muscle, sometimes as its principal manifestation – e.g., in the form of a quadriceps myopathy. Muscle biopsy reveals the typical giant-cell granulomas.

■ **Giant-Cell Myositis**
Giant-cell myositis without sarcoidosis has also been described. It may appear together with myocarditis in patients with myasthenia gravis and thymoma.

■ **Granulomatous Myositis**
Another kind of granulomatous myositis afflicts patients with Crohn's disease.

■ **Myositis Ossificans**
This disorder (also called fibrodysplasia ossificans) is characterized by bone formation in the subcutaneous tissue and along muscle fasciae (183). It usually appears before age 2 and may cause considerable deformity and limitation of movement.

■ **Myosclerosis**
This disorder (also called myositis fibrosa generalisata) involves hardening of the muscles and contractures (128). Biopsy reveals a marked increase of connective tissue and sometimes also inflammatory changes.

Treatment
Success has been reported with *D-penicillamine* in doses up to 750 mg/day.

Infectious Myositides

Viral infections. Various viruses can cause myalgia with elevation of the serum creatine kinase concentration, among them influenza, coxsackievirus, echovirus, and herpesvirus.

HIV infection. HIV can cause various types of myopathy. One type is clinically indistinguishable from polymyositis (202), usually appears in an early stage of HIV infection, and is painless. Steroid treatment is effective in roughly half of patients. On the other hand, severe myalgia is characteristic of the toxic myopathy that can develop after 6–18 months of treatment with zidovudine, in which muscle biopsy reveals the presence of ragged red fibers, as in a mitochondrial myopathy (357). Discontinuation of zidovudine improves myalgia, and often strength as well. HIV-associated myopathy must be carefully differentiated from polyradiculitis or chronic inflammatory demyelinating polyneuropathy (CIDP).

Bacterial infections. These only rarely cause myositis. *Staphylococcus aureus* and streptococci can produce more or less localized muscle infections or abscesses. Myalgia-like pain in the limbs is characteristic of acute *borre-* *liosis* (Lyme disease), but this type of pain is more commonly due to neuritis or arthritis than to myositis.

Other pathogens. *Systemic toxoplasmosis* produces fever, lymphadenopathy, headache, pharyngitis, and myalgia, but probably does not cause isolated myositis. *Worms*, particularly trichinae and cysticerci, can cause isolated myositis, which may be visible as muscle calcifications on radiographs and can be diagnosed by serology and muscle biopsy. Antihelminthic treatment is effective (p. 109 ff.).

▎Myopathy in Endocrine Diseases

Hyperthyroidism

Chronic thyrotoxic myopathy involves mainly proximal weakness. Hyperthyroidism can also rarely cause acute myopathy (p. 319), periodic paralysis (p. 884), endocrine ophthalmoplegia (p. 661), or a disturbance of neuromuscular transmission (p. 911). Moreover, the abuse of thyroid hormone preparations, too, can lead to myopathy.

Hypothyroidism

Hypothyroidism can cause mainly proximal weakness (p. 315), myotonia, and a disturbance of neuromuscular transmission (p. 911).

Hyperparathyroidism

The manifestations of hyperparathyroidism in muscle are described on p. 319.

Hypoparathyroidism

The muscular symptoms and proximal weakness caused by hypoparathyroidism and hypocalcemia are usually overshadowed by tetany (p. 318). The serum creatine kinase concentration may be elevated.

Cushing's Disease and Steroid Myopathy

Steroid myopathy is not uncommon. It usually consists of proximal weakness of the muscles of the lower limb and pelvic girdle, with preserved deep tendon reflexes. Atrophy is present in severe cases. Patients who take more than 30 mg of prednisone daily are at elevated risk, as are those who take steroids in combination with substances causing neuromuscular blockade (cf. myopathy with myosin deficiency in muscle fibers, p. 911). A dosage of 10 mg of prednisone daily, however, can suffice to produce steroid myopathy. The serum creatine kinase concentration remains normal. The EMG shows signs of myopathy. Histologic study reveals selective atrophy of type II fibers. Physical activity limits the extent of atrophy; patients who take steroids should be encouraged to remain physically active.

Conn Syndrome

Primary hyperaldosteronism (Conn syndrome) causes hypokalemia, which, in turn, may manifest itself primarily as muscle weakness. Arterial hypertension is typically also present.

Addison's Disease

Addison's disease causes muscle weakness, but it does not cause a true myopathy. The weakness is largely attributable to electrolyte abnormalities and an abnormality of carbohydrate utilization.

Acromegaly (513)

This disease often causes carpal tunnel syndrome (p. 773). It can also cause mild proximal muscle weakness, with a myopathic pattern on EMG, but normal serum enzymes and muscle biopsy findings.

Diabetes Mellitus

The muscular manifestations in diabetes mellitus are neurogenic, rather than due to primary involvement of muscle. The traditional term "diabetic amyotrophy" is a misnomer, as the pathogenetic mechanism is actually a mononeuropathy.

Muscular Manifestations of Electrolyte Disturbances

Either hypo- or hyperkalemia can cause muscle weakness. The periodic paralyses are described on p. 877. *Hyponatremia* usually causes fatigue and weakness, but these are less prominent than the cerebral manifestations (p. 335). Hypernatremia only rarely causes muscular manifestations. *Hypophosphatemia* can induce or aggravate neuromuscular disturbances, sometimes leading to rhabdomyolysis – e.g., in cachexia or alcoholism (787). The muscle weakness associated with *hypo- and hypercalcemia* was discussed in an earlier chapter (p. 318). *Hypomagnesemia*, too, can cause muscle weakness and tetany (p. 318).

Muscular Manifestations Due to Medications, Intoxications, and Nutritional Deficiencies (433, 980)

Overview:
Medications, intoxications, and nutritional deficiencies can harm muscle in many ways. There can be direct systemic injury to muscle cells, secondary muscle injury due to endocrine, metabolic, electrolyte, or immunologic disturbances or excessive energy consumption, local trauma (e.g., from injections), or crush injury under the weight of the body during episodes of unconsciousness ("self-crush" injury). These processes cause symptoms such as myalgia and cramps and signs such as weakness, myasthenia, and rhabdomyolysis with myoglobinuria.

A number of classic drug-induced disorders have already been discussed elsewhere in this text, including malignant neuroleptic syndrome (p. 307), malignant hyperthermia (genetic predisposition and succinylcholine, p. 893 ff), zidovudine-induced mitochondrial dysfunction in patients under treatment for HIV (p. 906), eosinophilia-myalgia syndrome after the consumption of denatured cooking oil (p. 906), steroid myopathy (p. 907), and the myopathy of thyroid hormone abuse (p. 315). The various possible causes of myoglobinuria were listed above in Table 14.7, and myotoxic substances (among others) in Table 2.73.

A few further situations and substances that can injure muscle are described in the following paragraphs.

"Self-Crush"

In a comatose patient, the weight of the body can mechanically compromise the blood supply, and thus the energy supply, of the muscle or muscles on which the patient lies, causing rhabdomyolysis. This may occur in substance-induced coma of any cause. Common causes are illicit drugs (opiates, cocaine), alcohol, diazepam and its derivatives, and other centrally active sedatives.

Cocaine

Cocaine-induced vasospasm can cause not only stroke and myocardial infarction, as discussed in an earlier chapter, but also necrosis of muscle, including in muscles that do not bear the weight of the comatose patient.

Vacuolar Myopathy due to Colchicine, Chloroquine, and Vincristine

These substances cause a vacuolar myopathy. They can also cause neuropathy. Chloroquine can impair neuromuscular transmission.

Gasoline Vapor, Toluene

Persons who sniff organic solvents or gasoline vapor are at risk for rhabdomyolysis (29). Toluene causes marked hypokalemia and hypophosphatemia, both of which promote rhabdomyolysis (pp. 910 ff.).

Antilipemic Drugs

Drugs such as clofibrate, lovastatin, simvastatin, gemfibrozil, and niacin cause structural damage in muscle, leading to rhabdomyolysis, perhaps because they impair cholesterol synthesis. This problem is common to all antilipemic drugs (fibrates and statins), but is worse among the HMG-CoA reductase inhibitors (statins). The latter have also been reported to have side effects that can be mistaken for polymyalgia rheumatica. The immune suppressant cyclosporine can also be myotoxic.

Hypokalemic Myopathy

Diuretics, laxatives, licorice, and alcohol (cf. hypokalemic myopathy in alcoholics) can cause hypokalemia, and thereby muscle damage.

Emetine and Ipecac

These substances can cause vacuolar myopathy with loss of mitochondria. Ipecac syrup is not uncommonly abused by persons with anorexia nervosa. Besides myopathy, it can also produce skin changes resembling those of dermatomyositis.

Inflammatory Myopathies

Penicillamine can cause inflammatory myopathy or a myasthenic syndrome; both of these are reversible if the medication is discontinued. The proton-pump inhibitor cimetidine can cause severe dose-limiting myalgia, and in rare cases a polymyositis-vasculitis syndrome with elevation of the serum creatine kinase concentration.

Types of Muscle Damage Due to Alcoholism

Rhabdomyolysis and "self-crush". Alcohol-induced generalized seizures can cause rhabdomyolysis, while alcohol intoxication can cause self-crush injuries.

Acute alcoholic myopathy. Chronic alcoholics may develop an impressively severe acute alcoholic myopathy (751). Pain and muscle cramps are the main symptoms. There may also be weakness. The serum creatine kinase concentration is elevated. The rise in lactate concentration in the ischemia test is inadequate, corresponding to diminished glycogen utilization that can be demonstrated by spectroscopy. Muscle biopsy often reveals tubular aggregates. This type of myopathy is seen almost exclusively in patients who also show other signs of chronic alcoholism. It reverses slowly if the patient abstains from alcohol.

Subacute or chronic alcoholic myopathy. Chronic alcoholism can also cause subacute or chronic myopathy, developing over weeks or months, respectively. The proximal muscles become weak and atrophic. This type of myopathy usually reverses with abstinence from alcohol. It may be due, not to alcohol per se, but to the nutritional deficiencies and electrolyte disturbances that often accompany alcoholism.

Hypokalemic myopathy in alcoholics. A further probable clinical entity is hypokalemic myopathy in alcoholics (810). Painless weakness arises and progresses rapidly (days). There is no swelling or myoglobinuria. The weakness is accompanied by hypokalemia and responds to potassium administration. Concomitant hypophosphate-mia should always be sought and, if necessary, corrected, especially in cases with rhabdomyolysis (373).

Muscular Manifestations of Nutritional Deficiencies

Long-standing inadequate nutrition, e.g., in maltreated prisoners of war, can cause myastheniform weakness, with prominent ptosis and weakness of the nuchal muscles (in Japanese, *kubisagari*, "one whose head hangs low"). Vitamin E deficiency can cause severe myopathy in experimental animals and in human beings. Weakness due to vitamin E deficiency has

been described (364, 1002), in addition to its other manifestations (p. 608 ff).

Myopathy with Myosin Deficiency in Muscle Fibers

Severely ill patients in intensive care units can develop a form of myopathy in which myosin is largely absent from the muscle fibers. The histochemical finding resembles that of critical illness neuropathy (19). Patients who are simultaneously treated with neuromuscular blocking agents and steroids are at elevated risk (804, 884). The weakness usually resolves over several months.

Disorders of Neuromuscular Transmission (280a)

Overview:

This category of diseases comprises myasthenia gravis (or, to give its full name, myasthenia gravis pseudoparalytica) and the myasthenic syndromes. The former is an acquired autoimmune disease in which the acetylcholine receptors on the postsynaptic membrane are destroyed. The latter are a heterogeneous group comprising the Lambert-Eaton myasthenic syndrome, congenital myasthenic syndromes, botulism, drug-induced myasthenias, organophosphate poisoning, and certain types of paralysis caused by snake venom (bungarotoxins).

Myasthenia Gravis (Myasthenia Gravis Pseudoparalytica, Erb-Goldflam Disease) (244, 278, 279, 416, 592, 686, 732)

Major Manifestations

The clinical features of myasthenia gravis are:

- Increasing fatigue of individual muscles with sustained activity.

Thus, the symptoms and signs tend to be worse in the evening.
- Recovery after a few minutes of rest.
- Onset typically in muscles whose motor units consist of relatively few fibers – i.e., the extraocular, palatal, and pharyngeal muscles.
- Fluctuating intensity of manifestations, with occasional crises.
- Involvement of muscles innervated by different peripheral nerves.

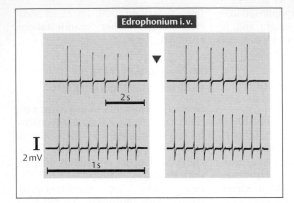

Fig. 14.**8** **Decrement in the EMG of a patient with myasthenia gravis.** The summed motor unit potential is recorded from the abductor digiti minimi on repetitive stimulation of the ulnar nerve. Note the marked decrement in amplitude (left), which then normalizes after edrophonium (Tensilon®) is given.

- Absence of sensory deficit and pain. Fasciculations and atrophy are seen only in exceptional cases.
- Immediate improvement or even full resolution of weakness upon injection of a cholinesterase inhibitor such as edrophonium chloride (Tensilon).
- The EMG shows a myasthenic reaction, with progressive diminution of amplitude on repeated contraction of a muscle (Fig. 14.**8**).
- Presence of serum antibodies directed against the acetylcholine receptors of the neuromuscular junction.

History

The earliest description of myasthenia gravis is attributed to Thomas Willis (1672). Erb (1879) and Goldflam (1893) provided detailed clinical descriptions of the syndrome. Jolly (1895) discovered the myasthenic reaction and named the disease myasthenia gravis pseudoparalytica (284, 354, 474). Weigert (1901) and Buzzard (1905) recognized the connection of this disease with thymoma and thymic hyperplasia. The first thymectomy was performed by Sauerbruch (1911), and Blalock (1936, 1944) demonstrated its therapeutic effectiveness. Anticholinesterase drugs, which had already been proposed by Jolly, came into use after their description in a publication by Walker (1934) (physostigmine, later neostigmine). The classic descriptions of the electrophysiologic features of the disease, including the progressive decline of the summed motor unit potential, were written by Lindsley (1935) and by Harvey and Masland (1941). In 1960, Simpson reported on the frequent association of myasthenia gravis with other autoimmune diseases and postulated that it was due to an immune attack on the motor end plate (882). The dysfunction of the acetylcholine receptor was demonstrated in 1973 (Fambrough, Drachman and Satyamurti), and, later in the 1970s, the antibodies to the acetylcholine receptor were directly demonstrated (Lindstrom 1976 in the serum, A.G. Engel 1977 at the motor end plate). The initial therapeutic results with prednisone were poor; its usefulness came to be realized only in

1970 (Warmolts, W.K. Engel, and Whitaker). Further forms of treatment (azathioprine since 1968, plasmapheresis since 1976, intravenous immunoglobulins since 1989) have broadened the therapeutic armamentarium significantly, so that, in many cases, the designation "gravis" fortunately no longer applies.

Epidemiology

Myasthenia gravis is relatively rare, with an incidence of ca. 10 cases per million persons per year and a prevalence of ca. 140 cases per million persons. It can arise at any age; it most frequently arises in the third decade in women, and in the sixth and seventh decades in men. The male-female ratio is 3 : 2; most younger patients are women, while most patients over 50 are men. The disease is not hereditary, but relatives of patients are at mildly elevated risk of developing the disease themselves.

Pathophysiology

The transmission of electrical impulses from the nerve terminal to the underlying muscle cells is the function of the neuromuscular junction (neuromuscular synapse). The action potential arriving at the nerve terminal causes acetylcholine packets

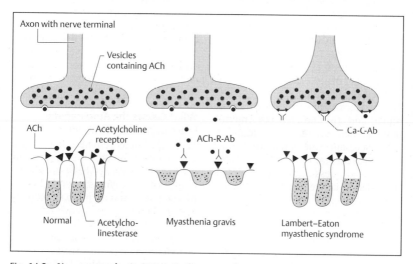

Fig. 14.**9** **Neuromuscular junction in the normal state, in myasthenia gravis, and in the Lambert-Eaton myasthenic syndrome.**
In myasthenia gravis, antibodies against the acetylcholine receptors on the postsynaptic membrane bring about the destruction of these receptors. The release of acetylcholine into the synaptic cleft functions normally, but, because there are fewer receptors, the end plate potential that is generated is insufficient to initiate an action potential. In the Lambert-Eaton myasthenic syndrome, antibodies against the calcium channels of the nerve terminal impair the release of acetylcholine.

Ach   Acetylcholine
Ach-R-Ab   Antibody against acetylcholine receptors
Ca-C-Ab   Antibody against calcium channels of the nerve terminal

(quanta) to be released: acetyl-choline-containing vesicles previously stored in the nerve terminal fuse with its membrane, liberating their contents into the synaptic cleft. Acetyl-choline molecules then bind to the acetylcholine receptors of the post-synaptic membrane, whereupon the cation channels in the receptors transiently open, generating an end-plate potential. If the summed end-plate potential from all of the activated receptors is sufficiently high (above a critical threshold), an action potential is generated that then travels down the muscle fiber and through the transverse tubular system, causing calcium to be released into the sarcoplasm, which then promotes the interaction of actin and myosin that causes the muscle cell to contract. Myasthenia gravis is due to an acquired disturbance of neuromuscular transmission. The number of acetylcholine receptors is substantially reduced (288, 753). The distance between the nerve terminal and the postsynaptic membrane is increased, and the folding of the postsynaptic membrane that contains the receptor molecules is coarsened and less extensive (278) (Fig. 14.**9**). The reduced number of acetylcholine receptors leads to diminution of the end plate potential, so that no action potentials can be generated in the affected fibers. If many fibers are affected, the muscle is weak. With repeated contraction of a muscle, neuromuscular transmission fails at an ever larger number of synapses, and the weakness becomes progressively more severe.

Why Are the Acetylcholine Receptors Fewer in Number?

Simpson's hypothesis of an autoimmune process attacking the motor end plate (882) was confirmed with the discovery of antibodies against the acetylcholine receptor both in the serum and on the postsynaptic membrane (277, 587). Further confirmation of an autoimmune pathogenesis was provided by the induction of myasthenic manifestations in animals by the administration of antibodies or immunization with the antigen (acetylcholine receptor) (949) and by clinical improvement upon lowering of the antibody titer. Finally, it was shown that the antibodies directed against the acetylcholine receptors indeed rendered them functionally inoperative or actually caused their destruction (244).

There is no correlation across patients between the serum antibody titer and the severity of disease manifestations, because the anti-receptor antibodies are very heterogeneous and affect the receptors to different degrees.

What Causes the Autoimmune Process, and How Is It Initiated?

These questions remain open. Only a few facts are known. Three out of four myasthenic patients have an abnormality of the thymus, thymic hyperplasia in 85% and thymoma in 15%. T- and B-lymphocytes recovered from the thymus of patients with myasthenia gravis are more reactive against acetylcholine receptors than those recovered from peripheral blood. The target of the immune attacks is not the acetylcholine receptors in muscle, but rather those on muscle-like (myoid) cells in the thymus itself. The generation of antibodies against acetylcholine receptors in muscle is presumably the result of a misdirected immune response. Genetic factors may play a role in the pathogenesis of myasthenia gravis, as they do in other autoimmune diseases. The disease is not hereditary, but it does tend to cluster in families, and certain HLA types are more common in persons suffering from myasthenia gravis and other autoimmune diseases.

Can damaged acetylcholine receptors be repaired?

The receptors are continually being destroyed and regenerated. Any lessening of synaptic transmission leads to increased transcription of the acetylcholine receptor gene and thus to increased generation of receptors. This process is an important prerequisite for clinical recovery once the autoimmune attack is brought under control.

Clinical Features

Patients complain of abnormal fatigability of individual muscles, which, when repeatedly activated, rapidly become weak. The weakness usually resolves after a few minutes of rest. The symptoms may arise over the course of the day or be present all day long with worsening toward evening. Muscles that function tonically are preferentially affected, especially muscles of the head that are composed of relatively small motor units (levator palpebrae, muscles of the soft palate, and extraocular muscles, particularly the superior rectus), as well as the nuchal musculature. Accordingly, the earliest manifestations of the disease are often ptosis, diplopia, nasal speech, dysphagia, and weakness of neck extension. There are also purely ocular forms of the disease. The muscles of the trunk and limbs generally do not become weak until later, though they may be weak at the onset of disease in exceptional

cases, even in the absence of weakness in other muscles.

In addition to the rapidly fluctuating severity of weakness, a further important point for diagnosis is that the affected muscles are innervated by different peripheral nerves. The deficits typically involve individual muscles or muscle groups in an asymmetric distribution, but may also be more or less symmetric on occasion.

Clinical examination usually reveals no more than the functional disturbance just described affecting individual muscle groups – i.e., a rapid and marked decrement in strength on repetitive muscle contraction. Unilateral or, frequently, bilateral ptosis is present and becomes worse after repeated forceful closing and opening of the eyes, or after the patient looks up for a prolonged period of time *(Simpson test)*. Weakness of the extraocular muscles is usually asymmetrical and often involves the muscles subserving convergence and vertical movement. Weakness of the muscles of facial expression may produce a mask-like facies, and the mouth often hangs open. A smile may be distorted into a grimace, because the corners of the mouth cannot be elevated. Weakness of the palatal veil causes nasal speech, and fluids may be regurgitated. Weakness of the larynx and pharynx causes dysphonia and dysphagia in which food and secretions "go down the wrong pipe." Dysphagia may worsen as the patient eats, accompanied by gradually worsening weakness of biting and chewing. The speech becomes increasingly nasal as the patient keeps speaking, and may finally become so slurred as to be unintelligible. Weakness of the muscles of respiration causes shortness of breath on exertion or even at rest. If the limb muscles are involved, the proximal muscles are usually more severely affected than the distal ones. Keeping the head erect is often difficult. Some 10% of patients develop muscle atrophy. The intrinsic muscle reflexes are normal or brisk, except in very weak muscles, where they may be diminished.

Comorbidity

Myasthenia gravis tends to appear in combination with other autoimmune diseases (Table 14.**13**). Concomitant hypo- or hyperthyroidism, systemic infection, or medications such as aminoglycosides, antiarrhythmics, anticonvulsants, or quinine can worsen the manifestations of myasthenia gravis.

Table 14.**13** Myasthenia in combination with other diseases (adapted from Jerusalem and Zierz)

Disease	Frequency (%)
Thymoma	10.0%
Hyperthyroidism	5.7%
Hypothyroidism	5.3%
Polyarthritis	3.6%
Pernicious anemia	0.9%
Systemic lupus erythematosus	0.2%
Sarcoidosis	0.2%
Sjögren syndrome, polymyositis, ulcerative colitis, pemphigus, Lambert-Eaton syndrome, Sneddon syndrome	Rare

Spontaneous Course without Treatment (732)

The signs and symptoms can fluctuate in severity from day to day, from week to week, and over longer times. Periods of complete remission lasting a considerable length of time can occur, but permanent, spontaneous remission is rare. In typical untreated cases, the manifestations of disease gradually spread from the eyes to the facial and bulbar muscles and then to the trunk and limbs. The first manifestation of the disease is in the eyes in half of all cases (equally divided between ptosis and diplopia), and the eyes are eventually involved in more than 90%. Generalization of manifestations practically always occurs within 3 years of onset and was, at one time, associated with 30% mortality. In 16% of untreated cases, however, the disease manifestations remain permanently confined to the extraocular muscles (363). Muscle relaxants such as curare can drastically worsen the clinical picture.

Grading the Severity of Myasthenia Gravis

Osserman scale. This scale divides cases of myasthenia into four varieties, one of which has two subtypes:

- **I:** *ocular myasthenia* – i.e., myasthenia confined to the eyes.
- **IIa:** *mild form* of generalized myasthenia.
- **IIb:** *moderately severe form* of generalized myasthenia. The muscles of respiration are not affected.
- **III:** *acute and rapidly progressive myasthenia.* Abrupt onset and progression, with involvement of the muscles of respiration within 6 months of onset.

- **IV:** *chronic, severe myasthenia.* Progression from groups I or II, after a relatively stable course lasting ca. 2 years. Patients in groups III and IV more often have a thymoma than those in groups I or II, and suffer a higher mortality.

Classification by age and thymoma. Alternatively, cases of myasthenia gravis can be classified according to the age of onset and the presence or absence of thymoma (278).

Ancillary Tests

Tensilon (edrophonium chloride) test. The test injection of an acetylcholinesterase inhibitor is easy to perform in the outpatient setting or at the hospital bedside. For example, one may inject 10 mg (i.e., 1 mL of a 1% solution) of edrophonium chloride (Tensilon) intravenously over 10 seconds. The effect appears about 30 seconds later, but lasts for only about 3 minutes. A previously severe ptosis may disappear with lightning speed and remains absent for a minute or two. The effect, however, is often not very impressive in patients with ocular and bulbar myasthenia. Atropine sulfate should always be at hand for administration as an antidote, if necessary (1 mg i.v., repeated if necessary). If the test is performed in a patient who is already being treated with a cholinesterase inhibitor to test whether a higher dose of medication is required, the initial injection is usually of 2 mg (i.e., 0.2 mL) i.v., given 1 hour after the last oral dose. The result will reveal whether more medication can be given with benefit, or whether, as in some cases, the weakness is actually compounded by the excessive cholinergic effect of the medication (see under "Treatment with cholinesterase inhibitors," below).

Electrophysiologic tests. Repetitive nerve stimulation with recording of the summed motor unit potential through a surface electrode has already been discussed in an earlier chapter (p. 744). The sensitivity of this test can be increased by the testing of multiple muscles, particularly those that are clinically affected. Single fiber electromyography is an even more sensitive test, though relatively cumbersome, technically demanding, and difficult to interpret. In myasthenia gravis, this test reveals increased jitter and more frequent blockades.

Antibodies against the acetylcholine receptor. These can be demonstrated by radioimmunoassay in about 85% of patients with myasthenia gravis, though they are not found in ca. 50% of cases of ocular myasthenia and in 10–20% of cases of generalized myasthenia. The reason may be either antibody heterogeneity or a serum titer that is too low to be detected by radioimmunoassay.

Chest radiography, CT, and MRI. CT or MRI should be performed to demonstrate or rule out a thymoma (71). The normal thymus is not visible in these studies after age 40.

Other ancillary tests. Further tests are used to detect or rule out the associated conditions listed in Table 14.**13**. In particular, the serum should be tested for antibodies against striated muscle, thyroid hormone, antithyroid antibodies, antinuclear antibodies, rheumatoid factor, and vitamin B_{12} and glucose concentrations. Baseline pulmonary function testing should also be performed as part of the initial evaluation of the patient. Further studies will depend on the particular clinical situation.

Diagnostic Evaluation

Myasthenia gravis is diagnosed on the basis of the history, clinical findings, electrophysiologic test results, and the demonstrations of antibodies against the acetylcholine receptor. Laboratory testing almost always confirms the diagnosis in cases of generalized myasthenia, even if no anti-receptor antibodies can be found. In ocular myasthenia, however, all ancillary tests are often negative. In such cases, the careful exclusion of other conditions in the differential diagnosis is more important than the diagnosis of myasthenia itself, because purely ocular myasthenia does not always need treatment. A falsely positive diagnosis may have the very unfortunate result of subjecting the patient to the discomfort, risk, and expense of protracted and unnecessary immunosuppressive therapy.

Treatment (203b, 244, 278, 465, 530a). The mortality of myasthenia gravis is now practically zero because of the multiple types of treatment that are available. Most patients can lead a normal life. They must, however, bear the risks associated with protracted, often lifelong immunosuppressive therapy. The therapeutic armamentarium currently consists of the following:

- cholinesterase inhibitors,
- thymectomy,
- corticosteroids and other immune suppressants,
- short-acting immune therapies (plasmapheresis, intravenous immunoglobulins).

Treatment with cholinesterase inhibitors (465)

Pyridostigmine (Mestinon) is the first line of treatment. Its effect begins 30–60 minutes after oral administration, reaches a maximum at 2 hours, and lasts 3–6 hours. It is available in 10 mg and 60 mg tablets, and in sustained-release tablets of 180 mg. The dose must be adjusted individually but is usually on the order of 300–600 mg/day. If the dose is raised beyond 120 mg every 3 hours (> 960 mg/day), any additional benefit is unlikely, and the risk of adverse side effects increases. Night-time or early morning weakness usually responds well to the administration of a single sustained-release tablet at bedtime.

Neostigmine (Prostigmin) is another cholinesterase inhibitor that is usually given intravenously or intramuscularly. A 0.5-mg i.v. bolus or an intramuscular dose of 1.0–1.5 mg is roughly as effective as 60 mg of pyridostigmine given orally.

Side effects:
High doses of cholinesterase inhibitors can cause unpleasant side effects, which are often referred to as a *cholinergic crisis,* as distinct from the *myasthenic crisis* of the disease. This is an oversimplification, in that the patient is generally still in a myasthenic crisis, upon which the nicotinic and muscarinic

side effects of high-dose medication are superimposed. The main nicotinic side effect is additional weakness due to depolarization block of whatever acetylcholine receptors remain functional on the postsynaptic membrane. Further effects include tremor, involuntary twitching, fasciculations, and painful muscle spasms. The muscarinic side effects are sweating, nausea, an epigastric pressure sensation, abdominal cramps, increased intestinal motility, copious respiratory secretions, and dyspnea. Patients are agitated and anxious and may suffer from insomnia, headache, and seizures through involvement of the central nervous system. (Agitation and anxiety may be components of a purely myasthenic crisis as well, for obvious reasons.) All of these side effects can be reduced by the temporary discontinuation of cholinesterase inhibitors, and the administration of atropine. Should there be uncertainty whether a higher dose of physostigmine might further improve the myasthenic weakness, a test injection of 1–2 mg of Tensilon may be given. Cholinesterase inhibitors hardly ever suffice as monotherapy and should be combined with other measures right from the outset of treatment.

Treatment with thymectomy

Thymectomy can result in a remission lasting months or years, or at least in improvement of the myasthenic manifestations. It is clearly indicated in adult patients below the age of 60. In children, thymectomy should be deferred, if possible, till after puberty, in order not to disturb the development of the immune system. Thymectomy is of questionable utility for patients over 60. In principle, it is primarily indicated for the treatment of generalized myasthenia. For purely ocular myasthenia, the indication is not compelling, and one may defer the procedure until the disease process becomes generalized, if it ever does. Yet good results of thymectomy for purely ocular myasthenia have been reported. In general, we recommend an early, active therapeutic approach, offering thymectomy to our patients with ocular myasthenia as well.

Thymomas should be *surgically excised* at any age, as these tumors can become locally invasive and, rarely, metastasize. If total resection cannot be achieved, the residual tumor must be dealt with by *radiotherapy* and possibly also be *chemotherapy.*

In general, thymectomy should only be performed in centers where a team of physicians and surgeons experienced in the treatment of myasthenia gravis is available. Endoscopic thymectomy was popular for some time, but at present surgeons are increasingly turning back to open surgery with splitting of the sternum, as it affords better exposure and a higher likelihood of total resection.

Treatment with corticosteroids and other immune suppressants

Immunosuppressive therapy is indicated when cholinesterase inhibitors alone provide insufficient benefit. This is, unfortunately, the case for most patients. Corticosteroids are the preferred initial method of immune suppression. When first given, they may cause a transient worsening of myasthenia; corticosteroid treatment is, therefore, usually begun on an inpatient basis. The initial dose is 10–20 mg of prednisone daily. The daily dose is then raised by 5 mg every 2–3 days until a target dose of 50–60 mg is reached. The beneficial effect usually does not appear till 2 weeks after the start of treatment and is not maximal till several months later. Once the myasthenic manifestations are under better control, the prednisone dose can be lowered, in similar fashion to that described above under polymyositis (p. 904). Prednisone can also be given every other day.

In general, prednisone should be continued for at least 1 or 2 years, though many patients require it for a longer time, or even for life. The dose must be individually titrated. *Azathioprine* (Imuran) can be used in patients who respond inadequately to steroids, or else as a primary alternative or supplement to steroid treatment. The initial dose of azathioprine is 50 mg per day. After one week of treatment, the dose is gradually raised up to the maintenance dose of 2–3 mg/kg/day. The daily maintenance dose is thus usually 150 mg or less; if it exceeds 200 mg for prolonged periods, leukopenia usually results, necessitating reduction of the dose. No effect at all should be expected for several months, and the maximal effect is usually not achieved till the second year of treatment. It thus makes no sense to give this drug for less than 2 years.

Cyclosporine (Sandimmune) is a further immunosuppressive agent. It is given at a dose of 125–250 mg twice a day (the dose must be titrated to the serum drug concentration). It requires several weeks to take effect, and the maximum effect is not reached for about six months. Cyclosporine is nephrotoxic and can raise the arterial blood pressure. It is therefore relatively contraindicated in patients with renal disease or hypertension.

The purine biosynthesis inhibitor *mycophenolate mofetil* (CellCept) is a new type of immunosuppressive agent that is used in organ transplant recipients in combination with steroids and cyclosporine. Initial studies have shown promising results of mono- or combination therapy with this drug in myasthenia gravis. The usual dose is 2 g/day. It should not, however, be given in combination with azathioprine (risk of severe leukopenia).

Short-acting immunotherapy (38, 216)

In a myasthenic crisis, *plasmapheresis* or *intravenous immunoglobulins* can bring significant relief within a few days. Typically, 3–4 L of plasma are exchanged two or three times per week for 2–3 weeks. The immunoglobulin dose is 400 mg/kg daily for 5 days. Either form of treatment can be used as intermittent long-term therapy for patients who respond inadequately to cholinesterase inhibitors, thymectomy, and immune suppression. Both are expensive and fraught with the risk of complications, but they can be very helpful if used selectively.

Transient Neonatal Myasthenia

Some 10–20% of children born to mothers with myasthenia gravis suffer at birth from hypotonia and difficulty swallowing liquids; a smaller percentage have respiratory difficulties as well. These problems last for a few days, rarely longer than 2 weeks, and never permanently. Neonatal myasthenia is explained, in part, as the result of passive transfer of maternal antibodies to the child.

Seronegative Myasthenia Gravis and Anti-MuSK Antibodies (287 f, 424 d, 763 b)

Autoimmune myasthenia gravis is said to be "seronegative" in the 10% to 20% of patients in whom antibodies to the acetylcholine receptor are not found. Nearly 70% of such patients do, however, have antobodies to muscle-specific receptor tyrosine kinase (MuSK). The remainder are thought to have another type of plasma factor interfering with the function of the acetylcholine receptor. Seronegative patients with anti-MuSK antibodies tend to be women, and also tend to be less than 40 years old at the onset of the disease. In seronegative patients, the cranial and bulbar muscles tend to be most severely affected, and respiratory crises are frequent. One-third of patients have a negative edrophonium test, and the response to oral pyridostigmine is often unsatisfactory, as it may bring only mild improvement or an actual worsening of symptoms. Immunosuppressive therapy is recommended; exacerbations occuring despite it can be treated with plasmapheresis. Thymectomy is no benefit.

Lambert-Eaton Myasthenic Syndrome (278, 717)

Overview:

This syndrome is an autoimmune condition caused by pathological antibodies directed against the voltage-sensitive calcium channels of the nerve terminal at the neuromuscular junction. Normally, an action potential arriving at the nerve terminal induces an influx of calcium into the terminal, which, in turn, leads to the release of acetylcholine into the synaptic cleft. If the number of functional calcium channels is diminished, this process is impaired. The reduced amount of acetylcholine that is released may be too low to generate a suprathreshold end plate potential, with the result that no action potential is fired in the muscle fiber.

Etiology

Some two-thirds of cases of Lambert-Eaton myasthenic syndrome are in the setting of malignant disease, 80% of the time a small-cell cancer of the lung (SCLC). Cases without malignancy are sometimes associated with other autoimmune diseases. Men are more frequently affected than women, in a ratio of 4.7 : 1.

The small cells of SCLC express voltage-sensitive calcium channels on their surface. Sensitization of the immune system to the cancer can result in the generation of antibodies to these channels and a consequent cross-reaction against channels on nerve terminals.

Clinical Features

The major manifestations are weakness and abnormal fatigability of the muscles of the limbs and trunk. The pelvic girdle and proximal leg muscles are typically severely affected. There may, however, be mild weakness in the upper limbs as well, and 70% of patients have transient ocular manifestations, such as ptosis. Muscular strength transiently increases on prolonged contraction, as may be demonstrated by having the patient clasp the examiner's hand firmly for several seconds. The intrinsic muscle reflexes are usually diminished or absent, in contrast to myasthenia gravis. Eighty percent of patients complain of a dry mouth or have other autonomic disturbances such as diminished lacrimation, orthostatic hypotension, impotence, or abnormal pupillary motility. Some complain of myalgias or paresthesiae.

Electromyography

The EMG reveals initially low muscle action potentials that increase in amplitude with repetitive nerve stimulation. The greater the frequency of stimulation, the higher the amplitude; thus, the amplitude is greatest on tetanic stimulation, or when the patient has voluntarily maximally contracted the muscle for several seconds before the beginning of nerve stimulation and recording.

Diagnostic Evaluation

The diagnosis is made on the basis of the clinical and electromyographic findings. If the patient is not already known to harbor a malignant tumor, one must be carefully sought. Lambert-Eaton myasthenic syndrome sometimes appears before the tumor does; thus, in cases where no tumor is found, repeated investigation for at least 3 years is recommended.

Differential Diagnosis

The differential diagnosis encompasses myasthenia gravis and other myasthenic syndromes, polymyositis and other diseases of muscle, polyradiculitis and other polyneuropathies, and hypermagnesemia and magnesium intoxication.

> **Treatment**
>
> Any accompanying malignancy or other autoimmune disease that is found should be treated. *Cholinesterase inhibitors* have only a weak effect, but should nevertheless be tried (p. 918). *3,4-Diaminopyridine* increases the calcium influx into the nerve terminal and can thereby lessen the disease manifestations. The same is true of guanidine and 4-aminopyridine, which, however, are no longer used because of their severe side effects. *Azathioprine* and *corticosteroids* can be of benefit in Lambert-Eaton syndrome just as they are in myasthenia gravis, and the same holds for *plasmapheresis* and *intravenous immunoglobulin therapy.*

Congenital Myasthenic Syndromes (278, 876, 876a)

The congenital myasthenic syndromes are a group of hereditary diseases whose pathophysiology is only partly understood. All of the ones that have been described to date are transmitted in an autosomal recessive inheritance pattern, with the exception of the autosomal dominant slow channel syndrome. The defective component(s) of neuromuscular transmission in a particular syndrome can be presynaptic, postsynaptic, or both. The presynaptic defects involve the synthesis, packaging, and release of acetylcholine quanta; the combined pre- and postsynaptic defects involve a deficiency of acetylcholinesterase; and the postsynaptic defects involve kinetic abnormalities of the acetylcholine receptors.

Congenital Myasthenia Gravis

All cases of congenital myasthenia gravis are hereditary except for the transient neonatal myasthenia described above that affects children of myasthenic mothers. Congenital myasthenia gravis is characterized by ocular manifestations, including ptosis, and, in some cases, lifelong generalized weakness.

> **Treatment**
>
> Cholinesterase inhibitors and, in occasional cases, 3,4-diaminopyridine are effective.

Familial Infantile Myasthenia

This disorder is due to a presynaptic defect of acetylcholine synthesis and of the packaging of acetylcholine in vesicles (quanta). Patients are hypotonic at birth and may develop respiratory failure in the setting of intercurrent illnesses such as respiratory tract infections.

> **Treatment**
>
> *Cholinesterase inhibitors* are effective. They are generally needed less and less as the patient grows older.

Slow Channel Syndrome

This disorder usually does not become apparent till adolescence, sometimes only in early adulthood. It is due to an excessively prolonged opening time of the cation channels of the acetylcholine receptor. Unlike in myasthenia gravis, muscle atrophy is present. The treatments that are beneficial in myasthenia gravis have no effect.

Other Myasthenic Syndromes

The aggravation of myasthenia gravis by aminoglycosides, quinine and other antimalarial agents, antiarrhythmics, and anticonvulsants has already been mentioned. Penicillamine can induce a myasthenic syndrome that is indistinguishable from autoimmune myasthenia gravis with positive antibodies but reverses when penicillamine is discontinued. The venom of certain types of snake contains bungarotoxin, an agent that binds to acetylcholine receptors, causing myasthenic weakness. Organophosphate poisoning can also impair neuromuscular transmission (p. 304).

Common Muscle Cramps (557)

Clinical Features and Etiology

Muscle cramps arise suddenly and involve visible and palpable contraction of a muscle or group of muscles. They are painful. The pain may last longer than the muscle contraction itself, and the serum creatine kinase concentration may rise. Cramps arise spontaneously or in response to certain types of movement; they often begin with intermittent twitching of the affected muscle. Passive stretching of the muscle terminates the cramp. The EMG during a muscle cramp shows a full interference pattern, in contrast to a contracture, which is electrically silent.

The etiology of common muscle cramps is not known with certainty, but most cramps are thought to have their origin in the distal portions of motor nerves. The more common types of cramp are ordinary nocturnal calf cramps in the elderly, and exercise-induced cramps of particular muscles during the daytime in healthy individuals. Cramps may be associated with benign fasciculations. They sometimes become bothersome during pregnancy.

Muscle cramps are of pathological significance in motor neuron diseases (e.g., amyotrophic lateral sclerosis), radiculopathies, and polyneuropathies. They may also be a sign of a metabolic disturbance (uremia, hypothyroidism, or hypocortisolism) or of an extracellular volume deficit (due to sweating, diarrhea, vomiting, or diuretic use).

Treatment

Membrane-stabilizing medications, such as *phenytoin* or *carbamazepine*, are often beneficial. *Quinine sulfate* at bedtime can be tried first for the treatment of nocturnal cramps. Some cramps respond favorably to *magnesium* supplementation.

15 References

Only the most important standard texts in neurology are included in the reference list below. The text of the book refers to approximately 2000 numbered reference sources, which can be accessed (usually along with an abstract) in the *complete reference list* from the publisher's Internet site:

- **http://www.thieme.com/mm-refs**

Other useful web sites:

Medical literature search:
- http://www4.ncbi.nlm.nih.gov/PubMed

Drug information in the English-speaking countries:

- United States
  http://www.nlm.nih.gov/medlineplus/druginformation.html

- Canada
  http://www.hc-sc.gc.ca/hpb-dgps/therapeut/htmleng/dpd.html

- United Kingdom
  http://www.ukmi.nhs.uk

- Ireland
  http://www.stjames.ie/ClinicalServices/NationalMedicinesInformation
  Centre/

- South Africa
  http://www.pharmnet.co.za

- Australia
  http://www.health.gov.au/tga/docs/html/artg.htm

Standard Reference Works

1. Aldrich MS. Sleep medicine. Oxford: Oxford University Press, 1999.
2. Appenzeller O. The autonomic nervous system: an introduction to basic and clinical concepts. 5th ed. New York: Elsevier, 1997.
3. Brandt T. Vertigo: its multisensory syndromes. 2nd ed. London: Springer, 1999.
4. Braunwald E, Fauci AS, Kasper DL, Hauser SL, Longo DL, Jameson JL. Harrison's principles of internal medicine, 15th ed. New York: McGraw Hill, 2001.
5. Brazis PW, Masdeu JC, Biller J. Localization in clinical neurology, 3rd ed. Boston: Little, Brown, 1996.
6. Compston A, Ebers G, Matthews B, et al. McAlpine's multiple sclerosis, 3rd ed. St. Louis: Mosby, 1998.
7. Duus P. Topic diagnosis in neurology, 3rd ed., tr. Lindenberg R. New York: Thieme, 1998.
8. Dyck PJ, Thomas PK, Griffin JW, et al. Peripheral neuropathy, 3rd ed. Philadelphia: Saunders, 1993.
9. Edelman RR, Hesselink JR, Zlatkin MB. Clinical magnetic resonance imaging, 2nd ed. Philadelphia: Saunders, 1996.
10. Engel AG. Myasthenia gravis and myasthenic disorders. Oxford: Oxford University Press, 1999.
11. Ginsberg MD, Bogousslavsky J. Cerebrovascular disease: pathophysiology, diagnosis and management. Oxford: Blackwell Science, 1998.
12. Glaser JS. Neuro-ophthalmology, 3rd ed. Philadelphia: Lippincott, 1999.
13. Greenberg HS, Chandler WE, Sandler HM. Brain tumors. Oxford: Oxford University Press, 1999.
14. Griggs RC, Mendell JR, Miller RG. Evaluation and treatment of myopathies. Philadelphia: Davis, 1995.
15. Jankovic J, Tolosa E. Parkinson's disease and movement disorders, 3rd ed. Baltimore: Williams & Wilkins, 1998.
16. Menkes J H, Sarnat HB. Textbook of child neurology, 6th ed. Philadelphia: Williams & Wilkins, 2000.
17. Miller NR, Newman NJ. The essentials: Walsh & Hoyt's clinical neuroophthalmology, 5th ed. Philadelphia: Williams & Wilkins, 1999.
18. Olesen S, Tfelt-Hansen P, Welch KMA. The headaches, 2nd ed. Philadelphia: Williams & Wilkins, 2000.
19. Osborn AG. Diagnostic neuroradiology. St. Louis: Mosby, 1994.
20. Paty DW, Ebers GC. Multiple sclerosis. Philadelphia: Davis, 1998.
21. Plum F, Posner JB. The diagnosis of stupor and coma, 3rd ed. Philadelphia: Davis, 1980.
22. Rowland LP. Merritt's neurology, 10th ed. Philadelphia: Williams & Wilkins, 2000.
23. Scheid WM, Whitley RJ, Durack DT. Infections of the central nervous system, 2nd ed. Philadelphia: Lippincott-Raven, 1997.
24. Victor M, Ropper AH, Adams RD. Principles of neurology, 7th ed. New York: McGraw-Hill, 2000.
25. Warlow CP, Dennis MS, van Gijn J, et al. Stroke: a practical guide to management, 2nd ed. Oxford: Blackwell Science, 2001.
26. Weir B. Subarachnoid hemorrhage: causes and cures. Oxford: Oxford University Press, 1999.

Appendix

Scales for the Assessment of Neurologic Disease

Last Name .... First name .... Date of birth ....

Unified Parkinson's Disease Rating Scale (UPDRS)

Date
Last medication
Examiner

I   Mentation, behavior, mood

   1 Intellectual impairment
   2 Thought disorder
   3 Depression
   4 Motivation/initiative

On Off	On Off	On Off	On Off	On Off	On Off

II Activities of daily living

   5 Speech
   6 Salivation
   7 Swallowing
   8 Handwriting
   9 Cutting food/handling utensils
  10 Dressing
  11 Hygiene
  12 Turning in bed/adjusting bedclothes
  13 Falling (unrelated to freezing)
  14 Freezing when walking
  15 Walking
  16 Tremor
  17 Sensory complaints

III Motor examination

Time of eximanation

  18 Speech
  19 Facial expression
  20 Tremor at rest
      Face
      Upper limbs   Right
                    Left
      Lower limbs   Right
                    Left

Unified Parkinson's Disease Rating Scale (UPDRS)

21 Action or postural tremor of hands	Right							
	Left							
22 Rigidity Neck	Right							
	Left							
Upper limbs	Right							
	Left							
Lower limbs	Right							
	Left							
23 Finger taps	Right							
	Left							
24 Hand movements	Right							
	Left							
25 Rapid alternating movements	Right							
	Left							
26 Leg agility	Right							
	Left							
27 Arising from chair	Right							
	Left							
28 Posture								
29 Gait								
30 Postural stability								
31 Body bradykinesia/hypokinesia								

IV. Complications of therapy

32 Dyskinesias (duration)						
33 Dyskinesias (disability)						
34 Dyskinesias (pain)						
35 Early morning dystonia						
36 Off periods: predictable						
37 Off periods: unpredictable						
38 Off periods: sudden onset?						
39 Off periods: total duration						
40 Anorexia, nausea, vomiting						
41 Sleep disturbances						
42 Symptomatic orthostatic hypotension						

V. Modified Hoehn and Yahr staging

VI. Schwab and England Activities of Daily Living Scale

Detailed Instructions for the Unified Parkinson's Disease Rating Scale (UPDRS)

I **Mentation, behavior, and mood** (to be assessed by interview)

1 Intellectual impairment

0 None

1 Mild. Consistent forgetfulness with partial recollection of events and no other difficulties

2 Moderate memory loss, with disorientation and moderate difficulty handling complex problems. Mild but definite impairment of function at home with need of occasional prompting

3 Severe memory loss with disorientation for time and often to place. Severe impairment in handling problems

4 Severe memory loss with orientation preserved to person only. Unable to make judgments or solve problems. Requires much help with personal care. Cannot be left alone at all

2 Thought disorder (due to dementia or drug intoxication)

0 None

1 Vivid dreaming

2 "Benign" hallucinations with insight retained

3 Occasional to frequent hallucinations or delusions; without insight; could interfere with daily activities

4 Persistent hallucinations, delusions, or florid psychosis. Not able to care for self

3 Depression

0 None

1 Periods of sadness or guilt greater than normal, never sustained for days or weeks

2 Sustained depression (1 week or more)

3 Sustained depression with vegetative symptoms (insomnia, anorexia, weight loss, loss of interest)

4 Sustained depression with vegetative symptoms and suicidal thoughts or intent

4 Motivation/initiative

0 Normal

1 Less assertive than usual; more passive

2 Loss of initiative or disinterest in elective (nonroutine) activities

3 Loss of initiative or disinterest in day to day (routine) activities

4 Withdrawn, complete loss of motivation

II Activities of daily living (for both "on" and "off")

5 *Speech*

   0 Normal

   1 Mildly affected. No difficulty being understood

   2 Moderately affected. Sometimes asked to repeat statements

   3 Severely affected. Frequently asked to repeat statements

   4 Unintelligible most of the time

6 *Salivation*

   0 Normal

   1 Slight but definite excess of saliva in mouth; may have nighttime drooling

   2 Moderately excessive saliva; may have minimal drooling

   3 Marked excess of saliva with some drooling

   4 Marked drooling, requires constant tissue or handkerchief

7 *Swallowing*

   0 Normal

   1 Rare choking

   2 Occasional choking

   3 Requires soft food

   4 Requires NG tube or gastrostomy feeding

8 *Handwriting*

   0 Normal

   1 Slightly slow or small

   2 Moderately slow or small; all words are legible

   3 Severely affected; not all words are legible

   4 The majority of words are not legible

9 *Cutting food and handling utensils*

   0 Normal

   1 Somewhat slow and clumsy, but no help needed

   2 Can cut most foods, although clumsy and slow; some help needed

   3 Food must be cut by someone, but can still feed slowly

   4 Needs to be fed

(Cont.) →

10 Dressing

0 Normal

1 Somewhat slow, but no help needed

2 Occasional assistance with buttoning, getting arms in sleeves

3 Considerable help required, but can do some things alone

4 Helpless

11 Hygiene

0 Normal

1 Somewhat slow, but no help needed

2 Needs help to shower or bathe; or very slow in hygienic care

3 Requires assistance for washing, brushing teeth, combing hair, going to bathroom

4 Foley catheter or other mechanical aids

12 Turning in bed and adjusting bed clothes

0 Normal

1 Somewhat slow and clumsy, but no help needed

2 Can turn alone or adjust sheets, but with great difficulty

3 Can initiate, but not turn or adjust sheets alone

4 Helpless

13 Falling (unrelated to freezing)

0 None

1 Rare falling

2 Occasionally falls, less than once per day

3 Falls an average of once daily

4 Falls more than once daily

14 Freezing when walking

0 None

1 Rare freezing when walking; may have start hesitation

2 Occasional freezing when walking

3 Frequent freezing. Occasionally falls from freezing

4 Frequent falls from freezing

15 Walking

0 Normal

1 Mild difficulty. May not swing arms or may tend to drag leg

2 Moderate difficulty, but requires little or no assistance

(Cont.) →

3 Severe disturbance of walking, requiring assistance

4 Cannot walk at all, even with assistance

16 *Tremor (symptomatic complaint of tremor in any part of body)*

0 Absent

1 Slight and infrequently present

2 Moderate; bothersome to patient

3 Severe; interferes with many activities

4 Marked; interferes with most activities

17 *Sensory complaints related to parkinsonism*

0 None

1 Occasionally has numbness, tingling, or mild aching

2 Frequently has numbness, tingling, or aching; not distressing

3 Frequent painful sensations

4 Excruciating pain

III Motor examination

18 *Speech*

0 Normal

1 Slight loss of expression, diction and/or volume

2 Monotone, slurred but understandable; moderately impaired

3 Marked impairment, difficult to understand

4 Unintelligible

19 *Facial expression*

0 Normal

1 Minimal hypomimia, could be normal "poker face"

2 Slight but definitely abnormal diminution of facial expression

3 Moderate hypomimia; lips parted some of the time

4 Masked or fixed facies with severe or complete loss of facial expression; lips parted ¼ inch/0.5 cm or more

20 *Tremor at rest (head, upper and lower extremities)*

0 Absent

1 Slight and infrequently present

2 Mild in amplitude and persistent. Or moderate in amplitude, but only intermittently present

3 Moderate in amplitude and present most of the time

4 Marked in amplitude and present most of the time

(Cont.) →

21 *Action or postural tremor of hands*

  0 Absent

  1 Slight; present with action

  2 Moderate in amplitude, present with action

  3 Moderate in amplitude with posture holding as well as action

  4 Marked in amplitude; interferes with feeding

22 *Rigidity* (judged on passive movement of major joints with patient relaxed in sitting position. Cogwheeling to be ignored)

  0 Absent

  1 Slight or detectable only when activated by mirror or other movements

  2 Mild to moderate

  3 Marked, but full range of motion easily achieved

  4 Severe, range of motion achieved with difficulty

23 *Finger taps* (patient taps thumb with index finger in rapid succession)

  0 Normal

  1 Mild slowing and/or reduction in amplitude

  2 Moderately impaired. Definite and early fatiguing. May have occasional arrests in movement

  3 Severely impaired. Frequent hesitation in initiating movements or arrests in ongoing movement

  4 Can barely perform the task

24 *Hand movements* (patient opens and closes hands in rapid succession)

  0 Normal

  1 Mild slowing and/or reduction in amplitude

  2 Moderately impaired. Definite and early fatiguing. May have occasional arrests in movement

  3 Severely impaired. Frequent hesitation in initiating movements or arrests in ongoing movement

  4 Can barely perform the task

25 *Rapid alternating movements of hands* (pronation-supination movements of hands, vertically and horizontally, with as large an amplitude as possible, both hands simultaneously)

  0 Normal

  1 Mild slowing and/or reduction in amplitude

(Cont.) →

2 Moderately impaired. Definite and early fatiguing. May have occasional arrests in movement

3 Severely impaired. Frequent hesitation in initiating movements or arrests in ongoing movement

4 Can barely perform the task

26 *Leg agility* (patient taps heel on the ground in rapid succession, picking up entire leg. Amplitude should be at least 3 inches/7.5 cm)

0 Normal

1 Mild slowing and/or reduction in amplitude

2 Moderately impaired. Definite and early fatiguing. May have occasional arrests in movement

3 Severely impaired. Frequent hesitation in initiating movements or arrests in ongoing movement

4 Can barely perform the task

27 *Arising from chair* (patient attempts to rise from a straight-backed chair, with arms folded across chest)

0 Normal

1 Slow; or may need more than one attempt

2 Pushes self up from arms of seat

3 Tends to fall back and may have to try more than one time, but can get up without help

4 Unable to arise without help

28 *Posture*

0 Normal erect

1 Not quite erect, slightly stooped posture; could be normal for older person

2 Moderately stooped posture, definitely abnormal; can be slightly leaning to one side

3 Severely stooped posture with kyphosis; can be moderately leaning to one side

4 Marked flexion with extreme abnormality of posture

29 *Gait*

0 Normal

1 Walks slowly, may shuffle with short steps, but no festination (hastening steps) or propulsion

2 Walks with difficulty, but requires little or no assistance; may have some festination, short steps, or propulsion

3 Severe disturbance of gait, requiring assistance

4 Cannot walk at all, even with assistance

(Cont.) →

30 Postural stability (response to sudden, strong posterior displacement produced by pull on shoulders while patient erect with eyes open and feet slightly apart. Patient is prepared)

0 Normal

1 Retropulsion, but recovers unaided

2 Absence of postural response; would fall if not caught by examiner

3 Very unstable, tends to lose balance spontaneously

4 Unable to stand without assistance

31 Body bradykinesia and hypokinesia (combining slowness, hesitancy, decreased arm swing, small amplitude, and poverty of movement in general)

0 None

1 Minimal slowness, giving movement a deliberate character; could be normal for some persons. Possibly reduced amplitude

2 Mild degree of slowness and poverty of movement which is definitely abnormal. Alternatively, some reduced amplitude

3 Moderate slowness, poverty or small amplitude of movement

4 Marked slowness, poverty or small amplitude of movement

IV Complications of therapy (in the past week, during "on" phase)

32 Dyskinesias (duration): What proportion of the waking day are dyskinesias present? (Historical information)

0 None

1 1–25% of day

2 26–50% of day

3 51–75% of day

4 76–100% of day

33 Dyskinesias (disability): How disabling are the dyskinesias? (Historical information; may be modified by office examination)

0 Not disabling

1 Mildly disabling

2 Moderately disabling

3 Severely disabling

4 Completely disabled

(Cont.) →

34 *Dyskinesias (painful):* How painful are the dyskinesias?

   0 No painful dyskinesias

   1 Slight

   2 Moderate

   3 Severe

   4 Marked

35 *Presence of early morning dystonia* (historical information)

   0 No

   1 Yes

36 *Are there predictable "off" periods (a given time after taking medication)?*

   0 No

   1 Yes

37 *Are there unpredictable "off" periods?*

   0 No

   1 Yes

38 *Do "off" periods come on suddenly, within a few seconds?*

   0 No

   1 Yes

39 *What proportion of the waking day is the patient "off" on average?*

   0 None

   1 1–25% of day

   2 26–50% of day

   3 51–75% of day

   4 76–100% of day

40 *Does the patient have anorexia, nausea, or vomiting?*

   0 No

   1 Yes

41 *Any sleep disturbances, such as insomnia or hypersomnolence?*

   0 No

   1 Yes

42 *Does the patient have symptomatic orthostatic hypotension?* (Record the patient's blood pressure, height and weight on the scoring form)

   0 No

   1 Yes

Simplified Scale for Evaluating the Severity of Individual Signs of Parkinson's Disease (Webster, 1968)

1 **Bradykinesia of hands, including handwriting**
0 Normal
1 Mild slowing
2 Moderate slowing, handwriting severely impaired
3 Severe slowing

2 **Rigidity**
0 None
1 Mild
2 Moderate
3 Severe, present despite medication

3 **Posture**
0 Normal
1 Mildly stooped
2 Arm flexion
3 Severely stooped; arm, hand, and knee flexion

4 **Arm swing**
0 Good bilaterally
1 Unilaterally impaired
2 Unilaterally absent
3 Bilaterally absent

5 **Gait**
0 Normal, turns without difficulty
1 Short steps, slow turn
2 Markedly shortened steps, both heels slap on floor
3 Shuffling steps, occasional freezing, very slow turn

6 **Tremor**
0 None
1 Amplitude < 2.5 cm
2 Amplitude > 10 cm
3 Amplitude > 10 cm, constant, eating and writing impossible

7 **Facies**
0 Normal
1 Mild hypomimia
2 Marked hypomimia, lips open, marked drooling
3 Mask-like facies, mouth open, marked drooling

8 **Seborrhea**
0 None
1 Increased sweating
2 Oily skin
3 Marked deposition on face

9 **Speech**
0 Normal
1 Reduced modulation, good volume
2 Monotonous, not modulated, incipient dysarthria, difficulty being understood
3 Marked difficulty being understood

10 **Independence**
0 Not impaired
1 Mildly impaired (dressing)
2 Needs help in critical situations, all activities markedly slowed
3 Cannot dress self, eat or walk unaided

Epworth Sleepiness Questionnaire

Last name _____ First name _____ Date _____

Date of birth_____

How likely are you to **doze off** or to **fall asleep** in the following situations, in contrast to just feeling tired? This refers to your usual way of life in the last 4 weeks. If you have not been in a particular situation recently, try to **imagine** what would have happened in that particular situation.

Use the following scale to choose the most appropriate number for each situation.

0 Would never doze

1 Slight chance of dozing

2 Moderate chance of dozing

3 High chance of dozing

Situation	*Chance of dozing*
• Sitting and reading	_____
• Watching TV	_____
• Sitting inactive in a public place (theater, movies, lecture, meeting)	_____
• As a passenger in a car for an hour	_____
• Lying down to rest in the afternoon	_____
• Sitting and talking to someone	_____
• Sitting quietly after a lunch without alcohol	_____
• In a car while stopped for a few minutes (red light, traffic)	_____

Barthel Index (of Disability)
(adapted from Granger et al.)

Feeding
0 Unable
5 Needs help cutting, spreading butter, etc., or needs modified diet
10 Independent

Bathing
0 Dependent
5 Independent (or in shower)

Grooming
0 Needs help with personal care
5 Independent face/hair/teeth/shaving (implements provided)

Dressing
0 Dependent
5 Needs help but can do about half unaided
10 Independent (including buttons, zips, laces, etc.)

Bowels
0 Incontinent (or needs to be given enemas)
5 Occasional accident
10 Continent

Bladder
0 Incontinent, or catheterized and unable to manage alone
5 Occasional accident
10 Continent

Toilet use
0 Dependent
5 Needs some help, but can do something alone
10 Independent (on and off, dressing, wiping)

Transfers (bed to chair and back)
0 Unable, no sitting balance
5 Major help (one or two people, physical), can sit
10 Minor help (verbal or physical)
15 Independent

Mobility (on level surfaces)
0 Immobile or < 50 meters
5 Wheelchair independent, including corners, > 50 meters
10 Walks with help of one person (verbal or physical) > 50 meters
15 Independent (but may use any aid; for example, stick) > 50 meters

Stairs
0 Unable
5 Needs help (verbal, physical, carrying aid)
10 Independent

Total Barthel index (0–100):

Modified Rankin Scale (for Stroke)
(adapted from van Swieten et al.)

Last name _____ First name _____ Date _____

Days since CVA _____

Description	Score
No symptoms at all	0
No significant disability despite symptoms (Able to carry out all usual duties and activities)	1
Slight disability (Unable to carry out all previous activities, but able to look after own affairs without assistance)	2
Moderate disability (Requiring some help, but able to walk without assistance)	3
Moderately severe disability (Unable to walk without assistance and unable to attend to own bodily needs without assistance)	4
Severe disability (Bedridden, incontinent and requiring constant nursing care and attention)	5
Dead	6

Rankin scale (0–6): _____

Modified NIH Stroke Scale
(adapted from Brett et al. and Lyden et al.)

Last name _____ First name _____ Date _____

Days since CVA _____

1a   Level of consciousness
   0   Alert; keenly responsive
   1   Not alert, but arousable by minor stimulation to obey, answer, or re-
       spond
   2   Not alert, requires repeated stimulation to attend, or is obtunded and
       requires strong or painful stimulation to make movements (not stereo-
       typed)
   3   Responds only with reflex motor or autonomic effects or totally unre-
       sponsive, flaccid, areflexic
                                                          Score _____/3

1b   LOC questions
       The patient is asked the month and his/her age. It is important that
       only the initial answer be graded and that the examiner not help the
       patient with verbal or nonverbal cues
   0   Answers both questions correctly
   1   Answers one question correctly *or* patient cannot speak because of
       dysarthria or intubation
   2   Answers neither question correctly *or* patient aphasic or stuporous
                                                          Score _____/2

1c   LOC commands
       The patient is asked to open and close the eyes and then to grip and
       release the nonparetic hand. Substitute another one-step command if
       the hands cannot be used. If the patient does not respond to com-
       mand, the task should be demonstrated (pantomime)
   0   Performs both tasks correctly
   1   Performs one task correctly
   2   Performs neither task correctly
                                                          Score _____/2

2   Eye movements
       Only horizontal eye movements are tested. Voluntary or reflexive (ocu-
       locephalic) eye movements are scored, but caloric testing is not per-
       formed
   0   Normal
   1   Partial gaze palsy (gaze is abnormal in one or both eyes, but there is
       no forced deviation or total gaze paresis)
   2   Forced deviation or total gaze paresis not overcome by the oculo-
       cephalic maneuver.
                                                          Score _____/2

(Cont.) →

3   Visual fields
(Test all quadrants)
0   No visual loss or only monocular visual loss
1   Partial hemianopsia
2   Complete hemianopsia
3   Bilateral hemianopsia (blind, including cortical blindness)

Score _____/3

4   Facial palsy
The patient is asked to show teeth or raise eyebrows and close eyes. Pantomime is used for patients who cannot follow verbal commands. For poorly responsive or noncomprehending patients, symmetry of grimace in response to noxious stimuli is scored
0   Normal symmetrical movement
1   Minor paresis (flattened nasolabial fold, asymmetric smile)
2   Total or nearly total paralysis of lower face
3   Total paralysis of one or both sides of the face (upper and lower portions)

Score _____/3

5–8 Motor arm and leg
The limb is placed in the appropriate position: extend the arms (palms down) 90° (if sitting) or 45° (if supine) and the legs 30° (always tested supine). Drift is scored if the arm falls within 10 seconds or the leg within 5 seconds

5   Right arm
0   No drift, limb holds 90° (or 45°) for full 10 seconds
1   Drift: limb holds 90° (or 45°), but drifts down before full 10 seconds; does not hit bed or other support
2   Some effort against gravity: limb cannot get to or maintain (if cued) 90° (or 45°), drifts down to bed, but has some effort against gravity
3   No effort against gravity, limb falls
4   No movement
x   Cannot be evaluated

Score _____/4

6   Left arm
0   No drift, limb holds 90° (or 45°) for full 10 seconds
1   Drift: limb holds 90° (or 45°), but drifts down before full 10 seconds; does not hit bed or other support
2   Some effort against gravity: limb cannot get to or maintain (if cued) 90° (or 45°), drifts down to bed, but has some effort against gravity
3   No effort against gravity, limb falls
4   No movement
x   Cannot be evaluated

Score _____/4

(Cont.) →

7   Right leg
0   No drift, leg holds 30° position for full 5 seconds
1   Drift, leg falls within 5 seconds but does not hit bed
2   Some effort against gravity; leg falls to bed by 5 seconds, but has
some effort against gravity
3   No effort against gravity, leg falls to bed immediately
4   No movement
x   Cannot be evaluated

Score _____/4

8   Left leg
0   No drift, leg holds 30° position for full 5 seconds
1   Drift, leg falls within 5 seconds but does not hit bed
2   Some effort against gravity; leg falls to bed by 5 seconds, but has
some effort against gravity
3   No effort against gravity, leg falls to bed immediately
4   No movement
x   Cannot be evaluated

Score _____/4

9   Limb ataxia
The finger-nose-finger and heel-shin tests are performed on both sides
with eyes open, and ataxia is scored only if present out of proportion
to weakness. A score of 0 is given in patients who cannot understand
or are paralyzed
0   No ataxia
1   Ataxia in one limb
2   Ataxia in two or more limbs
x   Cannot be evaluated

Score _____/2

10   Sensation
Sensation or grimace to pinprick, or withdrawal from noxious stimulus
in the obtunded or aphasic patient. Testing on arms, legs, trunk, face
0   Normal; no sensory loss
1   Mild to moderate sensory loss; pin-prick is dull, or less sharp, on the
affected side, *or* there is a loss of superficial pain to pinprick, but patient is aware of being touched
2   Severe or total sensory loss; patient is not aware of being touched in
the face, arm, and leg

Score _____/2

11   Language
0   Normal
1   Mild to moderate aphasia (paraphasia), communication still possible
2   Severe aphasia, communication barely possible
3   Mute, global aphasia

Score _____/3

(Cont.) →

12 Dysarthria
0   Normal articulation
1   Mild to moderate dysarthria (some words slurred)
2   Severe dysarthria (speech barely intelligible)
x   Cannot be evaluated

Score _____/2

13 Neglect
0   None (perception/attention intact on both sides)
1   Neglect in one modality (e.g., visual or tactile) or hemineglect
2   Bilateral neglect, or hemineglect in more than one modality (does not perceive own hand or orients self to one side only)

Score _____/2

Total NIH Stroke Scale score   Score _____/42

Expanded Disability Status Scale (DSS)
for Multiple Sclerosis (adapted from Kurtzke) (549)

0.0	No neurologic deficit
1.0	No disability, minimal symptoms in one functional system (FS)
1.5	No disability, minimal signs in more than one FS
2.0	Minimal disability in one FS
2.5	Minimal disability in two FSs
3.0	Moderate disability in one FS or minimal disability in 3–4 FSs, but still fully ambulatory
3.5	Moderate disability in one FS and more than minimal disability in several others, but still fully ambulatory
4.0	Fully ambulatory without aid, self-sufficient, up and about some 12 hours a day despite relatively severe disability; able to walk without aid or rest some 500 meters
4.5	Fully ambulatory without aid, up and about much of the day, able to work a full day, may otherwise have some limitation of full activity or require minimal assistance; characterized by relatively severe disability; able to walk without aid or rest some 300 meters
5.0	Ambulatory without aid or rest for about 200 meters; disability severe enough to impair full daily activities
5.5	Ambulatory without aid or rest for about 100 meters; disability severe enough to preclude full daily activities
6.0	Intermittent or unilateral constant assistance (cane, crutch, brace) required to walk about 100 meters with or without resting
6.5	Constant bilateral assistance (canes, crutches, braces) required to walk about 20 meters without resting
7.0	Unable to walk more than 5 meters even with aid, essentially restricted to wheelchair; wheels self in standard wheelchair, transfers unaided
7.5	Unable to take more than a few steps; restricted to wheelchair; may need aid in transfer; wheels self but cannot carry on in standard wheelchair a full day
8.0	Essentially restricted to bed or chair; retains many self-care functions; generally has effective use of arms
8.5	Essentially restricted to bed much of day; has some effective use of arms, retains some self-care functions
9.0	Helplessly bed-bound; can communicate and eat
9.5	Totally helpless, unable to communicate effectively, eat, or swallow
10.0	Death due to MS

Major Neurogenetic Diseases

Reproduced here with kind permission from the authors of the position paper of the German Neurological Society's Committee on Neurogenetics (Gasser T, Molekulare Diagnostik erblicher neurologischer Erkrankungen, **Nervenarzt** 2000; 71: 774–96, Table 1).

Disease	Symbol	Inheritance pattern	Locus	Gene	Mutation	Status	Remarks
Ataxias							
• Friedreich's ataxia	FRDA	AR	9q13-21.1	Frataxin	Trinucleotide/Pm	A	Most common recessive inherited spinocerebellar ataxia
• Spinocerebellar ataxias	SCA1	AD	6q21.3	Ataxin 1	Trinucleotide	A	SCA1, 2, and 3 together account for ca. 60% of dominant inherited spinocerebellar ataxias
	SCA2	AD	12q23-24.1	Ataxin 2	Trinucleotide	A	
	SCA3/MJD	AD	14q24	Ataxin 3	Trinucleotide	A	
	SCA4	AD	16q22.1	Unknown	Unknown	D	Rare families
	SCA5	AD	11cen	Unknown	Unknown	D	Rare families
	SCA6	AD	19p13	Ca channel	Trinucleotide	A	Allelic to FHM and EA2
	SCA7	AD	3p12-21.1	Ataxin 7	Trinucleotide	A	With pigmentary retinal degeneration
	SCA8	AD	13q21	Unknown	Trinucleotide	A	CTG prolongation in untranslated region
	SCA10	AD	22q13	Unknown	Unknown	D	Pure cerebellar ataxia, epilepsy

(Cont.)

Disease	Symbol	Inheritance pattern	Locus	Gene	Mutation	Status	Remarks
	SCA12	AD	5q31-q33	Protein phosphatase 2	Trinucleotide	A	
• Episodic ataxia with myokymia	EA1	AD	12p13	K channel	Pm	C	
• Episodic ataxia without myokymia	EA2	AD	19p13	Ca channel	Pm	C	Allelic to FHM and SCA6
• Ataxia with vitamin E deficiency	AVED	AR	8q13.1-13.3	α-Tocopherol transfer protein	Pm	C	Rare, mainly in N. Africa
Dystonias and other nondegenerative movement disorders							
• Primary torsion dystonia	DYT1	AD	9q34	Torsin A	GAG deletion	A	Early onset, generalized, rarely isolated writer's cramp
• X-chromosomal dystonia-parkinsonism	DYT3	XL	Xq11.2	Unknown	Unknown	D	Only in the Philippines
• Primary dystonia, mixed type	DYT6	AD	8cen	Unknown	Unknown	D	Only 2 families described
• Primary dystonia, focal type	DYT7	AD	18p13.1	Unknown	Unknown	D	
• Dopa-responsive dystonia	DRD	AD	14q22	GTP-cyclo-hydrolase 1	Pm	B	5% of idiopathic dystonias
• Dopa-responsive dystonia	DRD	AR	11p15.5	Tyrosine hydroxylase	Pm	C	Rare case reports
• Rapid-onset dystonia-parkinsonism	RDP	AD	19q13	Unknown	Unknown	D	Few families known
• Paroxysmal dystonia	FPD1	AD	2q33-35	Unknown	Unknown	D	

Disease	Symbol	Inheritance	Locus	Gene/Protein	Mutation	Class	Comments
• Myoclonus-dystonia syndrome	DYT11	AD	7q	Unknown	Unknown	D	
• Essential tremor	ETM1	AD	3q13	Unknown	Unknown	D	
	ETM2	AD	2p25-22	Unknown	Unknown	D	
• Familial hyperekplexia	STHE	AD	5q32	Glycine receptor	Pm	C	
• Wilson's disease	WND	AR	13q14.1	Copper transport protein	Pm/Del	B	
Neurodegenerative diseases							
• Huntington's disease	HD	AD	4p16.3	Huntingtin	Trinucleotide	A	
• Familial Parkinson's disease	PARK1	AD	4q21	α-Synuclein	Pm	C	Very rare, Mediterranean founder effect
• Autosomal recessive juvenile Parkinson's disease	PARK2, ARJP	AR	6q25-27	Parkin	Del	C	No Lewy body pathology
• Familial Parkinson's disease	PARK3	AD	2p13	Unknown	Unknown	D	North German founder effect?
• Familial Alzheimer's disease	AD1	AD	21q21	Amyloid precursor protein	Pm	B	Very rare
	AD2	AD	19q13.2	ApoE[1]	Pm	A	Susceptibility allele
	AD3	AD	14q24.3	Presenilin 1	Pm	B	Most common cause of dominant form
• Frontotemporal dementia and parkinsonism	AD4	AD	1q31-q42	Presenilin 2	Pm	B	Very rare
	FTDP-17	AD	17q21	MAPTAU	Pm	C	
• Familial amyotrophic lateral sclerosis	SOD1	AD	21q22	Superoxide dismutase 1	Pm	C	20% of hereditary ALS
• Dentato-rubro-pallido-subthalamic atrophy	DRPLA	AD	12p13.31	DRPLA protein	Pm	A	Rare in Europe

(Cont.) →

(Cont.)

Disease	Symbol	Inheritance pattern	Locus	Gene	Mutation	Status	Remarks
• Familial spastic paraplegia	SPG1	XL	Xq28	L1CAM	Pm	C	Complicated form
	SPG2	XL	Xq22	Proteolipid protein	Pm	B	Uncomplicated form
	SPG3	AD	14q11.2-24.3	Unknown	Unknown	D	
	SPG4	AD	2p24-p21	Spastin	Pm	C	Most common dominant form (45%)
	SPG5	AR	8p12-q13	Unknown	Unknown	D	
	SPG6	AD	15q11.1	Unknown	Unknown	D	
	SPG7	AR	16q24.3	Paraplegin	Del/Ins	C	
	SPG8	AD	8q23-24	Unknown	Unknown	D	One family described
Neurogenic muscular atrophies and neuropathies							
• Spinal muscular atrophy, infantile (Werdnig-Hoffmann)	SMA I	AR	5q11.2-13	Survival motoneuron (SMN)	Del	A	Deletion of exon 7 of the SMN gene in > 95% of cases. SMA I, II, and III are allelic
• Intermediate	SMA II	AR	5q11.2-13	SMN	Del	A	
• Juvenile (Kugelberg-Welander)	SMA III	AR	5q11.2-13	SMN	Del	A	
• Adult	SMA IV	?	?	?	?	D	
• Charcot-Marie-Tooth disease, type Ia	CMT1a	AD	17p11.2	PMP-22	Dupl/Pm	A	Duplication of a 1.5-Mb fragment in 70%
• Charcot-Marie-Tooth disease, type Ib	CMT1b	AD	1q22-23	MPZ	Pm	B	
• Charcot-Marie-Tooth disease, type II (axonal)	CMT2a	AD	1p36	Unknown	Unknown	C	PMP-22 and MPZ mutations in rare cases

Disease	Abbrev.	Inheritance	Locus	Gene product	Mutation		Comments
• Charcot-Marie-Tooth disease, type IV	CMT2b	AD	3q13-q22	Unknown	Unknown	D	Rare families
	CMT2d	AD	7p14	Unknown	Unknown	D	Rare Tunisian families
	CMT4a	AR	8q	Unknown	Unknown	D	
• Charcot-Marie-Tooth disease, X-chromosomal	CMT4b	AR	11q23	Unknown	Unknown	D	One family
	CMTX	XL	Xq13.1	Connexin-32	Pm	C	
• Hereditary sensory neuropathy	HSN I	AD	pq22.1-22.3	Unknown	Unknown	D	
• Hereditary motor neuropathy	HMN II	AD	12q24	Unknown	Unknown	D	
	HMN V	AD	7p	Unknown	Unknown	D	
• Tomaculous neuropathy (liability to pressure palsies)	HNPP	AD	17p11.2	PMP-22	Del/Pm	A	Usually due to deletion of a 1.5-Mb fragment (complementary to CMT I)
• Hereditary neuralgic amyotrophy	HNA	AD	17q24-25	Unknown	Unknown	D	
• Bulbospinal neuronopathy	XBSN	XL	Xq13-22	Androgen receptor	Trinucleotide	A	
Myopathies							
• Duchenne muscular dystrophy	DMD	XL	Xp21.2	Dystrophin	Del/Dupl/Pm	A	Most common hereditary myopathy (1/3300 male births), has rarer and more benign allelic variant
• Becker muscular dystrophy	BMD	XL	Xp21.2	Dystrophin	Del/Dupl/Pm	A	
• Emery-Dreifuss muscular dystrophy	EDMD	XL	Xq28	Emerin	Del/Ins/Pm	B	Early contractures, cardiac conduction disturbances
• Facioscapulohumeral muscular dystrophy	FSH-MD	AD	4qter	Unknown	Unknown	A	Association with a shortened DNA fragment

(Cont.) →

(Cont.)

Disease	Symbol	Inheritance pattern	Locus	Gene	Mutation	Status	Remarks
• Limb girdle muscular dystrophy	LGMD-1a	AD	5q31	Myotilin	Pm	C	
	LGMD-1b	AD	1q11-21	Lamin A/C	Pm	C	
	LGMD-1c	AD	3p25	Caveolin-3	Pm	C	
	LGMD-2a	AR	15q15-q21	Calpain-3	Pm/Del	C	
	LGMD-2b	AR	2p16-p13	Dysferlin	Pm	C	
	LGMD-2c	AR	13q12	γ-Sarcoglycan	Pm	C	
	LGMD-2d	AR	17q12-q21	Adhalin	Pm	C	
	LGMD-2e	AR	4q12	β-Sarcoglycan	Pm	C	
	LGMD-2f	AR	5q33-q34	δ-Sarcoglycan	Pm	C	
	LGMD-2g	AR	17q11-q12	Unknown	Unknown	D	Clinically similar to Kugelberg-Welander spinal muscular atrophy
	LGMD-2h	AR	9q31-q33	Unknown	Unknown	D	
• Oculopharyngeal muscular dystrophy	OPMD	AD	14q11.2-q13	Poly-(A)-binding protein 2	Trinucleotide	A	Relatively benign course
• Myotubular myopathy	MTM1	XL	Xq28	Myotubularin	Pm	C	Congenital myopathy with structural anomalies
• Myotonic dystrophy (Curschmann-Steinert)	DM	AD	19q13.3	Myotonin protein kinase	Trinucleotide	A	
• Central core disease	CCO	AD	19q12-q13	Ryanodin receptor	Pm	C	

(Cont.) →

Disease	Gene	Inheritance	Locus	Protein	Mutation	C	Comments
• Malignant hyperthermia	MHS1	AD	19q12-q13	Ryanodin receptor	Pm		Genetically heterogeneous
Ion channel diseases							
• Potassium-sensitive myotonia	SCN4A	AD	17q23-25	α subunit of Na channel	Pm	B	
• Hyperkalemic paresis	SCN4A	AD	17q23-25	α subunit of Na channel	Pm	B	
• Paramyotonia congenita	SCN4A	AD	17q23-25	α subunit of Na channel	Pm	B	
• Hypokalemic paresis	CACNA1S	AD	1q31-32	α1 subunit of dihydropyridine receptor	Pm	B	
• Myotonia congenita (Thomsen type)	CLCN1	AD	7q35	Cl channel	Pm	B	
• Myotonia congenita (Becker type)	CLCN1	AR	7q35	Cl channel	Pm/Del/Ins	B	
Hereditary tumor syndromes							
• Neurofibromatosis I (von Recklinghausen's disease)	NF1	AD	17q11.2	Neurofibromin	Del/Pm	B	
• Neurofibromatosis II	NF2	AD	22q12.2	Merlin	Del/Pm	B	
• Von Hippel-Lindau disease	VHL	AD	3p25		Pm/Del	B	
• Tuberous sclerosis	TSC1	AD	9q34	Hamartin		B	
•	TSC2	AD	16p13	Tuberin	Del	B	
Prion diseases							
• Familial Creutzfeldt-Jakob disease	PRNP	AD	20pter-p12	Prion protein	Pm/Ins	B	5–10% of cases of CJD
• Gerstmann-Sträussler-Scheinker syndrome	PRNP	AD	20pter-p12	Prion protein	Ins/Pm	B	Part of CJD spectrum

(Cont.) →

(Cont.)

Disease	Symbol	Inheritance pattern	Locus	Gene	Mutation	Status	Remarks
• Fatal familial insomnia	PRNP	AD	20pter-p12	Prion protein	Pm	B	Part of CJD spectrum
Epilepsies							
• Benign neonatal epilepsy	EBN1	AD	20q13	Pm	Pm	C	80 % of cases
	EBN2	AD	8q24	Pm	Pm	C	
• Nocturnal frontal lobe epilepsy	ADNFLE	AD	20q13	Pm	Pm	C	2 families to date
• Febrile seizures plus	GEFS+	AD	19q13.1	Pm	Pm	C	1 family to date
• Febrile seizures	FEB1	AD	8q13	Unknown	Unknown	D	
	FEB2	AD	19p13.3	Unknown	Unknown	D	Possibly Na channel SNC1B
• Progressive myoclonus epilepsy (Unverricht-Lundborg)	EPM1	AR	21q23.3	Cystatin B	Pm, 12 bp repeat expansion	B	12 bp repeat expansion in 80 % of cases
• Progressive myoclonus epilepsy (Lafora body disease)	EPM2	AR	6q24	Laforin (PTP)	Del	B	
• Juvenile neuronal ceroid lipofuscinosis	CLN3	AR	16p12.1	CLN3	Unknown	B	
• Juvenile myoclonic epilepsy	EJM1	AD	6p21.3	Unknown	Unknown	D	Clinically variable
	EJM2	AD	6p11	Unknown	Unknown	D	Classic JME
	EJM3	AR	15q14	Unknown	Unknown	D	Candidate gene: CHRNA7
• Benign centrotemporal epilepsy	ECT	AR	15q14	Unknown	Unknown	D	
• Childhood absence epilepsy	ECA1	AD	8q24	Unknown	Unknown	D	
• Idiopathic generalized epilepsy	EGI	AR	8q24	Unknown	Unknown	D	

(Cont.) →

Neurovascular diseases						
• CADASIL	CADASIL	AD	19p13.1	Notch3	Pm	B
• Hereditary cerebral hemorrhages with amyloid angiopathy	HCHWA-D	AD	21q21	Amyloid precursor protein	Pm	B
• Familial cavernomas	HCHWA-I	AD	20p11.2	cystatin C	Pm	B
	CCM1	AD	7q21-22	KRIT1	Pm/Del/Ins	C
	CCM2	AD	7p13-15	Unknown	Unknown	D
	CCM3	AD	3q25.2-27	Unknown	Unknown	D
• Familial hemiplegic migraine	FHM1	AD	19p13	Ca channel	Pm	C	Allelic to SCA6 and EA2, cf. ion channel diseases
	FHM2	AD	1q21-31	Unknown	Unknown	D
Neurolipidoses						
• Gaucher's disease	GBA	AR	1q21	Glucocerebrosidase	Pm/Del/Ins	B	Saposin gene mutation in ca. 1%
• Niemann-Pick disease type C	NPC-1	AR	18q11	NPC-1 gene	Pm/Ins	C
• Niemann-Pick disease type A/B	SMPD1	AR	11p15.4	Sphingomyelinase	Pm/Del/Ins	B
• Fabry's disease	GLA	XL	Xq22	α-Galactosidase	Pm/Del/Ins	C
• Tay-Sachs disease	HEXA	AR	15q23-24	Hexosaminidase	Pm/Del/Ins	C
Mitochondrial diseases						
• Myoclonic epilepsy with ragged red fibers	MERRF	Mat	nt8344	tRNA^{Lys}	Pm	A
• Mitochondrial encephalomyopathy with lactic acidosis and stroke-like episodes	MELAS	Mat	nt3243 (nt3271)	tRNA^{Leu}	Pm	A

(Cont.) →

Disease	Symbol	Inheritance pattern	Locus	Gene	Mutation	Status	Remarks
• Leber's hereditary optic neuropathy	LHON	Mat	nt11778	Complex 1 subunit ND4	Pm	A	
• Chronic progressive external ophthalmoplegia	CPEO	Spor		Common deletion of mtDNA	Del >> Pm	A	
• Kearns-Sayre syndrome	KSS	Spor	dermtDNA	Common deletion	Del >> Pm	A	

[1] Vulnerability locus: the presence of the e4 allele of the apolipoprotein gene (ApoE) increases the risk of developing Alzheimer's disease, but is, in itself, neither a necessary nor a sufficient condition for it.

Abbreviations

A	Molecular diagnosis available on a routine basis	AR	Autosomal-recessive
B	Molecular diagnosis available on a routine basis; because labor-intensive sequence analysis is required, discussion of indications with the laboratory performing the test is recommended	Del	Deletion
		Dupl	Duplication
		Ins	Insertion
		Mat	Maternal
C	Molecular diagnosis possible in principle	Pm	Point mutation
D	Molecular diagnosis not yet available	Spor	Sporadic
AD	Autosomal-dominant	trinucleotide	Trinucleotide repeat expansion
		XL	X-linked

Note:

The information provided here regarding genetic loci, mutations, and gene products in the more important neurogenetic diseases, as far as these are known, is incomplete, and the selection of diseases included in the table is relatively arbitrary. The purpose of the table is to provide the reader with an initial guide to the subject. Rapid progress in molecular genetic research soon renders any such table out of date. In case of doubt, current publications should be searched for, or specialized centers consulted. Mutations in other, as yet unidentified, genes can probably cause many, or perhaps most, of the diseases listed here.

A list of literature references for the above table is available on the publisher's Internet site: http://www.thieme.com/mm-refs

Glossary of Common Abbreviations in Neurology

a., aa.	Artery, arteries
ACA	Anterior cerebral artery
AChA	Anterior choroidal artery
ACommA	Anterior communicating artery
AD	Autosomal dominant
AEP	Auditory evoked potentials
AICA	Anterior inferior cerebellar artery
ALS	Amyotrophic lateral sclerosis
AMAN	Acute motor axonal neuropathy
AMSAN	Acute motor and sensory axonal neuropathy
ANCA	Antineutrophilic cytoplasmic antibody
ANS	Autonomic nervous system
ap	Anteroposterior
AR	Autosomal recessive
ARAS	Ascending reticular activating system
ATP	Adenosine triphosphate
AVM	Arteriovenous malformation
BAEP	Brainstem auditory evoked potentials
CADASIL	Cerebral autosomal dominant arteriopathy with subcortical infarcts and leukoencephalopathy
CIDP	Chronic inflammatory demyelinating polyneuropathy
CJD	Creutzfeldt-Jakob disease
CK	Creatine kinase
CMV	Cytomegalovirus
CNS	Central nervous system
COX	Cytochrome C oxidase
CRP	C-reactive protein
CPA	Cerebellopontine angle
CT	Computed tomography
CTS	Carpal tunnel syndrome
CVA	Cerebrovascular accident

CW	Continuous wave
DAD	Deafness and diabetes
DBS	Deep brain stimulation
DLP	Dorsolateral pontine nucleus
DSS	Expanded Disability Status Scale
EAE	Experimental allergic encephalomyelitis
ECG	Electrocardiogram (-ography)
EDTA	Ethylenediaminetetraacetic acid
EEG	Electroencephalogram (-ography)
EMG	Electromyogram (-ography)
ENG	Electroneurogram (-ography)
EOG	Electrooculogram (-ography)
EPSP	Excitatory postsynaptic potential
ESR	Erythrocyte sedimentation rate
fMRI	Functional magnetic resonance imaging
FTA-ABS test	Fluorescent treponemal antibody absorption test
GAD	Glutamic acid decarboxylase
GANS	Granulomatous angiitis of the nervous system
HIV	Human immunodeficiency virus
HMSN	Hereditary motor and sensory neuropathy
HNPP	Hereditary neuropathy with liability to pressure palsies ("tomaculous neuropathy")
h.s.	*Hora somni*, at bedtime
HSV	Herpes simplex virus
HTLV	Human T-cell lymphotropic virus
INO	Internuclear ophthalmoplegia

i.m.	Intramuscular
IPSP	Inhibitory postsynaptic potential
i.v.	Intravenous
IVIG	Intravenous immunoglobulin
KSS	Kearns-Sayre syndrome
LCMV	Lymphocytic choriomeningitis virus
LHON	Leber's hereditary optic neuropathy
lig.	Ligament
m., mm.	Muscle, muscles
MAG	Myelin-associated glycoprotein
MDMA	Methylenedioxymethamphetamine ("Ecstasy")
MEG	Magnetoencephalogram (-ography)
MELAS	Syndrome consisting of mitochondrial myopathy, encephalopathy, lactic acidosis, and stroke-like episodes
MEP	Motor evoked potentials
MERRF	Myoclonic epilepsy with ragged red fibers
MLF	Medial longitudinal fasciculus
MMN	Multifocal motor neuropathy
MNGIE	Myoneurogastrointestinal encephalopathy syndrome
MPTP	1-Methyl-2-phenyl-1,2,3,6-tetrahydropyridine
MRA	Magnetic resonance angiography
MRI	Magnetic resonance imaging
mRS	Modified Rankin scale
MS	Multiple sclerosis
MSA	Multisystem atrophy
MST	Medial superior temporal visual area
MT	Medial temporal visual area
mtDNA	Mitochondrial deoxyribonucleic acid
MTT	Mean transit time
n., nn.	Nerve, nerves
NARP	Neuropathy, ataxia, and retinitis pigmentosa syndrome
nDNA	Nuclear deoxyribonucleic acid
NIHSS	National Institutes of Health Stroke Scale
pa	Posteroanterior
PAN	Polyarteritis nodosa (= periarteritis nodosa)
PCA	Posterior cerebral artery; patient-controlled analgesia
PChA	Posterior choroidal artery
PCommA	Posterior communicating artery
PCR	Polymerase chain reaction
PDS	Paroxysmal depolarization shift
PET	Positron emission tomography
PICA	Posterior inferior cerebellar artery
PLEDS	Periodic lateralized epileptiform discharges
PLMS	Periodic limb movements in sleep
PML	Progressive multifocal leukoencephalopathy
PNET	Primitive neuroectodermal tumor
PNS	Peripheral nervous system; peripheral nerve stimulation
p.o.	*Per os*, by mouth
PPRF	Paramedian pontine reticular formation
p.r.	*Per rectum*, by rectum
PROMM	Proximal myotonic myopathy
PRPE	Progressive rubella panencephalitis
PW	Pulsed wave
r., rr.	Ramus, rami
REM	Rapid eye movement
riMLF	Rostral interstitial nucleus of the medial longitudinal fasciculus (= Büttner-Ennever nucleus)
RIND	Reversible ischemic neurological deficit
rt-PA	Recombinant tissue plasminogen activator

SAH	Subarachnoid hemorrhage	**SUNCT**	Short-lasting unilateral neuralgiform headache with conjunctival injection and tearing
s.c.	Subcutaneous		
SCA	Superior cerebellar artery		
SDAT	Senile dementia of Alzheimer type (earlier designation of Alzheimer's disease in the elderly)	**TGA**	Transient global amnesia
		TIA	Transient ischemic attack
		TMJ	Temporomandibular joint
		TOS	Thoracic outlet syndrome
SEP/SSEP	Somatosensory evoked potentials	**TPHA**	*Treponema pallidum* hemagglutination
SLE	Systemic lupus erythematosus	**TST**	Triple stimulating technique
		vCJD	Variant Creutzfeldt-Jakob disease
SPECT	Single photon emission computed tomography		
		VEP	Visual evoked potentials
SSPE	Subacute sclerosing panencephalitis	**VZV**	Varicella-zoster virus

Index

Page numbers in **red** refer to major references, figures, or tables.